Articulation and
Phonological Disorders

SIXTH EDITION

Articulation and Phonological Disorders
Speech Sound Disorders in Children

JOHN E. BERNTHAL
University of Nebraska–Lincoln

NICHOLAS W. BANKSON
James Madison University

PETER FLIPSEN JR.
Idaho State University

Boston   New York   San Francisco
Mexico City   Montreal   Toronto   London   Madrid   Munich   Paris
Hong Kong   Singapore   Tokyo   Cape Town   Sydney

Executive Editor and Publisher: *Stephen D. Dragin*
Editorial Assistant: *Anne Whittaker*
Executive Marketing Manager: *Krista Clark*
Production Editor: *Janet Domingo*
Editorial Production Service: *Publishers' Design and Production Services, Inc./Lynda Griffiths*
Composition Buyer: *Linda Cox*
Manufacturing Buyer: *Megan Cochran*
Electronic Composition: *Publishers' Design and Production Services, Inc.*
Interior Design: *Publishers' Design and Production Services, Inc.*
Cover Administrator: *Linda Knowles*

For related titles and support materials, visit our online catalog at www.pearsonhighered.com.

Between the time website information is gathered and then published, it is not unusual for some sites to have closed. Also, the transcription of URLs can result in typographical errors. The publisher would appreciate notification where these errors occur so that they may be corrected in subsequent editions.

ISBN-13: 978-0-205-56926-7   ISBN-10: 0-205-56926-9

Printed in the United States of America

10 9 8 7 6 5 4 3 2 1   RRD-VA   12 11 10 09 08

Allyn & Bacon
is an imprint of

Contents

8 Language and Dialectal Variations   331

by Brian A. Goldstein and Aquiles Iglesias

9 Phonological Awareness: Description, Assessment, and Intervention   357

by Laura M. Justice, Gail T. Gillon, and C. Melanie Schuele

Preface

As with the five previous editions of this book, we once again present information we regard as essential for students who are learning about the nature and treatment of disorders of the speech sound system. Since the publication of our last edition, knowledge in the area of clinical phonology has advanced, and in this revision we reflect state-of-the-art ideas, research, and practice components that are important for knowledge of and practice with these types of communication impairments.

This book reflects both theoretical and practical information, recognizing that elements of both are essential to the understanding of the literature and to clinical practice. Readers have continued to indicate that they appreciate the breadth and depth of the synthesis of the literature that this text provides, and we have in this edition again endeavored to provide this to the student so that clinical phonology may be viewed from a broad perspective. We have maintained our "eclectic" perspective relative to the nature and treatment of articulation and phonological disorders, but in the assessment and treatment chapters you will again see some of our own biases regarding clinical management. In general, however, we defer to clinician judgment in deciding which assessment and treatment procedures are most useful to them and the clients they serve.

Of particular significance in this sixth edition is the addition of Peter Flipsen Jr. as a coauthor. Dr. Flipsen is among the cadre of promising and productive young scholars in the area of clinical phonology, and he brings a very knowledgeable and fresh perspective to the topics we cover and the information presented. This book is the recipient of his outstanding expertise and communication skills in the area of speech sound disorders. We have also added a new subtitle "Speech Sound Disorders in Children" to reflect a recent shift in preferred terminology.

We are indebted to several people who have contributed immeasurably to this text. Ray Kent has once again shared his expertise on normal aspects of articulation in Chapter 2. Sharynne McLeod, an Australian speech-language pathologist with a broad range of knowledge and experience in the field, has provided a new chapter on normal speech sound acquisition. Brian Goldstein and Aquiles Iglesias have revised their chapter on language and dialectal variations, and Laura Justice and Melanie Schuele have added Gail Gillon as a coauthor in their revision of the phonological awareness chapter. Each of these authors is a highly recognized expert in the areas in which they are writing, and we feel fortunate to have them as contributors to this effort.

We also thank the following reviewers for their comments: Brenda L. Beverly, University of South Alabama; Gina Keene, University of Mississippi; and Michael J. Moran, Auburn University

As authors, we assume all responsibility for errors, oversights, and misconceptions that may appear in this book. Our hope is that this text will provide you with a comprehensive source of information on speech sound disorders, and that it will be a valuable resource as you learn about and practice clinical phonology.

Introduction

This edition has the same goal as the five previous editions: to present a comprehensive review of information important to the study of clinical phonology. You will note that there is an addendum to the previous title, with the new title being *Articulation and Phonological Disorders: Speech Sound Disorders in Children.* This title includes traditional terminology (i.e., articulation; phonological disorders), as well as the label more recently endorsed by the American Speech-Language-Hearing Association (ASHA) to identify this population: speech sound disorders. While focused on clinical management of phonological disorders, the book includes an introductory summary of the production and linguistic organization of speech sounds; the typical process of speech sound development in children; factors related to the presence of disorders, including the classification of disorders; the assessment and treatment of speech sound disorders; speech sounds as they relate to language and dialectal variations; and finally a presentation that relates speech sound productions to literacy acquisition. Discussion questions are included at the end of each chapter, and a case study is included in the assessment and remediation chapters.

This book continues to be focused primarily on the pediatric population, and those whose speech sound disorders are not etiologically associated with known or obvious sensory, structural, or neuromotor disorders. Although these topics are briefly discussed in this text, the reader is referred to other literature that addresses each of these topics in an in-depth fashion. It is recognized, however, that a speech sound disorder with no apparent etiology may be caused by one or more subtle organic, genetic, learning, or environmental factors. Thus, it is important that this book provide basic information in these areas to the student.

Those acquainted with previous editions of this text will notice some changes in organizational structure, authorship, and updated information concerning topics covered in previous editions. Once again we have tried to synthesize the literature, and discuss topics of current as well as traditional interest.

Articulation and Phonological Disorders is divided into nine chapters, with three chapters reflecting significant changes. A new Chapter 1 has been added, and it is designed to succinctly introduce students to the realm of clinical phonology, terminology used to designate this type of communication impairment, basic information related to how speech sounds are a part of the overall language system, and the nature and incidence of speech sound disorders in children. The intent is for this chapter to prepare students for the chapters that follow. The former Chapter 1 has now become Chapter 2, which reviews normal aspects of articulation and provides an introduction to the phonological system of American English. This information is typically covered in courses other than clinical phonology; however, for those who lack such coursework or, as is more frequently the case, need this review, this content is presented.

Chapter 3 is an entirely new chapter, and it presents a comprehensive review of normal speech sound acquisition. The author of this chapter has made the information highly applicable to the speech-language pathology student. For example, after a description of each model of phonological acquisition, a section entitled "Application to Speech-Language Pathology Practice" is included. The chapter includes 11 tables with normative and descriptive information that is highly relevant to clinical decision making, particularly in the area of assessment.

Chapter 4 again includes the comprehensive review of factors related to speech sound disorders that many readers have regarded as a strength of the book. The chapter, however, has been significantly expanded. For example, since the knowledge base on classification of speech sound disorders has evolved significantly in recent years, this chapter now includes an entire new section devoted to the question of classification, including both organic disorders and disorders of unknown etiology. A genetic syndromes section has been added, along with significant updates and modifications in sections that discuss the relevance of hearing loss to speech sound disorders. The expanded chapter also includes discussion of ASHA's new position statement on childhood apraxia of speech.

The procedures for speech sound sampling and interpretation are addressed in Chapter 5. Screening procedures, a battery of measures that comprise a comprehensive phonological assessment, and related procedures are reviewed and discussed. The chapter discusses how one can determine the need for intervention, and how target behaviors are selected for therapy. A case study is presented in which topics covered in the chapter are applied to a specific client.

Chapter 6 reviews basic concepts and considerations related to how one goes about doing "speech therapy" with clients who have speech sound difficulties. Included in this chapter is the framework for an overall treatment program, a framework for individual therapy sessions, a discussion of treatment style, and a review of generalization and how this psychological construct relates to the way one organizes treatment. A new section on measuring clinical change has been added.

The discussion of intervention continues in Chapter 7, which focuses on procedures for engaging in traditional motor-oriented therapy, as well as procedures for what are sometimes referred to as linguistic approaches to intervention. Differences, similarities, and how the two may both be used with a client are included in the discussion. Procedures for treating childhood apraxia of speech clients are presented, as well as a discussion of using oral-motor activities as part of intervention. The case study from Chapter 5 is again reviewed from the standpoint of how the treatment procedures discussed in this chapter would be applied to this child.

Chapter 8 presents updated information critical to increasing the professional's competence in serving a multicultural society. Common dialectical variations found in society are reviewed, including African American English, Spanish- and Asian-influenced English, and Eastern, Southern Appalachian, and Ozark English. Acquisition of speech sounds in these populations is also discussed.

Chapter 9 is concerned with the broad area of literacy acquisition, with an emphasis on phonological awareness. The chapter has been expanded in terms of its discussion of the relationship between speech sound disorders and phonological awareness, and how speech-language pathologists can include phonological awareness activities in their therapy. Detailed information is presented about phonological awareness, including its description, how it is assessed, and how deficiencies in that area are remediated. Given that children with significant speech sound disorders often have difficulty in the area of learning to read, the material in Chapter 9 is highly relevant to contemporary practice with the pediatric population.

Introduction to the Study of Speech Sound Disorders

NICHOLAS W. BANKSON

James Madison University

JOHN E. BERNTHAL

University of Nebraska–Lincoln

PETER FLIPSEN JR.

Idaho State University

Welcome to the world of clinical phonology! You are about to enter a detailed presentation and discussion of one of the most frequently occurring communication disorders that speech-language pathologists encounter. You may be wondering why we say "clinical phonology" rather than "speech sound disorders," "articulation disorders," or "phonological disorders." We use the term *phonology* as a synonym for speech sound disorders (we will elaborate on terminology in paragraphs that follow), and we use the term *clinical* to indicate that this book is focused on how you, as a clinician, will treat disorders related to speech sound production. This is in contrast to studying speech sounds from the standpoint of phonetics, linguistics, or acoustics—any one of which is often a course in and of itself. Although knowledge from each of these areas is important background information in our study of speech sound disorders, the distinguishing characteristic of this text is that it is focused on individuals, primarily children, who have difficulty learning to produce and appropriately use the speech sounds of the language.

The term presently accepted by the American Speech-Language-Hearing Association to identify those persons who have disorders related to saying the sounds of the language is *speech sound disorders*. Historically, these disorders were referred to as *articulation disorders*—a term still in widespread use. From the time the profession of speech-language pathology came into existence in the 1920s, until the 1970s, the prevailing viewpoint related to speech sound disorders was that they reflected a client's inability to motorically produce one or more speech sounds. The role of the speech clinician was to teach a client to say a sound, and then practice the sound until the new motor behavior became habitual.

When the first edition of this text was published in 1981, *Articulation Disorders* was used as the title of the book, since that was still the prevailing term used to identify speech sound disorders. Beginning in the 1970s, as the first edition of this book was being written, the field of linguistics began to influence the perception of how our field viewed speech sound disorders. Linguists, who study how speech sounds are used in various languages, provided information that indicated that speech sound disorders may not be only related to motor production difficulties, but they could also reflect a child's lack of knowledge regarding where to appropriately use sounds that he or she can produce. Said another way, the child might be having difficulty acquiring the phonological rules of the language. For example, a child may have difficulty learning to use sounds contrastively (e.g., /s/ and /z/ are contrasted in *sue* versus *zoo*), or in learning that certain sounds need to be placed at the beginning or ends of words in order to communicate effectively (e.g., *at* versus *hat; go* versus *goat*). Disorders related to learning the phonological rules of the language were referred to as *phonological disorders*, thus the term *phonology* was the second term (in addition to articulation) that moved into our vocabulary to identify speech sound disorders.

From the second edition of this book (1988) through the fifth edition (2004) the terms *articulation* and *phonological* were used in the title of the book (i.e., *Articulation and Phonological Disorders*). Some speech-language pathologists (SLPs) have differentiated these two terms for purposes of assessment and treatment of speech sound disorders. *Articulation* refers to production-based speech sound disorders and *phonological* denotes speech sound errors that are rule based. However, in reality, it may be difficult to determine which of these concepts is most appropriate in describing a particular client's error pattern. We must also recognize that there may be variables beyond motor production and rule acquisition that we need to attend to when we try to understand speech sound disorders. Presently, the term *speech sound disorder* is used as the umbrella term to refer to disorders that may be found in clients who have difficulty producing speech sounds. In this book we use the terms *articulation, phonology,* and *speech sound disorders* somewhat interchangeably, but will hold to the traditional differentiation we have referred to between *articulation* and *phonology* when we talk about assessment and treatment.

Speech sound disorders may be described as ranging from something as "mild" as a lisp (interdentalizing the /s/ sounds; sometimes identified as substituting a voiceless *th* sound for an /s/) to a disorder as significant as that found in an individual who is completely unintelligible. Typically, these disorders are found in children, and the pediatric population is the focus of this text. Data provided by various U.S. federal agencies related to education and health have indicated that 5 percent of the school-age population may be expected to have a communication impairment, with 10 to 15 percent occurring in the preschool population. Of these groups, speech sound disorders are the most frequent disorder observed, often co-existing with other aspects of language impairment. Most speech sound disorders occur in children under the age of 8 years, but disorders may persist past that point and also occur in adults. Information contained in this book is relevant to the treatment of any client who faces difficulties producing speech sounds; however, adult speech sound disorders are often related to organic conditions, and thus you will need to review other materials in planning treatment for most adult clients.

As we begin our discussion of speech sound disorders, it is important to recognize that for most children, the cause of the disorder is unknown. Often it is assumed that many children do not say their sounds properly because of difficulty in language development that is reflected in learning speech sounds. In some instances the problem may be related to difficulty with other aspects of language (e.g., vocabulary, syntax). As will be discussed later, a number of variables have been studied as they relate to such learning problems (e.g., familial history, tongue thrust, speech sound discrimination). Research focused on providing a better understanding of speech sound disorders where causality is difficult to establish is ongoing. Certainly, the effort to categorize or classify various types of speech sound disorders (e.g., speech delay, otitis media with effusion, motor speech involvement) is a step in the direction of helping clinicians better understand those children with speech sound disorders of unknown origin. For some children, the cause of their disorder may be more obvious (e.g., hearing loss, cleft palate); however, even then the impact of an organic condition does not necessarily determine the type of speech sound disorder a client may have, nor how he or she will respond to treatment.

In order to better understand and appreciate the contents of this book, it is assumed that you, the student, will already have obtained skills related to phonetic transcription of the speech sounds of the language, knowledge related to the physiological production of various sounds, an introduction to the acoustical characteristics of speech sounds, and knowledge of speech sound development in children. Many of you will already have taken a separate course that covers each of these areas, or perhaps a course that covers two areas (e.g., physiology of sound productions and their transcription). If this is the case, the information we present in our introductory chapters may serve as a review for you. If you have not had courses in these areas, information included in the next two chapters of this text ("Normal Aspects of Articulation" and "Speech Sound Acquisition") will be especially helpful. These chapters will provide background information that you may wish to study further by consulting other texts and/or sources. For all students, the information will be something that you may want to refer to when you encounter some of the concepts included in these chapters as you delve into assessment and treatment of speech sound disorders.

In addition to the background information referred to in the last paragraph, it is important to recognize that speech sounds are a part of language. In this instance the sounds are identified as the phonology of the language. Other aspects of language include semantics (meaning attached to words, vocabulary); morphology (minimum meaningful units in the language), or the words and attachments to words such as plural markers (e.g., /s/ in *dogs*) and tense markers (e.g., ed in *walked*, indicating past tense), or parts of words (e.g., *doghouse* has two minimum meaningful units); syntax (grammatical rules for putting words together in phrases and sentences); pragmatics (using language appropriately in a social context); and discourse (ability to string sentences together in a meaningful manner when communicating with others). Each of these areas is acquired gradually and simultaneously by young children. Initially we are concerned that children learn to use meaningful utterances to express themselves, but soon thereafter we become concerned about how accurate sounds are, because it is through accurate use of speech sounds that the child is understood by the listener, or, in other words, becomes intelligible. Speech-language pathologists are initially concerned with a young child's acquisition of semantics, phonology, and grammatical rules (morphology and syntax). Concern over the other areas comes later, since pragmatics and discourse are based on vocabulary and syntax. Thus, it is often older children for whom pragmatics and discourse may be targeted for instruction.

Increasingly it is being recognized that a normal sound system is important in learning to read and spell. Children's phonological awareness skills (or their ability to mentally manipulate the sounds and syllables in words) have been shown to impact literacy skills, and children with speech sound disorders are at risk for appropriate development of phonological awareness. For this reason, clinicians have been drawn into using their knowledge of phonology as part of a child's literacy development. Chapter 9 will provide information related to the role of the clinician in terms of developing phonological awareness in children.

In our discussion of speech sound disorders, we need to recognize that some children use different speech sounds than those found in their environment because perhaps their first language is different from English, or maybe they are a part of a regional or cultural group that uses a less common dialect of English. Certainly, the increasing multicultural nature of the United States makes us acutely aware of the fact that linguistic differences are a part of everyday communication. As speech-language pathologists, we are primarily focused on disorders that individuals may have in their speech sound productions. It is challenging to determine what is a disorder and what is a difference when the clinician does not speak the language or dialect. Fortunately, there are some guidelines to help us, but the reality is there is a need for clinicians who are bilingual and/or represent different language/dialect groups. All sound systems, whether they are part of a separate language or dialect, are legitimate and deserve acceptance. In some instances, however, the clinician may help an individual learn the sound system of mainstream English when a client elects to do this, often for educational, business, or social reasons. Chapter 8 will present language variations often found in the United States, and outline the role of speech-language pathologists as they assess and treat disorders, as well as provide instruction to those who wish to enhance their mainstream English speaking skills.

Often, Speech Sound Disorders is an early disorders course to which students are exposed. This is perhaps wise, since speech sounds are discrete entities that can be more easily identified and described than other communication entities such as voice quality or fluency characteristics. The study of speech sound disorders lends itself to helping students come to recognize the processes involved in formulating assessment and treatment protocols. Thus, the knowledge and skills that you will acquire in the process of studying speech sound disorders can provide the basis for learning how to proceed with other types of communication disorders. Speech sound disorders and all the complexities they encompass are a challenging study but one that is critical to how individuals who for one reason or another need assistance in learning the speech sounds of the language. For many children, learning to talk, including the learning of speech sounds, is difficult. For this reason, you need to be in a position to assist them so that communication is both effective and satisfying to them.

Normal Aspects of Articulation

RAY KENT

University of Wisconsin–Madison

This book is focused on the ability of humans to produce sounds that are used to convey a message. The act of producing such sounds is identified as *articulation*, and this activity is a major component of *speech*, as distinguished from the term *language*. *Speech* consists of an organized set or system of sounds that are used to convey meaning. Meaning itself is based in *language*, which includes the collection of words that are used in phrases and sentences and the grammar or rules of the language that we use to create those phrases and sentences. More formally, *language* may be described as an arbitrary system of signs or symbols used according to prescribed rules to convey meaning within a linguistic community. Of course, once an arbitrary association of symbol with meaning has been developed, the users of that language must learn and use this association of symbols if they want to communicate with one another. The word *dog* has a certain meaning in the English language, and this word can be communicated to other users of English through speaking, writing, or signing it with symbols used by the deaf.

Speech is but one modality for the expression of language; however, speech has special importance because it is the primary, first-learned modality for hearing language users. Speech is a system in the sense that it consistently and usefully relates the meanings of a language with the sounds by which the language is communicated.

Not all sound variations in speech are related to meaning. When a person suffers from a cold, he or she has a different way of talking, but so long as the cold is not so severe as to make speech unintelligible, the relation of sound to meaning is basically the same as when the person is healthy. The acoustic signal of speech—that is, the vibrations of air molecules in response to the energy source of human speech—carries more information than just the expression of meaning. As we listen to a speaker, we often make judgments not only about the intended meaning but also about the speaker's age and sex (if the speaker isn't visible), the speaker's mood, the speaker's state of health, and perhaps even the speaker's dialectal background. Thus, on hearing a simple question—"Could you tell me the time, please?"— we might deduce that the speaker is a young southern woman in a hurry, an elderly British gentleman in a cheerful mood, or a young boy quite out of breath.

▪ STRUCTURE OF LANGUAGE

Speech sounds, then, may be viewed from two perspectives: (1) as motor production (speech) and (2) as units that facilitate the expression of meaning (language). When sounds are studied as part of the language system, they are called *phonemes*.

To derive a speaker's meaning, the listener is basically concerned with the phonemes in the speech message. From a linguistic perspective, phonemes are sound units related to decisions about meaning. In the list *cat hat mat bat sat fat that chat,* each word rhymes with every other word because all end with the same sound. However, the words differ in their initial sounds, and these differences can change the meaning of the syllables. In fact, the linguist identifies the phonemes in a given language by assembling lists of words and then determining the sound differences that form units of meaning. The layperson usually thinks of words as the units of meaning, but the linguist recognizes a smaller form called the *morpheme*. For example, the linguist describes the words *walked* and *books* as having two morphemes: *walk + past tense* for *walked*, and *book + plural* for *books*. If two sounds can be interchanged without changing word meaning, or if they never occur in exactly the same combination with other sounds, then they are not different phonemes. Hence, phonemes are the minimal sound elements that represent and distinguish language units (words or morphemes).

A *phonemic transcription* (which is always enclosed in virgules / /) is less detailed than a *phonetic transcription* (which is enclosed in brackets [ ]). A phonetic transcription is sensitive to sound variations within a phoneme class. An individual variant of this kind is called an *allophone*. Thus, a phoneme is a family of allophones. Phonemes are the minimal set of sound classes needed to specify the meaningful units (words or morphemes) of the language. Allophones are a more numerous set of distinct sounds, some of which may belong to the same phoneme family. As a very simple example, the word *pop* begins and ends with the same phoneme but often begins and ends with a different allophone. If the final /p/ is produced by holding the lips together after they close, then this sound is the unreleased allophone of the /p/ phoneme. However, the initial /p/ must be released before the vowel is formed, so this sound is the released allophone of the /p/ phoneme. The /p/ phoneme also includes a number of other allophones, though perhaps not as obvious as these two.

To understand more clearly the difference between phonemes and allophones, say the following word-pairs to yourself as you try to detect a difference in the production of the italicized sounds.

> *k*eep - *c*oop   (phoneme /k/)
> m*a*n - b*a*t   (phoneme /æ/)
> te*n* - te*n*th   (phoneme /n/)

In the first pair of words, the phoneme /k/ is articulated toward the front of the mouth in the first word and toward the back of the mouth in the second. Despite the differences in the place of tongue contact, the two sounds are heard by speakers of English to be the same phoneme. Speakers of other languages, such as Arabic, may hear the two sounds as different phonemes. The tongue-front and tongue-back versions are allophones of the /k/ phoneme in English.

In the next pair of words, *man* and *bat*, the pertinent difference might be more easily heard than felt through articulation. In the word *man*, the vowel is nasalized (produced with sound transmission through the nose) owing to the influence of the surrounding nasal consonants. But in the word *bat*, the vowel /æ/ is not normally nasalized. The phonetic environment of the vowel—that is, its surrounding sounds—determines whether the vowel is nasalized. The nasal and nonnasal versions of the vowel are allophones of the /æ/ phoneme.

Finally, in comparing /n/ in the words *ten* and *tenth*, you might notice that your tongue is more toward the front (just behind the upper front teeth) in the word *tenth*. The final *th* sound exerts an articulatory influence on the preceding /n/, causing it to be dentalized or produced at the teeth. Again, the two types of /n/ are simply allophones of the /n/ phoneme.

Allophonic variation is of two types: complementary distribution and free variation. In *complementary distribution*, two (or more) allophones never occur in exactly the same phonetic environment, so that the occurrence of one is complementary (nonoverlapping) to the occurrence of the other. For example, the front and back /k/ discussed above are in complementary distribution. The front /k/ occurs in the environment of vowels made in the front of the mouth, and the back /k/ occurs in the environment of vowels made in the back of the mouth. Similarly, the nasal and nonnasal allophones of /æ/ are in complementary distribution, determined by the presence or absence of nasals in the phonetic environment. The nasalized /æ/ occurs only when this vowel is preceded or followed by nasal sounds. Allophones are said to be in *free variation* when they can occur in the same phonetic context. For example, the released /p/ and the unreleased /p/ are in free variation in word-final position in words like *pop* or *map*. As previously indicated, the final /p/ can be released audibly with a small burst as the lips open or it can be unreleased if the lip closure is maintained.

The discipline of linguistics is concerned primarily with the structure of language. The disciplines of psychology and speech-language pathology are concerned primarily with the processing of language—with its formulation and its reception. The linguistic study of language structure has influenced the study of language processing, and, to some degree, the reverse is true as well. Descriptions of language processing often use terms, such as *syntax, semantics, phonology*, and *phonetics*, that denote traditional areas of linguistic study. These terms have come to have a dual usage, one referring to structure and another to processing.

To briefly round out our discussion of the structure of language, we need to mention phonemes and morphemes. *Phonemes* are combined to produce meaningful units, called *morphemes*, which we usually identify as words. However, it should be recognized that a given word, such as *walked*, may actually be comprised of two or more morphemes—in the case of *walked*, the morphemes are the verb *walk* and the past tense marker *ed. Morphemes* are combined into phrases and sentences according to the grammatical rules of the language, and these combinations are referred to as the *syntax* of the language. Thus, language includes a set of phonemes and morphemes that are combined according to certain rules to reflect the syntax of the language. Meaning that is ascribed to individual words is identified as the *semantics* of the language. In a sense, the components of language (phonology, morphology, syntax) are one side of the coin, with semantics being the other side.

Figure 2.1 is a diagram of an information-processing model of verbal formulation and utterance production. The diagram attempts to show how different types of information are

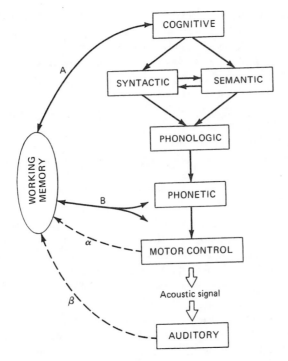

■ **FIGURE 2.1**   Information processing model of verbal formulation and utterance production.

Source: Adapted from Bock (1982).

processed in the act of speaking. The cognitive level is where a thought is initiated. This is a prelinguistic, propositional level that involves decisions such as the identification of participants and actions. For example, the cognitive processing that preceded formulation of the sentence, *The dog chased the cat*, involved the identification of a dog and a cat as participants and chasing or pursuit as an action. However, the words *dog*, *cat*, and *chased* were not actually selected. Rather, propositions or relations associated with these words were established.

Information from the cognitive level is used to make decisions at the syntactic and semantic levels. Syntax involves the ordering of words in a sentence and semantics involves the selection of words. Research on verbal formulation indicates that syntactic and semantic processing are interactive (hence, the arrows between them in the diagram). Deciding on a particular syntactic structure for a sentence can influence word selection, and selection of particular words can limit or direct syntactic decisions. The semantic level is sometimes called *lexicalization*, or the choice of lexical units. Lexicalization appears to be a two-stage process. The first stage is selection of a lexical concept, not a phonologically complete word. Phonologic specification—that is, specification of the word's sound pattern—is accomplished in the second stage of the process. The phonologic level in Figure 2.1 is the level at which the evolving sentence comes to have phonologic structure. Various decisions are made at this level to ensure that a sound pattern accurately represents the syntactic and semantic decisions made earlier. The phonologic information then directs decisions at the phonetic level, where the details of the sound pattern are worked out. We might think of the phonetic level as producing a detailed phonetic representation of the utterance.

The output of the phonetic level is sufficient to specify the phonetic goals to be satisfied in speech production. Actual motor instructions are determined by a motor control level. This level selects the muscles to be activated and controls the timing and strength of the muscle contractions. This is no small task. Speech requires rapid changes in the activation of about 100 muscles. Once the muscles have done their work, the acoustic speech signal is produced. This signal is then processed by the speaker and the listener(s) as auditory information. For the speaker, the auditory processing completes a feedback loop.

One component that remains to be explained in Figure 2.1 is working memory and its connections to other parts of the diagram. Working memory is a speaker's operational memory, the memory that is used to keep track of the information involved in sentence production. But this memory is limited, so it is in the interest of efficient processing to minimize demands on it. Therefore, the theory goes, two kinds of processing are involved in utterance production. One is *controlled processing*; this kind makes demands on working memory. The other is *automatic processing*, which does not require allocation of working memory. Verbal formulation is performed with both controlled processing and automatic processing. Controlled processing can be identified in Figure 2.1 by the arrows labeled A and B. Note that syntactic, semantic, and phonologic processing are automatic; that is, the speaker does not have direct access to these operations. It is for this reason that slips of the tongue are not detected until they are actually spoken.

Feedback is provided by two channels, labeled α and β in Figure 2.1. Channel α represents information from touch and movement. Channel β represents auditory feedback.

Researchers have concluded that when a person ordinarily produces a sentence, he or she doesn't make all of the syntactic, semantic, and phonologic decisions before beginning to speak. Rather, it is likely that the individual will utter a few words and then formulate the remainder of the utterance.

According to this view of verbal formulation, producing a sentence involves highly interactive levels of processing and a complex time pattern for this processing. It would not be surprising, then, to discover that articulation is affected by syntactic, semantic, and phonologic variables.

The following discussion of articulatory phonetics presents basic information on speech sound production. For the student who has had a course in phonetics, this chapter will serve as a summary review. The student without such background should be able to acquire at least the basics of articulatory phonetics. The topics to be discussed are these:

The Speech Mechanism

Vowels

  Monophthongs (single vowels)

  Diphthongs

Consonants

  Stops

  Nasals

Fricatives

Affricates

Liquids

Glides

Suprasegmentals

Coarticulation

Aerodynamics

Acoustics

Sensory Information

Phonology

FUNDAMENTALS OF ARTICULATORY PHONETICS

The Speech Mechanism

The anatomy of the speech production system is not within the scope of this chapter, but some general anatomical descriptions are needed to discuss the fundamentals of articulatory phonetics. The basic aspects of speech production can be understood by an examination of six principal organs or subsystems, illustrated in Figure 2.2. The *respiratory system*,

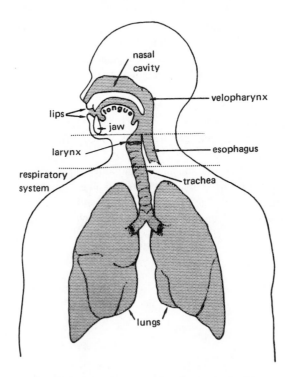

■ **FIGURE 2.2** Organs of speech production.

consisting of the lungs, airway, rib cage, diaphragm, and associated structures, provides the basic air supply for generating sound. The *larynx,* composed of various cartilages and muscles, generates the voiced sounds of speech by vibration of the vocal folds, or it allows air to pass from lungs to the vocal tract (the oral and nasal cavities) for voiceless sounds. The *velopharynx*—the soft palate (or velum) and associated structures of the velopharyngeal port—joins or separates the oral and nasal cavities so that air passes through the oral cavity, the nasal cavity, or both. The *tongue*, primarily a complex of muscles, is the principal articulator of the oral cavity; it is capable of assuming a variety of shapes and positions in vowel and consonant articulation. For articulatory purposes, the tongue is divided into five major parts: the tip or apex, the blade, the back or dorsum, the root, and the body. These divisions are illustrated in Figure 2.3. The *lips*, along with the jaw, are the most visible of the articulators; they are involved in the production of vowels and consonants. The *jaw*, the massive bony structure and its associated muscles, supports the soft tissues of both tongue and lower lip. It participates in speech production by aiding tongue and lip movements and by providing skeletal support for these organs.

Other anatomical features shown in Figure 2.2 provide general orientation or are relevant in a significant way to the processes of speech and hearing.

The respiratory system and larynx work together to provide the upper airway with two major types of air flow: a series of pulses of air created by the action of the vibrating vocal folds (for voiced sounds like the sounds in the word *buzz*), and a continuous flow of air that can be used to generate noise energy in the vocal tract (for voiceless sounds like the *s* in *see*). The basic function of the respiratory system in speech is to push air into the airway composed of the larynx and the oral and nasal cavities. The basic function of the larynx is to regulate the air flow from the lungs to create both voiced and voiceless segments. The upper airway, often called the vocal tract, runs from the larynx to the mouth or nose and is the site of what is commonly called speech articulation. For the most part, this process is accomplished by movements of the *articulators*: tongue, lips, jaw, and velopharynx. The vocal

■ **FIGURE 2.3** Divisions of tongue into five functional parts for speech articulation.

tract may be viewed as a flexible tube that can be lengthened or shortened (by moving the larynx up and down in the neck or by protruding and retracting the lips) and constricted at many points along its length by actions of tongue, velopharynx, and lips. Speech articulation is thus a matter of lengthening, shortening, and constricting the tube known as the vocal tract.

This entire process is controlled by the nervous system, which must translate the message to be communicated into a pattern of signals that run to the various muscles of the speech mechanism. As these muscles contract, a variety of things can happen: Air may be pushed out of the lungs, the vocal folds may start to vibrate, the velopharynx may close, the jaw may lower, or the lips may protrude. The brain has the task of coordinating all the different muscles so that they contract in the proper sequence to produce the required phonetic result. The margin for error is small; sometimes an error of just a few milliseconds in the timing of a muscle contraction can result in a misarticulation.

It is appealing to suppose that speech production is controlled at some relatively high level of the brain by discrete units, such as phonemes. However, a major problem in the description of speech articulation is to relate the discrete linguistic units that operate at a high level of the brain to the muscle contractions that result in articulatory movements. For example, to say the word *stop*, a speaker's brain must send nerve instructions, in the proper sequence, to the muscles of the respiratory system, larynx, tongue, lips, and velopharynx. The full understanding of speech production therefore involves a knowledge of *phonology* (the study of how sounds are put together to form words and other linguistic units), *articulatory phonetics* (the study of how the articulators make individual sounds), *acoustic phonetics* (the study of the relationship between articulation and the acoustic signal of speech), and *speech perception* (the study of how phonetic decisions are made from the acoustic signal).

Vowel Articulation: Traditional Phonetic Description

A vowel sound is usually formed as sound energy from the vibrating vocal folds escapes through a relatively open vocal tract of a particular shape. Because a syllable must contain a vowel or vowel-like sound, vowels sometimes are called *syllable nuclei*. Each vowel has a characteristic vocal tract shape that is determined by the position of the tongue, jaw, and lips. Although other parts of the vocal tract, like the velum, pharyngeal walls, and cheeks, may vary somewhat with different vowels, the positions of the tongue, jaw, and lips are of primary consequence. Therefore, individual vowels can be described by specifying the articulatory positions of tongue, jaw, and lips. Furthermore, because the jaw and tongue usually work together to increase or reduce the mouth opening (Figure 2.4), for general phonetic purposes vowel production can be described by specifying the positions of just two articulators, tongue and lips. Usually, the vocal folds vibrate to produce voicing for vowels, but exceptions, such as whispered speech, do occur.

The two basic lip articulations can be demonstrated with the vowels in the words *he* and *who*. Press your finger against your lips as you say first *he* and then *who*. You should feel the lips push against your finger as you say *who*. The vowel in this word is a rounded vowel, meaning that the lips assume a rounded, protruded posture. Vowels in English are described as being either rounded, like the vowel in *who*, or unrounded, like the vowel in *he*. Figure 2.5 illustrates the lip configuration for these two vowels.

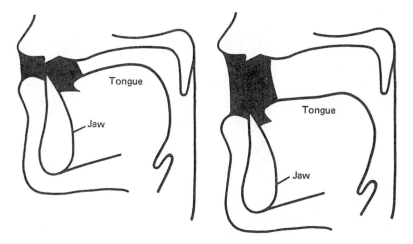

■ **FIGURE 2.4** Variations in mouth opening (darkened area) related to lowering of jaw and tongue.

■ **FIGURE 2.5** Vocal tract configurations for /i/ and /u/. Note lip rounding for /u/.

The tongue moves in essentially two dimensions within the oral cavity, as shown in Figure 2.6. One dimension, front-back, is represented by the motion the tongue makes as you alternately say *he*, *who* or *map*, *mop*. The other dimension, high-low, is represented by the motion the tongue makes as you say *heave-have* or *who-ha*. With these two dimensions of tongue movement, we can define four extreme positions of the tongue within the oral cavity, as shown in Figure 2.7. The phonetic symbols for these four vowels also are shown in the illustration. With the tongue high and forward in the mouth, the high-front vowel /i/ as in *he* is produced. When the tongue is low and forward in the mouth, the low-front vowel /æ/ as in *have* is produced. A tongue position that is high and back in the mouth yields the

■ FIGURE 2.6   The two major dimensions of tongue position, front-back and high-low.

high-back vowel /u/. Finally, when the tongue is low and back in the mouth, the vowel is the low-back /ɑ/. The four vowels, /i/, /æ/, /u/, and /ɑ/, define four points that establish the *vowel quadrilateral*, a four-sided figure against which tongue position for vowels can be described. In Figure 2.8, the vowels of English have been plotted by phonetic symbol and key word within the quadrilateral. As an example, notice the vowel /ɪ/ as in *bit* has a tongue position that is forward in the mouth and not quite as high as that for /i/. The tongue position for any one vowel can be specified with terms such as low-high, front for /ɪ/ as in *bit*, low-mid, front for /ɛ/ as in *bet*, mid-central for /ɝ/ as in *Bert*, and low-mid, back for /ɔ/ as in *bought*.

The vowels of English can be categorized as follows with respect to tongue position:

Front vowels:	/i/	/ɪ/	/e/	/ɛ/	/æ/		
Central vowels:	/ɝ/	/ʌ/	/ɚ/	/ə/			
Back vowels:	/u/	/ʊ/	/o/	/ɔ/	/ɑ/		
High vowels:	/i/	/ɪ/	/u/	/ʊ/			
Mid vowels:	/e/	/ɛ/	/ɝ/	/ʌ/	/ɚ/	/ə/	/o/ /ɔ/
Low vowels:	/æ/	/ɑ/					

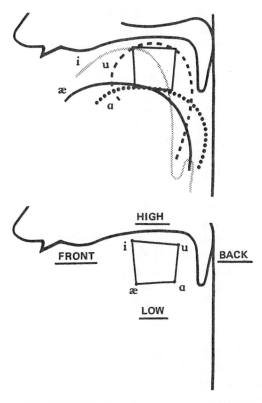

■ **FIGURE 2.7** The four corner vowels /i/, /u/, /ɑ/, and /æ/ are shown at the top as tongue positions in the oral cavity and at the bottom as points of a quadrilateral.

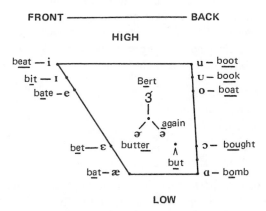

■ **FIGURE 2.8** English vowels, identified by phonetic symbol and key word and plotted within vowel quadrilateral.

The vowels can also be categorized with respect to lip rounding, with the following being rounded: /u/, /ʊ/, /o/, /ɔ/, and /ɝ/. All other vowels are unrounded. Notice that, in English, the rounded vowels are either back or central vowels; front rounded vowels do not occur.

Vowel production is also commonly described as *tense (long)* or *lax (short)*. Tense vowels are longer in duration and supposedly involve a greater degree of muscular tension. Lax vowels are relatively short and involve less muscular effort. One way of demonstrating the distinction between tense and lax is to feel the fleshy undersurface of your jaw as you say /i/ as in *he* and /ɪ/ as in *him*. Most people can feel a greater tension for /i/ (a tense vowel) than for /ɪ/ (a lax vowel). The tense vowels are /i/, /e/, /ɝ/, /u/, /o/, /ɔ/, and /ɑ/. The remaining vowels are considered lax, but opinion is divided for the vowel /æ/ as in *bat*.

In standard production, all English vowels are voiced (associated with vibrating vocal folds) and nonnasal (having no escape of sound energy through the nose). Therefore, the descriptors *voiced* and *nonnasal* usually are omitted. However, it should be remembered that vowels are sometimes devoiced, as in whispering, and nasalized, as when they precede or follow nasal consonants. For phonetic purposes it is usually sufficient to describe a vowel in terms of the three major characteristics of tenseness—laxness, lip configuration, and tongue position. Examples of vowel description are given as follows:

/i/	tense, unrounded, high-front
/o/	tense, rounded, high-mid, back
/ɝ/	tense, rounded, mid-central
/ʊ/	lax, rounded, low-high, back

Closely related to the vowels are the *diphthongs*, which, like vowels, are produced with an open vocal tract and serve as the nuclei for syllables. But unlike vowels, diphthongs are formed with an articulation that gradually changes during production of the sound. Diphthongs are dynamic sounds, because they involve a progressive change in vocal tract shape. An example of the articulation of /aɪ/ is shown in Figure 2.9. Many phoneticians regard diphthongs as combinations of two vowels, one called the *onglide* portion and the other called the *offglide* portion. This vowel + vowel description underlies the phonetic symbols for the diphthongs, which have the *digraph* (two-element) symbols /aɪ/, /aʊ/, /ɔɪ/, /eɪ/, and /oʊ/. Key words for these sounds are as follows:

/aɪ/	*I, buy, why, ice, night*
/aʊ/	*ow, bough, trout, down, owl*
/ɔɪ/	*boy, oil, loin, hoist*
/eɪ/	*bay, daze, rain, stay*
/oʊ/	*bow, no, load, bone*

Whereas the diphthongs /aɪ/, /aʊ/, and /ɔɪ/ are truly phonemic diphthongs, /eɪ/ and /oʊ/ are not; they are variants of the vowels /e/ and /o/, respectively. The diphthongal forms /eɪ/ and /oʊ/ occur in strongly stressed syllables, whereas the monophthongal (single-vowel) forms /e/ and /o/ tend to occur in weakly stressed syllables. For example, in the

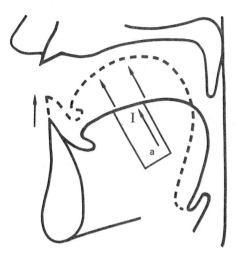

■ **FIGURE 2.9** Articulation of diphthong /aɪ/ (as in *eye*), represented as onglide (/a/) and offglide (/ɪ/) configurations.

word *vacation*, the first syllable (weakly stressed) is produced with /e/ and the second syllable (strongly stressed) is produced with /eɪ/. Stressed syllables tend to be long in duration and therefore allow time for the articulatory movement of the diphthong. The diphthongs /aɪ/, /aʊ/, and /ɔɪ/ do not alternate with monophthongal forms. To produce a recognizable /aɪ/, /aʊ/, or /ɔɪ/, a speaker must use a diphthongal movement.

    As shown in Figure 2.10, the onglide and offglide segments of the diphthongs are roughly located by the positions of the digraph symbols on the vowel quadrilateral. For example, in diphthong /aɪ/, the tongue moves from a low-back to nearly a high-front position. However, it should be noted that these onglide and offglide positions are only approximate and that substantial variation occurs across speakers and speaking conditions.

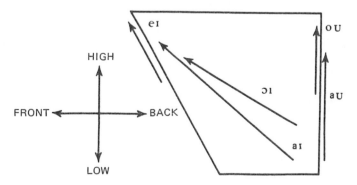

■ **FIGURE 2.10** Diphthong articulation shown as onglide to offglide arrows in the vowel quadrilateral.

Vowel Articulation: Description by Distinctive Features

The phonetic descriptions considered to this point are one method of classifying vowel sounds. An alternative is a method relying on *distinctive features*, as defined by the linguists Noam Chomsky and Morris Hallé (1968). The distinctive features are a set of binary (two-valued) features designed to describe the phonemes in all languages of the world. A convenient example of a binary feature is nasality. In general terms, a given speech sound is either nasal or nonnasal, meaning that sound energy is transmitted through the nose (nasal) or is not (nonnasal). If nasality is described as a binary feature, then sounds can be classified as +nasal (indicating the nasal transmission of sound) or −nasal (indicating the absence of nasal transmission). Hence, a positive value (+nasal) means that the property is present or is relevant to description of the sound. In some ways, distinctive feature analysis is similar to the guessing game of Twenty Questions in which the participants have to identify an object by asking questions that can be answered with only yes or no. Chomsky and Hallé proposed a set of 13 binary features, which, given the appropriate yes (+) or no (−) answers, can describe all phonemes used in the languages of the world.

In the Chomsky-Hallé system, the voiced vowels are specified primarily with the features shown in Table 2.1. First, notice the three major class features of *sonorant, vocalic,* and *consonantal.* A sonorant sound is produced with a vocal cavity configuration in which spontaneous voicing is possible. Essentially, the vocal tract above the larynx is sufficiently open so that no special laryngeal adjustments are needed to initiate voicing. For nonsonorants, or *obstruents,* the cavity configuration does not allow spontaneous voicing. Special mechanisms must be used to produce voicing during the nonsonorant sounds. Vocalic sounds are produced with an oral cavity shape in which the greatest constriction does not exceed that associated with the high vowels /i/ and /u/ and with vocal folds that are adjusted so as to allow spontaneous voicing. This feature, then, describes the degree of opening of the oral cavity together with the vocal fold adjustment. Finally, consonantal sounds have a definite constriction in the *midsagittal,* or midline, region of the

■ **TABLE 2.1** Distinctive Features for Selected Vowel Sounds (The Class Features Distinguish Vowels from Various Consonants; Therefore, All Vowels Have the Same Values for These Features)

Class Features	i	ɪ	ɛ	æ	ʌ	ɝ	u	ʊ	ɔ	ɑ
Sonorant	+	+	+	+	+	+	+	+	+	+
Vocalic	+	+	+	+	+	+	+	+	+	+
Consonantal	−	−	−	−	−	−	−	−	−	−
Cavity Features										
High	+	+	−	−	−	−	+	+	−	−
Low	−	−	−	+	−	−	−	−	+	+
Back	−	−	−	−	−	−	+	+	+	+
Rounded	−	−	−	−	−	+	+	+	+	−
Nasal	−	−	−	−	−	−	−	−	−	−
Manner of Articulation Feature										
Tense	+	−	−	+	−	+	+	−	+	+

vocal tract; nonconsonantal sounds do not. Vowels are described as +sonorant, +vocalic, and −consonantal. Taken together, these three features indicate that vowels are produced with a relatively open oral cavity, with no severe constriction in the midsagittal plane, and with a vocal fold adjustment that allows for spontaneous vocal fold vibration.

Vowels are also described with respect to cavity features and manner of articulation features, some of which are shown in Table 2.1 (the others will be discussed with respect to consonants later in this chapter). The cavity features of primary concern in vowel description are:

Tongue Body Features: High-Nonhigh; Low-Nonlow; Back-Nonback
(see Figure 2.11a, b, c)

High sounds are produced by raising the body of the tongue above the level that it occupies in the neutral (or resting) position, as shown in Figure 2.11a.

Low sounds are produced by lowering the body of the tongue below the level that it occupies in the neutral position; see Figure 2.11b.

Back sounds are produced by retracting the body of the tongue from the neutral position, as shown in Figure 2.11c.

Rounded–Nonrounded. Rounded sounds have a narrowing or protrusion of the lips.

Nasal–Nonnasal. Nasal sounds are produced with a lowered velum, so that sound energy escapes through the nose.

Table 2.1 shows that most vowels can be distinguished using the cavity features. For example, /i/ and /u/ differ in the back and rounded features, and /æ/ and /i/ differ in the high and low features. Most other distinctions can be made by referring to a manner of articulation called tense–nontense. Tense sounds are produced with a deliberate, accurate, maximally distinct gesture that involves considerable muscular effort. The tense–nontense distinction is best illustrated with the vowel pairs /i/–/ɪ/ and /u/–/ʊ/. Vowels /i/ and /u/ are tense vowels because they are lengthened and are produced with marked muscular effort. As mentioned earlier, the difference in muscular effort can be felt by placing your fingers in the fleshy area just under the chin, saying alternately /i/–/ɪ/. A greater tension occurs during production of the tense vowel /i/ than during the nontense vowel /ɪ/.

Consonant Articulation: Traditional Phonetic Description

The consonants generally differ from the vowels in terms of the relative openness of the vocal tract and the function within the syllable. Vowels are produced with an open vocal tract; most consonants are made with a complete or partially constricted vocal tract. Within a syllable, vowels serve as a nucleus, meaning that a syllable must contain one and only one vowel (the only exceptions to this rule are the diphthongs, which are like vowels plus vowel glides, and certain syllabic consonants to be discussed later). Consonants are added to the vowel nucleus to form different syllable shapes, such as the following, where V represents a vowel and C represents a consonant.

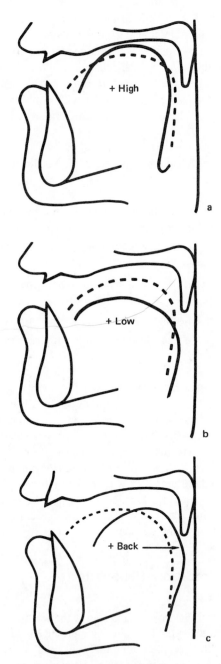

FIGURE 2.11 Vocal tract drawings illustrating the tongue body features *(a)* high, *(b)* low, and *(c)* back relative to the neutral tongue position (broken line).

VC shape: *on, add, in*
CV shape: *do, be, too*
CVC shape: *dog, cat, man*
CCVC shape: *truck, skin, clap*
CCVCC shape: *screams, squint, scratched*

Consonants are described by degree or type of closure and by the location at which the complete or partial closure occurs. The *manner* of consonant articulation refers to the degree or type of closure, and the *place* of consonant articulation refers to the location of the constriction. In addition, consonants are described as *voiced* when the vocal folds are vibrating and *voiceless* when the vocal folds are not vibrating. Thus, an individual consonant can be specified by using three terms: one to describe *voicing*, one to describe *place*, and one to describe *manner*. Tables 2.2 and 2.3 show combinations of these terms used to specify the consonants of English.

▦ **TABLE 2.2** Classification of Consonants by Manner and Voicing within Place

Place of Articulation	Phonetic Symbol and Key Word	Manner of Articulation	Voicing
Bilabial	/p/ (pay)	Stop	−
	/b/ (bay)	Stop	+
	/m/ (may)	Nasal	+
Labial/velar	/ʍ/ (which)	Glide (semivowel)	−
	/w/ (witch)	Glide (semivowel)	+
Labiodental	/f/ (fan)	Fricative	−
	/v/ (van)	Fricative	+
Linguadental (interdental)	/θ/ (thin)	Fricative	−
	/ð/ (this)	Fricative	+
Lingua-alveolar	/t/ (two)	Stop	−
	/d/ (do)	Stop	+
	/s/ (sue)	Fricative	−
	/z/ (zoo)	Fricative	+
	/n/ (new)	Nasal	+
	/l/ (Lou)	Lateral	+
	/ɾ/ (butter)	Flap	+
Linguapalatal	/ʃ/ (shoe)	Fricative	−
	/ʒ/ (rouge)	Fricative	+
	/tʃ/ (chin)	Affricative	−
	/dʒ/ (gin)	Affricative	+
	/j/ (you)	Glide (semivowel)	+
	/r/ (rue)	Rhotic	+
Linguavelar	/k/ (back)	Stop	−
	/g/ (bag)	Stop	+
	/ŋ/ (bang)	Nasal	+
Glottal (laryngeal)	/h/ (who)	Fricative	−
	/ʔ/	Stop	+(−)

■ **TABLE 2.3**　Classification of Consonants by Place and Voicing within Manner

Manner	Place	Voiced	Voiceless
Stop	Bilabial	b	p
	Alveolar	d	t
	Velar	g	k
	Glottal	------?------------------	
Fricative	Labiodental	v	f
	Linguadental	ð	θ
	Alveolar	z	s
	Palatal	ʒ	ʃ
	Glottal		h
Affricative	Palatal	dʒ	tʃ
Nasal	Bilabial	m	
	Alveolar	n	
	Velar	ŋ	
Lateral	Alveolar	l	
Rhotic	Palatal	r	
Glide	Palatal	j	
	Labial/Velar	w	ʍ

Table 2.2 contains four columns, showing place of articulation, phonetic symbol and key word, manner of articulation, and voicing. The terms for place of articulation usually signify two opposing structures that accomplish a localized constriction of the vocal tract. Notice in the following definitions the two structures involved for the place terms.

Bilabial: two lips (*bi = two* and *labia = lip*)

Labial/velar: lips, and a constriction between the *dorsum* or back of the tongue and the velum

Labiodental: lower lip and upper teeth

Linguadental or interdental: tip of tongue and upper teeth (*lingua = tongue*)

Lingua-alveolar: tip of tongue and the *alveolar ridge*

Linguapalatal: blade of tongue and palatal area behind the alveolar ridge

Linguavelar: dorsum or back of tongue and roof of mouth in the velar area

Glottal: the two vocal folds

Each of these places of articulation is discussed more fully on the next several pages. To get a feeling for these different places of consonant articulation, concentrate on the first sounds in each word as you say the sequence: *pie, why, vie, thigh, tie, shy, guy, hi*. Notice from Figure 2.12 that the initial sounds constitute a progression from front to back in place of articulation.

Table 2.3 provides a breakdown of English consonants by place and voicing within manner classes. The manner of production associated with complete closure is the *stop*,

■ **FIGURE 2.12** Places of articulation are marked by location of the phonetic symbols for the initial sounds in *pie, why, vie, thigh, tie, shy, guy, hi.*

which is formed when two structures completely block the passage of air from the vocal tract, building up air pressure behind the closure. Usually, when the closure is released, the air pressure built up behind the constriction causes a burst of escaping air. The burst is audible in words like *pie* and *two.*

Fricatives, like the initial sounds in *sue* and *zoo*, are made with a narrow constriction so that the air creates a noisy sound as it rushes through the narrowed passage.

Affricates, as in *church* and *judge*, are combinations of stop and fricative segments; that is, a period of complete closure is followed by a brief fricative segment. The stop + fricative nature of the affricates explain why these sounds are represented by the digraph symbols /tʃ/ and /dʒ/.

Nasals, as in the word *meaning* /minɪŋ/, are like stops in having a complete oral closure (bilabial, lingua-alveolar, or linguavelar) but are unlike stops in having an open velopharyngeal port so that sound energy passes through the nose rather than the mouth.

The *lateral* /l/ as in *lay* is formed by making a lingua-alveolar closure in the midline but with no closure at the sides of the tongue. Therefore, the sound energy from the vibrating folds escapes laterally, or through the sides of the mouth cavity.

The *rhotic* (or *rhotacized*) /r/ as in *ray* is a complex phoneme sometimes called *retroflex* in the phonetic literature. *Retroflex* literally means "turning" or "turned back" and refers to the appearance of the tongue tip, as viewed in X-ray films, for some /r/ productions. But in other productions of /r/, the tongue has a bunched appearance in the center or near the front of the mouth cavity. Because /r/ is produced in at least these two basic ways, the general term *rhotic* (Ladefoged, 1975) is preferable to the narrower term *retroflex*. This issue is discussed in more detail later in this chapter.

The /ʍ/, /w/, and /j/ sounds are said to have a *glide* (semivowel) manner of production. These sounds are characterized by a gliding, or gradually changing, articulatory shape. For example, in /ʍ/ and its voiced counterpart /w/, the lips gradually move from a rounded and narrowed configuration to the lip shape required by the following vowel simultaneously with a change in tongue position from high-back (like that for /u/) to the position for the following vowel. The glides always are followed by vowels.

In the following summary, manner of articulation is discussed for different places of articulation, proceeding from front to back.

Bilabial Sounds

In American English, the only consonant phonemes produced with a complete or partial closure (bilabial production) are the voiceless and voiced stops /p/ as in *pay* and /b/ as in *bay*, the nasal /m/ as in *may*, and the voiced and voiceless glides /w/ as in *witch* and /ʍ/ as in *which*. The vocal tract configurations for /p/, /b/, and /m/ are shown in Figure 2.13. These three sounds share a bilabial closure but differ in voicing and nasality. The stops /p/ and /b/ are called voiced and voiceless *cognates*, which means that they differ only in voicing. The production of these bilabial sounds is usually marked by a closed jaw position because the jaw closes somewhat to assist the constriction at the lips. The tongue is virtually unconstrained for /p/, /b/, and /m/, so that these bilabial sounds often are made simultaneously with the tongue position for preceding or following vowels. In other words, when we say words like *bee*, *pa*, and *moo*, the tongue is free to assume the required shape for the vowel during the closure for the bilabial, as illustrated in Figure 2.14.

■ **FIGURE 2.13** Vocal tract configurations for /p/, /b/, and /m/. Note labial closure for all three sounds and the open velopharynx for /m/.

■ **FIGURE 2.14**   Variation in tongue position during a bilabial closure: (*top*) tongue position during *pea*; (*bottom*) tongue position for *pa*.

The glides /w/ and /ʍ/ have a specified tongue position, roughly like that for the high-back vowel /u/, so these sounds cannot interact as freely with preceding or following sounds. Students (and even some practicing clinicians) sometimes fail to appreciate the importance of tongue articulation for /w/ and /ʍ/; for these sounds, both the tongue and lips execute gliding movements, as shown for the word *we* in Figure 2.15.

Labiodental Sounds

The voiceless and voiced *fricatives* /f/ as in *fan* and /v/ as in *van* are the only labiodental sounds in American English. The articulation is illustrated in Figure 2.16. Frication noise is generated by forcing air through the constriction formed by the lower lip and the upper teeth, principally the incisors. The noise is quite weak, very nearly the weakest of the fricatives. Like the labial sounds /p/, /b/, and /m/, the labiodentals allow the tongue to assume its position for preceding or following sounds. The jaw tends to close to aid the lower lip in its constricting gesture.

■ **FIGURE 2.15**   Illustration of gliding motion of tongue and lips for the word *we* (/wi/).

■ **FIGURE 2.16**   Vocal tract configuration for /f/ and /v/. Note labiodental constriction.

Interdental Sounds

There are only two interdentals, both fricatives: the voiceless /θ/ (e.g., *thaw*) and voiced /ð/ (e.g., *the*). They are illustrated in Figure 2.17. The frication noise is generated as air flows through the narrow constriction created by the tongue tip and the edge of the incisors. The weak frication noise is not much different from that for /f/ or /v/. The weak intensity of these sounds should be remembered in articulation testing, and the clinician should include both visual and auditory information in evaluating this pair of sounds. Jaw position for /θ/ and /ð/ usually is closed to aid the tongue in making its constriction. These sounds may be produced with either an interdental projection of the tongue or tongue contact behind the teeth.

/θ/ /ð/

■ **FIGURE 2.17** Vocal tract configuration for /θ/ and /ð/. Note linguadental constriction.

Alveolar Sounds

The alveolar place of production is used for two stops: the voiceless /t/ (e.g., *too*) and the voiced /d/ (e.g., *do*); a nasal: /n/ (e.g., *new*); a lateral: /l/ (e.g., *Lou*); and two fricatives: the voiceless /s/ (e.g., *sue*) and the voiced /z/ (e.g., *zoo*). Not surprisingly, given the frequent and diverse movements of the tongue tip in the alveolar region, motions of the tongue tip are among the fastest articulatory movements. For example, the major closing and release movement for the stops /t/ and /d/ is made within about 50 milliseconds, or a twentieth of a second. For /t/ and /d/, an airtight chamber is created as the tongue tip closes firmly against the alveolar ridge and the sides of the tongue seal against the lateral oral regions. The site of tongue tip closure actually varies to a limited degree with phonetic context. When /t/ or /d/ are produced before the dental fricatives /θ/ and /ð/, the stop closure is made in the dental region. This context-dependent modification of alveolar consonant production is termed *dentalization* and is illustrated for /t/ in Figure 2.18.

The nasal /n/ is similar in basic tongue shape and movement to the stops /t/ and /d/. But /n/ differs from both /t/ and /d/ in having an open velopharyngeal port, making /n/ nasalized. But /n/ further differs from /t/ in that /n/ is voiced; /t/ is not. Because /n/ and /d/ are very similar in lingual articulation and voicing, failure to close the velopharyngeal port for /d/, as might happen with some speech disorders, results in /n/. Like /t/ and /d/, /n/ is dentalized when produced in the same syllable and adjacent to a dental sound like /θ/; compare, for example, the /n/ in *nine* /naɪn/ with the /n/ in *ninth* /naɪnθ/.

The lateral /l/ is a *liquid* formed with midline closure and a lateral opening, usually at both sides of the mouth (see Figure 2.19). Because of the midline closure made by the tongue tip against the alveolar ridge, sound energy escapes through the sides of the oral cavity. Although /l/ is the only lateral sound in English, there are at least two major allophones. Historically, these allophones are termed *light* and *dark*, but phoneticians disagree as to exactly how these allophones are formed. Wise (1957a, 1957b) explained that the light

■ **FIGURE 2.18** Dentalization of /t/. The normal alveolar closure is shown by the solid line and the dental closure is shown by the broken line.

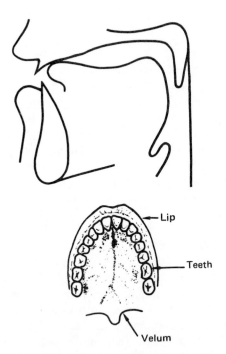

■ **FIGURE 2.19** Articulation of /l/, shown in side view of a midline section (*top*) and as regions of tongue closure (*shaded areas*) against roof of mouth.

/l/ is made with linguadental contact, whereas the dark /l/ is made with a lingua-alveolar contact. However, Kantner and West (1960) contend that the light /l/ has a greater lip spread and a lower and flatter tongue position than the dark /l/. An important feature of /l/, presumably, is a raising of the tongue toward the velum or palate. Giles (1971) concluded from X-ray pictures of speech that for allophonic variations of /l/, the position of the tongue dorsum falls into three general groups regardless of phonetic context: prevocalic, postvocalic, and syllabic (with syllabic being similar to postvocalic /l/). The postvocalic allophones had a more posterior dorsal position than the prevocalic allophones. Tongue tip contact occasionally was not achieved for the postvocalic allophones in words like *Paul*. Otherwise, the only variation in tongue tip articulation was dentalization influenced by a following dental sound. Apparently, then, /l/ can be produced with either a relatively front (light /l/) or back (dark /l/) dorsal position, but the light and dark variants are perhaps just as well termed prevocalic and postvocalic. Lingua-alveolar contact is not essential at least for /l/ in postvocalic position, which explains why postvocalic /l/ in words like *seal* may sound like /o/ or /ʊ/. The fricatives /s/ and /z/ are made with a narrow constriction between the tongue tip and the alveolar ridge (see Figure 2.20).

Palatal Sounds

The palatal sounds include the voiceless and voiced fricatives /ʃ/ (e.g., *shoe*) and /ʒ/ (e.g., *rouge*), the voiceless and voiced affricates /tʃ/ (e.g., *chin*) and /dʒ/ (e.g., *gin*), the glide /j/ (e.g., *you*), and the rhotic or retroflex /r/ (e.g., *rue*). For these sounds, the blade or tip of the tongue makes a constriction in the palatal region, the area just behind the alveolar ridge (see Figure 2.21).

The fricatives /ʃ/ and /ʒ/, like /s/ and /z/, are sibilants associated with intense noisy energy. For /ʃ/ and /ʒ/, this noise is generated as air moves rapidly through a constriction formed between the blade of the tongue and the front palate. Similarly, the affricates /tʃ/ and /dʒ/ are made in the palatal area as stop + fricative combinations. The airstream is first interrupted during the stop phase and then released during the fricative phase that immediately follows. In English, the only affricates are the palatal /tʃ/ and /dʒ/.

Constriction
Site

■ **FIGURE 2.20** Vocal tract configuration for /s/ and /z/. Note lingua-alveolar constriction.

■ FIGURE 2.21 Vocal tract configuration for /ʃ/ and /ʒ/. Note linguapalatal constriction.

The glide /j/ is similar to the high-front vowel /i/ (as in *he*). The tongue is initially far forward and high in the mouth and subsequently moves toward the position for the following vowel. The similarity between /j/ and /i/ can be demonstrated by saying the biblical pronoun *ye* while noting the tongue position. Because the glide /j/ must be followed by a vowel, its articulation involves a gliding motion from the high-front position to some other vowel shape. The gliding motion can be felt during articulation of the words *you, yea, ya*.

As mentioned previously, the articulation of /r/ is highly variable. It sometimes is produced as a retroflexed consonant, in which case the tongue tip points upward and slightly backward in the oral cavity. But /r/ also can be produced with a bunching of the tongue, either in the middle of the mouth or near the front of the mouth. These basic articulations are illustrated in Figure 2.22. Some speakers also round their lips for /r/, and some constrict the lower pharynx by pulling the root of the tongue backward. Because /r/ is variably produced, it seems advisable to use *rhotic* or *rhotacized* (Ladefoged, 1975) rather than *retroflex* as a general articulatory descriptor. Given the complicated articulation of /r/, it is not surprising that it should present a major problem to children learning to talk. The variation in tongue shape and position also complicates a speech clinician's attempts to teach /r/ articulations to a child who misarticulates the sound.

■ FIGURE 2.22 The two major articulations of /r/: (*left*) the retroflexed articulation; (*right*) the bunched articulation.

Velar Sounds

A velar constriction, formed by elevation of the tongue dorsum toward the roof of the mouth, occurs for the voiceless and voiced stops /k/ and /g/ and for the nasal /ŋ/. This articulation is illustrated in Figure 2.23, which shows that the constriction can be made with the tongue relatively toward the front or relatively toward the back. The tongue placement is generally determined by the vowel context, with a front placement for velars adjacent to front vowels (e.g., /g/ in *geese*) and a back placement for velars adjacent to back vowels (e.g., /g/ in *goose*). The nasal /ŋ/ has a tongue constriction similar to that for /k/ and /g/ but has an open velopharyngeal port for nasalization. The velar and bilabial places of articulation are similar in that both are used in English only for stops and nasals.

Glottal Sounds

The glottis, or chink between the vocal folds, is primarily involved only with two sounds, the voiceless fricative /h/ and the stop /ʔ/ (a stoppage of air at the vocal folds). The fricative is produced with an opening of the vocal folds so that a fricative noise is generated as air moves at high speed through the glottis. A similar vocal fold adjustment is used in whisper.

It can be seen from Tables 2.2 and 2.3 that more types of sounds are made at some places of articulation than at others. Moreover, some sounds occur more frequently in the English language than others, contributing to a further imbalance in the use of places of articulation. Actual data on the frequency of occurrence of English consonants, grouped by place of articulation, are shown in Figure 2.24. In this circle graph, based on data from Dewey (1923), the relative frequencies of occurrence of different places of articulation are

■ **FIGURE 2.23** Vocal tract configurations for velar consonants. Note variation in site of closure.

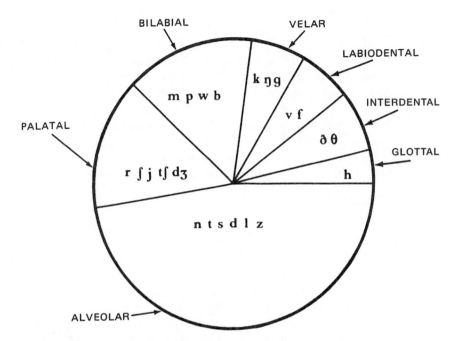

■ FIGURE 2.24   Circle graph showing relative frequency of occurrence of consonants made at different places of articulation.

Source: Based on data from Dewey (1923).

shown by the relative sizes of the pieces of the graph. Notice that alveolar sounds account for almost 50 percent of the sounds in English. The rank order of frequency of occurrence for place of articulation, from most to least frequent, is: alveolar, palatal, bilabial, velar, labiodental, interdental, and glottal. Within each place-of-articulation segment in Figure 2.24, the individual consonants are listed in rank order of frequency of occurrence. For example, /n/ is the most frequently occurring alveolar consonant (in fact, it is the most frequently occurring of all consonants). Because of the differences in frequency of occurrence of consonants, a misarticulation affecting one place of articulation can be far more conspicuous than a misarticulation affecting another place. Therefore, statistical properties of the language are one consideration in the assessment and management of articulation disorders.

Consonant Articulation: Description by Distinctive Features

Distinctive features, discussed earlier with respect to vowels, can be used as an alternative to the place-manner chart to describe consonants. One simple example is the feature of voiced: All voiced consonants can be assigned the feature value of +voiced, and all voiceless consonants can be assigned the value of −voiced. Some important features for consonants are defined briefly below and are used for consonant classification in Table 2.4. These definitions are based on Chomsky and Hallé (1968).

◼ **TABLE 2.4** Distinctive Feature Classifications for Selected Consonants

Feature	p	b	m	t	d	n	s	l	θ	k
Consonantal	+	+	+	+	+	+	+	+	+	+
Vocalic	−	−	−	−	−	−	−	−	−	−
Sonorant	−	−	+	−	−	+	−	+	−	−
Interrupted	+	+	−	+	+	−	−	−	−	+
Strident	−	−	−	−	−	−	+	−	−	−
High	(−)	(−)	(−)*	−	−	−	−	−	−	+
Low	(−)	(−)	(−)	−	−	−	−	−	−	−
Back	(−)	(−)	(−)	−	−	−	−	−	−	+
Anterior	+	+	+	+	+	+	+	+	+	−
Coronal	−	−	−	+	+	+	+	+	+	−
Rounded	−	−	−	−	−	−	−	−	−	−
Distributed	+	+	+	−	−	−	−	−	+	−
Lateral	−	−	−	−	−	−	−	+	−	−
Nasal	−	−	+	−	−	+	−	−	−	−
Voiced	−	+	+	−	+	+	−	+	−	−

*Feature values enclosed in parentheses indicate that the feature in question may not be specified for this sound. For example, tongue position for /p/, /b/, and /m/ is not really specified, as it is free to assume the position required for the following vowel.

Consonantal sounds have a radical or marked constriction in the midsagittal region of the vocal tract. This feature distinguishes the "true" consonants from vowels and glides.

Vocalic sounds do not have a radical or marked constriction of the vocal tract and are associated with spontaneous voicing. The voiced vowels and liquids are vocalic; the voiceless vowels and liquids, glides, nasal consonants, and obstruents (stops, fricatives, and affricates) are *nonvocalic* (that is, −vocalic).

Sonorant sounds have a vocal configuration that permits spontaneous voicing, which means that the airstream can pass virtually unimpeded through the oral or nasal cavity. This feature distinguishes the vowels, glides, nasal consonants, and lateral and rhotacized consonants from the stops, fricatives and affricates (the class of obstruents).

Interrupted sounds have a complete blockage of the airstream during a part of their articulation. Stops and affricates are +interrupted, which distinguishes them from fricatives, nasals, liquids, and glides. Sometimes the feature *continuant* is used rather than interrupted, with opposite values assigned, that is, +continuant sounds are −interrupted and vice versa.

Strident sounds are those fricatives and affricates produced with intense noise: /s/, /z/, /ʃ/, /ʒ/, /tʃ/, /dʒ/. The amount of noise produced depends on characteristics of the constriction, including roughness of the articulatory surface, rate of air flow over it, and angle of incidence between the articulatory surfaces.

High sounds are made with the tongue elevated above its neutral (resting) position (see Figure 2.11a).

Low sounds are made with the tongue lowered below its neutral position (see Figure 2.11b).

Back sounds are made with the tongue retracted from its neutral position (see Figure 2.11c).

Anterior sounds have an obstruction that is farther forward than that for the palatal /ʃ/. Anterior sounds include the bilabials, labiodentals, linguadentals, and lingua-alveolars.

Coronal sounds have a tongue blade position above the neutral state. In general, consonants made with an elevated tongue tip or blade are +coronal.

Rounded sounds have narrowed or protruded lip configuration.

Distributed sounds have a constriction extending over a relatively long portion of the vocal tract (from back to front). For English, this feature is particularly important to distinguish the dental fricatives /θ/ and /ð/ from the alveolars /s/ and /z/.

Lateral sounds are coronal consonants made with midline closure and lateral opening.

Nasal sounds have an open velopharynx allowing air to pass through the nose.

Voiced sounds are produced with vibrating vocal folds.

The feature assignments in Table 2.4 are for general illustration of the use of features. The features should be viewed with some skepticism, as several different feature systems have been proposed, and any one system is subject to modification. It should be understood that distinctive features are one type of classification system. It should also be realized that distinctive features have an intended linguistic function that may not always be compatible with their application to the study of articulation disorders. The issue is beyond the scope of this chapter, but the interested reader is referred to Walsh (1974) and Parker (1976).

The relationship between the traditional place terms of phonetic description and the distinctive features is summarized here. For each traditional place term, the associated features are listed. As an example, a bilabial stop is +anterior, −coronal, and +distributed. (The placement of both features within brackets indicates that they are considered together in sound description.)

$$
\text{Bilabial} \quad
\begin{bmatrix}
+\text{anterior} \\
-\text{coronal} \\
+\text{distributed}
\end{bmatrix}
$$

$$
\text{Labiodental} \quad
\begin{bmatrix}
+\text{anterior} \\
-\text{coronal} \\
-\text{distributed}
\end{bmatrix}
$$

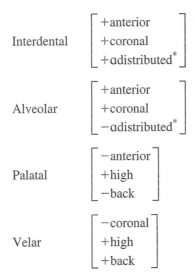

$$\text{Interdental} \quad \begin{bmatrix} +\text{anterior} \\ +\text{coronal} \\ +\alpha\text{distributed}^* \end{bmatrix}$$

$$\text{Alveolar} \quad \begin{bmatrix} +\text{anterior} \\ +\text{coronal} \\ -\alpha\text{distributed}^* \end{bmatrix}$$

$$\text{Palatal} \quad \begin{bmatrix} -\text{anterior} \\ +\text{high} \\ -\text{back} \end{bmatrix}$$

$$\text{Velar} \quad \begin{bmatrix} -\text{coronal} \\ +\text{high} \\ +\text{back} \end{bmatrix}$$

Suprasegmentals

The phonetic characteristics discussed to this point are *segmental*, which means that the units involved in the description are the size of phonemes or phonetic segments. *Suprasegmentals* are characteristics of speech that involve larger units, such as syllables, words, phrases, or sentences. Among the suprasegmentals are stress, intonation, loudness, pitch level, juncture, and speaking rate. Briefly defined, the suprasegmentals, also called *prosodies*, or *prosodic features*, are properties of speech that have a domain larger than a single segment. This definition does not mean that a single segment cannot, at times, carry the bulk of information for a given suprasegmental; on occasion, a segment, like a vowel, can convey most of the relevant information. Most suprasegmental information in speech can be described by the basic physical quantities of amplitude (or intensity), duration, and fundamental frequency (f_0) of the voice. Stated briefly, amplitude refers to the perceptual attribute of loudness; duration, to the perceptual attribute of length; and fundamental frequency, to the perceptual attribute of vocal pitch.

Stress

Stress refers to the degree of effort, prominence, or importance given to some part of an utterance. For example, if a speaker wishes to emphasize that someone should take the *red* car (as opposed to a blue or green one), the speaker might say "Be sure to take the *red* car," stressing *red* to signify the emphasis. There are several varieties of stress, but all generally

---

*The symbol α is a "dummy variable" and is used here to indicate that the Chomsky-Hallé features can distinguish the interdental and alveolar consonants only if they differ with respect to the feature *distributed*. Thus, if interdentals are regarded as −distributed, then alveolars must be +distributed. (See Ladefoged [1971] for development of this issue.)

involve something akin to the graphic underline used to denote emphasis in writing. Although underlining is seldom used in writing, stress is almost continually used in speech. In fact, any utterance of two or more syllables may be described in terms of its stress pattern. Because stress has influences that extend beyond the segment, stress usually is discussed with respect to syllables. The pronouncing guide of a dictionary places special marks after individual syllables to indicate stress. For example, the word *ionosphere* is rendered as (i-ɑn′ ə-sfer′), with the marks ′ and ′ signifying the primary and secondary stress for the syllables.

The International Phonetic Alphabet (IPA) uses a different stress notation from that commonly found in dictionaries. In IPA the stress mark precedes the syllable to which it refers, and the degree of stress is indicated by whether *any* stress mark is used and by the *location* of the stress mark in the *vertical* dimension. The strongest degree of stress is indicated by a mark above the symbol line: ′ɑn (rather like a superscript); the second degree of stress is indicated by a mark below the symbol line: ˌaɪ (like a subscript); and the third degree of stress is simply unmarked: ə. The word *ionosphere* is rendered as /ˌaɪ′ ɑn ə ˌsfɪr/, with three degrees of stress marked.

Acoustically, stress is carried primarily by the vowel segment within a syllable. The acoustic correlates, roughly in order of importance, are fundamental frequency (especially with a rise in fundamental frequency on or near the stressed syllable), vowel duration (greater duration with increased stress), relative intensity (greater intensity with increased stress), sound quality (reduction of a vowel to a weaker, unstressed form, like /ɑ/ to /ə/, vowel substitution, and consonant changes), and disjuncture (pauses or intervals of silence) (Rabiner, Levitt, and Rosenberg, 1969).

Another form of unstressed (or weakly stressed) syllable is the syllabic consonant. This type of consonant, usually an /l/, /m/, or /n/ (but infrequently /r/), acts like a vowel in forming a syllable nucleus. Examples of syllabic consonants are the final sounds in the words *battle* /bætl̩/, *something* /sʌmʔm̩/, and *button* /bʌtn̩/. The syllabic function of a consonant is designated by a small vertical mark placed under the phonetic symbol. Syllabic consonants are most likely to occur when the consonant is *homorganic* (shares place of articulation) with a preceding consonant because it is economical or efficient simply to maintain the articulatory contact for both sounds. Additional information on stress will be provided following some basic definitions of related terms.

Intonation

Intonation is the vocal pitch contour of an utterance, that is, the way in which the fundamental frequency changes from syllable to syllable and even from segment to segment. Fundamental frequency can be affected by several factors, including the stress pattern of an utterance, tongue position of a vowel (high vowels have a higher f_0), and the speaker's emotional state.

Loudness

Loudness is related to sound intensity or to the amount of vocal effort that a speaker uses. Although loudness is ordinarily thought to be related to the amplitude or intensity of a sound, some evidence suggests that a listener's judgments of loudness of speech are related more directly to the perceived vocal effort, essentially the amount of work that a speaker does (Cavagna and Margaria, 1968). There is some evidence (Hixon, 1971; MacNeilage, 1972) that intensity variations in speech result mostly from respiratory activity, but variations of f_0 are easily accomplished at the level of the vocal folds.

Pitch Level

Pitch level is the average pitch of a speaker's voice and relates to the mean f_0 of an utterance. A speaker may be described as having a high, low, or medium pitch.

Juncture

Juncture, sometimes called "vocal punctuation," is a combination of intonation, pausing, and other suprasegmentals to mark special distinctions in speech or to express certain grammatical divisions. For example, the written sentence "Let's eat, Grandma," has a much different meaning than the same sentence without the comma, "Let's eat Grandma!" A speaker can mark a comma vocally with a short pause and an adjustment in intonation. Juncture is also used to make distinctions between similar articulations, such as between the word *nitrate* and the phrase *night rate*. Intonation and pausing enable a speaker to indicate which alternative he or she wants to express.

Speaking Rate

The rate of speaking is usually measured in words per second, syllables per second, or phonemes per second. As speaking rate increases, segment durations generally become shorter, with some segments affected more than others. The segments most vulnerable to contraction as a speaker talks more rapidly are pauses, vowels, and consonant segments involving a sustained articulation (like fricatives). Apparently, most speakers do not really increase the rate of individual articulatory movement as they increase their rate of speaking. Rather, they reduce the duration of some segments and reduce the overall range of articulatory movement (Lindblom, 1963). As a result, the articulatory positions normally assumed during a slow rate of speaking may be missed at a faster rate. The "missing" of articulatory positions as speaking rate increases is called *undershoot*. This is why a speaker's words are apt to sound less distinct to you as the rate of speaking increases.

Vowel Reduction

Vowels are particularly susceptible to articulatory change as speaking rate is increased or stress is decreased. Such articulatory alterations are termed *reduction* and are schematized in Figure 2.25. The arrows between pairs of vowels show directions of reduction; for example, /i/ reduces first to /ɪ/ and then to /ə/, the ultimate reduced vowel. The scheme shows that, with reduction, all vowels tend toward /ə/ or /ʌ/.

Clear versus Conversational Speech

There is considerable evidence to show that speakers alter their patterns of speech production depending on situation and listener. One variation is clear versus conversational speech. Clear speech is what speakers use when they are trying to be as intelligible as possible. Compared to more casual conversational speech, clear speech is (1) slower (with longer pauses between words and a lengthening of some speech sounds), (2) more likely to

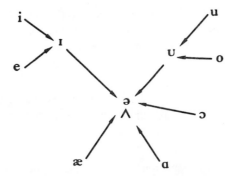

■ **FIGURE 2.25**   A scheme of vowel reduction. The arrows between vowel symbols show vowel changes resulting from reduction. For example, /i/ and /e/ reduce to /ɪ/, and /ɪ/ reduces to /ə/, which is the ultimate reduced vowel. Note that these changes occur within the quadrilateral defined by the corner vowels /i/, /æ/, /ɑ/, and /u/.

avoid modified or reduced forms of consonant and vowel segments (such as the vowel reduction described earlier), and (3) characterized by a greater intensity of obstruent sounds, particularly stop consonants (Picheny, Durlach, and Braida, 1986). When talkers want to be easily understood, they modify their speech to make it slower and more acousti-cally distinctive. Whereas vowels in conversational speech often are modified or reduced, therefore losing some of their acoustic distinctiveness, these sounds in clear speech are produced in distinctive forms. Similarly, word-final stops in conversational speech frequently are not released, so that the burst cue for their perception is eliminated. But in clear speech, stop consonants (and consonants in general) tend to be released and this feature enhances their perception.

These differences are central to a hypothesis proposed by Lindblom (1990) that speakers vary their speech output along a continuum from *hypospeech* to *hyperspeech* (the H&H hypothesis). The basic idea is that speakers adapt to the various circumstances of communication, to match their production patterns to communicative and situational factors. When a speaker believes that special care is required to be understood, he or she alters articulation accordingly. In Lindblom's view, clear speech (hyperspeech in his H&H hypothesis) is not simply loud speech but reflects an articulatory reorganization (Moon and Lindblom, 1989). Adams (1990), however, reported contrary evidence. He concluded from an X-ray microbeam study of speech movements that changes in speech clarity did not seem to reflect a reorganization of speech motor control. Adams observed that in clear speech, articulatory movements tended to be both larger and faster but there was no general indication that the speech patterns were organized differently than in conversational speech. The important point for clinical purposes is that speech articulation can be controlled by a speaker to enhance intelligibility when conditions warrant such deliberate effort. The primary articulatory change appears to be in the magnitude and speed of movement.

New versus Given Information

New information in a discourse is information that the listener would not be expected to know from the previous conversation or from the situation. Given information is predictable, either from the previous discourse or from the general situation. New information often is highlighted prosodically. For example, Behne (1989) studied prosody in a mini-discourse such as the following:

> "Someone painted the fence."
> "Who painted the fence?"
> "Pete painted the fence."

In this exchange, the new information ("Pete") is lengthened and produced with a higher fundamental frequency. In effect, the speaker uses prosody to highlight the new information.

Contrastive Stress in Discourse

Another discourse-related prosodic effect is *contrastive stress*. Such stress can be given to almost any word, phrase, or clause which the speaker considers to contradict or contrast with one that was previously expressed or implied. For instance, a speaker who wants to emphasize that she took the red ball rather than the green or blue one, might say, "I took the *red* ball" (where the italicized word receives contrastive stress). Contrastive stress is sometimes used clinically to give prosodic variation to an utterance or to elicit a stressed form of a target element.

Phrase-Final Lengthening

At the syntactic level, juncture and pause phenomena are used to mark multiword units. For example, in English, *phrase-final lengthening* operates to lengthen the last stressable syllable in a major syntactic phrase or clause. For example, if we contrast the following two sentences:

1. Red, green, and blue are my favorite colors.
2. Green, blue, and red are my favorite colors.

the word *blue* will be longer in (1) than in (2) because in the former this word is at the end of the subject noun phrase and is therefore subject to phrase-final lengthening. This regularity can be exploited clinically to obtain durational adjustments for a target word. In addition, Read and Schreiber (1982) showed that phrase-final lengthening is helpful to listeners in parsing (that is, to recognize the structure of) spoken sentences. They also suggested that children rely more on this cue than adults do, and, moreover, that prosody assists the language-learner by providing structural guides to the complex syntactic structures of language.

Declination

Another effect at the syntactic level is *declination*, or the effect in which the vocal fundamental frequency contour typically declines across clauses or comparable units. Why this tilt in the overall fundamental frequency pattern occurs is a matter of debate (Cohen, Collier, and t'Hart, 1982), but it is a robust feature of prosody at the sentence or clause level. This pattern is helpful to listeners in recognizing the structure of discourse, such as in identifying sentence units.

Lexical Stress Effects

These effects operate at the level of the word. For example, English has many noun–verb pairs like *'import* versus *im'port*, or *'contrast* versus *con'trast*, in which the difference between the members of a pair is signaled primarily by stress pattern. Another common effect at the word level occurs with a distinction between compounds and phrases. For example, the compound noun *'blackbird* contrasts with the noun phrase *black 'bird* (a bird that is black).

Although the lay listener often thinks stress in English is just a matter of giving greater intensity to part of an utterance, laboratory studies have shown that stress is signaled by duration, intensity, fundamental frequency, and various phonetic effects (Fry, 1955). It is important to remember that stress affects segmental properties such as the articulation of vowels and consonants (Kent and Netsell, 1972; de Jong, 1991). Segments in stressed syllables tend to have larger and faster articulatory movements than similar segments in unstressed syllables. For this reason, stressed syllables often are favored in some phases of articulation therapy.

Because suprasegmentals like stress and speaking rate influence the nature of segmental articulation, some care should be taken to control suprasegmental variables in articulation tests and speech materials used in treatment. Vowels carry much of the suprasegmental information in speech, but stress, speaking rate, and other suprasegmentals can influence consonant articulation as well. The suprasegmental features of speech have been discussed by Crystal (1973), Lehiste (1970), and Lieberman (1967), and the reader is referred to these accounts for a more detailed consideration of this complex area.

COARTICULATION: INTERACTIONS AMONG SOUNDS IN CONTEXT

Convenient though it might be to consider phonemes as independent, invariant units that are simply linked together to produce speech, this simplistic approach does not really fit the facts. When sounds are put together to form syllables, words, phrases, and sentences, they interact in complex ways and sometimes appear to lose their separate identity. The influence that sounds exert on one another is called *coarticulation*, which means that the articulation of any one sound is influenced by a preceding or following sound. Coarticulation makes it impossible to divide the speech stream into neat segments that correspond to phonemes. Coarticulation implies nonsegmentation, or, at least, interaction of the presumed linguistic segments. Hockett (1955) provided a colorful illustration of the transformation from phoneme to articulation:

> Imagine a row of Easter eggs carried along a moving belt; the eggs are of various sizes, and variously colored, but not boiled. At a certain point, the belt carries the row of eggs between the two rollers of a wringer, which quite effectively smashes them and rubs them more or less into each other. The flow of eggs before the wringer represents the series of impulses from the phoneme source. The mess that emerges from the wringer represents the output of the speech transmitter. (p. 210)

Although this analogy makes the process of articulation sound completely disorganized, in fact the process must be quite well organized if it is to be used for communication. Phoneme-sized segments may not be carried intact into the various contractions of the speech muscles, but some highly systematic links between articulation and phonemes are maintained. Research on speech articulation has provided a clearer understanding of what the links are although the total process is far from being completely understood.

It often is possible to describe coarticulation in terms of articulatory characteristics that spread from one segment to another. Examine the following examples of coarticulation:

1a. He sneezed   /h i s n i z d/ (unrounded /s/ and /s/)
1b. He snoozed   /h i s n u z d/ (rounded /s/ and /n/)
2a. He asked   /h i æ s k t/ (nonnasal /æ/)
2b. He answered /h i æ n s ɚ d/ (nasal /æ/)

The only phonemic difference between the first two items is the appearance of the unrounded vowel /i/ in 1a and the appearance of the rounded vowel /u/ in 1b. The lip rounding for /u/ in *He snoozed* usually begins to form during the articulation of the /s/. You might be able to feel this *anticipatory lip rounding* as you alternately say *sneeze* and *snooze* with your finger lightly touching your lips. In articulatory terms, the feature of lip rounding for the vowel is assumed during the /sn/ consonant cluster as the consequence of anticipating the rounding. The contrast between *sneeze* and *snooze* shows that the /sn/ cluster acquires lip rounding only if it is followed by a rounded vowel. This example of sound interaction is termed *anticipatory lip rounding* because the articulatory feature of rounding is evident before the rounded vowel /u/ is fully articulated as a segment.

Another form of anticipatory coarticulation occurs in 2b. Perhaps you can detect a difference in the quality of the /æ/ vowel in the phrases *He asked* and *He answered*. You should be able to detect a nasal quality in the latter because the vowel tends to assume the nasal resonance required for the following nasal consonant /n/. In this case, we can say that the articulatory feature of velopharyngeal opening (required for nasal resonance) is anticipated during the vowel /æ/. Normally, of course, this vowel is not nasalized. The contrasts between 1a and 1b and between 2a and 2b illustrate a type of coarticulation called *anticipatory*. Another type, *retentive*, applies to situations in which an articulatory feature is retained after its required appearance. For example, in the word *me* the vowel /i/ tends to be nasalized because of a carry-over velopharyngeal opening from the nasal consonant /m/. The essential lesson to be learned is that coarticulation occurs frequently in speech, so frequently in fact that the study of articulation is largely a study of coarticulation.

Phonetic context is highly important in understanding allophonic variation. For example, you should be able to detect a difference in the location of linguavelar closure for the /k/ sounds in the two columns of words below.

keen	*coon*
kin	*cone*
can	*con*

The point of closure tends to be more to the front of the oral cavity for the words in the first column than it is for the words in the second column. This variation occurs because, in English, the velar stops /k/ and /g/ do not have a narrowly defined place of articulation; all that is required is that the dorsum, or back, of the tongue touch the ceiling of the mouth. Therefore, the tongue is simply elevated at the position needed for the following vowel. When the tongue is in the front of the mouth (note that the vowels in the left column are front vowels), the dorsal closure is made in the front of the mouth, and when the tongue is in the back of the mouth (as it would be for the vowels in the right column), the point of closure is to the back of the velar surface.

Coarticulation arises for different reasons, some having to do with the phonology of a particular language, some with the basic mechanical or physiological constraints of the speech apparatus. Hence, some coarticulations are learned and others are the inevitable consequences of muscles, ligaments, and bones of the speech apparatus that are linked together and unable to move with infinite speed. Consider, for example, the closing and opening of the velopharyngeal port. This articulatory gesture is rather sluggish (compared to movements of the tongue tip), so it is not surprising that the velopharyngeal opening for a nasal consonant carries over to a following vowel, as in the word *no*. The extent of this carryover nasalization, however, varies with the phonologic characteristics of a particular language. In French, vowel nasalization is phonemic (that is, it can make a difference in meaning), but in English, vowel nasalization is only allophonic. Some aspects of coarticulation reflect universal properties of the human speech mechanism and hence affect all languages. Other coarticulations are governed by the phonemic structure of a particular language and are therefore learned with that language. Many coarticulatory effects are assimilatory in that a feature from one segment is adopted by an adjacent segment. For example, the nasalization of vowels by neighboring nasal consonants is nasal assimilation. Such effects may make speech production easier and faster because articulatory movements can be adapted to a particular phonetic and motor sequence. Assimilation is a general process in spoken language and will be taken up later in discussions of phonology.

Another aspect of coarticulation is the overlapping of articulations for consonants in clusters. Quite often, the articulation for one consonant is made *before* the release of a preceding consonant in any two-consonant cluster. For example, in the word *spy* /spaɪ/, the bilabial closure for /p/ is accomplished shortly (about 10 to 20 msec) before the release of the constriction for /s/. This overlapping of consonant articulations makes the overall duration of the cluster shorter than the sum of the consonant durations as they occur singly; that is, the duration of /sp/ in *spy* is shorter than the sum of the durations of /s/ in *sigh* /s aɪ/ and /p/ in *pie* /p aɪ/. The overlapping of articulation contributes to the articulatory flow of speech by eliminating interruptions. The temporal structure of a /spr/ cluster, as in the word *spray*, is pictured schematically in Figure 2.26. Notice that the constrictions for /s/ and /p/ overlap by 10 to 20 milliseconds and that the closure for /p/ overlaps with the tongue position for /r/ by a similar amount. Because consonants in clusters frequently present special difficulties to children (and adults) with articulation disorders, clinicians must know how such clusters are formed. Because clusters have overlapping articulations of the constituent consonants, in general, the cluster is a tightly organized sequence of articulatory gestures. The articulation of clusters is further complicated by allophonic variations, such as those listed in Table 2.5. In English, unaspirated released stops occur only when stops follow /s/, as in the words *spy*, *stay*, and *ski*. Otherwise, released stops are aspirated, meaning that the release is followed by a brief interval of glottal frication (an

■ **FIGURE 2.26** Schematic drawing of the articulatory organization of a /spr/ consonant cluster (as in the word *spray*), showing overlapping of consonantal articulations.

Source: Based on data from Kent and Moll (1975).

■ **TABLE 2.5** Examples of Context-Dependent Modifications of Phonetic Segments

Modification	Context Description
Nasalization of vowel	Vowel is preceded or followed by a nasal, e.g., [ɔ̃n]—*on* and [m̃æ̃n]—*man*
Rounding of consonant	Consonant precedes a rounded sound, e.g., [k̫win]—*queen* and [t̫ru]—*true*
Palatalization of consonant	Consonant precedes a palatal sound, e.g., [kɪʃ ju]—*kiss you*
Devoicing of obstruent	Word-final position of voiced consonant, e.g., [dɔg̥]—*dog* and [liv̥]—*leave*
Devoicing of liquid	Liquid follows word-initial voiceless sound, e.g., [pl̥eɪ]—*play* and [tr̥i]—*tree*
Dentalization of coronal	Normally alveolar sound precedes a dental sound, e.g., [wɪd̪θ]—*width* and [naɪn̪θ]—*ninth*
Retroflexion of fricative	Fricative occurs in context of retroflex sounds, e.g., [harʂɚ]—*harsher* and [pɝʂɚ]—*purser*
Devoicing of sound	Consonant or vowel in voiceless context, e.g., [sɪ̥stɚ]—*sister*
Lengthening of vowel	Vowel preceding voiced sound, especially in stressed syllable, e.g., [ni : d]—*need*
Reduction of vowel	Vowel in unstressed (weak) syllable, e.g., [tæbjuleɪt] [tæbjəleɪt]—*tabulate*
Voicing of sound	Voiceless in voiced context, e.g., [æbz̬ɝd]—*absurd*
Deaspiration of stop	Stop follows /s/, e.g., [sp = aɪ]—*spy* vs. [pʰaɪ]—*pie*

/h/-like noise). Similarly, the devoiced /l/ and /r/ normally occur only after voiceless consonants, as in the words *play* and *try*.

The examples of context-dependent articulatory modifications in Table 2.5 show the variety of influences that sounds exert on adjacent sounds. For a given sound, place of articulation, duration, voicing, nasalization, and rounding may vary with phonetic context, and these variations are noted with the special marks shown in Table 2.5.

Some aspects of coarticulation can be understood by knowing the extent to which individual sounds restrict the positions of the various articulators. Table 2.6 summarizes degrees of restriction on lips, jaw, and parts of the tongue for the different places of consonant articulation. A strong restriction is indicated by an X, a slight to moderate restriction by a −, and a minimal restriction by an O. Because this table shows which parts of the vocal

■ **TABLE 2.6** Coarticulation Matrix, Showing for Each Place of Consonant Articulation Those Articulators That Have Strong Restrictions on Position (Marked with X), Those That Have Some Restriction on Position (Marked with —), and Those That Are Minimally Restricted (Marked with O). For Example, the Bilabials /b/, /p/, and /m/ Strongly Restrict the Lips, Moderately Restrict the Jaw, and Leave the Tongue Essentially Free to Vary. The Glides /w/ and /ʍ/ Are Not Included Because They Involve Secondary Articulations. Lip Rounding, as Often Occurs for /r/, Has Been Neglected

Tongue Place	Lip	Jaw	Tip	Blade	Dorsum	Body
Bilabial /bpm/	X	—	O	O	O	O
Labiodental /vf/	X	—	O	O	O	O
Interdental /ðθ/	O	—	X	X	—	—
Alveolar /dtzsln/	O	—	X	X	—	—
Palatal /ʃ ʒ dʒ tʃ j r/	O	—	—	X	X	X
Velar /gkŋ/	O	O	O	—	X	X
Glottal /h/	O	O	O	O	O	O

tract are free to vary during articulation of a given consonant, it can be used to predict certain aspects of coarticulation. For example, because bilabial sounds do not restrict the tongue as long as it does not close off the tract, Os are indicated for all parts of the tongue. Jaw position is shown as moderately restricted for most places of articulation because some degree of jaw closing usually aids consonant formation. The ability of jaw movement to aid tongue movement declines as place of articulation moves back in the mouth, so a velar consonant may not restrict jaw position as much as more frontal articulation (Kent and Moll, 1972). The only sound that allows essentially unrestricted coarticulation is the glottal /h/. Thus, /h/ usually is made with a vocal-tract configuration adjusted to an adjacent sound, such as the following vowel in the words *he* /hi/, *who* /hu/, *ham* /hæm/, and *hop* /hɑp/.

Investigators of speech articulation (Daniloff and Moll, 1968; Moll and Daniloff, 1971; Kent and Minifie, 1977) have shown extensive overlapping of articulatory gestures across phoneme-sized segments, causing debate about the size of unit that governs behavior. Some investigators propose that the decision unit is an allophone, others argue for the phoneme, and still others for the syllable. A popular syllable-unit hypothesis is one based on CV (consonant-vowel) syllables, with allowance for consonant clustering (CCV, CCCV, and so on). This hypothesis states that articulatory movements are organized in sequences of the form CV, CCV, CCCV, and the like, so that a word like *construct* would be organized as the articulatory syllables /kɑ/ + /nstrʌkt/. Notice the odd assembly of the second syllable. This issue is of more than academic importance. Discovery of the basic decision unit would have implications for speech remediation—for example, enabling a speech clinician to choose the most efficient training and practice items for correcting an error sound. In addition, syllabic structures may explain certain features of speech and language development as discussed by Branigan (1976).

Coarticulation also has clinical relevance, in that a sound might be more easily learned or more easily produced correctly in one context than in others. In other words, the phonetic context of a sound can facilitate or even interfere with correct production of the sound. The effect of phonetic context could explain why misarticulations are often inconsistent, with correct production on certain occasions and incorrect productions on others. By judiciously selecting the phonetic context where an error sound is initially corrected, the clinician can sometimes enhance the efficiency of speech remediation. Such examples show why a thorough knowledge of articulatory phonetics is important to decisions in the management of articulation disorders.

AERODYNAMIC CONSIDERATIONS IN SPEECH PRODUCTION

Because the production of speech depends on the supply and valving of air, a knowledge of air pressure, flow, and volume is essential to an understanding of both normal and disordered speech. Many abnormalities of speech production are caused by irregularities or deficiencies in the supply and valving of air, and a number of clinical assessment techniques rely on measures of air pressure, flow, or volume. To understand the regulation of air pressures and flows in speech, it is important to recognize that (1) air flows only in one direction—from a region of greater pressure to one of lesser pressure; and (2) whenever the vocal tract is closed at some point, the potential exists for the buildup of air pressure behind the closure.

English speech sounds are normally *egressive*, meaning that, in sound production, air flows from the inside (usually the lungs) to the outside (the air around us). The basic energy needed to produce sound is developed in the lungs. After air is inspired by enlargement of the lung cavity, the muscle activation changes so that the lung cavity returns to a smaller size. If the airway above is closed, the same volume of air is enclosed in a smaller space. Because the same amount of air is contained in a smaller cavity, the air pressure within the lungs increases. This overpressure (relative to atmosphere) in the lungs is the source of the regressive air flow for all speech sounds. It is a fact of clinical importance that the air flow requirements for speech are not much greater than the requirements for ordinary breathing; that is, the volume of air inspired and expired in speaking is not much different from that in quiet respiration.

The regulation of air pressure and flow for speech is diagrammed in Figure 2.27, a simple model of the vocal tract. This model, in the form of the letter F, shows the three general areas where constriction (narrowing or closure) can occur: the laryngeal, oral, and nasal sections. The first site of constriction for egressive air is in the larynx. If the vocal folds close tightly, no air can escape from the lungs. If the folds are maximally open, then air passes through the larynx readily. If the folds are closed with a moderate tension, then the buildup of air pressure beneath them eventually blows them apart, releasing a pulse of air. After the folds are blown apart, they quickly come together again through the action of various physical restoring forces. This alternation of closed and open states, occurring many times per second, is called voicing. Successive pulses of air from the vocal folds are a source of acoustic energy for all voiced sounds, such as vowels.

The F-shaped vocal tract model shown in Figure 2.27a illustrates the air flow for vowel sounds. The vocal folds are shown as being partly closed to represent the vibratory pattern of opening and closing. The nasal tube is tightly closed because vowels in English are nonnasal unless they precede or follow nasal consonants. The oral tube is widely open to represent the open oral cavity in vowel articulation. Because the nasal tube is closed, the acoustic energy from the vibrating vocal folds passes through the oral tube.

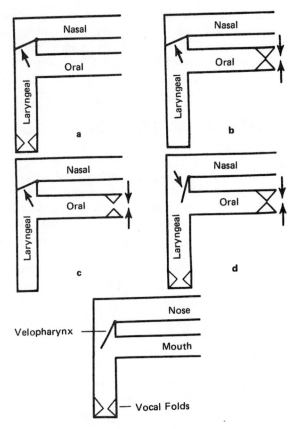

■ FIGURE 2.27 Simple models of vocal tract for major sound classes: (*a*) vowels, liquids, and glides; (*b*) voiceless stops; (*c*) voiceless fricatives; (*d*) nasals. The major parts of the model are shown at the bottom of the figure.

The configuration of the vocal tract for a voiceless stop like /p/, /t/, or /k/ is diagrammed in Figure 2.27b. The constriction at the larynx is shown as completely open because air from the lungs passes readily through the larynx and into the oral cavity. The constriction at the velopharynx is shown as closed to indicate that no air flows through the nasal tube. The oral constriction is closed to represent the period of stop closure. After this period, the oral constriction opens rapidly to allow a burst of air to escape from the oral pressure chamber. Assuming a stop closure of suitable duration, the air pressure developed within the oral cavity can be nearly equal to that in the lungs because the open vocal folds permit an equalization of air pressure in the airway reaching from the lungs up to the oral cavity. Therefore, voiceless stops have high intraoral air pressures. Also, it should be noted that children may use *greater* intraoral air pressures than adults (Subtelny, Worth, and Sakuda, 1966; Bernthal and Beukelman, 1978; Netsell, Lotz, Peters, and Schulte, 1994).

The model for voiceless fricatives in Figure 2.27c is like that for voiceless stops, but instead of a complete oral constriction, the model has a very narrow constriction, required for fricative noise. Because the velopharyngeal constriction is tightly closed and the laryngeal constriction is open, voiceless fricatives like /s/ and /ʃ/ have high intraoral air pressures. The voiceless stops and fricatives are sometimes called *pressure consonants*.

Voiced stops and fricatives differ from voiceless stops and fricatives in having vibrating vocal folds. Therefore, the models in Figures 2.27b and 2.27c would have a partial laryngeal constriction to represent voicing of these sounds. Because a certain amount of air pressure is lost in keeping the vocal folds vibrating (that is, pressure across the glottis drops), the voiced stops and fricatives have smaller intraoral air pressures than their voiceless cognates.

Finally, the model for nasal consonants is depicted in Figure 2.27d. A partial constriction at the larynx represents the vibrating vocal folds, and a complete oral constriction represents the stop-like closure in the oral section of the vocal tract. For nasal consonants, the acoustic energy of voicing is directed through the nasal cavity. Very little air pressure builds up within the oral chamber.

Liquids and glides can be modeled in essentially the same way as vowels (Figure 2.27a). Because the oral constriction for these sounds is only slightly greater than that for vowels, there is very little intraoral air pressure buildup.

Pressures and flows can be used to describe the function of many parts of the speech system. For example, a normal efficient operation of the larynx can often be distinguished from inefficient pathological states by the excessive air flow in the latter conditions. This excessive flow, or air wastage, may be heard as breathiness or hoarseness. Velopharyngeal incompetence can be identified by recording air flow from the nose during normally nonnasal segments. Frequently, velopharyngeal incompetence is signaled both by inappropriate nasal air flow (for example, air flow during stops or fricatives) and by reduced levels of intraoral air pressure. Sometimes, more than one pressure or flow must be recorded to identify the problem. For example, reduced levels of intraoral air pressure for consonants can be related to at least three factors: (1) respiratory weakness, resulting in insufficient air pressure; (2) velopharyngeal dysfunction, resulting in a loss of air through the nose; or (3) an inadequacy of the oral constriction, allowing excessive air to escape.

Clinically, aerodynamic assessment is especially important when dealing with a structural defect (such as cleft palate) or a physically based control problem (as in cerebral palsy, vocal fold paralysis, and other neurologic disorders). Young children may use greater intraoral air pressure than adults for constant production, so normative pressure data obtained from adults should be used with caution in clinical evaluation of children. Moreover, the higher pressures in children's speech mean that children must close the velopharyngeal port even more tightly than adults to prevent nasal loss of air during stop or fricative consonants. Speech and language clinicians who do not possess equipment for aerodynamic recordings of speech should nonetheless be aware of the pressure and flow requirements in speech production. These requirements have important implications for the diagnosis and evaluation of communicative problems and for the design of remediation programs.

ACOUSTIC CONSIDERATIONS OF SPEECH

It is far beyond the scope of this chapter to consider in any detail the acoustic structure of speech sounds, but it is possible to draw here a few major conclusions about the acoustic signal of speech. Acoustic signals can be described in terms of three fundamental physical variables—frequency, amplitude, and duration. *Frequency* refers to the rate of vibration of a sound. Generally, the faster the rate of vibration, the higher the pitch heard. In other words, frequency is the most direct physical correlate of pitch. *Amplitude* refers to the strength or magnitude of vibration of a sound. The higher the magnitude of vibration, the louder the sound heard. Amplitude is the most direct physical correlate of loudness. Because the actual amplitude of vibration is minute and, therefore, difficult to measure, sound intensity or sound pressure level is used instead when making actual speech measurements. *Duration* refers to the total time over which a vibration continues. Duration is the most direct physical correlate of perceived length.

Virtually all naturally occurring sounds, speech included, have energy at more than a single frequency. A tuning fork is designed to vibrate at a single frequency and is one of the very few sound sources with this property. The human voice, musical instruments, and animal sounds all have energy at several frequencies. The particular pattern of energy over a frequency range is the *spectrum* of a sound. Speech sounds differ in their *spectra*, and these differences allow us to distinguish sounds perceptually.

Table 2.7 is a summary of the major acoustic properties of several phonetic classes. The table shows the relative sound intensity, the dominant energy region in the spectrum, and the relative sound duration for each class. Vowels are the most intense speech sounds, have most of their energy in the low to mid frequencies, and are longer in duration than other sounds (although the actual duration of vowel sounds may range from about 50 milliseconds to half a second). Because vowels are the most intense sounds, they typically determine the overall loudness of speech. The most intense vowels are the low vowels and the least intense, the high vowels.

The glides and liquids are somewhat less intense than the vowels and have most of their energy in the low to mid frequencies. The duration of the glides /w/ and /j/ tends to be longer than that of the liquids /l/ and /r/.

The strident fricatives and affricates (/s, z, ʃ, ʒ, tʃ, dʒ/) are more intense than other consonants but considerably weaker than vowels. The stridents have energy primarily at the high frequencies and, therefore, are vulnerable to high-frequency hearing loss. A good tape recording of the stridents requires a recorder with a wide frequency response. Stridents tend to be relatively long in duration, especially compared to other consonants, and fricatives typically are longer than affricates.

The nasals are sounds of moderate intensity, low-frequency energy, and brief to moderate duration. The nasals have more energy at very low frequencies than do other sounds.

■ **TABLE 2.7** Summary of Acoustic Features for Six Phonetic Classes

Sound Class	Intensity	Spectrum	Duration
Vowels	Very strong	Low frequency dominance	Moderate to long
Glides and liquids	Strong	Low frequency dominance	Short to moderate
Strident fricatives and affricates	Moderate	High frequency dominance	Moderate
Nasals	Moderate	Very low frequency dominance	Short to moderate
Stops	Weak	Varies with place of articulation	Short
Nonstrident fricatives	Weak	Flat	Short to moderate

The stops are relatively weak sounds of brief duration. The burst that results from release of a stop closure can be as short as 10 milliseconds. The primary energy for stops varies over a wide range of frequencies—from low to high; bilabials have relatively low-frequency energy, while velars and alveolars have most of their energy in, respectively, the mid and mid to high frequencies.

The nonstrident fricatives /f, v, θ, ð/ are weak sounds of typically moderate duration. They tend to have a flat spectrum, meaning that the noise energy is distributed fairly uniformly over the frequency range. Of all sounds, /θ/ usually is the weakest—so weak that it can barely be heard when produced in isolation at any distance from a listener.

Finally, two points should be made concerning acoustic implications for clinical assessment and management. First, the absolute frequency location of energy for speech sounds varies with speaker age and sex. Men have the lowest overall frequencies of sound energy, women somewhat higher frequencies, and young children the highest frequencies. This relationship follows from the acoustic principle that an object's resonance frequency is inversely related to its length. The longest pipe in a pipe organ has a low frequency (or low pitch) and the shortest pipe a high frequency (high pitch); similarly the adult male vocal tract is longer than a woman's or a child's and therefore has resonances of lower frequency. This difference has practical implications. Most acoustic data have been collected for men's speech; much less is known about women's or children's speech, and the data for men may not be directly applicable to either. Moreover, the recording and analysis of women's and children's speech requires a wider frequency range than that suitable for men's speech. This issue can be particularly important for fricatives and affricates.

Second, because speech sounds vary widely in intensity, dominant energy region, and duration, they are not equally discriminable under different listening situations. The acoustic differences summarized in Table 2.7 should be kept in mind when testing articulation or auditory discrimination.

SENSORY INFORMATION IN SPEECH PRODUCTION

As speech is produced, a number of different kinds of sensory information is generated. The types of information include tactile (touch and pressure), proprioceptive (position sense), kinesthetic (movement sense), and auditory. The total sensory information is genuinely plurimodal—that is, available in several modalities. Most authorities agree that the rich sensory information associated with speech production is particularly important in speech development and in the management of some speech disorders, as when a child must learn a new articulatory pattern. A clinician therefore should be knowledgeable about the kinds and characteristics of sensory, or afferent, information.

The major characteristics of the sensory systems in speech were reviewed by Hardcastle (1976) and later by Kent, Martin, and Sufit (1990). Tactile receptors, which consist of free nerve endings and complex endings (for example, Krause end-bulbs and Meissner corpuscles), supply information to the central nervous system on the nature of contact (including localization, pressure, and onset time) and direction of movement. Remarkably, the oral structures are among the most sensitive regions of the body. The tongue tip is particularly sensitive and can therefore supply detailed sensory information. Tactile receptors belong to a more general class of receptors called mechanoreceptors (which respond to mechanical stimulation). These receptors respond not only to physical contacts of articulatory structures but also to air pressures generated during speech.

The proprioceptive and kinesthetic receptors include the muscle spindles, Golgi tendon organs, and joint receptors. Muscle spindles provide rich information on the length of muscle fibers, degree and velocity of stretch, and the direction of movement of a muscle. Golgi receptors relay information on the change of stretch on a tendon caused by muscular contraction or by other influences, including passive movement. Joint receptors, located in the capsules of joints, inform the central nervous system on the rate, direction, and extent of joint movement. Even a relatively simple movement, such as closing the jaw and raising the tongue, supplies a variety of afference to the central nervous system.

The auditory system supplies information on the acoustic consequences of articulation. Because the purpose of speech is to produce an intelligible acoustic signal, auditory feedback is of particular importance in regulating the processes of articulation. Interestingly, when an adult suffers a sudden and severe loss of hearing, speech articulation usually does not deteriorate immediately, but only gradually. The other types of sensory information are probably sufficient to maintain the accuracy of articulation for some time.

Many tactile receptors are comparatively slow acting because the neural signals travel along relatively small fibers in a multisynaptic pathway (a pathway composed of several neurons). Much of the tactile information is available to the central nervous system after the event to which it pertains. This information is particularly important to articulations that involve contact between articulatory surfaces, such as stops and fricatives. Obviously, prolonging an articulation helps to reinforce its sensory accompaniment. When the mucosal surfaces of the articulators are anesthetized, one of the most disturbed class of sounds is the fricatives.

▪ PHONOLOGY AND PHONOLOGICAL THEORY

Phonology has been defined as the part of linguistics concerned with "putting sounds together" or "putting sounds into words." Somewhat more precisely, Sloat, Taylor, and Hoard define phonology as "the science of speech sounds and sound patterns" (1978; 1). These authors note that each language has its own sound pattern, which is (1) the set of sounds used by a certain language, (2) the acceptable arrangement of these sounds to form words, and (3) the various processes by which sounds are added, deleted, or changed. Thus, the sound patterns of different languages can differ in the sounds available for use, the permissible ordering of these sounds, and the rules or processes that operate on the sounds. Phonological rules are prescriptions that convert abstract phonological representations into phonetic representations. An example from Hyman (1975) is the pronunciation of the verb *miss*. The word is pronounced /mis/ in the phrase *we miss it* but /mɪʃ/ in the phrase *we miss you*. In English, the /s/ often is palatalized when it is followed by a palatal /j/ (which itself may be deleted). Thus, the morpheme *miss* has these two pronunciations determined by the phonology of English.

The idea that there are rules that determine which pronunciation is to be expressed assumes that phonemes are abstract mental (sometimes called *phonological*) representations.

It also assumes that these representations must then be converted into context-sensitive forms before being expressed. A number of different theories have evolved that have attempted to explain how this might work. The more widely known of these theories are discussed next. A more thorough review can be found in Ball and Kent (1997).

Although this chapter is not directly concerned with linguistics, you should at least recognize the relevance of some phonological principles to the study of normal and disordered articulation. The study of phonology offers many important insights into the interactions among sound segments and the interactions between speech articulation and higher levels of linguistic organization. In a sense, phonological analysis is a key to the door between articulation and the various levels of language structure. Many aspects of articulation—such as the duration of constriction for an /s/, the duration of a vowel sound, the occurrence of palatalization for consonants, or the devoicing of a normally voiced segment—can be understood through the study of phonology.

Generative Phonology

The most widely studied phonological theory is generative phonology, which emerged largely out of the classic work *The Sound Pattern of English* by Chomsky and Hallé (1968). It is based largely on the idea that some of the interactions among units in the oral expression of language can be described and perhaps even explained through phonological rules. A *phonological rule* is a formal expression of a regularity that occurs in the phonology of a language or in the phonology of an individual speaker. These rules are either *context-free* or *context-sensitive*. A context-free rule is not dependent on a specific context. For example, if a child always substitutes (replaces) stops for fricatives (e.g., *sees* /siz/ becomes /tid/), we can formulate a rule that states simply that fricatives become stops:

Fricative $\rightarrow$ Stop

In this example, the word *fricative* represents the category of fricatives and the word *stop* represents the category of stops and the arrow means "is replaced by." Thus, the rule means that a fricative unit is replaced by a stop unit. Because this change or replacement always occurs, it is not necessary to state any context restriction on its operation.

On the other hand, assume that a child replaces fricatives with stops only in the initial position of a syllable; for example, /si/ (*see*) becomes /ti/ and /zu/ (*zoo*) becomes /du/. The restriction to syllable-initial position is a context restriction, or a constraint on the operation of the rule. To formalize this operation, the following rule can be used:

Fricative $\rightarrow$ Stop / # ___

This rule states that a fricative unit is replaced by a stop unit if the fricative is in the context such that it initiates a syllable. The slash / means "in the environment such that," the # represents a syllable boundary, and the underline ___ indicates the location of the fricative segment. Hence, the /#___ means that the fricative immediately follows the syllable boundary (that is, begins the syllable).

A general form of a phonological rule is the following:

$X \rightarrow Y / a$ ___ b

This rule expresses a modification in which X becomes Y whenever X occurs following a and preceding b. The rule structure is decomposed as follows:

$$X \rightarrow Y \quad / \quad a \underline{} b$$

A unit of the phonological system ⌐
is replaced by
another unit of the phonological system
in the environment such that
the original unit X follows a and precedes b

For example, imagine an allophonic modification in which a vowel is nasalized if it occurs between two nasal consonants (as in the word *man*). A rule of the form given above could be used to describe this change as follows:

Vowel → Nasal vowel / Nasal consonant ___ Nasal consonant

But a nasal consonant can be regarded as a sound having the features +nasal and +consonant. When features such as nasal and consonant apply together, it is convenient to place them in brackets so that the rule above becomes:

$$\text{Vowel} \rightarrow \begin{bmatrix} +\text{Nasal} \\ +\text{Vowel} \end{bmatrix} \; / \; \begin{bmatrix} +\text{Nasal} \\ +\text{Consonant} \end{bmatrix} \; \underline{} \; \begin{bmatrix} +\text{Nasal} \\ +\text{Consonant} \end{bmatrix}$$

Some additional examples of rules are given below. By studying these rules, the student should be able at least to interpret phonological rules, if not to devise them. The basic advantage of a phonological rule is that it expresses in a formal or mathematical fashion a regularity of the phonological system and allows for an accurate, compact description of various context dependencies.

Example of deletion rule.   Consonants following nasal consonants are deleted.

$$C \rightarrow \emptyset \qquad / \begin{bmatrix} +\text{Nasal} \\ C \end{bmatrix} \; \underline{}$$

(Ex.: [ænt] → [æn])

Explanation.   As an abbreviatory convenience, C stands for consonant, and a nasal consonant is C with the feature +nasal. Deletion is represented by the null element ø so that the rule literally reads "a consonant is replaced by a null element (nothing) when the consonant follows a nasal consonant."

Example of insertion rule.   A schwa vowel is inserted following syllable-final voiced stops.

$$\emptyset \rightarrow /\ni/ \qquad / \begin{bmatrix} +\text{Voiced} \\ +\text{Stop} \end{bmatrix} \; \underline{} \; \#$$

(Ex.: [dɔg] → [dɔgə])

Explanation.   The rule literally reads "a null element (nothing) is replaced by a schwa vowel when the null element occurs at the end of a syllable following a voiced stop."

Example of feature-changing rule.   Syllable-final voiced obstruents are devoiced.

$$\begin{bmatrix} -\text{Sonorant} \\ +\text{Voiced} \end{bmatrix} \rightarrow [-\text{Voiced}] \, / \, \underline{\quad} \, \#$$

(Ex.: [bɪg] → [bɪk])

Explanation.   Obstruents are stops, fricatives, and affricates, all of which are represented by the feature –sonorant. Thus, the rule states literally that "voiced nonsonorants (i.e., obstruents) are replaced by their voiceless counterparts at the end of syllables."

Example of feature-assimilation rule.   A normally voiceless consonant is voiced when it occurs between two voiced sounds.

$$\begin{bmatrix} \text{C} \\ -\text{Voiced} \end{bmatrix} \rightarrow [+\text{Voiced}] \, / \, [+\text{Voiced}] \, \underline{\quad} \, [+\text{Voiced}]$$

(Ex.: [æbsɝd] → [æbzɝd])

Explanation.   A voiceless consonant becomes voiced if the preceding and following segments are voiced.

Natural Phonology

A topic of considerable interest and importance in phonology is that of naturalness. A natural class, property, process, or rule is one that appears to be preferred or is frequently used in phonologic systems (Sloat et al., 1978; Stampe, 1979; Ingram, 1976). Evidence of naturalness is generally taken from developmental studies (early appearance or acquisition in a child's language), from cross-linguistic studies (universality across languages), or from studies of sound change in a language. One phonological property is more natural than another if the first appears before the second in language development and if the first is attested to in a greater number of languages. *Markedness* is a term sometimes used in this connection. An *unmarked* sound is one that appears to be natural. Unmarked sounds are acquired earlier than marked sounds in children's language, tend to be established in a language before marked sounds can be added, and tend to occur in different languages more frequently than marked sounds. By these criteria, voiceless stops are an example of unmarked (more natural) sounds, whereas voiced obstruents are marked (less natural).

Studies of natural phonology have shown that certain *assimilatory* and *nonassimilatory* processes occur commonly enough to be regarded as natural (Sloat et al., 1978). An assimilatory process is one in which a sound changes to assimilate (become similar) to another sound. A nonassimilatory process does not appear to be based on similarity between sounds.

Examples of Assimilatory Processes

Voicing changes.   These are intervocalic voicing and voicing and devoicing of obstruents. In intervocalic voicing, an obstruent (stop, fricative, or affricate) becomes voiced when it occurs between two vowels (hence, intervocalic). For example, *puppy* /pʌpɪ/ becomes /pʌbɪ/. The voiceless obstruent is assimilated to the voiced elements that surround it. The pattern of obstruent voicing or devoicing varies with languages, but one common process is word-final devoicing, in which an obstruent loses its voicing when it occurs at the end of the word. This change sometimes is considered assimilatory because it is thought that the voiced segment is assimilated to the voiceless pause at the end of the word. For example, *dog* /dɔg/ becomes /dɔk/.

Nasalization.   As already discussed in this chapter, vowels and, occasionally, other resonants are assimilated to nasal consonants by becoming nasal themselves. Thus, in the word *lamb* /læm/, the vowel often is nasalized.

Nasal assimilation.   Nasal consonants tend to assume the place of articulation of a neighboring sound. In English, this process is amply illustrated by the large number of homorganic nasal-stop combinations: *impolite, imbue, improper, indelicate, unturned, endeared, anchor, anger, congress.*

Palatalization.   Nonpalatal consonants become palatal when followed by a front vowel or a glide. For example, the /n/ in *news* and the /k/ in *cute* become palatalized when these words are produced with the glide + vowel /ju/ (/njuz/ and /kjut/). As mentioned earlier, /s/ often is palatalized when it is followed by the glide /j/ in phrases such as *miss you.*

Examples of Nonassimilatory Processes

Deletion or loss of segments.   Sometimes a segment or number of segments at the end of a word are dropped in a process known as *apocope*. For example, in the Eastern dialect of English, speakers often drop the /r/ in words such as *car, store,* and *stair*, pronouncing *car* /kar/ as /ka:/. Young children also frequently delete the final consonants of words. Final consonant omission is noted by speech clinicians more often than initial consonant omission. When segments are lost at other than the end of a word, the process is sometimes called *syncope*. Apocope and syncope frequently simplify (or reduce) clusters; *extra*, for example, may become /ɛktrə/ and *asks* may become /æks/.

Insertion of segments.   In one type of insertion process, called *prosthesis*, a segment is added in the initial position. In another type, called *epenthesis*, a segment is added elsewhere in the word. Children frequently will break up clusters by inserting vowels (often the schwa /ə/): *blue* becomes /bəlu/ and *clock* becomes /kəlak/.

Metathesis.   The order of segments is reversed in this process. For example, a child may say /nets/ for *nest* /nɛst/ and /mjukis/ for music /mjusik/ (the second example also involves final-segment devoicing).

Breaking. By this process, long vowels become diphthongs, as in the examples *fast* /fæɪst/, *pass* /pæɪs/, *bag* /bæɪg/, and *cat* /kæɪt/. Breaking often may be heard in the speech of young children.

Natural phonology offers some valuable perspectives on the acquisition of phonology by children. Some authors believe that natural phonological processes are innate or are acquired early and rather easily by children and that whenever a natural process opposes a phonological property of the language the child is learning, some resistance may be expected. Stampe (1969) viewed natural processes as innate processes that simplify the adult target word. One interesting implication of naturalness is that children tend to exhibit strong biases or preferences in their sound formations and sound sequences. It has been proposed that some such preferences are based on phonetic grounds. For example, obstruent devoicing (or the tendency for stops, fricatives, and affricatives to be devoiced) may be related to the fact that it is difficult to maintain laryngeal vibrations during a period of vocal tract closure. To maintain voicing during closure of the tract, special measures must be taken to enable air flow to continue through the vocal folds. This can be done through an expansion of the oral air chamber (Perkell, 1969; Kent and Moll, 1969), accomplished by expanding the pharynx or by depressing the larynx. However, not all natural processes have a simple phonetic basis, and, most likely, other factors will have to be considered in reaching a full explanation. Whatever this explanation may be, it behooves the speech clinician to be aware that speech and language learning may be influenced by phonological forces that occur commonly enough to be called natural. Such preferences or predispositions in speech production may be a substrate for the process of acquisition. Furthermore, the maintenance of natural processes beyond their usual survival time in learning a particular phonological system could result in articulation disorders.

Nonlinear Phonology

Nonlinear phonology was developed as an alternative to linear generative phonology because the latter was perceived to have certain shortcomings. The basic goals of generative phonologies are to (1) describe phonological patterns in natural languages, (2) formulate the rules that account for these systems, and (3) identify universal principles that apply to phonological systems. A particular reason why nonlinear phonologies were introduced was to account for the influence of stress (as in weak and strong clusters in English stress systems) and the description of tone and stress features in levels of representation independent of the segmental representation. Linear generative phonology was regarded by some to be inadequate in dealing with prosodic effects in general. Early generative phonologies regarded phonological representation as "linear strings of segments with no hierarchical organization other than that provided by syntactic phrase structure" (Clements and Keyser, 1983, p. 1). This kind of generative phonology was characterized by rules that operated in a domain of linear strings of segments. But this approach encountered some difficulties in regard to the effects of stress and other prosodic variables. More generally, linear generative phonology failed to account satisfactorily for the relationships among various sizes of units because phonological operations were constrained to act on linear sequences.

There are several different versions of nonlinear phonology, but two particularly influential theories are autosegmental theory (Goldsmith, 1976, 1990; Hayes, 1988) and metrical theory (Goldsmith, 1990; Hayes, 1988). *Autosegmental theory* divides phonological features into parallel tiers of quasi-independent sequences. The tiers are like interconnected but independent levels. The term *autosegment* refers to a unit in a given tier. An autosegment can be realized in one or more ways; for example, a tonal tier may allow realizations such as high, mid, or low tones. The sequences in each tier are time-aligned with association lines that indicate simultaneity across tiers. In this way, stress and segmental representations are coordinated. A detailed discussion cannot be given here for this complex development in phonological theory, but the central idea is fairly simple: Phonological patterns evolve from connections across different representations, and not, as linear generative phonology maintained, from operations across a single linear sequence of phonological units. Nonlinear phonology is a significant break from an earlier theoretical view. It accommodates interactions across various sizes and types of phonological representation.

Metrical theory organizes phonological units into hierarchies—for example, feet, syllables, and segments. Unlike linear generative phonology, metrical theory gives a special definition to stress. Stress patterns arise from rhythm (an alternating prominence, such as strong–weak) and syllable weight. Stress assignments are made across the various levels of the hierarchy (such as syllables, feet, and words). This treatment of stress is very different from that of linear generative phonology.

Hierarchy also is important to theories of feature geometry, another development in nonlinear phonology. Two influential accounts of feature geometry are McCarthy (1988) and Sagey (1986). In systems such as that shown in Figure 2.28, syllable, consonant, and

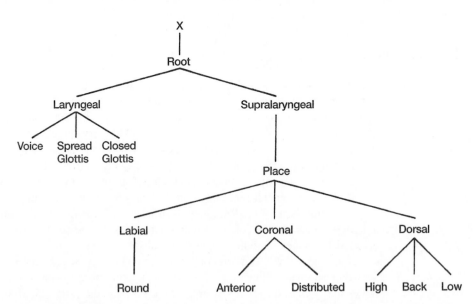

■ **FIGURE 2.28**   Hierarchical tree structure for one version of feature geometry. The features under the supralaryngeal node have been defined previously. The features under the laryngeal node refer to vocal fold configurations.

vowel appear as superordinate nodes that govern other nodes specifying laryngeal and supralaryngeal articulations. That is, the features are arranged hierarchically. Linear phonology, such as that of Chomsky and Hallé (1968), typically specified features in a matrix where orthogonality or independence among features was desirable if not always attainable. In contrast, feature geometry exploits nonorthogonality among features. The hierarchical patterns implied by nonorthogonality become organizing principles in feature geometry.

The three nonlinear phonological theories just reviewed—autosegmental theory, metrical theory and feature geometry—all represent major departures from what had been the standard phonological theory. Not surprisingly, these theories are now being considered with respect to phonological development (Schwartz, 1992; Spencer, 1988) and phonological disorders in children (Bernhardt, 1990; Chiat, 1989; Chin and Dinnsen, 1991; Gandour, 1981; Spencer, 1984).

Optimality Theory

Optimality theory is a relatively new and highly influential account of phonology. It resembles some other phonological theories in maintaining that internal (innate) mechanisms govern phonological decisions. In generative phonology, these mechanisms were the distinctive features, which are thought to apply universally across languages. In natural phonology, the innate mechanisms were phonological processes. In optimality theory, the innate mechanisms are *constraints*, which act to select the most optimal output from a set of alternatives. Where do the alternatives arise? These are produced by a mechanism called a *generator* that provides a set of potential output forms for a given input representation. Say, for example, that the input is the word /kæt/. Suppose that the generator supplies the following output forms: /kæt/, kætl/, /æt/, /kæts/. All of these are potential matches to the input representation, but only one should be selected. A mechanism called an *evaluator* uses language-specific constraints to select the most optimal output from the set of outputs supplied by the generator. That is, the evaluator selects the most appropriate (harmonious or optimal) output. Because the ranking of constraints is language specific, a particular ranking reflects learning of a given language. In this way, optimality theory can account for developmental changes in phonology.

As with the nonlinear theories, there have been some recent attempts to apply optimality theory to both normal phonological development (Barlow and Gierut, 1999; Bernhardt and Stemberger, 2000) and phonological disorders in children (Barlow, 2001; Stemberger and Bernhardt, 1997).

Which Phonological Theory to Select?

There is no lack of phonological theories. Only a few have been discussed here; see Ball and Kent (1997) for a more complete discussion. How can we choose among them? This decision depends, in part, on how the theory is to be applied. If the intention is to apply the theory to the development of speech or to phonological/articulatory disorders, the following criteria may guide the selection.

1. Does the theory account for common patterns observed in the development of spoken language in children?
2. Does the theory account for individual differences in the acquisition of speech?
3. Can the theory deal effectively and reasonably with continuity (developmental change)?
4. Is the theory helpful in designing treatment programs for children with phonological/articulatory disorders?
5. Does the theory relate to readily observable events or behaviors?
6. Does the theory provide an index of severity of disorder or disability?
7. Does the theory have elegance and parsimony?

■ SUMMARY OF LEVELS OF ORGANIZATION OF SPEECH

Various levels of organization of speech are shown in Table 2.8, beginning with the syllable and working down to the acoustic sequence that might be seen on a spectrogram or

■ **TABLE 2.8**   Levels of Organization of Speech

SYLLABIC INTEGRITY:	/p a/
	SYL
PHONEMIC COMPOSITION:	/p/ + /a/
PHONETIC PROPERTIES:	[pʰa:]
Note: stop /p/ is aspirated and vowel /a/ is lengthened	
SEGMENTAL FEATURES:	[p] — +Stop
	+Labial
	+Consonantal
	−Nasal
	−Voice
	[a] — +Syllabic
	−Consonantal
	−Front
	+Low
	−Round
	−Nasal
	+Voice
ARTICULATORY SEQUENCE:	Closure of velopharynx
	Abduction of vocal folds
	Adjustment of tongue for /a/
	Closure of lips
	Opening of lips and jaw
	Adduction of vocal folds
	Final abduction of vocal folds
ACOUSTIC SEQUENCE:	Silent period during /p/ closure
	Noise burst for /p/ release
	Aspiration period as folds close
	Voiced period after folds close, with distinct resonant shaping

visual representation of sounds. Although *syllable integrity* is the highest level shown, the table could have begun with an even higher level, such as a phrase or a sentence. However, for our purposes here, it is sufficient to consider only the levels presented in the table. The syllable is an organizational unit that consists of one or more phonemes; in this case, the syllable /pa/ includes the phonemes /p/ and /a/. Because phonemes are abstract, a phonemic description does not touch on a number of details of phonetic organization and speech behavior. Some of these details are shown in the level of *phonetic properties*. The phoneme /p/ has as its phonetic representation the aspirated [ph], and the phoneme /a/ has as its phonetic representation the lengthened [a:]. These phonetic representations are, of course, allophones of the /p/ and /a/ phonemes. The English phoneme /p/ is always aspirated in syllable-initial position, and the phoneme /a/ frequently is lengthened when uttered in an open monosyllable (that is, a CV syllable).

Segmental features comprise the next level of the table. These features are phonetic dimensions or attributes by which sounds may be described. For example, the consonant [p] is defined by its inclusion in the classes of *stops, labials,* and *consonantals* and by its exclusion from the classes of *nasals* and *voiced sounds*. These features are similar to the distinctive features discussed earlier in this chapter, but they are intended to be more phonetic in character. Even without rigorous definitions of the features suggested, it should be clear that each feature defines an articulatory property of the sound in question; for example, vowel [a] is a syllable nucleus, is not a consonant, is low-back and unrounded, and is a voiced nonnasal sound.

The features are less abstract than phonemes but still must be interpreted by the motor control system of the brain to provide proper neural instructions to the speech muscles; that is, the features listed for [p] and [a] must be translated into a pattern of muscle contractions that yields the articulatory sequence shown in the next to last level of the table. The −*nasal* feature of [p] requires that the velopharynx be closed, and the −*voice* feature of the same segment requires that the vocal folds be abducted (open). In this way, each feature requirement is given an articulatory interpretation, accomplished by the contraction of muscles.

Finally, as the consequence of muscle contractions, a series of speech sounds is uttered. In this *acoustic sequence*, the last level of the table, one can see acoustic segments of the kind visible on a spectrogram. Notice that one acoustic segment does not necessarily correspond to a single phoneme. The phoneme /p/ is associated with at least three acoustic segments: a silent period corresponding to the bilabial closure, a noise burst produced as the lips are rapidly opened, and an aspiration interval related to a gradual closure of the vocal folds in preparation for voicing the following vowel.

Although Table 2.8 is fairly detailed, it represents only part of the complexity of speech. In the linguistic-phonetic organization of speech behavior, we need to consider three major components: the *segmental* (or *phonetic*) component, the *suprasegmental* (*prosodic*) component, and the *paralinguistic* component. The first two already have been discussed in this chapter. The paralinguistic component is similar to the prosodic component in that it might be called nonsegmental. This component includes those aspects of speech represented by terms such as *emotion* and *attitude*. A speaker who plans an utterance must decide not only about phonetic sequencing but also about prosodic structure and emotional and attitudinal content (that is, the "tone of voice"). The segmental component includes words, syllables, phonemes, and features. The suprasegmental or prosodic component includes stress, intonation, juncture, rate, loudness, and pitch level. The paralinguistic component is made up of tension, voice quality, and voice qualifications (Crystal, 1969).

The complexity of speech behavior can be illustrated by listing the various types of information represented in the speech signal. A *partial* listing (mostly from Branigan, 1979) is

1. A set of articulatory targets or goals corresponding to the intended phonetic sequence
2. Assignment of stress to the syllables that make up the sequence
3. Adjustments of syllable duration to stress, phonetic composition, and position of the syllable in the utterance
4. Specification of junctural features, including transitions between elements and terminal juncture at the end of the utterance
5. Internal ordering of words as it reflects syntactic form to convey semantic intentions (meaning)
6. Determination of other prosodic features such as speaking rate, pitch, level, and loudness
7. Use of paralinguistic features to convey emotion or attitude

It is important to remember that even an apparently simple aspect of speech behavior can be influenced by a host of variables. For example, the duration of a vowel is determined by tongue height, tenseness or laxness, consonant context, stress pattern, frequency of occurrence of the word in which the vowel occurs, syntactic ordering of the word in which the vowel appears, and rate of speaking (Klatt, 1976).

CONCLUDING NOTE ON IMPLICATIONS FOR SPEECH ACQUISITION

Speech articulation has its early roots in the vocalizations of infants. Just how the coos and babbles of the first year of life relate to the development of speech is not well understood, but there is growing evidence that early vocalizations prepare the child for acquisition of a phonetic system. The syllable appears to be an important unit in early sound patterns, and the development of syllabic organization of sounds may be a major framework of speech development. If so, it is of interest to chart the way in which syllabic structures develop during the first year of life. The following account is based on several chapters in *Precursors of Early Speech Development*, edited by Bjorn Lindblom and Rolf Zetterström (1986) and *The Emergence of the Speech Capacity* by Oller (2000).

The major phases in syllable development are as follows: (1) Continuous phonation in a respiratory cycle provides the basic phonatory pattern from which refinements in articulation can develop; (2) intermittent phonation within a respiratory cycle breaks the basic pattern of continuous phonation and, thus, is a precursor of syllable units; (3) articulatory (supraglottal) movements interrupting or combined with phonation provide early experience in the control of co-occurring phonation and articulation; (4) marginal syllables (in isolation or in sequence) are early syllabic forms that, although lacking the detailed structure of adult syllables, prefigure the basic syllable shape; (5) canonical syllables (in isolation or in sequence) anticipate important structural properties of adult speech and may be particularly important in relating an infant's perceptions of adult speech with his or her own productive patterns; and (6) reduplicated babble (repeated syllable patterns) gives the infant experience with both prosody (especially rhythm) and sequences of articulations. It is on this vocal bedrock that speech develops. For a time, babbling and early words coexist, sharing some phonetic properties but, perhaps, differing in others.

The CV syllable, occurring in virtually all of the world's languages, has long been recognized as a preferred basic unit of speech articulation. It appears to be an optimal unit for learning perceptual discriminations in infancy. Infants younger than 4 months old can discriminate segments contained in sequences of the form CV, CVC, VCV, and CVCV (Bertoncini and Mehler, 1981; Jusczyk and Thompson, 1978; Trehub, 1973); and an alternating CV pattern seems to enhance the infant's ability to discriminate variations in place, manner, and voicing. Since redundant syllable strings, such as [ba ba ba ba] (Goodsitt, Morse, and Ver Hoeve, 1984), further enhance this performance, we can conclude that the CV syllable train characterizing reduplicated babble is an excellent perceptual training ground for the infant.

The advantage of the CV syllable applies to production as well. This syllable form is one of the earliest syllables to be identified in infant vocalizations; the vocalizations of 1-year-olds are, predominantly, simple V or CV syllables and their elaborations, for example, VCV or CVCV (Kent and Bauer, 1985). Branigan (1976) regarded the CV syllable as a training ground for consonant formation. Most consonants are produced first in the initial position of CV syllables and then, later, in postvocalic (e.g., VC) position.

The importance of the canonical CV syllable as a unit for perceptuomotor integration is indicated by its long-delayed appearance in the vocal development of infants with hearing impairments (Kent, Osberger, Netsell, and Hustedde, 1987; Oller, 1986). There is also evidence that early CV syllable production is linked, in a developmental chain, to the early word production and to the articulation of word-final consonants (Menyuk, Liebergott, and Schultz, 1986).

Speech acquisition is a complex process, one that involves learning a language (its syntax, semantics, and phonology)—a speech code that relates meaning to sound, and a motor skill by which the speech organs are controlled to produce rapid and overlapping movements. The layperson often characterizes developing speech in the child by reference to frequently occurring substitutions (as when the child says *wabbit* for *rabbit* or *thee* for *see*) or other common misarticulations. But developing speech differs from adult speech in other ways.

First, children's speech generally is slower than adult speech. For example, McNeill (1974) reported speaking rates of slightly over 3 words per second for adults, about 2.5 words per second for 4- to 5-year-olds, and 1.6 words per second for children of about age 2. Not surprisingly, then, the durations of individual segments are longer in children's speech (Naeser, 1970; Smith, 1978; Kent and Forner, 1980). Smith reported that the durations of nonsense utterances were 15 percent longer for 4-year-olds than for adults and 31 percent longer for 2-year-olds than for adults. Similarly, when Kent and Forner measured durations of phrases and short sentences, they found them to be 8 percent longer for 12-year-olds than for adults, 16 percent longer for 6-year-olds than for adults, and 33 percent longer for 4-year-olds than for adults. Some individual segments, such as the duration of stop closure, were observed by Kent and Forner to be twice as long in children's speech as in adult speech. The speaking rates of children have implications for both the production and perception of speech. It has been shown that children more successfully imitate sentences spoken at a rate nearer their own than at slower or faster rates (Bonvillian, Raeburn, and Horan, 1979).

Second, children's speech differs from adult speech in its variability. When children make the same utterance several times, the duration of individual segments varies more than for adults (Eguchi and Hirsh, 1969; Tingley and Allen, 1975; Kent and Forner, 1980). This difference in reliability of production may be an index of the child's linguistic and neuromotor immaturity. In general, a young child's speech patterns are less well controlled than an adult's, and there is evidence that the control continues to improve until the child reaches puberty (Kent, 1976).

A third difference between the speech of children and adults is in patterns of coarticulation. Data on this difference are not abundant, but Thompson and Hixon (1979) reported that with increasing age, a greater proportion of their subjects showed nasal air flow beginning at the midpoint of the first vowel in /ini/. They interpreted this to mean that anticipatory coarticulation occurred earlier for progressively older subjects. In other words, more mature speakers show increased anticipation in producing a phonetic sequence.

In summary, young children differ from adults not only in their obvious misarticulations, but also in their slower speaking rates, greater variability (error) in production, and reduced anticipation in articulatory sequencing.

■ QUESTIONS FOR CHAPTER 2

1. Discuss the relationship among the following concepts: *morpheme, phoneme, allophone.* For example, explain why a morpheme is relevant to identifying phonemes and why phonemes are relevant to identifying allophones.

2. This chapter summarized two ways of describing vowel articulation: traditional phonetic description and distinctive features. Discuss the similarities and differences between these two approaches.

3. Using Table 2.2 as a guide, classify all of the consonants in the phrase *Good morning, take a ticket, and get in line,* according to place of articulation, manner of articulation, and voicing. Note that in all of the words containing two or more consonants, the consonants share a phonetic feature. What is this feature for each word?

4. What is coarticulation and why does it occur?

5. Compare and contrast any two of the theories of phonology discussed in this chapter.

Speech Sound Acquisition

SHARYNNE McLEOD

Charles Sturt University, Australia

From the moment children are born they vocalize. Refinement of this vocalization into intelligible speech takes many years while children's body structures develop, and their perception and production systems become more sophisticated and attuned to their ambient language. This chapter explores typical or normal speech sound acquisition. At the beginning of the chapter we consider the reasons it is important for speech-language pathologists (SLPs) to understand typical speech sound acquisition, models of speech sound acquisition, and the research methods that have been employed to understand how children learn to produce speech sounds. The remainder of the chapter examines children's speech sound acquisition of English, from infancy to the school years. A comprehensive appendix summarizes data on speech sound acquisition of English. Since this chapter addresses only the acquisition of English speech sounds, the symbol /r/ is used to indicate /ɹ/ following the convention of Ladefoged (2005).

■ RELEVANCE OF UNDERSTANDING TYPICAL SPEECH SOUND ACQUISITION FOR SLPS

A sound understanding of typical speech sound acquisition is akin to having solid foundations under a house. In pediatric SLP practice, decision making occurs daily as to whether children's speech is typical or not. This decision making is guided by knowledge of research data as well as clinicians' experience. Studies of children's typical speech sound acquisition are the primary research data used by SLPs to make these decisions.

There are seven main areas of SLP practice that are informed by a comprehensive understanding of speech sound acquisition:

1. *Referral.* Providing advice to parents, educators, and health professionals regarding whether a child should be referred for a speech assessment.
2. *Assessment.* Deciding which assessment tools will appropriately examine the range of speech behaviors that are relevant for the age of the child. For example, if the child is 1;6, then an inventory of consonants, vowels, and syllable shapes should be determined. If the child is 7;0 then polysyllabic words and phonological awareness skills also should be assessed.

3. *Analysis.* Analyzing the speech sample in order to decide whether the child's speech is age-appropriate on a range of measures.
4. *Diagnosis.* Determining whether a child has a delay or disorder and whether his or her areas of difficulty warrant speech sound intervention.
5. *Selection of intervention targets.* There are two major schools of thought regarding how to use knowledge of typical speech sound acquisition to select intervention targets. Proponents of the *traditional developmental approach* suggest focusing on errors on the production of early developing sounds as intervention targets (cf. Davis, 2005; Shriberg and Kwiatkowski, 1982). Proponents of the *complexity approach* (also called nontraditional approach and least knowledge approach) select later developing sounds; the aim of such an approach is to produce a systemwide change (cf. Gierut, Morrisette, Hughes, and Rowland, 1996).
6. *Intervention.* Adapting teaching and feedback to an age-appropriate level, and determining that a child has achieved his or her goals to the expected level.
7. *Dismissal/discharge.* Deciding whether a child's speech is within normal limits (Tyler, 2005), and whether his or her speech sound intervention should be concluded.

The goal of this chapter is to assist SLPs in all these areas by providing basic or foundational knowledge for working with children with speech sound disorders.

MODELS OF SPEECH ACQUISITION

The acquisition of speech and language is a complex process and many models of acquisition have been proposed. Each model provides a different insight into how the process might work. Thus, it is useful for SLPs working with children to consider a range of models in their practice. Barlow and Gierut (1999, p. 1482) recommend that when considering models of speech acquisition, an adequate model must account for: "(a) the actual facts of children's productions and the mismatches between a child's output and the adult input forms; (b) the generalities that span children's sound systems, as well as associated variability within and across developing systems; and (c) the changes that occur in children's grammars over time." They also indicated that an adequate model must be "testable and falsifiable." With these premises in mind, a range of models of speech acquisition will be presented. For a comprehensive account, see Ball and Kent (1997).

Traditionally, SLPs used a behaviorist model to explain how children learn the sounds of the language. More recently, linguistic-based models have evolved based on theories of generative phonology, natural phonology, nonlinear theory, optimality theory, and sonority. Such approaches not only provided SLPs with greater insight into children's developing speech systems but they also extended and enhanced guidelines for assessment, analysis, and intervention. Most linguistic theories maintain that innate or natural mechanisms govern a child's phonological system. In generative phonology these are expressed as *distinctive features,* in natural phonology these are expressed as *phonological processes* (or *patterns*), in nonlinear phonology these are expressed as *multitiered* representations, and in optimality theory these are expressed as *constraints*. However, although linguistic-based models provided descriptions of children's phonology, they failed to provide explanations of the underlying cognitive mechanisms involved in the perception and production of speech. Consequently, the most recent explanations are psycholinguistic models of speech development.

Traditional Models of Speech Acquisition

Behaviorist Models

Behaviorism focused on describing overt and observable behaviors. Behaviorism was proposed by Watson (1913/1994, p. 248) in his article "Psychology as a Behaviorist Views It" and was described as an "objective experimental branch of natural science that can be studied without references to consciousness." The most influential proponent of behaviorism was B. F. Skinner. Skinner's operant conditioning can be traced back to the stimulus-response psychology of the Russian physiologist, Pavlov, who trained a dog to respond by salivating when hearing the stimulus of a bell ringing. Skinner created the concept of operant or instrumental conditioning to focus on controlling acts by changing the consequences that occur immediately following the act (Skinner, 1972; Thomas, 2000). In a behaviorist approach, consequences can be described either as positive or negative, reinforcement or punishment. Skinner's behaviorism has been applied to a wide range of ages, cultures, and behaviors (including physical, social, and emotional). Behaviorist principles have been applied throughout SLP practice, particularly from the 1950s to the 1970s.

Application to Typically Developing Children. When behaviorist models have been applied to speech acquisition, the focus has been on observing environmental conditions (stimuli) that co-occur and predict overt verbal behaviors (responses). For example, Olmsted (1971) suggested that sounds that were easy to discriminate would be learned first; however, his order of discrimination has not been supported by subsequent research. Behaviorist approaches documented normative behaviors of large groups of children during the speech acquisition period. Speech-language pathologists described speech development as correct pronunciation of speech sounds. Age-of-acquisition data were collected to provide descriptive normative information (e.g., Templin, 1957). Evaluation of phonological learning, articulatory mastery, and maturation were not the primary focus.

A major criticism of the application of behaviorism to children's speech acquisition is that children master speech and language acquisition more quickly than they could if they had to depend on stimulus-response mechanisms to learn each element. That is, there is no capacity for parental/environmental reinforcement of all speech behaviors, leading to mastery of such a complex skill as speech and language. Another criticism is that acquisition of speech and language is too complex to be explained solely by reinforcement.

Application to Speech-Language Pathology Practice. Although behaviorism as an explanation for sound acquisition has not been supported, behavioral principles have had a significant impact on SLP practice for children with speech sound disorders. Speech production was considered a motor activity and analysis of speech was conducted using segmental error analysis. Speech was analyzed as a series of sounds, and the function of sound differences to signal meaning differences was not taken into consideration (e.g., Van Riper and Irwin, 1958). The stimulus-response paradigm was the basis of traditional articulation intervention. Using this behavioral approach, a child was presented with a sound or word that he or she was required to say, then received positive reinforcement in the form of praise, a sticker, or a token on a set schedule (cf. Winitz, 1969).

Linguistic Models of Speech Acquisition

In the traditional models of speech acquisition there was limited consideration of the patterns, structures, and contexts of mispronunciations (with exceptions such as McDonald, 1964b) or of the cognitive dimension of linguistic knowledge. This gave rise to the linguistic models of speech development.

Generative Phonology

Generative phonology is a theory of the sound structure of human languages and was developed by Noam Chomsky. The key principles of generative phonology were illustrated in the landmark study of English phonology presented in Chomsky and Hallé's (1968) book, *The Sound Pattern of English*. Generative phonology moved away from the traditional phonemic analysis and introduced two major concepts:

1. Phonological rules map underlying representations onto surface pronunciations.
2. Phonological descriptions are dependent on information from other linguistic levels.

Although generative phonology incorporates consideration of semantic and syntactical aspects of language (concept 2), most phonology texts focus on concept 1. The area of generative phonology that has received the most attention is the description of phonological relationships that are expressed by proposing an abstract underlying representation and a set of phonological rules. To provide an example, generative phonology can be used to explain the way that English-speaking adults nasalize vowels before nasal consonants. In generative phonology, this concept is written as the following rule:

$$\begin{bmatrix} +\text{Vowel} \\ -\text{Consonant} \end{bmatrix} \rightarrow [\text{Nasal}] / - \begin{bmatrix} +\text{Consonant} \\ +\text{Nasal} \end{bmatrix}$$

The information to the left of the arrow indicates the segments that conform to the rule. The arrow means "is realized as." Only the relevant rules are included to the right of the arrow. Other features are assumed to remain as they were. The diagonal slash means "in the context of." The dash and information that follows provide the context of the segment described by the rule. Thus, this generative phonology rule reads: Vowels are realized as nasal in the context of (in this case, specifically just before) nasal consonants.

Application to Typically Developing Children.   Generative phonology has been applied to the understanding of children's speech acquisition (cf. Grunwell, 1987) as it enabled description of the relationship of children's productions to adult pronunciation in terms of phonological rules. Grunwell (1987) indicated that generative phonology has been readily applied to children's speech since generative phonological rules can explain substitutions, distortions, omissions, additions, metathesis, and coalescence (for examples, see Grunwell, 1987, pp. 176–197).

Some of the premises of generative phonology have received criticism in subsequent research. For example, there has been criticism of the premise that the child's underlying representation of the sound is adult-like (this viewpoint will be discussed later when we consider psycholinguistic theories). Additionally, there has been criticism of the premise that the rules that were applied had a corresponding reality to the processing and production systems of the child (i.e., it is not clear that we actually apply such rules in our heads when we comprehend and produce speech).

Application to Speech-Language Pathology Practice. As a theory, generative phonology has not seen broad application in the field of speech-language pathology. Hodson (2007b) describes generative phonology as the "first steps into phonologically based clinical analysis" (p. 55); however, additional knowledge gained from the theory of natural phonology (below) lead to the identification of patterns in phonological analysis procedures.

Natural Phonology

The theory of natural phonology (Stampe, 1969, 1979) formed the basis of the phonological process approach to assessment and treatment of speech sound disorders, and is regarded as the phonological model that has had the greatest impact on the field of SLP (Edwards, 2007). *Natural processes* (or *patterns*) are those that are preferred or frequently used in phonological systems and are identified in two ways: those that are universal across languages, and those that are frequently used by young children. According to Stampe, a phonological process is a "mental operation that applies in speech to substitute for a class of sounds or sound sequences presenting a common difficulty to the speech capacity of the individual, an alternative class identical but lacking the difficult property" (Stampe, 1979, p. 1) and phonological processes merge "a potential opposition into that member of the opposition which least tries the restrictions of the human speech capacity" (Stampe, 1969, p. 443).

In Stampe's view, the child's underlying representations are akin to adult forms. Natural (or innate) phonological processes apply to these underlying representations resulting in the child's productions (or surface forms). For example, it is assumed that children have the adult form of a word, such as *tree* /tri/, in their underlying representation. However, natural processes such as cluster reduction are applied because the child (at least temporarily) has some limitation to produce a particular sound or group of sounds. In this case, the surface form (child's production) would most likely be [ti]. Later, in the discussion of psycholinguistic models, we will critique the notion that children's underlying representations are akin to the adult form.

Application to Typically Developing Children. Natural phonology has provided great insight to the understanding of typical speech acquisition. Natural processes are described as innate rules that are systematically applied to speech production until children learn to suppress them. Since these rules are universal, they are meant to apply to all children speaking all languages. Thus, speech acquisition is a progression from these innate speech patterns to the pronunciation system of the language(s) learned by the child. By applying natural phonology to English speech acquisition, Grunwell (1987) presented a table of the ages of suppression of phonological processes by typically developing children, such as cluster reduction, fronting, and stopping. Other researchers have also provided lists of natural phonological processes (e.g., Ingram, 1976; Shriberg and Kwiatkowski, 1980). One of the most comprehensive lists of such processes is provided by Edwards and Shriberg (1983).

Application to Speech-Language Pathology Practice.   The phonological pattern/process approach to assessment and intervention based on natural phonology transformed the way that SLPs viewed children's speech sound errors. Since Ingram's (1976, 1989a) seminal work on phonological impairments in children, SLPs increasingly have applied descriptive linguistic-based models to their clinical activities. Ingram's application of natural phonology was widely accepted by SLPs in the 1970s and 1980s and remains popular for directing the assessment, analysis, and intervention of children with speech sound disorders (Bankson and Bernthal, 1990a; Khan, 1982; Shriberg and Kwiatkowski, 1980; Weiner, 1979). Assessment approaches were developed to specifically assess subgroups of sounds within a given phonological pattern (e.g., *Bankson-Bernthal Test of Phonology* (*BBTOP*, Bankson and Bernthal, 1990a). Phonological processes were also described as part of a broader analysis procedure for several speech sampling tools (e.g., *Phonological Assessment of Child Speech* (*PACS*, Grunwell, 1995) and as stand-alone analyses to be applied to conversational speech (e.g., *Natural Process Analysis*) (Shriberg and Kwiatkowski, 1980). One of the goals of intervention based on natural phonology is "to teach children to suppress innate simplification processes" (Hodson, 2007b, p. 55).

Limitations of the application of natural phonology to SLP practice have been identified. First, although most SLPs can readily describe children's nonadult productions using phonological process terms such as *cluster reduction* and *fronting*, SLPs' use of phonological processes are descriptive rather than an application of the theoretical tenets of natural phonology. Shriberg (1991, p. 270) described this as an "atheoretical use of process terminology." Second, natural phonology does not account for "nonnatural" simplifications in children's speech (Hodson, 2007). Many children with highly unintelligible speech produce speech sounds in a way that cannot be classified using natural phonology. Terms such as *backing* and *initial consonant deletion* are in the literature to describe phonological processes that are not seen in children with typical speech acquisition (Dodd, 1995b).

One question that remains unresolved with natural phonology is whether the process labels being applied actually represent mental operations going on inside the head of the child. However, because such labels do capture "patterns" of errors being observed, the term *phonological patterns* is frequently used in place of "phonological processes." For example, the title of the most recent version of a popular assessment tool in this area is now the *Hodson Assessment of Phonological Patterns* (Hodson, 2004).

Nonlinear Phonology

Nonlinear phonology refers to a collection of theories that focus on the hierarchical nature of the relationships between phonological units. Nonlinear phonology was first introduced by Goldsmith in his doctoral dissertation (see Goldsmith, 1990). These theories include autosegmental theory, metrical theory, moraic theory, feature geometry theory, and underspecification theory. Nonlinear phonology attempts to account for the idea that production of speech involves more than just production of a line of phonemes; it takes many elements into account (features, segments, syllables, feet, words, and phrases) both independently and in relation to one another, hence the term *non*linear. There are two main tiers in nonlinear phonology:

1. The *prosodic tier* focuses on words and the structure of words and includes a number of levels: word tier, foot tier, syllable tier, onset-rime tier, skeletal tier, and segmental tier (see Figure 3.1).
2. The *segmental tier* focuses on the segments or speech sounds and the features that make up those sounds (see Figure 2.28).

In the prosodic tier, the *word tier,* simply denotes words. Immediately below the word tier is the *foot tier*, which refers to grouping of syllables, and syllables may either be strong (S) or weak (w). A foot can contain only one strong syllable (but can also contain other weak syllables). A foot that includes a weak syllable can be either Sw (left prominent or trochaic), or wS (right prominent or iambic). Below the foot is the *syllable tier*. A syllable consists of one prominent phoneme (the peak), which is usually a vowel and less prominent phonemes

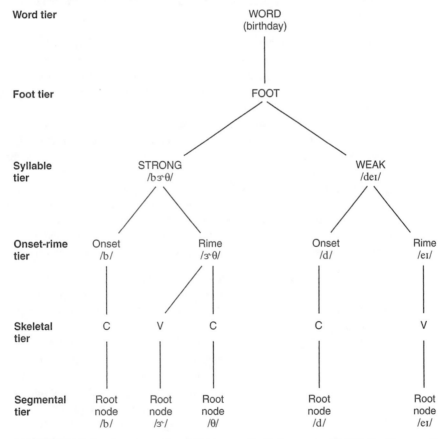

■ **FIGURE 3.1** An example of the prosodic tier representation for the word *birthday*.

(generally consonants) that can appear before or after the peak. Consonants that appear before the vowel are known as *onsets,* and consonants that appear after the vowel are *codas.* The peak and the coda together make up the *rime.* All languages allow syllables without a coda (e.g., CV), but some do not allow a syllable to have a coda (e.g., CVC). A syllable with a coda is called a *closed syllable.* Across the world's languages open syllables occur more often than closed. Below the syllable tier is the *skeletal tier*, which includes slots for the individual speech sounds.

In the *segmental tier*, features are described according to three nodes: the root node, the laryngeal node, and the place node (the segmental tiers were outlined in Chapter 2; see Figure 2.28). The root node [sonorant] and [consonantal] defines the segment as a vowel/glide or a consonant. The features [continuant] and [nasal] define the classes of stops, fricatives, and nasals. The laryngeal node includes the features of [voice] and [spread glottis] and differentiate vowels as well as voiced from voiceless consonants. The place node designates the oral cavity characteristics of the segment and includes labial [round], coronal [anterior], [distributed], and dorsal [high], [low], [back]. Default nodes are generally the most frequent features (unmarked) and the easiest features for a child to use. In English, the default consonant is /t/ because it is coronal, but not continuant, not lateral, not nasal, and not voiced.

Application to Typically Developing Children.   Two of the major benefits of nonlinear phonology to the understanding of typical phonological development are (1) the concept of links between the segmental and suprasegmental tiers and prosodic variables that highlight the interaction between speech sounds and other speech-language domains and (2) the view that development is progressive or additive, which is in contrast to the negative progression suggested by a phonological process approach whereby children learn to "undelete" deleted final consonants (Bernhardt and Stoel-Gammon, 1994). Bernhardt (1992a) discussed these developmental implications of nonlinear phonology and highlighted the importance of considering children's representations instead of the negative progression of rules of generative grammar. Bernhardt (1992a) suggested that children's representations (or simple syllable templates such as CV units and stop consonants) account for a large proportion of young children's speech production and that children add to these representations as they mature. Nonlinear phonology also enables consideration beyond the acquisition of consonants, as it also addresses vowels, syllable shapes, words, and stress.

Application to Speech-Language Pathology Practice.   Bernhardt, Stemberger, and colleagues have been major proponents of the use of nonlinear phonology in SLP practice. Bernhardt and Stoel-Gammon (1994) presented an excellent overview of the benefits of nonlinear phonology to SLPs. Bernhardt and Stemberger developed a theoretical text (Bernhardt and Stemberger, 1998), a workbook for clinicians (Bernhardt and Stemberger, 2000), and a computerized assessment and analysis (*CAPES: Computerized Articulation and Phonology Evaluation System*) (Masterson and Bernhardt, 2001). Additionally, they have applied principles of nonlinear phonology to goal setting and intervention for children with speech sound disorders (Bernhardt, 1992b; Bernhardt, Stemberger, and Major, 2006). In the assessment of children's speech using nonlinear phonology, attention is not only paid to production of consonants, but vowels, syllables, word shapes, and stress patterns are also important. Nonlinear intervention goals focus on utilizing established sounds in new syllable shapes and new sounds in established syllable shapes.

Optimality Theory

Optimality theory was first described by Prince and Smolensky (1993) in their report titled *Optimality Theory: Constraint Interaction in Generative Grammar*. Optimality theory originally was developed to describe adult languages. The basic units of optimality theory are constraints, and there are two major types:

1. *Markedness constraints* (also called *output constraints*) capture limitations on what can be produced (or the output). Output is simplified by markedness constraints that are motivated by the frequency and distribution of sounds in the ambient language as well as perceptual and articulatory characteristics of the sounds. Sounds that are difficult to pronounce or perceive are marked.
2. *Faithfulness constraints* capture the features to be "preserved," prohibiting addition and deletion that violates the ambient language.

Constraints are assumed to be universal to all languages (Barlow and Gierut, 1999). There is a reciprocal relationship between faithfulness and markedness constraints (Kager, 1999). Faithfulness can result in the inclusion of phonological features, whereas markedness can result in their exclusion.

Application to Typically Developing Children and Speech-Language Pathology Practice. Optimality theory has been applied to the understanding of the typical development of children's speech (see Barlow and Gierut [1999] for an overview). The aim during development is for the output to match the adult target, and this is achieved by promoting faithfulness constraints and demoting markedness constraints. One example of the application of optimality theory has been to develop a model of children's acquisition of polysyllabic words (James, van Doorn, and McLeod, 2008). The model proposes five stages each of which elucidates relevant faithfulness constraints. In stage 1 (ages 1;0 to 2;3), children are faithful to the stressed syllable and the duration of the whole word. Stage 2 (ages 2;4 to 3;11) foregrounds faithfulness to the number of syllables in a word. That is, during this stage children reduce the occurrence of weak syllable deletion, cluster reduction, and final consonant deletion. Stage 3 (ages 4;0 to 6;11) highlights faithfulness to all the phonemes in the words and can co-occur with a period of dysprosody (e.g., word rhythm is disrupted). Stage 4 (ages 7;0 to 10;11) emphasizes faithfulness to word rhythm with accurate delineation between stressed and unstressed syllables. The final stage (age 11;0 and older) represents adult-like production of polysyllabic words.

Optimality theory also has been applied to SLP practice with children with speech sound disorders (Barlow and Gierut, 1999). Children's possible productions of words are placed into a constraint table and violations of constraints are identified. Fatal violations (involving a highly ranked constraint) are also identified. The optimal constraint (the form most likely to be produced by the child) is the one that violates the least number of constraints, or the lowest ranking constraints. As children's speech systems mature, they re-rank constraints until eventually their productions match the adult form (Edwards, 2007).

Sonority Hypothesis

Sonority was first described in 1865 (see Clements, 1990) and refers to the relative loudness of a sound relative to other sounds with the same pitch, stress, and length (Ladefoged,

1993). The sonority of a sound is dependent on the degree of voicing and the amount of opening (stricture) involved in producing the sound. Voiced sounds are more sonorous than voiceless sounds. Sounds with open articulation (e.g., vowels and liquids) are highly sonorous, whereas sounds with closed articulation (e.g., stops and fricatives) are less sonorous. Phonemes are allocated a numerical value to represent their degree of sonority. A number of different value hierarchies have been proposed, with the hierarchy by Steriade (1990) being the one most commonly used within SLP (e.g., Gierut, 1999; Ohala, 1999). Steriade proposes that voiceless stops (value of 7) are the least sonorous phonemes and vowels (value of 0) are the most sonorous sounds.

The Sonority Sequencing Principle (SSP) is a "presumed universal which governs the permissible sequence of consonants within syllables" (Gierut, 1999, p. 708). Thus, phonemes with low sonority values are found at the syllable margins, and sounds with high sonority values are located toward the center of the syllable (Clements, 1990; Roca and Johnson, 1999). In the word *drink*, for example, the vowel /ɪ/ has high sonority, therefore it is found in the middle of the syllable. The next most sonorous sounds are liquids (such as /r/) and nasals (such as /n/), hence they are found on either side of the vowel. The least sonorous sounds are stops (such as /d/ and /k/). These are found at the syllable margins.

Application to Typically Developing Children.   In accordance with the SSP, it has been proposed that children reduce word-initial consonant clusters in a manner that produces a maximal rise in sonority, and that word-final consonant clusters are reduced to produce a minimal fall in sonority. This pattern of reduction is termed the *sonority hypothesis.* Ohala (1999) considered the application of the sonority hypothesis when he described the productions of consonant clusters in nonsense words produced by 16 typically developing children ages 1;9 to 3;2. When the children reduced word-initial fricative + stop clusters (e.g., /sp/) and word-initial fricative + nasal clusters (e.g., /sn/), the remaining consonant was consistently the least sonorous element. Additionally, when the children reduced word-final fricative + stop consonant clusters (e.g., /-st/), the remaining consonant was consistently the most sonorous element. Wyllie-Smith, McLeod, and Ball (2006) analyzed the production of word-initial consonant clusters of 16 typically developing 2-year-old children over two occasions for each child. Overall, the sonority hypothesis was adhered to when the children reduced a consonant cluster by producing one of the target elements; however, reductions to nontarget consonants were inconsistent (some adhered to and some violated the sonority hypothesis). Recently, Yavaş (2006) led an international study to examine children's use of the sonority hypothesis. The hypothesis was upheld across children with typical speech acquisition who spoke languages as diverse as Turkish, Norwegian, and Israeli Hebrew.

Application to Speech-Language Pathology Practice.   Sonority has been used as a theoretical basis for making clinical decisions regarding target selection with children who have impaired speech (Anderson, 2000; Baker, 2000; Ball and Müller, 2002; Gierut, 1998, 1999; Gierut and Champion, 2001). It has been used to analyze children's phonemic awareness skills (Yavaş, 2000; Yavaş and Core, 2001; Yavaş and Gogate, 1999) and to analyze productions of consonant clusters of children with speech impairment (Anderson, 2000; Baker, 2000; Chin, 1996; Gierut, 1998, 1999; Gierut and Champion, 2001; Wyllie-Smith et al., 2006).

Psycholinguistic Models

While linguistic applications are useful for the *description* of children's phonological systems, psycholinguistic applications provide the potential for the *explanation* of children's phonology. A psycholinguistic model draws on the fields of psychology and linguistics and attempts to account for psychological processes or mental mechanisms involved in the "perception, storage, planning and production of speech as it is produced in real time in real utterances" (McCormack, 1997, p. 4). At the simplest level, a psycholinguistic model describes the distinction between underlying representations of words and their production (Fee, 1995). It is used to map interactions between auditory input, underlying cognitive-linguistic processes, and speech production output (Dodd, 1995a). In doing so, psycholinguistic models attempt to provide explanations for the descriptive or symptomatic information derived from linguistic-based assessments (Stackhouse and Wells, 1993). An example of such a model is presented in Chapter 4 (Figure 4.1).

Application to Typically Developing Children.   Numerous authors have been involved in the construction of psycholinguistic models of speech development. These include Smith (1973, 1978), Menn and colleagues (Kiparsky and Menn, 1977; Menn, 1971, 1978; Menn and Matthei, 1992; Menn, Markey, Mozer, and Lewis, 1993), Macken (1980a, 1980b), Spencer (1986, 1988), Hewlett and colleagues (Hewlett, 1990; Hewlett, Gibbon, and Cohen-McKenzie, 1998), and Stackhouse and colleagues (Pascoe, Wells, and Stackhouse, 2006; Stackhouse and Wells, 1993, 1997). A number of useful historical accounts and critiques of psycholinguistic models exist (e.g., Bernhardt and Stemberger, 1998; Maxwell, 1984; Menn and Matthei, 1992; Vihman, 1996).

In a psycholinguistic model, the first point of the speech process is the *input,* which is the speech signal heard by the child. The final point of the speech process is the *output,* which is the speech signal (usually words) actually produced/spoken by the child. The possible events that occur between input and output are the focus of psycholinguistic models. Menn (1994) describes psycholinguistic modeling as a "black box approach," whereby input and output are examined to construct a mechanism, which can explain the effects seen.

input → black box → output

Within the "black box" different levels of representation of knowledge are hypothesized. *Underlying representation* refers to "the basic unaltered pronunciation before any processes have had a chance to operate" (Spencer, 1996, p. 50). Thus, the underlying representation is the phonological information that is stored in the speaker's mind about the words known and used.

input → underlying representation → output

The child's underlying representation is stored in the *lexicon* or "mental dictionary" (Maxwell, 1984, p. 18). Depending on the theoretical model being considered, the lexicon may contain semantic or meaning-based information (Bernhardt and Stemberger, 1998) and/or phonological information (e.g., Menn, 1978; Smith, 1973). Stackhouse and Wells (1997) suggest the lexicon contains phonological, semantic, grammatical, orthographic, and motor programming information. Definitions of the storage, nature, and number of underlying representations differ among researchers.

Initially, *single-lexicon models* of the speech process were posited, whereby children were considered to have an adult-like underlying representation of speech (e.g., Smith, 1973). The lexicon was synonymous with the underlying representation and contained information about the adult pronunciation of words. Development of single-lexicon models continued through the 1970s (Braine, 1979; Macken, 1980a; Smith, 1978). Much of the revision was focused around evidence that did not support Smith's (1973) assumption that the child's perception was always adult-like. Consequently, Smith (1978) revised his model by adding a perceptual filter to account for the possibility that the child may have inaccurate perception.

Early single-lexicon models could not account for variable pronunciations, in particular, for instances where different tokens of a word could be pronounced in different ways, and where one phoneme could be pronounced differently in different words (Bernhardt and Stemberger, 1998). Consequently, *two-lexicon models* were proposed where two levels of underlying representation exist: the input and output lexicons. The *input lexicon* refers to the perceptually based phonological representations that enable the child to perceive speech, or "all the child's knowledge that permits him or her to recognize a word" (Menn and Matthei, 1992, p. 214). The *output lexicon* refers to the articulatorily based phonological representations that enable the child to produce speech. Menn (1983) described the output lexicon as "ways-to-say-words." If it exists independently, the input lexicon is almost certain to be richer in contrasts than the output lexicon (Hewlett, 1990), and some suggest that the input lexicon contains the same information as the adult surface representations (Spencer, 1988).

$$\text{input} \rightarrow \text{input lexicon} \rightarrow \text{output lexicon} \rightarrow \text{output}$$

Two-lexicon models allowed for the notion that young children may have underlying representations that are unique to their own system. That is, the output (production) lexicon was able to hold underlying representations that were not adult-like. This notion was contrary to Smith's ideas that children have underlying representations that were similar to adult surface forms (for a complete discussion, see Maxwell, 1984).

In a two-lexicon account, the child stores underlying adult-like perceptual representations in the input lexicon. These perceptual representations are then modified off-line through the application of rules or processes to create underlying production representations in the output lexicon. Once a child has stored a word in the output lexicon, subsequent productions are accessed from the output lexicon rather than being accessed from the input lexicon and modified on-line.

Although two-lexicon models provided a way of accounting for the variability in children's speech, there are three primary criticisms of the two-lexicon accounts (Bernhardt and Stemberger, 1998; Chiat, 1994; Menn and Matthei, 1992; Vihman, 1996). First, with the potential for duplication of lexical items, particularly in the output lexicon, the models fail to explain how children select one representation over another, or how representations change to being more adult-like. That is, the models do not explain when and how old forms are deleted (Bernhardt and Stemberger, 1998; Dinnsen, Barlow, and Morrisette,

1997; Vihman, 1996). A second criticism concerns the "continuity hypothesis" (Bernhardt and Stemberger, 1998; Menn, 1994). Developmentalists argue that there should not be one model that applies to children and another for adults, because accounting for the shift between the two models is difficult. It has been suggested that a child's output lexicon will eventually match his or her input lexicon because the forms within the output lexicon will become adult-like; thus, adults may only have a single lexicon. The third major criticism is that both single- and two-lexicon models were designed to describe single-word production and do not take into account constraints that occur between words in connected speech (Hewlett, 1990; Vihman, 1996).

Hence, two-lexicon accounts, thus have a number of limitations. Consequently, single-lexicon theories are currently being postulated with the notion that input and output forms are represented in some way (e.g., Hewlett et al., 1998). Furthermore, the hard-walled "boxes" of the two-lexicon accounts are now being represented by connectionist models (Bernhardt and Stemberger, 1998; Menn and Matthei, 1992; see Baker et al. [2001] for a description). Connectionist models use computer modeling to test a cognitive task, such as speech production. Networks of nodes connect the input and output, and during computer simulations, the probability of the activation of each node is tested. Connectionist models can be run many times to provide the probability of a specific output occurring, thus enabling testing of hypotheses of speech and language acquisition.

Application to SLP Practice.   The earliest authors in the field of speech-language pathology to suggest consideration of children's underlying representation were Shriberg and Kwiatkowski (1980) and Edwards (1983). Since then, consideration of underlying representation has been presented in speech-language pathology intervention case studies (e.g., Bryan and Howard, 1992; McGregor and Schwartz, 1992; Stackhouse, Pascoe, and Gardner, 2006). Baker, Croot, McLeod, and Paul (2001) provide a tutorial of the application of psycholinguistic models to SLP practice, and an important series of books have been written for speech-language pathologists on assessment and intervention for speech and literacy within a psycholinguistic framework (Stackhouse and Wells, 1997, 2001; Pascoe, Wells, and Stackhouse, 2006; Stackhouse, Vance, Pascoe, and Wells, 2007).

We have presented several models of speech sound acquisition and have related them to clinical practice. As stated earlier, each has its strengths, with some perhaps being more helpful than others to one's understanding of how sounds are acquired. If nothing else, we certainly gain an appreciation of how complex the process is, and how difficult it may be to explain it to parents and clients. In the section that follows we will shift our attention from theories, to how to gather data to inform us about how speech sound acquisition has been observed, recorded, and analyzed.

HOW SPEECH ACQUISITION DATA ARE OBTAINED

At the beginning of this chapter, we identified how important it is for SLPs to be well acquainted with typical speech sound development. Later in this chapter, a wide range of speech acquisition data will be presented. It is beneficial to understand how these speech acquisition data are obtained, since some are based on small samples of children taken over a long period of time, whereas other data are based on large groups of children seen once. There are three major techniques that have been used for collecting speech acquisition data: diary studies, large cross-sectional group studies, and longitudinal studies.

Historically, research into typical speech sound acquisition was conducted using *diary studies*. Famous historical diary studies include descriptions of the speech of children such as Amahl (Smith, 1973), Hildegarde (Leopold, 1947), and Joan (Velten, 1943). With the influence of behaviorism, *large cross-sectional group studies* became prevalent. The earliest of these studies relating to English-speaking children's speech sound acquisition were conducted by Poole (1934), Wellman, Case, Mengurt, and Bradbury (1931), and Templin (1957). More recently, *longitudinal studies* comprising a smaller group of participants have complemented the large-scale cross-sectional studies to enhance the understanding of speech acquisition (e.g., Carroll, Snowling, Hulme, and Stevenson, 2003; Dodd, 1995a; McLeod, van Doorn, and Reed, 2001b; Watson and Scukanec, 1997a, 1997b; Walker and Archibald, 2006). Each of these methodologies has their strengths and weaknesses. A primary difference is in the trade-off between the extent of data analyzed and reported versus the number of participants.

To contextualize this discussion of research methods, an overview of key studies into typical English speech sound acquisition is summarized at the back of this book in Appendix A. The appendix provides information about the authors, year of publication, country in which the study was conducted, number and age of the children studied, sample type, and method of data collection. You are encouraged to access the original sources in order to utilize the full range of information offered by these researchers. For a wide-ranging overview of speech acquisition in a range of English dialects and languages other than English, see *The International Guide to Speech Acquisition* (McLeod, 2007a). Note that most studies listed in Appendix A have used either cross-sectional or longitudinal data collection methods. Those that used a cross-sectional design typically used single-word sampling. Those that used a longitudinal design typically used connected speech sampling. Each of these research techniques will now be described in detail.

Diary Studies of Typical Speech Sound Acquisition

Diary studies were the initial major source of data about children's speech and language development. Typically, a parent who was a linguist or psychologist kept a comprehensive diary of his or her child's speech and/or language development over a period of time. An early diary study of a child's language development was that of Humphreys (1880). Famous diary studies which have focused on speech development include Leopold's (1939–49) four-volume account of his daughter, Velten's (1943) study of his daughter, and Smith's (1973) extensive analysis of his son's speech.

The parental diary study has continued to be used as a method for data collection, but more specifically to collect data on a specific issue, rather than general speech and language development. For example, Berg (1995) collected data from his German-speaking daughter on a daily basis from the age of 3;4 to 4;3. He presented data on interword variation in the development of velars. Other examples of diary studies of typical phonological development include Menn's (1971) report on her son's early constraints on sound sequences, the account by Elbers and Ton (1985) of Elbers's son's words and babbling within the first-word period, Stemberger's (1988) account of his eldest daughter's between-word processes and his (1989) account of both daughters' nonsystemic errors within and across phrases, French's (1989) account of her son's acquisition of word forms in the first 50-word stage, and Lleo's (1990) report of her daughter's use of reduplication and homonymy as phonological strategies.

The diary study methodology also has been used to study typical speech acquisition of children where the researchers are not the parents (e.g., Bernstein-Ratner, 1993; Fey and Gandour, 1982). An extension of diary studies is the single case study methodology that has been particularly beneficial for the documentation of intervention effects on children with speech impairment (see Crystal, 1987) (e.g., Camarata, 1989; Camarata and Gandour, 1985; Crosbie, Pine, Holm, and Dodd, 2006; Grunwell and Yavaş, 1988; Leonard and Leonard, 1985; McGregor and Schwartz, 1992; Pascoe, Stackhouse, and Wells, 2005).

Advantages and Disadvantages of Diary Studies

The primary advantage of diary studies is that they contain some of the most detailed accounts of speech acquisition. The depth and breadth of detail enables examination of descriptive, exploratory, and explanatory intent. The detail places change into context, since diary studies allow for the retention of the holistic and meaningful characteristics of the child's real-life events (Yin, 1989).

Although general trends about speech acquisition cannot be derived from diary study data, the rich source of data (often contained in appendices) has been used to test and retest statements and hypotheses long after the original reason for collecting the data has been superseded. For example, the extensive data provided by Smith (1973) in his appendices have been reexamined by Braine (1979) and Macken (1980a) to find evidence against Smith's earlier conclusion that the child's underlying representations must be adult-like. Similarly, Greenlee (1974) reexamined data from a number of cross-linguistic diary studies to describe a sequence of development for consonant clusters.

There are a number of disadvantages of using diary studies as the only means to understand children's speech acquisition. First, it is easy to assume that the single child under study is typical unless reference is made to other normative studies. An example can be seen with Leopold's daughter Hildegarde, who replaced word-initial /f/ with a [w] or [v] (Leopold, 1947). These substitutions are atypical according to Ingram, Christensen, Veach, and Webster (1980), who did not find a single such instance in their study of the typical acquisition of fricatives in 73 children. Second, the fact that the children studied are primarily those of linguists suggests that these children may be precocious or at least different in their acquisition from the general population, whether as a result of genetic endowment or environment. Other disadvantages of using diary studies include randomness of data collection, lack of structure in data collection and potential observer bias since the parent is often the researcher (Ingram, 1989b). Until recently, many diary studies relied on on-line transcription, making it impossible to determine transcription reliability. Some of these problems were overcome with the introduction of the large-group cross-sectional study and the longitudinal study.

Large-Group Cross-Sectional Studies of Typical Speech Sound Acquisition

From the 1950s to 1970s, behaviorism was a major theoretical paradigm for considering speech sound acquisition, and the emphasis in data collection in the fields of psychology, linguistics, and speech-language pathology moved from diary studies to cross-sectional methodology. Using this methodology, researchers attempted to describe typical behavior by establishing developmental norms through the observation of large numbers of children. Commonly, children were placed into selected age groupings, and each child underwent the same testing procedure. Possible confounding influences such as gender, socioeconomic status, and intelligence were carefully controlled. The results of these experiments were presented as proportions and percentages, often in large tables indicating the age of acquisition of phonemes or the age of decline of certain phonological processes.

The majority of research describing the typical acquisition of English speech sounds uses large-group cross-sectional methodology (Anthony, Bogle, Ingram, and McIsaac, 1971; Arlt and Goodban, 1976; Bankson and Bernthal, 1990; Chirlian and Sharpley, 1982; Dodd, Hua, Crosbie, Holm, and Ozanne, 2002; Flipsen, 2006a; Haelsig and Madison, 1986; Ingram, Pittman, and Newman, 1985; Irwin and Wong, 1983; Kilminster and Laird, 1978; Lowe, Knutson, and Monson, 1985; Olmsted, 1971; Paynter and Petty, 1974; Poole, 1934; Prather, Hedrick, and Kern, 1975; Preisser, Hodson, and Paden, 1988; Smit, 1993a, 1993b; Smit, Hand, Freilinger, Bernthal, and Bird, 1990; Templin, 1957; Wellman et al., 1931) (see Appendix A).

The pioneering large-group studies of typical speech acquisition were conducted by Wellman and colleagues (1931) and Poole (1934). In 1957, Templin undertook a comprehensive study of the speech development of 480 children aged 3;0 to 8;0. She provided comprehensive text, 71 tables, and 9 figures to explain children's acquisition of articulation, discrimination, sentence development, and vocabulary. Templin presented the age of acquisition at which 75 percent of children could produce each speech sound in initial, medial, and final word positions. Templin's classic study has been quoted as an authoritative source on speech development by researchers (e.g., Powell and Elbert, 1984; Smit, 1986; Stockman and Stephenson, 1981; Young, 1987) and speech-language pathologists (e.g., Stewart and Weybright, 1980) for many years. Templin's study was considered in need of updating in 1976 by Arlt and Goodban who noted "expanding effects of television, earlier schooling . . . the accelerating effects of developments in education" and suggested that "for purposes of revalidation it seems appropriate to update or examine such norms at 10-year intervals" (Arlt and Goodban, 1976, p. 173). Their suspicions possibly were confirmed when they found that "33% of the sounds tested in this investigation were produced correctly by 75% of the children at least 1 year earlier than would be expected from previously established norms" (p. 176).

The most recent, largest, and heavily cited cross-sectional study of American English was undertaken by Smit and colleagues (1990), who studied 997 children's productions of consonants and consonant clusters. They not only reported age of acquisition of phonemes but they also presented graphical data (cf. Sander, 1972) that indicated the progression of development from age 3;0 to 9;0. These graphs described the trajectory for boys' and girls' speech acquisition. As shown in Table 3.3 on page 96, the data collected by Smit and associates either mirror Arlt and Goodban's data, or fall between their data and the data of

Templin, possibly indicating the relevance of data collection methods and context. Other large cross-sectional studies of speech acquisition include Kilminster and Laird (1978), who studied the speech acquisition of 1,756 Australian English-speaking children; Nagy (1980), who studied the speech acquisition of 7,602 Hungarian children; and Nakanishi, Owada, and Fujita (1972), who studied the speech acquisition of 1,689 Japanese children. The largest studies of Spanish-speaking children were conducted by Acevedo (1993) and Jimenez (1987), who each studied 120 Mexican children.

Advantages and Disadvantages of Large-Group Cross-Sectional Studies

The primary advantage of large-group cross-sectional studies is that they provide normative information by which children can be compared. Such norms are beneficial to SLPs in the identification of impairment. It is assumed that if enough participants are selected for each age group, then typical behavior is observed. Consequently, general trends are ascertained from summary tables provided by such studies. Another advantage of large-group cross-sectional studies is that the emphasis on methodology encourages systematic observation of behavior (Ingram, 1989b). All participants are studied for the same amount of time for the same behaviors using the same experimenters. The third advantage of large-group cross-sectional studies is that there is an emphasis on standardized measurement tools so that studies can be replicated.

Disadvantages of such studies include (1) they typically are collected using single-word, not connected, speech samples; (2) both imitated and spontaneous productions are elicited; (3) they collect data in specific geographical regions that may have dialectical variants; and (4) the experience and reliability of examiners is not always reported (Smit, 1986). Additionally, Peña, Spaulding, and Plante (2006) recently questioned the assumptions behind the selection of children for participation in large-group cross-sectional studies. They argued that, traditionally, children were excluded from cross-sectional studies if they were not experiencing typical development. However, Peña and colleagues indicated that this strategy was akin to "shooting ourselves in the foot." They concluded that if the purpose of a normative study is to identify children who are not developing typically, then the normative sample should include children who are not developing typically. Although their study addressed the area of children's language, their claims are likely to be true for children's speech also.

To conclude, the major strengths of the large-group cross-sectional studies are also a weakness. The grouping of data for statistical analyses means that the data collected for individual children are not reported. The only glimpse of individual variation can be found in the standard deviations from the mean. Longitudinal studies, a third approach, can elucidate individual variability and provide additional insights into children's speech acquisition.

Longitudinal Studies of Typical Speech Sound Acquisition

The possibility that children follow different paths and strategies in typical speech and language acquisition prompted a shift in focus from the large-group studies to longitudinal studies of smaller groups of children. Ingram (1989b) expressed the concern that many of the diary and large-group studies considered only superficial issues, such as the timing of the occurrence of particular features in children's speech. Quotes such as this from Khan (1982, p. 78) occur commonly within the literature from the mid-1970s, expressing a need for "controlled, longitudinal examination of large numbers of children."

Longitudinal studies of speech sound acquisition are characterized by the study of groups of children at repeated intervals. These studies are usually conducted for specific purposes that are beyond describing the age of acquisition of phonemes, to writing rules and explaining the acquisition process. Longitudinal studies share a number of characteristics with diary case studies, in that they study the same children over time. However, there are three primary differences. First, the researcher is independent (recall that diary studies often were conducted by the parent of the child). Second, instead of only one or two children, typically a small group is studied. Third, children in longitudinal studies usually are studied for a set period of time each week or month, instead of daily or at random intervals. Thus, longitudinal studies have the potential to capitalize on the strengths of both diary and large-group studies.

Ferguson and Farwell (1975) conducted one of the earliest and most influential longitudinal studies of speech development. They studied the emergence of words and sounds in early language development, plotting the progress of three young children and the point of 50 words in the children's vocabularies. The data for one of the children were extracted from the diary of Leopold's (1947) Hildegarde; the other two children were personally studied by Ferguson and Farwell. Ferguson and Farwell presented phone trees of data to demonstrate individual learning strategies undertaken by these children.

Since Ferguson and Farwell's original work, there have been a number of longitudinal studies considering different aspects of the development of young children's phonology (e.g., Anderson, 2004; Dodd, 1995b; Dyson, 1986, 1988; Dyson and Paden, 1983; Fee and Ingram, 1982; McLeod et al., 2001b; Otomo and Stoel-Gammon, 1992; Robb and Bleile, 1994; Schwartz, Leonard, Wilcox, and Folger, 1980; Stoel-Gammon, 1985; Vihman and Greenlee, 1987; Walker and Archibald, 2006; Watson and Scukanec, 1997a, 1997b). For example, Robb and Bleile (1994) conducted a comprehensive longitudinal study of the consonant inventories of seven children aged 8 to 25 months. They were able to present valuable individualized data on the sequence of development over time. Similarly, Selby, Robb, and Gilbert (2000) studied the development of vowels in five children aged 15, 18, 21, 24, and 36 months of age.

Advantages and Disadvantages of Longitudinal Studies

There are two major advantages of conducting longitudinal studies of a select group of children. First, studying a small group of children allows researchers to capture individual variations in approaches to learning that may be masked by a large-group study. Knowing about these individual differences increases the likelihood of creating successful, individualized teaching and learning experiences for SLP clients. Second, longitudinal studies allow for the reporting of developmental trends (Macken, 1995). For example, Lleo and Prinz (1996) reported that German- and Spanish-speaking children produced word shapes in the following developmental sequence: CV → CVC → CVCC → CCVCC. Knowing about typical developmental sequences enhances the ability of SLPs to assess whether their clients are delayed or disordered, and may yield a more accurate understanding of the learning process, which could be replicated in intervention strategies.

Interestingly, despite the unique data that result from longitudinal studies, not all such studies report individual developmental information. For example, Dyson and Paden (1983) conducted a longitudinal study of 40 children and reported grouped findings from the first and eighth observations; however, they did use their data to propose sequences of development.

There are three major disadvantages of longitudinal studies. First, longitudinal studies frequently use small numbers of children. As a result, the findings may not be representative of the general population. Second, longitudinal studies generally have regularly scheduled intervals of weeks or months between visits. Such scheduling may allow the child to show considerable change between observations. On the other hand, possible crucial periods of change may occur over a day or two, and a flexible schedule may be more appropriate to allow "emergency visits" when alerted by parental reports of change (Ingram, 1989b). Finally, researchers using longitudinal methodology often prepare stimulus materials for elicitation; thus, a picture of the child's natural speech may not be obtained (French, 1989).

Combined Data-Collection Procedures

In order to obtain the advantages of both cross-sectional and longitudinal methodologies, a number of researchers have developed combined methodologies. Some fundamentally cross-sectional studies have assessed children more than once, thus gaining some longitudinal continuity in their data. For example, Roberts, Burchinal, and Footo (1990) utilized a combination of cross-sectional and longitudinal methodology in their examination of 145 children between the ages of 2;6 and 8;0. Over the six-year period, 13 of these children were examined six times, 24 were tested five times, and so on, with 32 being tested only once. Similarly, Stoel-Gammon (1985) studied 33 children's development of phonetic inventories; 7 children were studied at age 15 months, 19 children at age 18 months, 32 children at age 21 months, and 33 children at age 24 months. Neither of these studies presented individualized longitudinal results.

Another approach is to undertake a longitudinal study in which children are studied over time, but different cohorts of children are studied at different ages (e.g., Chervela, 1981; Dyson, 1988). For example, Chervela (1981) conducted a "longitudinal and cross-sectional study" (p. 63) of the development of medial consonant clusters in four children ages 1;6 to 3;0. He selected one child at each of the ages of 1;6, 2;0, 2;6, and 3;0. The data were collected once a month for six months for each child. A combination of data-collection methodologies enables researchers to manipulate the advantages and disadvantages of each methodology in order to provide more comprehensive findings about the typical developmental sequence. As Stokes, Klee, Carson, and Carson (2005, p. 828) recommend: "Large-scale longitudinal studies, combined with statistical analyses, would provide the best possible view of the nature of phonemic development." With this understanding of data-collection procedures, we will now explore data that have been collected on children's speech acquisition.

◾ OVERALL SEQUENCE OF SPEECH SOUND ACQUISITION

It takes a child many years to progress from the first cries at birth to being able to produce intelligible speech incorporating adult-like production of vowels, consonants, syllable structures, and prosody (including tones, if applicable). There are four phases of speech acquisition (adapted from Bleile, 2004):

> Phase 1: Laying the foundations for speech (birth to 1 year)
>
> Phase 2: Transitioning from words to speech (1 to 2 years)
>
> Phase 3: The growth of the inventory (2 to 5 years)
>
> Phase 4: Mastery of speech and literacy (5+ years)

During the first year, the child produces sounds, first reflexively then more purposefully. Children cry, coo, and babble during their first year, and toward the end of this time they produce their first words. Within phase 2, children's communicative focus is on transitioning from words to speech. During their second year they can produce a small vocabulary with a simplified phonological structure. During phase 3, from 2 to 5 years of age, children learn to produce the majority of speech sounds and syllable structures as well as grammatical and syntactical structures. Finally, phase 4 is a period of mastery that includes sophistication of timing, prosody, and accurate production of polysyllabic words and consonant clusters. Additionally, sounds are conveyed through writing (reading and spelling) and are no longer only in the spoken domain. An expanded description of children's acquisition of speech follows and an age-by-age summary is found in Appendix A.

◾ PHASE 1: LAYING THE FOUNDATIONS FOR SPEECH

Development of the Structure and Function of the Oral Mechanism

There is an interrelationship between the ability to produce intelligible speech and the development of a child's oromotor, neurological, respiratory, and laryngeal systems (Kent, 1976). The development of oral structure and function begins in the fetus, starts to approximate the adult configuration at age 6 years, and is finished at approximately 18 years of age (Kent and Tilkens, 2007). The development of the anatomical structures and functions that support speech acquisition are described next.

Anatomical Structures Supporting Speech Acquisition

The vocal tract of the newborn differs both in size and shape from the vocal tract of an adult. The vocal tract of the newborn is three times smaller than that of the adult and is considered to be similar to a single tube to facilitate coordination between breathing, sucking, and swallowing (Kent and Tilkens, 2007; Vorperian, Kent, Gentry, and Yandell, 1999). The adult vocal tract is considered to be akin to two tubes, with the oral tube enabling a wide variety of articulations and the laryngeal tube facilitating coordination between breathing and swallowing. The newborn's larynx is located between the first and fourth cervical vertebrae; however, by 6 years of age, it has descended to the adult-like position: between the fourth and seventh vertebrae (Kent and Tilkens, 2007). From puberty onward, there is a significant sex difference in the overall vocal tract length and the proportions of the pharyngeal and oral cavities (Fitch and Giedd, 1999).

In infancy, the respiratory system consists of a "bellows-like displacement of the diaphragm" (Kent and Tilkens, 2007, p. 9) and infants' breathing rate at rest is between 30 to 80 breaths per minute. By age 6 months, the infant's rib cage is horizontal and by 1 year of age, respiration for speech and breathing is differentiated. Respiration matures at approximately 7 years of age, when the lung architecture is similar to that of an adult (Kent and Tilkens, 2007). However, during speaking tasks children still have greater subglottal air pressure than adults. Low birth weight is a major factor in poor adult respiratory function, as identified in a large prospective longitudinal birth cohort study conducted by Canoy and associates (2007).

Neurological development is also important for speech acquisition, and significant neurological development occurs over the lifespan (Sowell, Thompson, and Toga, 2004). Ruben (1997) described flexibility of the central auditory nervous system and stated, "The critical/sensitive period of phonology is from the 6th month of fetal life through the 12th month of infancy" (p. 202). Between infancy and adolescence, brain weight and intracranial space grows by approximately 25 percent, then declines to brain volumes similar to those of young children in late adulthood (Courchesne et al., 2000). In a longitudinal study, Sowell, Thompson, Leonard, Welcome, Kan, and Toga (2004) studied children between the ages of 5 and 11 years and found that brain growth progressed at a rate of between 0.4 to 1.5 mm per year. They also found that significant thickening was restricted to left Broca's and Wernicke's areas; gray matter thickness was correlated with changing cognitive abilities. Additionally, rapid myelination occurs during the first year of life (Barkovich, Kjos, Jackson Jr., and Norman, 1988) and is important for gross- and fine-motor movements, including speech (Bleile, 2007).

Anatomical Functions Supporting Speech Acquisition

Precision of articulatory movements of the lip, jaw, and tongue commence in infancy and continue to develop well into adolescence (Walsh and Smith, 2002). Green, Moore, and Reilly (2002) examined vertical movements of the upper lip, lower lip, and jaw during speech for children and adults. They found that jaw movements matured before lip movements, with 1- and 2-year-old children's jaw movements being similar to adults' jaw movements. However, the upper and lower lip movements were more variable and became more adult-like with maturation. Cheng and colleagues have conducted a number of studies of the maturation of tongue control for speech in children, adolescents, and adults using electropalatography (EPG) and electromagnetic articulography (EMA) (Cheng, Murdoch, and Goozee, 2007; Cheng, Murdoch, Goozee, and Scott, 2007a, 2007b). Using EPG, Cheng and colleagues (2007a) found that children's tongue/palate contact for the sounds /t/, /l/, /s/, and /k/ largely resembled those of adults; however, the children ages 6 to 11 years old displayed increased palatal contact and an excessively posterior tongue placement compared with adults. The researchers also indicated that the maturation of the speech motor system was nonuniform and that significant changes in the maturation of tongue control occurred until 11 years of age.

During adolescence tongue control was continually refined. The coordination of tongue and jaw was considered by Cheng and associates (2007b) using EMA. They found that maturation continued until 8 to 11 years of age, with continual refinement into adolescence. There was a differing relationship between the tongue-tip and tongue-body movement with the jaw. The tongue-tip became increasingly synchronized with jaw movement, but the tongue-body retained movement independence with the jaw.

Speech and articulation rates also have been studied in children (Flipsen, 2002a; Ozanne, 1992; Robb, Gilbert, Reed, and Bisson, 2003; Robb and Gillon, 2007; Robbins and Klee, 1987; Williams and Stackhouse, 1998, 2000) and are relevant to our consideration of the maturation of oral functioning. Increasing rate may serve as an indicator of improving control over the articulators. Williams and Stackhouse (1998) suggested that typically developing children ages 3 to 5 years increased their accuracy and consistency but not the rate during diadochokinetic (DDK) tasks. Williams and Stackhouse (2000) suggested that rate was not as useful a predictor as accuracy and consistency of response. Similarly, Walker and Archibald (2006) conducted a longitudinal study of articulation rates in children 4, 5, and 6 years old. They found that articulation rate did not increase significantly with age. However, Flipsen (2002a) reviewed a series of studies of articulation rate and concluded that rate does increase across the developmental period.

Infant Perception

Another important foundation of speech acquisition is infant perception.

Infants' Auditory Perception

Humans are able to perceive sound well before birth (Lasky and Williams, 2005). For example, in a study of 400 fetuses at 16 weeks gestation it was found that they were able to respond to pure tone auditory stimuli at 500Hz (Shahidullah and Hepper, 1992). In a follow-up study, Hepper and Shahidullah (1994) described the progression of the fetuses' responses to different sound frequencies:

- 19 weeks gestation: fetuses responded to 500Hz
- 27 weeks gestation: fetuses responded to 250 and 500Hz (but not 1,000 and 3,000Hz)
- 33 to 35 weeks gestation: fetuses responded to 250, 500, 1,000, and 3,000Hz

As the fetuses matured, they required a lower intensity of sound (20 to 30 dB) in order to respond. Hepper and Shahidullah (1994, p. F81) concluded that "the sensitivity of the fetus to sounds in the low frequency range may promote language acquisition." Another study demonstrated that fetuses not only demonstrate the ability to hear but also to perceive differences in sounds. DeCasper, LeCanuet, Busnel, Granier-Deferre, and Maugeais (1994) asked mothers to recite a nursery rhyme to their fetus three times a day for 4 weeks between 33 and 37 weeks gestation. They found that the fetuses responded with a change in heart rate when presented with a recorded version of the nursery rhyme, but not when presented with an alternative rhyme. They concluded that by the third trimester, "fetuses become familiar with recurrent, maternal speech sounds" (DeCasper et al., 1994, p. 159).

After birth, infants demonstrate sophisticated perceptual skills. Traditionally, the main experimental technique that was used to ascertain infants' ability to discriminate sounds is called the *high amplitude sucking technique* developed by Siqueland and Delucia (1969). Using this technique, infants sucked on a nonnutritive nipple that was equipped to detect changes in pressure. Experimenters found that infants sucked vigorously when a new sound was played, but as they became familiar with the sounds their sucking decreased in frequency and intensity. When a new sound was played, their sucking again became vigorous, then diminished with familiarity with the signal. More recently, *event-related potentials (ERPs)* have been used to determine infants' ability to discriminate aspects of communication (e.g., Shafer, Shucard, Shucard, and Gerken, 1998). Event-related potentials are low-amplitude neurophysiological responses that follow presentation of a stimulus and are typically recorded via electrophysiological instrumentation such as electroencephalograms (EEG) or electromyograms (EMG). They are suitable for studying infants' perceptions, as ERPs are noninvasive and require no overt response. Using both of these techniques, researchers have discovered that infants prefer voices and have the ability to discriminate speech sounds.

The fact that infants demonstrate a preference for voices, particularly their mothers' voices has been shown by a number of researchers (Augustyn and Zuckerman, 2007). For example, DeCasper and Fifer (1980) demonstrated that by 3 days of age, children can distinguish their mothers' voices from a stranger's voice and show a preference for their mothers' voices. Infants appear to prefer child-directed speech (also called *motherese*) to adult-directed speech. Cooper and Aslin (1990) found that this held true for children as young as 2 days old and was still apparent in children who were 1 month old.

Infants also have been shown to be able to discriminate both place and voicing features of consonants. For example, Eimas (1974b) showed that children who were 2 months old could discriminate between the place contrast of /d/ and /g/. Similarly, Aslin and colleagues (1983) showed that children could discriminate between /f/ and voiceless *th* phonemes that also differ by place. A number of authors have demonstrated that infants can discriminate between voiced and voiceless consonants. Eimas, Siqueland, Jusczyk, and Vigorito (1971) showed that infants who were 1 and 4 months old could discriminate between synthesized voiced and voiceless contrasts such as in the stimuli /pa/ and /ba/. Similarly, Eilers, Wilson and Moore (1977) demonstrated that 6-month-old infants can discriminate /sa/ and /za/.

As children are exposed to their native language and reach the end of their first year, some authors suggest that their ability to discriminate nonnative sounds diminishes. For example, Ruben (1997, p. 203) describes this juxtaposition: "By at least 2 days of age, the neonate has an ability to discriminate language specific acoustic distinctions. . . . The 12 month old human has developed the capacity to categorize only those phonemes which are in its native language." However, some researchers believe that more research is needed prior to confirming this view (Rvachew, 2007a), since we do not know whether all infants can discriminate all phonetic inputs; nor do we know that all infants lose the ability to discriminate language-specific inputs. Recent research indicates that infants may retain the ability to discriminate vowels without supporting input (Polka and Bohn, 2003), whereas other children may lose the ability to perceive contrasts despite receiving supporting input (Nittrouer, 2001).

Infants' Visual Perception

In addition to auditory perception, visual speech perception plays a critical role in infants' learning of language. It has long been known that infants prefer looking at faces compared with objects and are even able to discriminate and imitate facial expressions (Field, Woodson, Greenberg, and Cohen, 1982). Recently, it has been discovered that infants are able to distinguish between familiar and unfamiliar languages using only visual cues (Weikum, Vouloumanos, Navarra, Soto-Faraco, Sebastián-Gallés, and Werker, 2007). Weikum and colleagues (2007) found that infants of 4 and 6 months of age were able to distinguish between English (familiar) and French (unfamiliar) using a video (without auditory input) of an adult; however, by 8 months of age this ability was lost.

Infant Production

Developmental Summaries of Early Speech Production

Infants enter the world being able to vocalize through crying. Throughout the first months the repertoire of sounds increases. Two developmental summaries of early speech production will be presented: one based on the work by Oller and colleagues and the other based on the work by Stark and colleagues.

Stark's Typology of Infant Phonations. The *Stark Assessment of Early Vocal Development–Revised* is based on work by Stark and colleagues (Nathani, Ertmer, and Stark, 2006; Stark, Bernstein, and Demorest, 1983). This typology includes five levels of development of infant vocalizations (see Box 3.1). The first level comprises *reflexive* sounds, including *quasi-resonant nuclei (Q)*, defined as "faint low-pitched grunt-like sounds with muffled resonance" (Nathani et al., 2006, p. 367). Reflexive vocalizations are common between 0 and 6 weeks of age (Stark, Bernstein, and Demorest, 1983) and include fussing and crying. McGlaughlin and Grayson (2003) indicated that the mean amount of crying within a 24-hour period fell from 90 minutes when children were 1 to 3 months of age, to 60 to 65 minutes from 4 to 9 months of age, then back to 86 minutes from 10 to 12 months of age. However, McGlaughlin and Grayson reported that other studies show a decrease in crying after 10 months of age.

The second level of the *Stark Assessment of Early Vocal Development–Revised* is called *control of phonation*. During this level, *fully resonant nuclei (F)* occur and are defined as "vowel-like sounds . . . that have energy across a wide range of frequencies (not restricted to low frequencies like Q)" (*Q* refers to the quasi-resonant nuclei as defined above) (Nathani et al., 2006, p. 367). Additionally, *closants* (consonant-like segments such as a raspberry, click, or isolated consonant) and *vocants* (vowel-like segments) are produced during the second level. During the third level, *expansion,* infants produce isolated vowels, two or more vowels in a row, vowel glide combinations, ingressive sounds, squeals, and marginal babbling. Marginal babbling comprises a series of closant and vocant segments.

The fourth level, *basic canonical syllables*, occurs between 5 and 10 months of age. Infants during this level produce canonical babbling, single consonant-vowel syllables, whispered productions, disyllables (CVCV) and a consonant-vowel combination followed

■ **BOX 3.1**   Two typologies of infants' vocalizations

Typology 1: *Stark Assessment of Early Vocal Development–Revised* **(Nathani, Ertmer, and Stark, 2006)**

1. *Reflexive (0 to 2 months):* Vegetative sounds, sustained crying/fussing, quasi-resonant nuclei (Q) ("faint low-pitched grunt-like sounds with muffled resonance"(p. 367))
2. *Control of phonation (1 to 4 months):* Fully resonant nuclei (F), two or more Fs, closants (consonant-like segments: raspberry, click, isolated consonant), vocants (vowel-like segments), closant-vocant combinations, chuckles or sustained laughter
3. *Expansion (3 to 8 months):* Isolated vowels, two or more vowels in a row, vowel glide, ingressive sounds, squeals, marginal babbling
4. *Basic canonical syllables (5 to 10 months):* Single consonant-vowel syllable, canonical babbling, whispered productions, a consonant-vowel combination followed by a consonant (CV-C), disyllables (CVCV)
5. *Advanced forms (9 to 18 months):* Complex syllables (e.g., VC, CCV, CCVC), jargon, diphthongs

Typology 2: Oller's typology of infant phonations (Oller, 2000; Oller, Oller, and Badon, 2006)

1. Non-speech-like vocalizations
   a. *Vegetative sounds:* Burps, hiccups
   b. *Fixed vocal signals:* Crying, laughing, groaning
2. Speech-like vocalizations (protophones)
   a. *Quasi-vowels (0 to 2 months):* Vowel-like productions without shaping of the articulators
   b. *Primitive articulation stage (2 to 3 months):* Vowel-like productions produced by shaping the articulators
   c. *Expansion stage (3 to 6 months):* Marginal babbling comprising a consonant-like and a vowel-like sound
   d. *Canonical babbling (6+ months):* Well-formed syllables such as [baba]

---

by a consonant (CV-C). *Canonical babbling* is seen as an important stage in the transition from babbling to speech. Nathani and associates (2006) define canonical babbling as including both reduplicated babbling (e.g., [baba]) and nonreduplicated babbling (e.g., [badu]). It is important for SLPs to pay attention to infants' babbling, since late onset of canonical babbling may be a predictor of later speech sound disorders. For example, Oller, Eilers, Neal, and Schwartz (1999) found children who had late onset of canonical babbling had smaller production vocabularies at 1;6, 2;0, and 3;0 years of age.

The fifth and final level of the *Stark Assessment of Early Vocal Development–Revised* is titled *advanced forms*. This level typically occurs between 9 and 18 months of age. During this time the children produce complex syllables (e.g., VC, CCV, CCVC), jargon, and diphthongs. Nathani and colleagues (2006) considered the application of the *Stark Assessment of*

Early Vocal Development–Revised to 30 infants in a mixed cross-sectional and longitudinal design spanning five age ranges from 0 to 20 months of age. They found that as the children increased in age, speech-like utterances increased in frequency while non-speech-like utterances decreased in frequency. Productions typically associated with Levels 1 and 2 decreased with age, whereas productions associated with level 4 was rarely produced before 9 months of age. Level 5 vocalizations occurred only 10 percent from 0 to 15 months, but jumped to 20 percent by 16 to 20 months of age.

Oller's Typology of Infant Phonations.   Oller and colleagues (Oller, 2000; Oller, Oller, and Badon, 2006) indicated that infants' vocalizations can be classified into being non-speech-like and speech-like (see Box 3.1). Non-speech-like vocalizations include *vegetative sounds*, such as burps and hiccups, and *fixed vocal signals*, such as crying, laughing, and groaning. Speech-like vocalizations are then classified into four phases of development: quasi-vowels, primitive articulation stage, expansion stage, and canonical babbling. From 0 to 2 months of age, children phonate and produce quasi-vowels (vowel-like productions) and glottals (Oller et al., 1999). The phase between 2 and 3 months of age (the primitive articulation stage) (Oller et al., 1999) is where children begin to produce vowel-like sounds that are sometimes called gooing (Oller et al., 1999) or cooing (Stark et al., 1983). From 3 to 6 months of age (the expansion stage), children expand their repertoires, producing full vowels and raspberries (Oller et al., 1999). They also begin to produce syllable-like vocalizations (Stark et al., 1983) or marginal babbling (Oller et al., 1999). From 6 months of age onward, infants produce canonical babbling—that is, well-formed canonical syllables (e.g., [babababa]) (Oller et al., 1999).

Babbling and Speech

The developmental typologies mentioned earlier indicate that children's babble consists of a series of consonants and vowels. However, over the years there have been differing views on the importance of babbling to children's speech acquisition. Some time ago, Jakobson (1968, p. 24) described babbling as "purposeless egocentric soliloquy" and "biologically oriented 'tongue delirium,'" and contrasted babbling with the production of words in the following way: "In place of the phonetic abundance of babbling, the phonemic poverty of the first linguistic stages appear, a kind of deflation which transforms the so-called 'wild sounds' of the babbling period into entities of linguistic value" (p. 25). Jackobson's extreme views that babbling and speech are discontinuous have been opposed by more recent researchers. Indeed, most researchers now believe that there is continuity between babbling and early speech (Davis and MacNeilage, 1995; Storkel and Morrisette, 2002) and suggest that babbling and early words share consonants (such as /m, n, p, b, t, d/) and vowels.

There are differences between the babbling of children who are typically developing and those who have additional learning needs. For example, researchers compared the babbling of children who were hearing impaired compared with children who were typically developing (Oller and Eilers, 1988; Stoel-Gammon and Otomo, 1986). They found that babies who were hearing impaired babbled later, babbled less frequently, used fewer syllables, were more likely to use single syllables than repeated syllable combinations, and used a disproportionate number of glides and glottal sequences. The babbling of late talkers has also been found to be different from typically developing children. Stoel-Gammon (1989) indicated that less canonical babbling was produced by late talkers from 9 to 21 months than for typically developing children.

As children near their first birthdays, they utter their first words. These words are to be distinguished from babbling and from phonetically consistent forms (PCF). Owens (1994) suggested two indicators that designate production of true words:

1. The child's utterance must have a phonetic relationship to an adult word (i.e., it sounds somewhat similar).
2. The child must use the word consistently in the presence of a particular situation or object.

Therefore, if a child babbled "mama," but his or her mother was not present, then this would not qualify as a word, since there was no referent. Similarly, phonetically consistent forms that children consistently produce that do not have a relationship to an adult word (e.g., "taka" for *dog*) are not true words, as they do not meet the first indicator.

PHASE 2: TRANSITIONING FROM WORDS TO SPEECH

Children's First Fifty Words

Children's pronunciation in the first 50-word stage appears to be constrained by their physiology, ambient language, and child-specific factors (Vihman, 1992). There is much individual and phonetic variability during this stage (Grunwell, 1982). First words typically consist of one or sometimes two syllables and are of the following shapes: CV, VC, CVCV. Consonants produced at the front of the mouth predominate (e.g., /p, b, d, t, m, n/) (Robb and Bleile, 1994). Final consonants are typically omitted or followed by a vowel (e.g., *dog* may be produced as "do" or "doggy"). Young children also produce a limited repertoire of vowels. According to Donegan (2002), children favor low, nonrounded vowels during their first year and produce height differences in vowels before they produced front-back differences. Common phonological processes (or patterns) produced by young children include reduplication, final consonant deletion, and cluster reduction.

It has been suggested that young children use selection and avoidance strategies in the words they produce. Possible selection patterns are the size and complexity of syllables and the sound types included (Ferguson, 1978). Early words are thought to be learned as "whole word patterns." Homonyms are common in children's early words (e.g., "tap" for *tap, cap, clap*; "no" for *no, snow, nose*). Researchers suggest that children can approach homonyms in two ways: Sometimes they use homonyms to increase their lexicon, and at other times they appear to aim to limit the number of homonyms in order to be intelligible. As children mature, the number of homonyms decreases (McLeod, van Doorn, and Reed, 1998, 2001a).

Two different learning styles have been suggested for children learning to speak. Vihman and Greenlee (1987) conducted a comprehensive longitudinal study comparing the speech development of 10 typically developing children between 9 and 17 months, then examined them again at age 3. They reported wide individual variation, particularly for specific segment substitutions and cluster reductions. The researchers described two differing learning styles that were evident in their children at 1 year and remained at 3 years of age. They proposed a continuum of "tolerance for variability" on which they could place their children as being either "systematic (and stable)" or "exploratory (and variable)" (Vihman and Greenlee, 1987, p. 519). These two learning styles are reminiscent of the research into the learning styles used by young children in language acquisition (Bates, Dale, and Thal, 1995). Bates and associates described children with learning style 1 as being word oriented, having high intelligibility, a segmental emphasis, and consistent pronunciation across word tokens. In contrast, children with learning style 2 were described as intonation oriented, having low intelligibility, a suprasegmental emphasis, and variable pronunciation across word tokens.

Young Children's Consonant Inventories

Children's early consonant inventories have nasal, plosive, fricative, approximant, labial, and lingual phonemes (Grunwell, 1981). As children grow, the number of consonants in their inventories increases. In a large study of over 1,700 children, Ttofari-Eecen, Reilly, and Eadie (2007) reported that by age 1;0, children had an average of 4.4 consonants in their inventories (median = 4; range = 0–16) and typically these were /m, d, b, n/. Robb and Bleile (1994) conducted a longitudinal study of seven children, examining phonetic inventories from ages 0;8 to 2;1. The most frequent manner of articulation was stops and the most frequent places of articulation were toward the front of the mouth: labials and alveolars. Their findings, summarized in Table 3.1, demonstrate the broader range of consonants produced

■ **TABLE 3.1**   Summary of Studies of English-Speaking Children's Consonant Inventories

Age	Robb & Bleile (1994) Number of Syllable-Initial Consonants	Robb & Bleile (1994) Number of Syllable-Final Consonants	Ttofari-Eecen et al. (2007) Total Number of Consonants
0;8	5	3	
0;9	5	2	
0;10	6	4	
0;11	4	2	
1;0	5	2	4.4
1;1	6	2	
1;2	10	2	
1;3	6	2	
1;4	6	2	
1;5	9	3	
1;6	6	3	
1;7	11	6	
1;8	10	5	
1;9	9	4	
1;10	11	3	
1;11	12	5	
2;0	10	4	
2;1	15	11	

in syllable-initial compared with syllable-final position. For example, at 8 months of age, the children produced 5 syllable-initial consonants (typically /d, t, k, m, h/) and 3 syllable-final consonants (typically /t, m, h/). By age 2;1, children produced 15 syllable-initial consonants and 11 syllable-final consonants.

Phonological Knowledge and Vocabulary Acquisition

There appears to be a close relationship between young children's phonological knowledge and their acquisition of vocabulary (Storkel, 2006). According to Storkel, phonological knowledge can be defined in terms of three phonotactic constraints:

1. *Inventory constraints.* Inventory of sounds that are produced by the child
2. *Positional constraints.* Sounds that are produced in different syllable positions
3. *Sequence constraints.* Restrictions on the co-occurrence of sounds

During the first year of life, children learn words that are consistent with phonotactic constraints within their babbling. According to Locke (2002, p. 249), "The sounds babbled most frequently are produced more accurately by English-learning 2-year-olds, and appear more often in the languages of the world, than other sounds."

Sounds within a child's inventory are sometimes described as IN sounds, and those not used within their inventories are described as OUT sounds. Much research has been conducted on the perception and production of IN and OUT sounds for infants who have learned fewer than 50 words. These young children appear to have opposite preferences for perception and production. Infants tend to listen to OUT sounds longer than to IN sounds (Vihman and Nakai, 2003, cited in Storkel, 2006). However, when infants are taught to produce new words, they tend to learn words containing IN sounds more quickly than OUT sounds (Schwartz and Leonard, 1982). Storkel (2005, 2006) extended this work by considering the role of and IN and OUT sounds in word learning for preschool children beyond the 50-word stage. She found that these older children were more accurate in learning words containing OUT sounds than they were in learning words containing IN sounds. This finding held for both typically developing children and children with speech impairment, and was counter to the finding for the younger children in the first 50-word stage.

PHASE 3: THE GROWTH OF THE INVENTORY

This section discusses the third phase of speech acquisition and focuses on typical acquisition of aspects of speech sound production beyond approximately 2 to 5 years of age. Traditionally, many speech-language pathologists' understanding of typical speech sound acquisition has been informed by normative data on the age of acquisition of phonemes (e.g., Smit et al., 1990) and the age at which phonological processes disappear (e.g., Grunwell, 1981). These measures typically address the final product—that is, the age of mastery of certain phonemes and phonological processes. In addition to such data, however, many other data on typical speech sound acquisition are available and should be used in clinical decision making (see Appendix A). For example, data on the route of development include typical range of "errors" of phonemic, phonetic, and syllable inventories. This shift in emphasis to include both the end-point and the route of development equips SLPs with information to identify children with impaired speech at a younger age than we have historically been able to.

A comprehensive overview of typical speech sound acquisition includes many facets (see Box 3.2). Each of these areas will be described in detail and speech sound acquisition data will be summarized according to children's ages (also see Appendix A). Additionally, under each heading in the next section, a table will highlight the findings from the available research studies. Data from a range of studies are presented in the columns to enable you to compare findings and encourage consideration of diversity and individuality across studies and children. Appendix A presents the available acquisition data in a different way. It is organized according to children's ages to reflect the typical developmental sequence. However, rates of development vary among typically developing children. Where possible, data from more than one study are presented for each category at each age to allow for comparison and to encourage consideration of diversity and individuality.

Intelligibility

Intelligibility has been described as "the single most practical measurement of oral communication competence" (Metz, Samar, Schiavetti, Sitler, and Whitehead, 1985, cited in Gordon-Brannan, 1994, p. 17). A speaker's intelligibility can be affected by articulatory, phonological, suprasegmental, and other linguistic features. For example, Vihman (1988) indicated that at 3 years of age, children who used more complex sentences were more difficult to understand. Additionally, intelligibility is affected by the speaker's relationship with the listener; for example, there are differences according to whether the listener is the child's parent, a stranger, or a person trained in phonetic transcription (e.g., see Flipsen, 1995).

Kent, Miolo, and Bloedel (1994) provide a comprehensive review of procedures for the evaluation of intelligibility, including a range of commercially available instruments. Recently, Flipsen (2006b) discussed several variations of the Intelligibility Index (II)

■ **BOX 3.2**   Components of a comprehensive overview of typical speech acquisition

---

1. Intelligibility
2. Comparison of the child's speech sounds with the adult target
   a. *Acquired sounds:* Consonants, consonant clusters, vowels
   b. *Percent correct (percent error):* Consonants, consonant clusters, vowels
   c. *Common mismatches:* Consonants, consonant clusters, vowels
   d. Phonological patterns/processes
3. Abilities of the child (without comparison to the adult target)
   a. *Phonetic inventory:* Consonants, consonant clusters, vowels
   b. *Syllable structure*
4. Prosody
5. Metalinguistic/phonological awareness skills

(Shriberg, Austin, Lewis, McSweeny, and Wilson, 1997a). The Intelligibility Index is "the percentage of words in the entire sample that the transcriber could reliably understand" (Flipsen, 2006b, p. 306). Flipsen reported data from 320 children ages 3;1 to 8;0 and found gradual increases across this age range (see Table 3.2).

The results of several studies of children's intelligibility, summarized in Table 3.2, demonstrate that, as children grow older, the percentage of intelligible words increases. The extent of intelligibility is also influenced by the children's relationship with the person to whom they are speaking. The largest study of 2-year-olds' intelligibility was conducted by Roulstone, Loader, Northstone, Beveridge, and the ALSPAC team (2002). As a result of their study of 1,127 children who were 25 months of age, they reported that "children were mostly intelligible to their *parents* with 12.7% parents finding their child difficult to understand and only 2.1% of parents reporting that they could rarely understand their child" (p. 264). In contrast, studies that considered children's intelligibility to *strangers* demonstrated that 2-year-old

TABLE 3.2 Summary of Studies of English-Speaking Children's Intelligibility

Age	Roulstone et al. (2002)	Weiss (1982)	Coplan & Gleason (1988)	Vihman (1988)	Gordon-Brannan, (1993, cited in Gordon-Brannan, 1994)	Flipsen (2006b)
	Intelligibility to the children's parents	Intelligibility	Parental estimates of intelligibility to strangers	Intelligibility judged by three unfamiliar listeners	Intelligibility in conversational speech with unfamiliar listeners	Percent of words that could be reliably understood by the transcriber*
2;0	87.3%	26–50%	50% (22 months)			
2;6		51–70%				
3;0		71–80%	75% (37 months)	73% (50–80%)		95.68% (88.89 − 100.00)
4;0			100% (48 months)		93% (73–100%)	96.82% (88.42 − 100.00)
5;0					Intelligible	98.05% (89.84 − 100.00)
6;0						98.43% (91.67 − 100.00)
7;0						99.51% (97.36 − 100.00)
8;0						99.01% (97.07 − 100.00

* = Intelligibility index − original (for more details, see Flipsen, 2006b).

children's speech was 50 percent intelligible to strangers (Coplan and Gleason, 1988; Vihman, 1988), and by 3 years of age, children's speech was around 75 percent intelligible to strangers (Coplan and Gleason, 1988; Vihman, 1988). Whereas at 3 years of age 95 percent of words could be reliably understood by a *transcriber* (Flipsen, 2006b), Bernthal and Bankson (1998, p. 272) concluded that "a client 3 years of age or older who is unintelligible is a candidate for treatment and intelligibility expectations increase with age." Between 4 and 5 years of age, children's speech is considered to be intelligible.

Age of Acquisition of Speech Sounds

One of the major techniques for considering speech sound acquisition has been to compare children's development with the adult target. *Age of acquisition* refers to the age at which a certain percentage of children have acquired a speech sound. Large-group cross-sectional studies have predominantly been used for this purpose. Consonants have been the primary focus of these studies; however, there are some studies that have examined consonant clusters and vowels. Age-of-acquisition data have had a long history of credence within the SLP profession. Well-known U.S. studies include those by Templin (1957) and, more recently, Smit, Hand, Frelinger, Bernthal, and Bird (1990). However, studies examining age of acquisition of speech sounds have been published for other English dialects and many languages around the world, including Arabic, Cantonese, Dutch, Finnish, German, Greek, Hungarian, Israeli Hebrew, Japanese, Korean, Maltese, Norwegian, Portuguese, Putonghua, Spanish, Thai, Turkish, and Welsh (see McLeod, 2007a).

When considering the age-of-acquisition findings for consonants, consonant clusters, and vowels, it is important to remember the methodological constraints of these data. The samples in these studies have been elicited from single words (not conversation) and often only one word has been elicited for each speech sound in each word position. Thus, the samples may not be fully representative of typical speaking situations, and variability in production has not been considered. Some studies have scored productions as either correct or incorrect and have not considered phonological development (hence, readers also need to consider additional data such as phonological processes, mismatches, etc.).

Another issue with these studies is that they vary in terms of the criterion for determining age of acquisition. For example, Templin (1957) indicated that a sound had to be acquired in the initial-, medial-, and final-word positions, whereas others have used only initial- and final-word positions (e.g., Prather et al., 1975; Smit et al., 1990). In addition, a range of standards (e.g., 50 percent, 75 percent, 90 percent, and 100 percent) have been used as criteria for age of acquisition. Tables 3.3 to 3.5 provide the criterion adopted by each researcher. In 1972, Sander emphasized the importance of presenting age-of-acquisition data using a continuum, rather than a definite age at which phonemes are acquired. Consequently, a number of more recent authors (e.g., Smit et al., 1990) have adopted this approach and have presented graphical displays of acquisition for each speech sound over the different ages.

Consonants

Table 3.3 (pages 96–97) provides a summary of studies of English-speaking children's age of acquisition of consonants. It includes studies of English dialects as spoken in the United States, England, Scotland, and Australia. As demonstrated by Table 3.3, the majority of

English consonants are acquired by the age of 3 to 4 years. As Porter and Hodson (2001, p. 165) indicated, "3-year-olds had acquired all major phoneme classes, except liquids . . . sibilant lisps were still common until the age of 7 years." However, the findings in Table 3.3 suggest that acquisition of all singleton consonants in English does not conclude until 8 or 9 years of age. It should be noted as well that in each study the youngest and oldest age of acquisition is affected by the age range that has been studied. For example, only three studies included in Table 3.3 assessed the speech of children who were 2 years old (Chirlian and Sharpley, 1982; Prather et al., 1975; Paynter and Petty, 1971); thus, it could be that children acquire some sounds even earlier, as evidenced by studies of languages other than English (e.g., Cantonese) (So and Dodd, 1995).

Looking at Table 3.3, notice the differences in the age of acquisition of consonants provided from these studies. Dodd, Holm, et al. (2003), for example, reported a greater number of consonants acquired by age 3;0 than most of the other studies. This finding was probably influenced by their inclusion of children's spontaneous *and imitated* productions of speech sounds in defining age-appropriate production, whereas many other studies have been based only on spontaneous productions. The age of acquisition for the fricatives /s/ and /z/ appears to vary more than any other speech sounds. For example, some authors suggest that /z/ is acquired at age 3 years (Dodd, Holm, et al., 2003), others at 4 years (Arlt and Goodban, 1976), others at 5 years (Kilminster and Laird, 1978; Anthony et al., 1971; Smit et al., 1990 [females]), others at 6 years (Smit et al., 1990 [males]), others at 7 years (Templin, 1957), and others after 9 years (Chirlian and Sharpley, 1982). Similarly, the age range for the acquisition of /s/ extends from age 3 (Dodd, Holm, et al., 2003; Prather et al., 1975) to age 7 (Poole, 1934). There are three possible reasons for the variability in the age of acquisition of /s/ and /z/. The first concerns whether children were included who had lost their central incisor teeth but had not yet acquired their adult dentition. Such an absence might well affect their ability to produce a fully correct /s/. The second possibility concerns differences in the definition of an adult-like /s/, particularly whether dentalized /s/ sounds are considered to be correct (Smit et al., 1990). The final possibility relates to the methodology employed within the studies, including the complexity of the words elicited and the criterion for acquisition.

Another approach to the consideration of the age of acquisition is that taken by Shriberg (1993), who created a "profile of consonant mastery" based on the average percent correct in continuous conversational speech. Using data from 64 children with speech delays, ages 3 to 6 years, Shriberg suggested that there were three stages of phoneme acquisition:

1. Early 8 [m, b, j, n, w, d, p, h]
2. Middle 8 [t, ŋ, k, g, f, v, tʃ, dʒ]
3. Late 8 [ʃ, θ, s, z, ð, l, r, ʒ]

Shriberg (1993) tested the validity of these three stages against four studies of speech sound acquisition (see Shriberg, 1993, table 8): Sander (1972), Prather and colleagues (1975), Hoffmann (1982) (articulation and connected speech samples), and Smit and colleagues (1990). He reported that there were a number of differences between studies of typical development and his speech-delay data. For example, in the comparison with the Sander (1972) data, 15 of the 24 consonant ranks fell within their assumed groups on the consonant mastery

■ **TABLE 3.3** Summary of Studies of English-Speaking Children's Age of Acquisition of Consonants

	Dodd, Holm, et al. (2003)	Smit et al. (1990) (females)	Smit et al. (1990) (males)	Chirlian & Sharpley (1982)	Kilminster & Laird (1978)	Arlt & Goodban (1976)	Prather et al. (1975)	Paynter and Petty (1974)	Anthony et al. (1971)	Templin (1957)
Age range tested	3;0–6;11	3;0–9;0	3;0–9;0	2;0–9;0	3;0–9;0	3;0–6;0	2;0–4;0	2;0–2;6	3;0–6;0	3;0–8;0
Criterion	90%	75%	75%	75%	75%	75%	75%	90%	90%	75%
Country	England & Australia	USA	USA	Australia	Australia	USA	USA	USA	Scotland	USA
2;0				m, n, h			m, n, ŋ, h, p	h, w		
2;4							j, d, k, f			
2;6				p, ŋ, w, d, g				p, b, t, m		
2;8							w, b, t			
3;0	p, b, t, d, k, g, m, n, ŋ, f, s, z, h, w, l, j	m, n, h, w, p, b, t, d, k, ŋ, f, s*	m, n, h, w, p, b, t, d, k, g	j, k, f, ʃ,	p, b, m, n, ŋ, h, w, j, t, d, k, g, ʒ*	p, b, t, d, k, g, m, n, ŋ, h, f, w	g, s		p, b, m, t, d, n, w, j	m, n, ŋ, p, f, h, w
3;4							l, r			
3;6		j	f, j	b, t, tʃ, dʒ	f	v			k, g, ŋ, f, j, v, h	
3;8							ʃ, tʃ			
4;0	ʒ, dʒ	v, ð, ʃ, tʃ	dʒ	l, ʒ, s	l, ʃ, tʃ,	s, z, ʒ, tʃ, dʒ, l	ð, ʒ			k, b, d, g, r

■ **TABLE 3.3** *(Continued)*

	Dodd, Holm, et al. (2003)	Smit et al. (1990) (females)	Smit et al. (1990) (males)	Chirlian & Sharpley (1982)	Kilminster & Laird (1978)	Prather et al. (1975)	Arlt & Goodban (1976)	Paynter and Petty (1974)	Anthony et al. (1971)	Templin (1957)
Age range tested	3;0–6;11	3;0–9;0	3;0–9;0	2;0–9;0	3;0–9;0	2;0–4;0	3;0–6;0	2;0–2;6	3;0–6;0	3;0–8;0
Criterion	90%	75%	75%	75%	75%	75%	75%	90%	90%	75%
Country	England & Australia	USA	USA	Australia	Australia	USA	USA	USA	Scotland	USA
4;6	ʃ	dʒ, l*	v	r,	dʒ, s*, z*	v, θ, z	ʃ		l	s, ʃ, tʃ
5;0		z*	s*, ʃ, tʃ		r	dʒ	θ, ð, r			
5;6		ŋ, θ,	ð, r						s, z, ʃ, ʒ	
6;0	r	r	ŋ, θ, z, l		v					t, θ, v, l
6;6	θ, ð								θ, ð, tʃ	
7;0	θ, ð								dʒ, r	ð, z, ʒ, dʒ
7;6				ð, θ						
8;0					ð					
8;6				v	θ					
9;0										
9;0+				z						
Not tested					j					

* = Reversal occurs at a later age group.

profile. However, overall Shriberg (1993, p. 122) concluded, "Thus, as a cross-sectional esti-mate of the rank-order of consonant mastery in speech-delayed children, the reference con-sonant mastery profile agrees quite well with estimates of the developmental order of consonant acquisition." Recently, Shriberg has begun referring to the preceding three group-ings as "developmental sound classes." Shriberg's profile of consonant mastery has received a large amount of attention within the SLP profession (e.g., Bleile, 2006), but it should be remembered that its basis is the mastery of phonemes by children with speech delays.

Consonant Clusters

The age of acquisition of consonant clusters for English-speaking children is summarized in Table 3.4, which includes three comprehensive studies (Anthony et al., 1971; Smit et al., 1990; Templin, 1957) and one more narrowly focused study that considered the acquisition of three /s/ clusters (Higgs, 1968). Data on the acquisition of consonant clusters also has been presented by Olmsted (1971); however, his data were not included as the definition of initial and final positions related to the sentence rather than a word. An extensive literature review of the acquisition of consonant clusters was presented by McLeod, van Doorn, and Reed (2001a) (see Box 3.3). McLeod and associates indicated that 2-year-olds are able to produce at least some consonant clusters correctly; however, complete mastery may take until 9 years of age. Typically, two-element consonant clusters (e.g., /sp, st, sk/) are mas-tered before three-element consonant clusters (e.g., /spr, str, skr/). Clusters containing frica-tives (e.g., /fl/) usually are more difficult than clusters containing stops (e.g., /kl/). To date, Templin (1957) and Anthony and associates (1971) are the only researchers to study the acquisition of word-final consonant clusters in English (see Table 3.4). It is important to consider the influence of morphological structures on the acquisition of word-final conso-nant clusters. For example, Templin reported that /kt/ was acquired at 8 years of age; how-ever, this consonant cluster occurs both in monomorphemic contexts such as *act* and morphophonemic contexts such as *lacked* created by the past tense morpheme. It is possi-ble that morphophonemic clusters may be acquired later due to their complexity.

Vowels

The description of the age of acquisition of vowels has received much less attention than that for consonants. One reason for this is that vowels are influenced by the accent or dialect spoken by the child. For example, in General American English there are either 18 or 19 vowels (depending on whether /ɔ/ is included) and 3 or 4 diphthongs (depend-ing on whether /ju/ is included) (Smit, 2007). In contrast, there are 12 vowels and 8 diphthongs in English spoken in England (Howard, 2007), Australia (McLeod, 2007b), and New Zealand (Maclagan and Gillon, 2007), although there are differences between the exact vowels produced in each dialect. There are only 10 vowels and 3 diphthongs in Scottish English (Scobbie, Gordeeva, and Matthews, 2007). Howard and Heselwood (2002) provide a discussion of the sociophonetic variation between vowel productions for speakers of different dialects.

There are two aspects of acquisition of vowels: paradigmatic and syntagmatic acqui-sition (James, van Doorn, and McLeod, 2001). The *paradigmatic* aspect to mastering vowel production refers to learning to produce vowel in isolation or in simple monosyllabic words. Children attempt the paradigmatic aspects of vowel production at a very young age.

■ **TABLE 3.4** Summary of Studies of English-Speaking Children's Age of Acquisition of Consonant Clusters

	Smit et al. (1990)	Smit et al. (1990)	Templin (1957)	Higgs (1968)	Anthony et al. (1971)	Templin (1957)	Anthony et al. (1971)
Age range tested	3;0–9;0 (females)	3;0–9;0 (males)	3;0–8;0	2;6–5;	3;0–5;	3;0–8;	3;0–5;6
Criterion	90%	75%	75%	75%	75%	75%	75%
Word position	Word-initial	Word-initial	Word-initial	Word-initial	Word-initial	Word-final	Word-final
3;0						ŋk	nt
3;6	tw, kw	tw, kw				rk, ks, mp, pt, rm, mr, nr, pr, kr, br, dr, gr, sm	
4;0	pl, bl, kl		pl, pr, tr, tw, kl, kr, kw, bl, br, dr, gl, sk, sm, sn, sp, st		kw	lp, rt, ft, lt, fr	
4;6	sp, st, sk, sw*, gl, fl, kr*, skw*	gl	gr, fr	sp, st, sk	kr, fl	lf	
5;0		sp, st, sn*, bl, dr*	fl, str		gl*, tr, kl, br	rp, lb, rd, rf, rn, ʃr, mbr	
5;6	sm, sn	pl, kl, fl, pr, tr, kr, gr, fr			sl		dz, mps, ŋgz
6;0	sl, pr, br, tr, dr, gr, fr, spl	sk, sw, br	skw		θr, sm, st, str, sp	lk, rb, rg, rθ, nt, nd, ðr, pl, kl, bl, gl, fl, sl, str, rst, ŋkl, ŋgl, rdʒ, ntθ, rtʃ	sk
7;0	θr	sm, sl, θr, skw, spl,	θr, ʃr, sl, sw, skr, spl, spr			lz, zm, tθ, sk, st, skr, kst, dʒd	
8;0	spr, str, skr	spr, str, skr				kt, tr, sp	
>8;0						lfθ tl	

*A reversal occurs in older age groups.

■ **BOX 3.3** Typical acquisition of consonant clusters

Observations of the following phenomena may indicate typical development of consonant clusters in children:

1. Two-year-old children can produce consonant clusters, but these clusters may not be of the same form as the ambient language.

2. Word-final consonant clusters generally appear in inventories earlier than word-initial clusters. Children's production of word-final consonant clusters is increased by the emergence of grammatical morphemes (e.g., plurals and past tense) and consequently the creation of morphophonological consonant clusters (e.g., [-ts] as in *cats*).

3. Two-element consonant clusters are generally produced and mastered earlier than three-element clusters. There is inconclusive evidence regarding whether phonemes are mastered in singleton contexts before they can be accurately produced in clustered contexts.

4. Consonant clusters containing stops (e.g., /pl/, /kw/) are acquired generally before consonant clusters containing fricatives (e.g., /st/, /θr/).

5. Young children typically delete one element of a consonant cluster (cluster reduction), and this deletion may be explained by principles of markedness and sonority.

6. Homonymy occurs in young children's attempts to produce consonant clusters. Homonymy frequently occurs as a result of cluster reduction; however, homonyms can also occur as a result of cluster creation.

7. There are a number of other non-adult realizations of consonant clusters; the most common is cluster simplification, with others including epenthesis and coalescence. Metathesis is rare.

8. The acquisition of consonant clusters is gradual, and there is a typical developmental sequence. It is not an all-or-nothing process. For word-initial clusters, children may initially delete a member of a consonant cluster (one-element realization), then preserve the members while producing one in a non-adult manner (two-element realization), and finally they will produce the consonant cluster correctly (correct realization). Other developmental sequences are possible, particularly for word-final consonant clusters.

9. There is an interrelationship between cluster reduction, cluster simplification, and correct productions of consonant clusters. Initially, most children reduce consonant clusters. Over time, the occurrence of cluster reduction diminishes, whereas the occurrence of cluster simplification increases. Simultaneously, the occurrence of correct productions increases, until eventually production is mastered.

10. Despite there being a typical developmental sequence, the acquisition of consonant clusters is marked by reversals and revisions with considerable individual variation.

Source: McLeod, van Doorn, and Reed (2001a), p. 107.

In the first year, low, nonrounded vowels are favored, and height differences appear before front-back vowel differences (Donegan, 2002). Otomo and Stoel-Gammon (1992) conducted a longitudinal study of six children's acquisition of the unrounded vowels between 22 and 30 months of age and found that /ɪ/ and /ɛ/ were mastered early, then /e/ and /æ/;

whereas /ɪ/ and /ɛ/ were least accurate. Children master the paradigmatic aspects of vowels by the age of 3 (Donegan, 2002; Selby, Robb, and Gilbert, 2000; Vihman, 1992) or 4 years (Dodd, Holm, et al., 2003). Statements such as the following are plentiful throughout the literature on typical speech acquisition:

- ■ "By the age of 3 years, all normal children have evolved a stabilized vowel system" (Anthony et al., 1971, p. 12).
- ■ "The literature on vowel development suggests that vowels are acquired early, both in production and perception. There is considerable variability in their production, but most studies suggest that vowel production is reasonably accurate by age 3, although some studies call this into question" (Donegan, 2002, p. 12).

However, these comments refer to the mastery of vowels in a paradigmatic context.

The second aspect of acquisition of vowels is called the *syntagmatic* acquisition (James et al., 2001). This refers to the ability to produce sequences of vowels within syllables and words in conjunction with other phonological variables such as stress. Knowledge of the syntagmatic aspect of vowel production is particularly apparent in the ability to produce schwa correctly in polysyllabic words. According to James and colleagues (2001), children acquire at least some of the syntagmatic aspects of vowels between 3 to 5 years of age; however, mastery of vowels in polysyllabic words and stressed syllables extends beyond 3 years of age (Allen and Hawkins, 1980; James et al., 2001; Selby, Robb, and Gilbert, 2000; Stoel-Gammon and Herrington, 1990). For example, Allen and Hawkins (1980) found that children mastered vowels in stressed syllables by 3 years of age but did not master vowels in unstressed syllables until they were 4 to 5 years old.

Percentage Sounds Correct/Percentage Sounds in Error

Consonants

Another index of speech sound acquisition is percentage of consonants correct (PCC), which considers the number of consonants produced correctly divided by the total number of consonants. Table 3.5 summarizes data from a range of studies detailing PCC at different ages. As can be seen, when children reach 2 years of age, it is typical for around 70 percent of their consonants to be produced correctly. For example, Watson and Scukanec (1997b) described longitudinal PCC data for 12 U.S. children. The mean PCC for the children at age 2;0 was 69.2 percent, and by age 3;0 it had climbed to 86.2 percent. As children grow older, their percentages of consonants correct increases. For example, Dodd, Holm, and associates (2003) found that children ages 5;6 to 6;6 produced 95.9 percent of consonants correctly.

Although Shriberg and Kwiatkowski's (1982a) original recommendations for computing PCC refers to connected speech samples, different sampling techniques have been applied to this metric. James and colleagues (2002) demonstrated that there are significant differences between PCC scores depending on the speech sampling task. Significantly higher PCCs were found for children's productions of monosyllabic versus polysyllabic words (see Table 3.5). The PCC will be discussed later in Chapter 5 as a data analysis procedure employed in speech sound assessment.

■ **TABLE 3.5**   Summary of Studies of English-Speaking Children's Percent of Consonants Correct (PCC)

	Pollock (2002)	Stoel-Gammon (1987)	Watson & Scukanec (1997b)	Dodd, Holm, Hua, & Crosbie (2003)	James, van Doorn, and McLeod (2002)	Waring, Fisher, & Atkin (2001)
1;6	53%					
2;0	70%	70%	69.2% (53–91)			
2;3			69.9% (51–91)			
2;6	81%		75.1% (61–94)			
2;9	92%		82.1% (63–96)			
3;0			86.2% (73–99)	82.11%	76.77% (MSW)	
3;6	93%				76.41% (PSW)	85.2%
4;0	93%			90.37%	83.97% (MSW)	88.5%
4;6	94%				82.45% (PSW)	
5;0	93%				89.54%(MSW)	93.4%
5;6	96%			95.86%	88.36% (PSW)	
6;0	97%				93.74% (MSW)	95.1%
6;6	93%				90.76% (PSW)	
7;0					93.93% (MSW)	98.4%
7;6					90.99% (PSW)	

MSW = monosyllabic words; PSW = polysyllabic words

Consonant Clusters

A few researchers have described children's percentage of consonant clusters correct at different ages (see Table 3.6). Roulstone and colleagues (2002) indicated that 1,127 children who were 25 months of age had an error rate of 78 percent (22 percent correct) for production of consonant clusters. In a longitudinal study of Australian 2-year-olds, McLeod, van Doorn, and Reed (2002) reported that overall 31.5 percent of consonant clusters were produced correctly in connected speech. Word-final consonant clusters (e.g., /nd/ in *hand*) were more likely to be correct (48.9 percent of the time), followed by word-initial fricative clusters (e.g., /sn/ in *snail*) (38.5 percent) and word-initial stop clusters (e.g., /bl/ in *blue*) (24.3 percent). Waring and colleagues (2001) presented cross-sectional data on Australian children's productions of consonant clusters in single words. They found that children ages 3;5 to 3;11 were able to produce 51 of a total of 59 (86 percent) consonant clusters correctly. By ages 7;0 to 7;11, most consonant clusters were produced correctly (58/59 to 98 percent).

Vowels

A summary of studies of the percentage of vowels produced correctly by children at different ages is provided in Table 3.7. Pollock and colleagues (Pollock and Berni, 2003; Pollock, 2002) have conducted the most extensive study of U.S. children's acquisition of

■ **TABLE 3.6**   Summary of Studies of English-Speaking Children's Percent of Consonant Clusters Correct (PCCC)

	Roulstone et al. (2002)	McLeod, van Doorn, & Reed (2002)	Waring, Fisher, & Atkin (2001)
2;0	22%*		
2;6		31.5%	
3;0			86.4%
3;6			
4;0			88.4%
4;6			
5;0			94.9%
5;6			
6;0			96.6%
6;6			
7;0			98.3%
7;6			

*Conversion from mean error rate of 78%.

■ **TABLE 3.7**   Summary of Studies of English-Speaking Children's Percent of Consonant Clusters Correct (PCCC)

	Pollock (2002)	Pollock and Berni (2003)	Dodd, Holm, et al. (2003)	James, van Doorn, & McLeod (2001)
	Rhotic	**Nonrhotic**	**Nonrhotic**	**Nonrhotic**
1;6	23.52%	82.19%		
2;0	37.54%	92.39%		
2;6	62.52%	93.90%		
3;0	79.24%	97.29%	97.39%	94.90% (MSW)
3;6	76.50%	97.19%		88.28% (PSW)
4;0	90.11%	98.06%	98.93%	95.20% (MSW)
4;6	86.80%	98.20%		92.08% (PSW)
5;0	88.21%	99.21%		94.80% (MSW)
5;6	80.31%	99.38%	99.19%	94.30% (PSW)
6;0	77.20%	98.5%		95.39% (MSW)
6;6		99.19%		94.86% (PSW)
7;0				95.10% (MSW)
7;6				95.44% (PSW)

MSW = monosyllabic words; PSW = polysyllabic words

rhotic (vowels with r-coloring such as ɝ) and nonrhotic vowels. They demonstrate that the nonrhotic vowels are more likely to be correct than rhotic vowels for a child of the same age. The studies by Dodd, Holm, et al. (2003) and James and associates (2001) were conducted on nonrhotic vowels since rhotic vowels are not present in English produced in England and Australia. The data from Australian and English children are similar to those from Pollock and Berni (2003) regarding nonrhotic vowels. James and associates (2001) indicated that the accuracy of vowel production decreased with an increase in the number of syllables in the word: There was greater accuracy for vowels in monosyllabic words compared with polysyllabic words.

Phonological Patterns/Processes

Phonological processes are defined by Bankson and Bernthal (1990b, p. 16) as "simplification of a sound class in which target sounds are systematically deleted and/or substituted." As mentioned in the section on natural phonology, the notion of systematicity was introduced to the field of linguistics by Stampe (1969) then adapted and called phonological processes by authors such as Ingram (1976). Since this time, many authors have provided differing lists of phonological processes. Table 3.8 provides a summary of definitions and examples of commonly occurring phonological processes. Recall, as mentioned earlier, that the term *pattern* is now more typically used than the term *process*.

In 1981, Grunwell presented a graphical display of the chronology of phonological processes that has been used widely as a means for identifying the age at which phonological processes are typically suppressed. Since this time a number of other researchers have presented the age of suppression of phonological processes (e.g., Bankson and Bernthal, 1990b; Dodd, 1995a; Haelsig and Madison, 1986; James, 2001; Roberts, Burchinal, and Footo, 1990; Pressier, Hodson, and Paden, 1988). A summary of these studies is presented in Table 3.9. Some of the findings from these studies indicate that the most prevalent processes for young children (18 to 29 months) were cluster reduction (e.g., *spoon* – [pun]) and liquid deviation (e.g., *leaf* – [wif]) (Pressier et al., 1988). According to Roberts and colleagues (1990) there was a marked decline in the usage of phonological processes between 2;6 and 4;0 years, with the most prevalent processes during these years being final consonant deletion, cluster reduction, fronting, stopping, and liquid gliding.

In 1999, James, McCormack, and Butcher presented data on 240 children's (ages 5; 0 to 7; 11) use of phonological processes. Among other findings, they reported four clusters of phonological process use, from those that were rarely present (cluster 1) to those that were present in a majority of possible occurrences (cluster 4):

Cluster 1.   Context sensitive voicing, early stopping, final consonant deletion, nasal assimilation

Cluster 2.   Later stopping, velar assimilation, velar fronting

Cluster 3.   Deaffrication and palatal fronting

Cluster 4.   Cluster reduction, cluster simplification, fricative simplification, liquid simplification, and liquid deletion

■ **TABLE 3.8** Definitions and Examples of Commonly Occurring Phonological Processes/Patterns

Overarching Description	Phonological Process	Definition	Example
Assimilation processes: When one sound in the word becomes similar to another sound in the word	Assimilation (consonant harmony)	One sound is replaced by another that is the same or similar to another sound within the word	*dod* instead of *dog*
Substitution processes: When one sound is substituted by another sound in a systematic fashion	Fronting	Velars are realized as sounds produced further forward in the oral cavity (typically alveolars)	*tar* instead of *car*
	Gliding	Liquids /l, r/ are replaced by a glide /w, j/ or another liquid	*wabbit* instead of *rabbit*
	Stopping	Fricatives and/or affricates are realized as stops	*tun* instead of *sun*
	Depalatization	Palatal sounds are realized as sounds produced further forward in the oral cavity (typically alveolars)	*fis* instead of *fish*
	Deaffrication	Affricates are realized as fricatives	*shursh* instead of *church*
Syllable structure processes: Phonological processes that affect the syllable structure	Final consonant deletion	Deletion of the final consonant in the word	*do* instead of *dog*
	Cluster simplification/ reduction	Deletion of one element of the cluster	*pane* instead of *plane*
	Weak syllable deletion	Deletion of the unstressed syllable	*nana* instead of *banana*

Source: Adapted from Bankson and Bernthal (1990 b), pp. 16–19.

James (2001) presented further data on the use of phonological processes by 365 children ages 2;0 to 7;11 years. She found that the major decline in the use of phonological processes was between the ages of 3 to 4 years. However, some processes had fluctuating distributions. For example, gliding declined by 50 percent or more between 2 and 3 years, then again between 4 and 5 years.

Common Mismatches

As well as the identification of the age at which children generally learn to produce sounds, it is useful to have data to describe the typical "errors," or mismatches, children make in their attempts to produce sounds. Phonological processes provide typical patterns

TABLE 3.9 A summary of Studies of Children's Use of Phonological Processes/Patterns

Age	Dodd, Holm, et al. (2003)	Grunwell (1981, 1987)	Preisser et al. (1988)	Watson & Scukanec (1997b)	Lowe, Knutson, & Monson (1985)	James (2001)	Haelsig & Madison (1986)
2;0		**Present:** Weak syllable deletion; final consonant deletion, cluster reduction, fronting of velars, stopping, gliding, context-sensitive voicing **Declining:** Reduplication, consonant harmony	**Most prevalent:** Cluster reduction, liquid deviations (gliding)	**Present:** Final consonant deletion, liquid simplification, later stopping, cluster reduction, vowelization			
2;6		**Present:** Weak syllable deletion; cluster reduction, fronting of velars, fronting of /ʃ/, stopping /v, θ, ð, tʃ, d, ʒ/, gliding, context-sensitive voicing **Declining:** Final consonant deletion			23% fronting	**Declining:** Affrication, depalatalization, gliding, meathesis, prevocalic voicing, vowel changes	

■ **TABLE 3.9** (*Continued*)

Age	Dodd, Holm, et al. (2003)	Grunwell (1981, 1987)	Preisser et al. (1988)	Watson & Scukanec (1997b)	Lowe, Knutson, & Monson (1985)	James (2001)	Haelsig & Madison (1986)
3;0	**Present:** Gliding, deaffrication, cluster reduction, fronting,* weak syllable deletion, stopping	**Present:** Weak syllable deletion; stopping /v, θ, ð/, fronting /ʃ, tʃ, dʒ/, gliding **Declining:** Cluster reduction		Later stopping, cluster simplification		**Declining:** Backing, cluster reduction, deaffrication, final consonant deletion, final devoicing, initial consonant deletion, labial assimilation, palatalization, stopping, unstressed syllable deletion, fricative simplification	Gliding of liquids, weak syllable deletion, glottal replacement, alveolar & labial assimilation, cluster reduction, stopping, vocalization, final consonant deletion
3;6	**Present:** Gliding, deaffrication, cluster reduction, fronting,** weak syllable deletion	**Present:** Stopping /θ, ð/					

■ **TABLE 3.9** *(Continued)*

Age	Dodd, Holm, et al. (2003)	Bankson & Bernthal (1990)	Grunwell (1981, 1987)	Preisser et al. (1988)	Watson & Scukanec (1997b)	Lowe, Knutson, & Monson (1985)	James (2001)	Haelsig & Madison (1986)
			Declining: Weak syllable deletion, cluster reduction, gliding					
4;0	**Present:** gliding, deaffrication, cluster reduction (3-element clusters)		**Present:** /θ/ → [ð], /ð/ → [d, v], depalatization of /ʃ, tʃ, dʒ/, gliding				**Declining:** Depalatalization, gliding, glottal replacement	**Declining:** Weak syllable deletion, vocalization, gliding of liquids (20% criterion)
			Declining: Cluster reduction					
4;6	**Present:** Gliding, deaffrication		**Declining:** stopping /θ, ð/, gliding /r/					
5;0	**Present:** Gliding		**Declining:** stopping /θ, ð/, gliding /r/				**Declining:** Deaffrication, epenthesis, metathesis, fricative simplification (v/ð)	
5;6	**Present:** Gliding							

* Voicing pattern not present at any age.

** Fronting of /k, g/ ended at age 3;11, whereas fronting of /ŋ/ continued until 5;0 in the word *fishing*.

of errors, but Smit (1993a, 1993b) has taken this further by presenting errors children make when attempting individual speech sounds. Smit reanalyzed the data from Smit and associates (1990) and provided many tables of data containing frequent to rare errors children make in their attempts to produce consonants (Smit, 1993a) and consonant clusters (Smit, 1993b) (for a summary, see Table 3.10). You are encouraged to consult Smit (1993a, 1993b) to make use of the exhaustive information provided therein. Anthony and associates (1971) also provided an analysis of the errors made by children in their Appendix B, but these were organized according to words rather than speech sounds.

■ **TABLE 3.10** Children's Common Errors in Producing Consonants and Consonant Clusters (Errors Occurred > 15%)

	Smit (1993a)	Smit (1993b)	Smit (1993b)
Age	Consonants	Two-element consonant clusters	Three-element consonant clusters
2;0	ŋ → n; j → Ø; l → w; r → w; v → b; θ → f; ð → d; s → dentalized* z → d; ʃ → s; tʃ → t/d; ʒ → d	pr → p, pw; br → b, bw; tr → t, tw; dr → d, dw; kr → k, kw; gr → g, gw; fr → f, fw; θr → f, θ w; sw → w; sm → m; sn → n; sp → p, b; st → t, d; sk → k	skw → k, t, kw, gw; spl → p, b, pl, pw; spr → p, pw, pr, sp; str → t, d, st, tw, sw; skr → k, w, kw, gw, fw
3;0	ŋ → n; r → w; v → b; θ → f; ð → d; s → dentalized	pr → pw; br → bw; tr → tw; dr → dw; kr → kw; gr → gw; fr → fw;	skw → θkw; spl → θpl, spw; spr → θpr, spw; str → θtr, stw; skr → θkr, skw

■ **TABLE 3.10**   *(Continued)*

Age	Smit (1993a) Consonants	Smit (1993b) Two-element consonant clusters	Smit (1993b) Three-element consonant clusters
		θr → fr; st → θt;	
4;0	θ → f; s → dentalized	pr → pw; br → bw; br → bw; tr → tw; dr → dw; kr → kw; gr → gw; fr → fw; θr → fr; st → θt	skw → θkw; spl → θpl, spw; spr → θpr, spw; str → θtr, stw; skr → θkr, skw;
5;0	Nil	pr → pw;	
5;6	Nil	br → bw; tr → tw; dr → dw; kr → kw; gr → gw	skw → θkw; spl → θpl, spw; spr → θpr, spw; str → θtr, stw; skr → θkr, skw
6;0	Nil	tr → tw	skw → θkw; spl → θpl; spr → θpr, spw; str → θtr, stw; skr → θkr, skw

* Smit (1993b) used dentalized (dnt); whereas /θ/ was used in the present table.

In Smit's analysis, two sounds warranted extra attention: /s/ and /r/. Smit (1993a) indicated that when the children were ages 2;0 and 2;6, they were more likely to produce word initial /s/ as [t] or [d]; however, for children from 3;0 to 9;0 years the most common error in the word-final context was dentalization. Lateralized [ş] productions were rare, which could be interpreted that SLPs should consider that lateral production of /s/ warrants intervention regardless of the child's age. Smit (1993a) also indicated that the most common error production for word-initial /r/ was [w]. Less commonly, children used derhotacized and labialized productions.

Perception

Earlier in this chapter we considered infants' perceptual capabilities. As children's speech develops, so does the link between their production and perceptual capabilities. This link was described in our consideration of the psycholinguistic models of speech acquisition. Although some authors believe that perception for speech is achieved in infancy, Rvachew (2007a, p. 28) suggests that there are three stages of development of "adult-like acoustic, phonological and articulatory representations" and that these stages are clinically relevant:

1. The child is unaware of the phonological contrast, and can produce realizations that are acoustically and perceptually similar.
2. The child is aware of the phonological contrast, and may produce acoustically different realizations that are not perceptible to adult listeners.
3. The child is aware of the phonological contrast, and can produce different realizations that are acoustically and perceptually accurate.

Rvachew (2007a) suggests that children's perceptual capabilities continue to develop into late childhood. For example, Hazan and Barrett (2000) found that children from 6 to 12 years of age showed increasing mastery in the ability to discriminate synthesized differences in place, manner, and voicing, but had not yet achieved adult-like accuracy.

Suprasegmentals/Prosody

Prosody refers to the suprasegmental aspects of speech production, including stress, intonation, and rhythm. Gerken and McGregor (1998) present a helpful overview of prosody and its development in children, and Wells and Peppé (2003) provide a helpful overview of prosody in children with speech and language impairment. There appears to be a close interaction between suprasegmentals, "motherese," and early language development.

Intonation develops before stress. For example, Snow (1994) found that young children acquire skills that control intonation earlier than final-syllable timing skills. At 6 months of age, children use intonation, rhythm, and pausing in their speech (Crystal, 1986). By 1 to 2 years of age, children use intonation and stress to reduce homonyms and to differentiate between commands, requests, and calling (Dore, 1975).

Kehoe (1997) studied the ability of 18 children, ages 22, 28, and 34 months, to produce three- and four-syllable words. She found that there was a significantly greater number of stress errors in SwS words (S = strong, w = weak), and a tendency for greater number of stress errors in SwSw words. Stress errors were more frequent in imitated than spontaneous productions. She suggested that stress errors may be associated with articulatory and phonetic-control factors. Omission of unstressed and nonfinal syllables is common in young children, whereas stressed and final syllables are usually preserved (Kehoe, 2001; James, 2007). Gerken and McGregor (1998) suggest that children leave an "acoustic trace" of the omitted syllable; that is, although changes cannot be detected by the human ear, spectrographic analysis can reveal changes in factors such as voice onset time and vowel length.

PHASE 4: MASTERY OF SPEECH AND LITERACY

Our interest in speech acquisition leads us to literacy acquisition, with phonological awareness being a logical extension or especially relevant to those of us interested in speech sound acquisition and disorders. When children attend school, refinement of their speech production and perception skills continues until eventually they reach adult-like mastery. This refinement occurs in a number of domains, including prosody, phonotactics, and their production of speech segments. As illustrated in the tables of speech acquisition earlier in this chapter, studies show continued growth in skill until 8 to 9 years of age. A major area of attention during the school years is the development of literacy—specifically, reading and spelling. In the psycholinguistic model, discussed earlier in this chapter, authors such as Stackhouse and Wells (1993) closely link speech and literacy in input–storage–output pathways. Phonological awareness is a skill that is closely associated with speech and literacy.

Phonological Awareness

Phonological awareness is "the ability to reflect on and manipulate the structure of an utterance as distinct from its meaning" (Stackhouse and Wells, 1997, p. 53) and is essential for the development of reading and spelling (Gillon, 2004). Children's phonological awareness skills also affect their perception of salient auditory cues (Mayo, Scobbie, Hewlett, and Waters, 2003). Children with speech difficulties typically find phonological awareness tasks difficult. Severity and type of speech impairment has been suggested as a significant predictor of performance of phonological awareness tasks (Holm, Farrier, and Dodd, 2007; Leitão and Fletcher, 2004; Rvachew, 2007b; Stackhouse and Wells, 1997; Sutherland and Gillon, 2007). Phonological awareness skills (particularly phoneme isolation) were improved during a randomized controlled trial for children with speech impairment (Hesketh, Dima, and Nelson, 2007).

Phonological awareness includes rhyme knowledge, blending and segmentation, and manipulation of syllables, clusters, and phonemes. Although syllable segmentation and knowledge of nursery rhymes has been found to be a good predictor of literacy outcome, the best predictors are suggested to be phoneme segmentation and phoneme manipulation.

Rhyme Knowledge

Rhyme knowledge reflects an understanding of the constituents of a syllable; that is, a syllable is created with an onset + rime (see earlier discussion of nonlinear phonology). Words that rhyme differ in their onsets (e.g., *cat, mat, brat, splat*). There are three main rhyme knowledge tasks: rhyme judgment (*fan-van; fan-fin*), rhyme detection (*fan-van-pin*), and rhyme production (words that rhyme with *fan*).

Blending and Segmentation

During blending tasks children are presented with elements of a word and are asked to put them together to produce a word. Thus, an example of syllable blending is *com-put-er* = *computer* and an example of phoneme blending is *f-i-sh* = *fish*. Segmentation tasks are the reverse, where a child is asked to segment a word into either syllables or phonemes.

Manipulation

Manipulation of syllables, clusters, and phonemes requires children to respond to tasks such as the following: "Say *clap*, now say it again without the 'l'" = *cap*. The ability to manipulate syllables, clusters, and phonemes requires sophisticated understanding of onsets, rimes, and codas.

Acquisition of Phonological Awareness

Children's acquisition of phonological awareness is said to consist of three stages. Goswami and Bryant (1990) proposed that the three stages are (1) awareness of syllables and words, (2) awareness of onsets and rimes, and (3) awareness of phonemes. Carroll and associates (2003) conducted a longitudinal study of 67 preschool-aged children and assessed them at the following average ages: 3;10, 4;2, and 4;9 years. They recommended a revised series of stages: (1) early implicit large-segment sensitivity (associated with vocabulary knowledge), (2) sound similarity, and (3) explicit awareness of phonemes.

A number of researchers have considered English-speaking children's acquisition of phonological awareness skills and their results are summarized in Table 3.11. The results listed in this table demonstrate that children have emerging skills from 3 to 4 years of age. As Dodd and Gillon (2001, p. 142) reported, "The majority of 4-year-old children . . . will not exhibit phonological awareness other than syllable segmentation and the emergence of rhyme awareness." By 5 years of age the following skills are established: syllable segmentation, rhyme awareness, alliteration awareness, phoneme isolation, and letter knowledge. Phoneme segmentation is one of the latest skills to be established when children are 6 to 7 years old.

FACTORS INFLUENCING TYPICAL ACQUISITION OF SPEECH

Many factors influence typical acquisition of speech. The tables in this chapter clearly indicate that one of the major influences is the age of the child. As children mature, so does their accuracy of all aspects of speech production. However, within the literature there is discussion of other aspects that may influence speech acquisition. These include gender, socioeconomic status, and concomitant language development.

■ **TABLE 3.11** Summary of Studies of English-Speaking Children's Acquisition of Phonological Awareness

	Lonigan, Burgess, Anthony, & Barker (1998)	Burt, Holm, & Dodd (1999)	Dodd & Gillon (2001)	Gillon & Schwarz (2001)	Carroll, Snowling, Hulme, & Stevenson (2003)
	USA	UK	UK & Australia	New Zealand	UK
2;0	Wide variability; some children could perform above the level of chance on rhyme oddity detection, alliteration oddity detection, blending, and elision				
3;0			Emerging skills		Easiest to most difficult: 1. Rime matching 2. Syllable matching 3. Initial phoneme matching
4;0		Showed awareness of the concepts of syllable, onset, and rime, but not awareness of individual phonemes	Showed awareness of syllable segmentation and rhyme awareness	Easiest to most difficult: 1. Generating rhyming words 2. Phoneme blending 3. Phoneme segmentation	Easiest to most difficult: 1. Rime matching 2. Syllable matching 3. Initial phoneme matching
4;6					Easiest to most difficult:

■ **TABLE 3.11** *(Continued)*

	Lonigan, Burgess, Anthony, & Barker (1998)	Burt, Holm, & Dodd (1999)	Dodd & Gillon (2001)	Gillon & Schwarz (2001)	Carroll, Snowling, Hulme, & Stevenson (2003)
	USA	UK	UK & Australia	New Zealand	UK
					1. Rime matching
					2. Initial phoneme matching
					3. Phoneme completion
					4. Phoneme deletion
5;0	Syllable blending established for middle-income, but not lower-income, children		Established skills: syllable segmentation, rhyme awareness, alliteration awareness, phoneme isolation, letter knowledge		
5;6			Established skills: phoneme segmentation		
6;0			**Australia 6;0–6;5** Established skills: syllable segmentation, rhyme awareness, alliteration awareness, phoneme isolation **Australia 6;6–6;11** Established skills: phoneme segmentation		

■ **TABLE 3.11**   *(Continued)*

Lonigan, Burgess, Anthony, & Barker (1998)	Burt, Holm, & Dodd (1999)	Dodd & Gillon (2001)	Gillon & Schwarz (2001)	Carroll, Snowling, Hulme, & Stevenson (2003)
USA	UK	UK & Australia	New Zealand	UK
		UK 6;0–6;11		
		Established skills: syllable segmentation, rhyme awareness, alliteration awareness, phoneme isolation, letter knowledge, phoneme segmentation		

Gender

There is a range of differing evidence regarding the effect of gender on the age of acquisition of speech sounds. However, one generalization can be made: If a gender difference is reported, girls are found to acquire speech more quickly than boys. Kenney and Prather (1986) found that boys made significantly more speech sound errors than girls at ages 3;0, 3;6, 4;0, 4;6, and 5;0, but not at 2;6. Smit and colleagues (1990) reported that boys and girls had different ages of acquisition for 11 sounds, with significant differences between genders at ages 4;0, 4;6, and 6;0. All consonants except for /dʒ/ were acquired earlier by the girls. Dodd, Holm, et al. (2003) found no gender differences in speech acquisition for children ages 3;0 to 5;5; however, girls outperformed the boys at ages 5;6 to 6;11 in areas such as production of interdental fricatives and consonant clusters. Similarly, Poole (1934) indicated that girls acquired sounds earlier than boys after 5;6 years, whereas their development was similar at younger ages. In a study of the occurrence of phonological processes, McCormack and Knighton (1996) reported that boys age 2;6 had more final consonant deletion, weak syllable deletion, and cluster reduction than girls. In a study of phonological awareness, Gillon and Schwarz (2001) found that 6-year-old girls performed significantly better than boys. The suggestion that boys differ from girls in speech acquisition is consistent with the reports of a greater number of boys than girls being identified as having a speech impairment (Campbell et al., 2003; Law, Boyle, Harris, Harkness, and Nye, 1998; McKinnon, McLeod, and Reilly, 2007)

Socioeconomic Status

The effect of socioeconomic status (SES) on speech sound acquisition is not straightforward due to the range of different ways that SES can be measured (income, education, occupation, urban/suburban/rural, etc.) and the level of inference that is made about factors such as home language environment (Dodd, Holm, et al., 2003). In some large-scale studies, SES has not been found to affect age of acquisition of speech (Dodd, Holm, et al., 2003; Smit et al., 1990); however, in others, children from a high SES background performed better than those from a low SES background (Templin, 1957). Socioeconomic status background has been found to have a significant effect on the acquisition of phonological awareness skills, with children from mid to high SES backgrounds outperforming children from low SES backgrounds (Burt et al., 1999; Gillon and Schwarz, 2001; Lonigan et al., 1998). For example, Lonigan and associates (1998) found that at 5 years of age, 89 percent of children from a middle-income background performed above chance on syllable blending tasks, whereas only 27 percent of children from a lower-income background performed above chance on the same task.

Language Development

Speech and language acquisition are intimately connected during the early stages of language acquisition (Paul and Jennings, 1992; Roulstone et al., 2002; Stoel-Gammon, 1991). For example, Roulstone and colleagues (2002) reported an interrelationship between speech and language for 1,127 children age 25 months. Although these children were of the same age, they had differing levels of expressive language. The number of phonological errors decreased as the level of language increased. For instance, for the production of velar consonants, children at the single-word stage had 57 percent errors, children at the two-word utterance stage had 37 percent errors, and children at the three- to four-word utterance stage only had 24 percent errors. This pattern was repeated for fricatives (single-word, 61 percent; two-word, 48 percent; three- to four-word, 30 percent); liquids (75 percent, 66 percent, 51 percent, respectively); postvocalic consonants (48 percent, 33 percent, 15 percent, respectively); and consonant clusters (88 percent, 80 percent, 66 percent, respectively).

Smith, McGregor, and Demille (2006) also studied the interaction between language and speech for 2-year-old children. In their study they compared the phonological development in lexically precocious (advanced vocabulary) 2-year-olds with age-matched and language-matched (2 1/2-year-old) peers. They found that the phonological skills of the lexically precocious 2-year-olds were similar to the language-matched peers and superior to the age-matched peers, again supporting the correlation between speech and language learning in the early years.

Individual Variability

Within the literature, variability is generally used in two ways: variability between individuals and variability within individuals. First, we will examine *variability between individuals*—that is, variability in individuals' rates and/or sequences of development. Variability between individuals is also referred to as "individual differences" (e.g., Bleile, 1991; Ferguson and Farwell, 1975) and occurs when different children of the same age or stage of development have different realizations for speech sounds for the same words. Variability between individuals also describes differing rates of development, different patterns of consistency in repetitions of words, and different styles of learning. Most researchers agree that no two children follow identical paths to development. Progress beyond the first 50 words has been understood as a period of significant transition for children developing language. For example, Vihman and Greenlee (1987) studied 10 typically developing children at 1 and 3 years of age. Significant differences were reported between the children's rate of vocabulary acquisition, phonological maturity, and general approach to learning.

Alternatively, variability is sometimes used to describe differences *within individuals* (e.g., Barlow, 1996; Berg, 1995; Bernhardt and Stemberger, 1998; French, 1989; Leonard, Rowan, Morris, and Fey, 1982) and occurs in two different forms. First, variability occurs when a child has different realizations of a particular speech sound for different lexical items. For example, /s/ may be realized as [s] in *sea*, but [t] in *seat*. Second, variability occurs when a child has different realizations for multiple productions of the same lexical item. For example, a child with variable repeated productions of *sleep* may realize /sl/ as [sl] in [sli:], simplify /sl/ by substituting [sw] in [swip], reduce /sl/ to [s] in [sip], and omit /sl/ entirely in [ip]. Leonard and colleagues (1982) described some of the reasons for variable productions of words: "Variable words are most often those which have more advanced canonical forms or sounds" and "Word shape as well as consonant composition may play a role in intra-word variability" (p. 56).

There are numerous examples of variability within the production of speech sounds by typically developing children. Ferguson and Farewell (1975) described a child who was age 1;3 who produced the word *pen* in 10 different ways. Vogel Sosa and Stoel-Gammon (2006) conducted a longitudinal study of four typically developing children between 1 and 2 years of age. They found high overall variability, as well as a peak in variability that corresponded to the onset of combinatorial speech. Stoel-Gammon (2004) conducted a longitudinal study and considered the speech of five children ages 21 to 33 months and found high rates of variability, even in CVC words. Dyson and Paden (1983) conducted a longitudinal study over a 7-month period to consider phonological acquisition strategies used by 2-year-olds. Comparisons of each child's productions of target words across time led them to comment, "This period of roughly two to three-and-one-half years of age seems to be one of extreme variability with subjects 'trying out' a variety of strategies to approximate the adult model" (Dyson and Paden, 1983, p. 16). Menn and Stoel-Gammon (1995, pp. 340–341) indicated that early words are "extremely variable in pronunciation." Similarly, in a longitudinal study of typically developing 2- to 3-year old children, McLeod and Hewett (in press) examined variability in the production of words containing consonant clusters produced in spontaneous speech. Half (53.7 percent, range = 42.4 to 77.6 percent) of all repeated words were produced variably. As the children reached age 3, they increased the accuracy and decreased the variability of their productions; however, variability between and within individuals continued to occur. Holm, Crosbie, and Dodd (2007) considered the variability of the speech of 405 typically developing children ages 3;0 and 6;11 on a single-word task that contained many polysyllabic words. The younger children demonstrated the highest levels of variability (13 percent) and their variable productions predominantly reflected maturational influences.

As will be noted in later chapters, variability has been considered a diagnostic marker of speech impairment (see, for example, the discussion in Chapter 4 on "Childhood Apraxia of Speech"; also see Holm et al., 2007). However, the presence of high degrees of variability in typically developing children's speech should be taken into account (Stoel-Gammon, 2007). If the speech of typically developing children is highly variable, then the extent and nature of variability must be defined when it is used as a diagnostic marker of speech impairment (McLeod and Hewett, in press). From the studies examined here, there is variability between children in the acquisition of speech. Additionally, there is variability within the speech of individuals. Variability within individuals is more likely to occur with younger children and in spontaneous speech contexts.

CONCLUSION: UNDERSTANDING AND APPLYING TYPICAL SPEECH ACQUISITION

As speech-language pathologists, we use information on typical speech acquisition as the foundation of our clinical decision making. Thomas (2000) suggests that there are two ways of understanding normal speech acquisition: knowledge of statistical similarity (typical acquisition) and understanding of attitudes and desirability within the child's context (acceptable acquisition). The majority of this chapter has examined the literature on typical speech acquisition and has described ages of attainment of a wide range of measures. These tables will be useful as a resource in your SLP practice. However, you are also encouraged to think as an anthropologist within the communities that you are working to understand notions of acceptability within the child's context. Chapter 8 will discuss this issue in more detail.

QUESTIONS FOR CHAPTER 3

1. Describe how the following models of speech acquisition add to our overall picture of how children acquire speech: behaviorism, generative phonology, natural phonology, nonlinear phonology, sonority, optimality theory, and psycholinguistic theory.

2. Describe the advantages and disadvantages of the three major research methods employed to examine speech acquisition.

3. Delineate the stages of infant vocal production from birth to age 1.

4. How do perception and production interact in infants?

5. Describe the characteristics and accomplishments of the transition stage of speech acquisition.

6. Review the large-scale normative data for English and identify early, mid, and late developing sounds.

7. What are phonological patterns/processes? Describe young children's use of phonological patterns.

8. How would a child at age 2 years and 5 years with typical speech say *cheese, hat, spoon, caterpillar, running,* and *three*? To answer this question consider:

   a. What phonemes are in the words? When are they normally mastered?

   b. Which word position are they in?

   c. What syllable shapes are represented? Would a child of this age typically produce these syllable shapes?

   d. What phonological patterns normally operate at this age?

   e. What are normal mismatches for a child of this age?

9. What is the importance of the acquisition of phonological awareness in school-age children?

10. How are children similar and different in speech acquisition?

Classification and Factors Related to Speech Sound Disorders

PETER FLIPSEN JR.
Idaho State University

NICHOLAS W. BANKSON
James Madison University

JOHN E. BERNTHAL
University of Nebraska–Lincoln

In Chapter 1 we defined in a broad sense what we mean by speech sound disorders. On examination of all the variations of these problems that are seen in children, speech-language pathologists wonder if there is some way to classify various types of disorders. Knowledge in this regard is still limited enough that in 2003 the U.S. National Institutes of Health issued a call for research proposals to study the classification of speech sound disorders in children. Some progress has been made on this issue, and in this chapter an attempt will be made to outline research in this area. Following that, we will also explore some of the factors that have been potentially linked to the presence of and/or nature of speech sound disorders.

Relative to classification, for many years speech-language pathologists have divided the population of children with speech sound disorders into two relatively large groups. The first, often referred to as the *organically based disorders,* includes those children whose difficulty with speech sounds can be readily linked to an obvious etiology or cause. This group includes subgroups based on specific causes. The second large group is those for whom *there is no obvious cause.* This latter group has been much more elusive and more difficult to understand. It has gone by many names over the years, including *functional articulation disorders, developmental phonological disorders, idiopathic speech sound disorders,* and *speech delay of unknown origin.*

▨ ORGANICALLY BASED SPEECH SOUND DISORDERS

The following discussion is not meant to be all-inclusive. The groups discussed are meant only to be a representative sample of organically based speech sound disorders. The information is also not intended as an exhaustive coverage of any of the particular groups that are identified. Entire textbooks have been devoted to discussions of the assessment and treatment of the speech sound problems experienced by some of these populations (e.g., Bzoch, 2004).

Major Structural Variations of the Speech Mechanism

Speech-language pathologists should recognize that significant anomalies of the oral structures are frequently associated with specific speech problems. Oral structural anomalies may be congenital (present from birth) or acquired. Cleft lip and/or palate is perhaps the most common congenital anomaly of the orofacial complex. Acquired structural deficits may result from trauma to the orofacial complex or surgical removal of oral structures secondary to oral cancers. For individuals with orofacial anomalies, the course of habilitation or rehabilitation often includes surgical and/or prosthetic management, and therefore the speech clinician must work closely with various medical and dental specialists.

Lips

Surgical repair of clefts of the lip can result in a relatively short immobile upper lip. Although this might be expected to adversely affect articulation skills, there is little evidence that this anomaly causes a speech problem for most speakers. Bloomer and Hawk (1973) reported the effects of ablative surgery on production of labial phonemes in a patient who underwent surgical removal of the external and internal nasal structures for treatment of cancer. Although surgery resulted in a relatively immobile and shortened upper lip, the patient maintained good overall speech intelligibility, producing labiodental approximations for all bilabial consonants. The development of compensatory articulatory gestures to achieve acoustically acceptable speech production is very common in many patients with structural anomalies.

Tongue

The tongue is a muscular structure capable of considerable changes in length and width. Because the tongue is such an adaptable organ, speakers are frequently able to compensate for extensive amounts of the tongue missing and still maintain intelligible speech. Clinical investigators have repeatedly reported intelligible speech production following partial glossectomies (surgical removal of the tongue) (see Leonard, 1994). One early case study (Backus, 1940) recorded the speech pattern of a 10-year-old boy with an undersized tongue after excision of the tongue tip and the left half of the tongue. Initially, the child's speech sound skills were characterized by numerous consonant substitutions, but after a period of treatment, he was able to produce all consonants with little identifiable deviation.

For many patients, however, speech production is affected in varying degrees when part of the tongue is excised. Skelly, Spector, Donaldson, Brodeur, and Paletta (1971) reported pre-treatment and post-treatment intelligibility scores for 25 glossectomy (14 total, 11 partial) patients. Intelligibility judgments were based on single-word productions audio tape-recorded and played back to listeners. Intelligibility scores for those who underwent partial glossectomy ranged from 6 to 24 percent on the pre-test and from 24 to 46 percent on the post-test. Intelligibility scores for those who underwent total glossectomy ranged from 0 to 8 percent prior to treatment and from 18 to 24 present after treatment. The investigators noted that the compensatory articulatory patterns of the two groups differed. Partial glossectomy patients utilized the residual tongue stump to modify articulation; total glossectomy patients made mandibular, labial, buccal, and palatal adjustments during speech production.

Massengill, Maxwell, and Picknell (1970) reported that speech intelligibility in three patients decreased as the amount of tongue excised increased. The patients demonstrated minimal difficulty in verbal communication, although speech distortion was present. Skelly and colleagues (1971) reported that unilateral tongue excision required fewer speech adaptations than tongue tip excisions.

Leonard (1994) reported a study where listeners were asked to evaluate consonants produced by 50 speakers with various types of glossectomy. She indicated that fricatives and plosives were most frequently judged to be inaccurate, while nasals and semivowels appeared more resistant to perceptual disruption.

For partial glossectomy patients, the specific surgical procedure used and/or the particular muscles removed may have different effects on speech outcomes (Bressmann, Sader, Whitehill, and Samman, 2004). Improvements in speech production skill have been reported for some post-surgical interventions. These include the use of a *palatal augmentation prosthesis (PAP)* in which "the palatal vault is re-established at a lower level than normal, requiring less bulk and mobility of the tongue for appropriate palatolingual contacts during speech" (Marunick and Tselios, 2004, p. 67) and the addition of artificial grafts (Terai and Shimahara, 2004).

Hard Palate

The removal of any part of the maxilla which includes the hard palate (e.g., necessitated by oral cancer), if not restored surgically or prosthetically, creates a serious problem for the speaker. Most patients receive palatal closure through a prosthetic (dental) appliance. Sullivan and colleagues (2002) reported results from 32 cancer patients who had palatal defects because of surgical removal of a portion of the palate as a result of cancer of the maxillar sinus and alveolar ridge. The maxillectomy patients had their defects obturated with a dental appliance. Testing was conducted one month after obturation on measures of speech intelligibility, speaking rate, nasality, and communication effectiveness. With the obturator removed, mean speech intelligibility was 61 percent, speaking rate was 138 words per minutes, and nasality was 5.8 on a 0–7 point scale. With the obturator inserted, mean speech intelligibility was 94 percent, speaking rate was 164 words per minute, and nasality was rated 1.6 The mean self-perception of communication effectiveness by patients was 75 percent of what it was prior to the cancer. The authors concluded that "obturation is an effective intervention for defects of the maxillary sinus and alveolar ridge on speech performance. Variations in effectiveness were noted based on site defect and patient satisfaction with the intervention."

For children born with clefts of the hard palate, the palate is typically repaired within the first 12 to 14 months of life. Scarring associated with the surgery has not been found to interfere with articulatory production in most cases.

Soft Palate

The relationship of the soft palate (velum) to articulation has been a topic of considerable research, much of it focusing on the sphincteral closure of the velopharyngeal port and the effect of velopharyngeal competence on articulation. *Velopharyngeal competence* refers to the valving that takes place to separate the nasal cavity from the oral cavity during non-nasal speech production. Inadequate velopharyngeal closure is frequently associated with (1) hypernasal (excessive nasal) resonance of vowels, vocalic consonants, and glides and liquids; (2) reduced or diminished intraoral breath pressure during production of pressure consonants (i.e., fricatives, stops, and affricates); and (3) nasal air emission accompanying production of pressure consonants (e.g., substitutions of glottal stops for stop consonants and pharyngeal fricatives for sibilants). Although velopharyngeal incompetence is often associated with individuals with clefts of the soft palate, some speakers without clefting also demonstrate such incompetence—for example, individuals with dysarthria related to neurogenic paresis or paralysis of the velopharyngeal muscles (Johns and Salyer, 1978).

The pharyngeal fricative and the glottal stop are two examples of compensatory articulatory gestures associated with velopharyngeal valving problems. The glottal stop is characterized by interruption of the airstream at the glottis, resulting in a glottal click, or cough-like sound. Glottal stops are generally substituted for stops, particularly velar stops, as well as fricatives and affricates. The pharyngeal fricative is produced with the source of friction in the pharyngeal area and is frequently substituted for fricatives and affricates. The presence of hypernasality, nasal emission of air, weak consonants, glottal stops, and pharyngeal fricatives are all signs of velopharyngeal valving difficulties.

When the oral cavity communicates (is open to) with the nasal cavity, for example, through palatal fistulae (openings), or following ablative surgery or velopharyngeal incompetence, varying degrees of hypernasality will usually result. On the other hand, hyponasality (denasality) may result when the nasopharynx or nasal cavity is obstructed during speech production. Inflammation of the mucous membranes of the nasal cavity or a deviated septum may also cause hyponasality.

In addition to immediate problems associated with speech production, children born with clefts of the soft palate also experience a higher frequency of middle ear infections (otitis media) (Sheahan, Miller, Sheahan, Earley, and Blayney, 2003) than children without clefts. The frequency of otitis media in children born with clefts appears to be the result of problems with either the structure or function of the Eustachian tube mechanism, which develops at about the same time in the embryo as the palate. Kemaloglou, Kobayashi, and Nakajima (1999) reported shorter and more horizontal Eustachian tubes in children with clefts of the palate compared to children without clefts. A higher incidence of otitis media may be important for speech because of its potential impact on speech sound acquisition. It is a reasonable inference that if a child has a hearing loss it may affect speech sound acquisition.

Nasopharynx

The nasopharyngeal tonsils (adenoids) are located at the upper or superior pharyngeal area. Hyperthrophied (enlarged) adenoids may compensate for a short or partially immobile velum, by assisting in velopharyngeal closure. Thus, their removal may result in hypernasality. But the adenoids may become sufficiently enlarged as to constitute a major obstruction of the nasopharynx, resulting in hyponasal speech. Enlarged adenoids may also interfere with Eustacian tube function in some individuals. When adenoids constitute an obstruction of the Eustacian tube, they may be removed for medical reasons.

Summary

Although individuals with major oral structural deviations frequently experience articulation problems, the relationship between structural deficits and articulation skills is not highly predictable. The literature cites many instances of individuals with structural anomalies who have developed compensatory gestures to produce acoustically acceptable speech. Why some individuals are able to compensate for relatively gross abnormalities and others are unable to compensate for lesser deficits has not been resolved. A speech-language clinician who evaluates or treats individuals with oral structural anomalies must work collaboratively with various medical and dental specialists during speech habilitation or rehabilitation. For an excellent review of the speech characteristics and treatment of individuals with glossectomy and other oral/oropharyngeal ablation, see Leonard (1994).

Genetic Syndromes

A number of genetic syndromes may include problems with speech sound acquisition or be associated with speech sound disorders. An excellent source of more detailed information is Shprintzen (1997). Two of the most common and well-documented genetic syndromes with speech consequences will be mentioned here as illustrations. The first is *Down syndrome (DS)*, which is thought to occur once in about every 700 births. In most cases, Down syndrome results from an extra copy of chromosome 21 (hence, it is often called *Trisomy 21*). Several features associated with this syndrome likely contribute to difficulties with speech in this population. First, DS includes varying degrees of *cognitive* impairment that may lead to an overall delay in speech sound acquisition. Second, individuals with DS are said to have *relative macroglossia*, or a normal sized tongue in a relatively small oral cavity; this results in less space for the tongue to maneuver during connected speech production. This might then explain why one of the most frequently cited problems reported for individuals with DS is reduced speech intelligibility in conversation (Kumin, 1994). Other problems for individuals with Down syndrome relative to speech include both generally *reduced muscle tone* and a *high frequency of otitis media* associated with Eustachian tube problems (Marder and Cholmain, 2006). There remains some controversy about whether the pattern of speech sound acquisition in DS is similar to what we see in typically developing children (but simply delayed) or actually follows a different course. A recent analysis by Roberts and colleagues (2005), which included 32 boys with DS and 33 typically developing boys matched for mental age, highlighted the difficulty in answering that question. Their findings showed an overall pattern of delayed speech sound development. However, these investigators also reported some examples of error patterns such as lateralization of sibilants and deletion of nasals, which are uncommon in even very young typically developing children. Additional discussion of speech sound problems in DS can also be found later in this chapter in the section titled "Language Development."

A second genetic syndrome that has been shown to include difficulty with speech sounds (without clefting) is *Fragile X syndrome (FXS)*. Somewhat less common than Down syndrome, Fragile X is thought to occur once in about every 4,000 births. In this case, there is a mutation that turns off a particular section of the X chromosome, resulting in failure to produce a particular protein. Males have only a single X chromosome and so are much more likely to be affected by FXS than females (for whom the mutation might be present on only one of their two X chromosomes). As with DS, FXS includes varying degrees of cognitive impairment that may delay speech sound acquisition. Another feature shared with DS is that the speech of individuals with FXS is noticeably difficult to understand. The study by Roberts and colleagues (2005) also included 50 boys with FXS. In this case, the findings suggested error patterns that were generally typical of much younger, typically developing children, suggesting a more straightforward diagnosis of delay (rather than deviance).

Hearing Loss

A third subgroup of organically based speech sound disorders includes those with significant hearing loss. One of the most important elements underlying the production and comprehension of speech, as well as the monitoring of one's own speech, is an auditory system that is sensitive to the frequency range where most speech sounds occur (500 to 4000 Hz). Individuals with more severe hearing loss will have difficulty decoding the incoming sound signal and will perceive words differently than individuals with normal hearing mechanisms.

The child who is hard of hearing or deaf faces the challenging task of learning how to produce speech without adequate auditory input. Learning to discriminate and produce speech must then be accomplished by watching how sounds look on the face, how they feel through vibrations, and what can be perceived from a distorted auditory signal. A certain level of hearing is required to learn and maintain normal speech production. Ling (1989) summarized this relationship by noting that the more normal a person's hearing, the more natural his or her speech is likely to be.

Several aspects of hearing loss have been shown to affect speech perception and production; these include the level of hearing sensitivity, speech recognition ability, and configuration of the hearing loss. Individual hearing losses range from mild to severe or profound (greater than 70 dB HL). Labels such as *hard of hearing* and *deaf* are frequently applied to persons with varying degrees of hearing impairment.

Hearing sensitivity typically varies somewhat from one frequency to another, with speech and language differentially influenced by the frequency configuration and severity of the hearing loss. Although information recorded on an audiogram is a useful prognostic indicator of speech reception ability, children with similar audiograms may not perceive speech sounds in the same way. A pure-tone audiogram cannot measure a person's ability to distinguish one frequency from another or to track formant transitions (a skill critical to speech perception). For these and other reasons (e.g., age of fitting and full-time use of amplification, concomitant factors, quality of early intervention programs), individuals with similar pure-tone audiograms can differ greatly in their understanding of speech.

A second hearing-related factor important to speech sound acquisition and maintenance is the age of onset and the age of detection of the hearing loss. If a severe loss has been present since birth, acquisition of language—including phonology, syntax, and semantics—is difficult, and specialized instruction is necessary to develop speech and language. Such instruction may rely on visual, tactile, and kinesthetic cues, and signing as well as whatever residual auditory sensation the person possesses or has been afforded via technology. For a discussion of the influence of hearing loss on infants and toddlers phonologic development, see Stoel-Gammon and Kehoe (1994). Children and adults who suffer a serious loss of hearing after language has been acquired usually retain their speech sound production patterns for a time, but frequently their articulatory skills deteriorate. Even those assisted with amplification may find it difficult to maintain their previous level of articulatory performance.

The most obvious characteristic of the speech of those with significant hearing loss is that it can often be very difficult to understand. Gold (1980) stated that for most listeners it may be possible to understand only 20 percent of what speakers with congenitally severe or profound hearing loss are attempting to say. The difficulty with understanding the speech of these individuals appears to be the product of problems at both the segmental and suprasegmental levels. At the segmental level, errors on both consonants and vowels can be observed (Levitt and Stromberg, 1983; Paterson, 1994).

At the suprasegmental level, persons who are deaf or hard of hearing generally speak at a slower rate than normal-hearing speakers because of longer duration of both consonants and vowels. They also use more frequent pauses and slower articulatory transitions. Stress patterns may also differ from those of normal-hearing speakers, as many persons who are deaf or hearing impaired do not distinguish duration associated with stressed and unstressed syllables. Persons who are deaf or hearing impaired sometimes use too high or too low a pitch, and nonstandard inflectional patterns. Harsh or breathy voice quality, and hypo- or hypernasal speech are also commonly reported (Dunn and Newton, 1986).

As noted previously, even in cases of severe and profound hearing impairment, the specific types of perception problems and speech production errors are difficult to predict. There is a great deal of individual variability. Less information however is available for individuals with mild to moderate hearing losses than for those with more severe losses.

Calvert (1982) reported that errors of articulation common to deaf children are not confined to productions of individual phonemes; errors also occur because of the phonetic context in which the phones are embedded. Calvert documented specific examples of omission, substitution, distortion, and addition errors relative to particular target phonemes, classes of phonemes, and phonetic contexts. These are highlighted in Table 4.1.

The preceding discussion is most relevant for those individuals with hearing loss who use hearing aids. The introduction of the cochlear implant has revolutionized the management of hearing loss, particularly for children who receive them early. These devices include a series of tiny wires (called *electrodes*) that are surgically implanted into the inner ear. The electrodes are connected to an external microphone and a speech processor.

■ **TABLE 4.1** Common Speech Errors Seen in Deaf Speech

1. Errors of Omission
   a. Omission of final consonants
   b. Omission of /s/ in all contexts
   c. Omission of initial consonants
2. Errors of Substitution
   a. Voiced for voiceless consonants
   b. Nasal for oral consonants
   c. Low feedback substitutions (substitution of sounds with easily perceived tactile and kinesthetic feedback for those with less; for example, /w/ for /r/ substitution)
   d. Substitution of one vowel for another
3. Errors of Distortion
   a. Degree of force (stop and fricative consonants are frequently made with either too much or too little force)
   b. Hypernasality associated with vowel productions
   c. Imprecision and indefiniteness in vowel articulation
   d. Duration of vowels (deaf speakers tend to produce vowels with undifferentiated duration, usually in the direction of excess duration)
   e. Temporal values in diphthongs (deaf speakers may not produce the first or the second vowel in a diphthong for the appropriate duration of time)
4. Errors of Addition
   a. Insertion of a superfluous vowel between consonants (e.g., /sʌnoʊ/ for /snoʊ/)
   b. Unnecessary release of final stop consonants (e.g., [stopʰ])
   c. Diphthongization of vowels (e.g., *mit* → [mɪʌt])
   d. Superfluous breath before vowels

Source: Calvert (1982).

Speech is received by the microphone and sent via the processor to the electrodes, which stimulate the auditory nerve via electrical pulses. A number of investigators (e.g., Allen, Nickolopoulos, and O'Donoghue, 1998; Flipsen and Colvard, 2006; Inscoe, 1998) have reported that the conversational speech produced by these children can be highly intelligible (up to 90 percent in some cases). However, studies have shown similar types of errors and error patterns (albeit less frequent) to those found in hearing impaired individuals who use hearing aids (Chin and Pisoni, 2000; Flipsen and Parker, 2007; Grogan, Barker, Dettmen, and Blamey, 1995). Table 4.2 presents a list of error patterns that have been observed in both children with hearing aids and cochlear implants.

In addition to errors on specific speech sounds or sound combinations, the suprasegmental aspects of speech may continue to be of concern for even the most successful

■ **TABLE 4.2** Speech Sound Error Patterns Observed in Both Children Who Use Hearing Aids and Children Who Use Cochlear Implants

Developmental Patterns[1]	Nondevelopmental Patterns[2]
Assimilation Errors	Initial Consonant Deletion
Consonant Cluster Reduction	Glottal Stop Substitution
Final Consonant Deletion	Backing
Liquid Simplification	Vowel Substitution
Palatal Fronting	Diphthong Simplification
Stopping	
Unstressed (weak) Syllable Deletion	
Velar Fronting	

[1]Error patterns seen in younger typically developing (normal hearing) children.
[2]Error patterns not usually seen in younger typically developing (normal hearing) children.
Source: Adapted from Parker (2005). Used by permission.

cochlear implant recipients. Abnormal resonance and difficulty with the use of syllable and word-level stress may continue to be a problem for these children (Lenden and Flipsen, 2007).

It should be noted, of course, that as with children fitted with hearing aids, outcomes for children fitted with cochlear implants can be quite variable (Geers, 2006). Age at implantation continues to be a crucial variable, with children receiving their implants at younger ages clearly evidencing better performance. Current criteria for implantation set by the U.S. Food and Drug Administration permit implantation in children as young as age 12 months, but there is ongoing debate about implantation at even younger ages. In some European countries, children are receiving implants as young as 4 months of age. Regardless of the age limit, however, it is still the case that not all children with hearing impairments are identified as early as they should be. Newborn Infant Hearing Screening is now widely conducted but is not yet truly universal. Other aspects of eligibility criteria for implantation are also changing. For example, more children with some degree of residual hearing in at least one ear are receiving implants. Preliminary data suggest that outcomes in such cases are better than for children with no residual hearing. Such children may especially benefit if a hearing aid is fitted in their nonimplanted ear. This arrangement (cochlear implant in one ear and hearing aid in the other) is referred to as *bimodal hearing*. In addition, many child implant candidates now receive cochlear implants in both ears *(bilateral implantation)*. Some recent studies have shown that bimodal hearing (Ching, Incerti, Hill, and van Wanrooy, 2006; Madell, Sislian, and Hoffman, 2004) and bilateral implantation (Biever and Kelsall, 2007; Galvin, Mok, and Dowell, 2007) both result in significant improvements in speech perception outcomes over a single implant alone. Data still appear to be lacking, however, on speech production outcomes for these groups.

Neuromotor Disorders

A fourth group of children with organically based speech sound disorders are those with identifiable impairments of speech movement control (i.e., those with neuromotor impairments). Speech production at a motor level requires muscle strength, speed of movement, appropriate range of excursion, accuracy of movement, coordination of multiple movements, motor steadiness, and muscle tone (Darley, Aronson, and Brown, 1975). Damage that impairs one or more of these neuromuscular functions may affect motor speech production, including phonation, respiration, or velopharyngeal function. Neuromotor speech disorders more typically occur in adults than children, since they are often associated with strokes or other forms of brain injury. Cerebral palsy is one example of a condition that results in a variety of neuromotor-based speech disorders in children.

Neurologists and speech-language pathologists have sought to understand the possible relationship between the clinical (behavioral) responses associated with neurologically impaired individuals and the site and extent of the neurological lesions (brain damage). The reason for such inquiry is to identify some potential commonality across patients between the specific brain damage and the concomitant cognitive language impairment.

Although as noted earlier, entire books are devoted to motor speech disorders, the following offers a brief introduction to this topic.

Dysarthrias

The *dysarthrias* are neurologic motor speech impairments characterized by slow, weak, imprecise, and/or uncoordinated movements of the speech musculature. Yorkston, Beukelman, Strand, and Bell (1999) state that "dysarthrias form a group of disorders marked by impaired execution of the movements of speech production." Because dysarthrias are caused by different types of lesions, trauma, or disease that cause central or peripheral nervous system damage, dysarthrias cannot be described by a single set of characteristics.

Dysarthrias are characterized by a paralysis, weakness, or incoordination of the speech musculature, which may result from localized injuries to the nervous system, various inflammatory processes, toxic metabolic disorders, vascular lesions or trauma of the brain, and lesion, disease, or trauma to the nervous system. The most significant characteristic of dysarthric speech is reduced intelligibility. Dysarthric speech can involve disturbances in respiration, phonation, articulation, resonance, and prosody. Phonemes misarticulated in spontaneous speech are also likely to be misarticulated in other situations, such as reading and imitation tasks.

Table 4.3 lists the types of dysarthrias and the most prominent speech characteristics associated with each. The most common of these characteristics is the production of imprecise consonants.

Apraxia

Apraxia is a motor speech disorder also caused by brain damage, but it is differentiated from the dysarthrias and described as a separate clinical entity. Apraxia of speech is characterized by an impairment of motor speech programming with little or no weakness, paralysis, or incoordination of the speech musculature. Whereas dysarthrias frequently affect all motor speech processes—respiration, phonation, articulation, resonance, and prosody—apraxia primarily affects articulatory abilities with secondary prosodic alterations.

■ **TABLE 4.3**   Dysarthrias and Associated Speech Deviations

Type	Discrete Neurological Group	Relative Prominence of Speech Deviations
Flaccid dysarthria—(disorders of the lower motor neuron)	Bulbar palsy	1. Hypernasality 2. Imprecise consonants 3. Breathiness (continuous)
Spastic dysarthria—(disorders of the upper motor neuron)	Pseudobulbar palsy	1. Imprecise consonants 2. Monopitch 3. Reduced stress
Ataxic dysarthria—(disorders of the cerebellar system)	Cerebellar lesions	1. Imprecise consonants 2. Excess and equal stress 3. Irregular articulatory breakdown
Hypokinetic dysarthria—(disorders of the extra-pyramidal system)	Parkinsonism	1. Monopitch 2. Reduced stress 3. Monoloudness
Hyperkinetic dysarthria—(disorders of the extra-pyramidal system)	Chorea	1. Imprecise consonants 2. Prolonged intervals 3. Variable rate
	Dystonia	1. Imprecise consonants 2. Distorted vowels 3. Harsh voice quality
Unilateral upper motor neuron—(disorders on right or left side)	Pseudobulbar palsy	1. Imprecise articulation 2. Hypernasality 3. Slow-labored rate
Mixed dysarthrias—	Amyotrophic lateral sclerosis with relative prominence in pseudobulbar palsy and bulbar palsy	1. Imprecise consonants 2. Hypernasality 3. Harsh voice quality

Source: Adapted from Darley, Aronson, and Brown (1975).

A description of some of the clinical characteristics of this disorder has been provided by Duffy (2005):

> Deviant speech characteristics . . . include a number of abnormalities of articulation, rate, prosody, and fluency. The characteristics that best distinguish it from other motor speech disorders (the dysarthrias) are distorted sound substitutions and additions, decreased phonemic accuracy with increased rate, attempts to correct articulatory errors that cross phonemic boundaries, groping for articulatory postures, greater difficulty on volitional than automatic speech tasks, and greater difficulty on SMR [sequential motion rate] and multisyllabic word tasks than AMR (alternate motion rate] and single syllable tasks. . . . Articulatory distortions, reduced rate, and various prosodic abnormalities help distinguish AOS from aphasic phonologic errors. (p. 330)

Some clients who demonstrate apraxia of speech (verbal apraxia) also demonstrate similar difficulty in volitional oral nonspeech tasks, a behavior described as oral apraxia

(Duffy, 2005). For example, an individual may protrude his or her tongue during eating but may be unable to perform this act voluntarily. Although oral apraxia often coexists with verbal apraxia, this is not always the case.

Johns and Darley (1970) compared apraxic and dysarthric speakers on tasks involving spontaneous speaking and reading at a "self-chosen rate" and at a rapid rate. They reported that (1) apraxic speakers were less consistent than dysarthric speakers in their speech sound errors; (2) apraxics made fewer speech sound errors and were more intelligible when reading at rapid rates rather than slow rates; (3) apraxics performed better on the spontaneous speaking tasks than on the reading tasks; (4) dysarthrics made fewer errors and were more intelligible when speaking at slow rates rather than fast rates; and (5) distortions accounted for 65 percent of the errors made by dysarthrics but only 10 percent of the errors made by apraxic speakers; substitutions accounted for 50 percent of the errors made by apraxic speakers but only 10 percent of the errors made by dysarthric speakers. Speech sound errors seen in apraxia have usually been identified as sound substitution errors and thereby differentiated from the speech sound distortions seen in dysarthrics. Itoh and Sasanuma (1984) have argued, however, that some of the substitutions seen in apraxia can better be described as distortions, and thus apraxia may be characterized by both substitution and distortion errors. Lapointe and Wertz (1974) described patients who demonstrated a "mixed" articulation disorder consisting of a combination of apraxic and dysarthric speech characteristics.

CHILDHOOD APRAXIA OF SPEECH

One of the more controversial speech sound disorder categories is *childhood apraxia of speech (CAS);* this condition is also known by several other names, including *developmental apraxia of speech* and *developmental verbal dyspraxia.* Two reasons appear to have spawned the controversy with this diagnosis. First, there have long been disagreements about the specific distinguishing characteristics of this condition, or even if such characteristics exist. One of the more complete attempts to reconcile this controversy was presented by Davis, Jakielski, and Marquardt (1998). The list of potential characteristics of CAS they generated is shown in Table 4.4.

It is important to note that many of the characteristics highlighted in Table 4.4 are not necessarily unique to CAS. Investigators who have looked for such characteristics don't always agree with one another. For example, Table 4.4 lists studies that show "poor non-speech praxis abilities" as well as other studies that suggest such abilities may be normal. Some have argued that such conflicts may simply reflect co-existing *oral apraxia* in some children with CAS. This is a similar issue in adult apraxia of speech.

The failure to identify the unique features of CAS has led some to suggest that this disorder may not exist as a unique "diagnostic entity"; those taking this position argue that it simply represents the most severe form of speech delay of unknown origin (to be discussed later). However, others argue that CAS itself can be manifested along the entire continuum from mild to severe. The failure to identify the unique features of CAS has also led some to use the label *suspected apraxia of speech* for these children (Shriberg, Aram, and Kwiatkowski, 1997a).

■ **TABLE 4.4**   Summary of Diagnostic Characteristics

Speech Production Characteristics

Restricted consonant inventory:
  Bloise and Marquardt, 1990; Chappell, 1973; Crary, 1984; Parsons, 1984

Restricted vowel inventory:
  Davis, Marquardt and Sussman, 1985: Marquardt, Smith, Rudrauff, Davis and Cannito, 1990; Pollock and Hall, 1991; Smith, Marquardt, Cannito and Davis, 1994

Lack of consistent production of misarticulations:
  Aram and Nation, 1982; Marquardt and Sussman, 1991; Parsons, 1984; Rosenbek, Hanson, Baughman and Lemme, 1974

Insufficiently characterized by phonological process analysis:
  Bloise and Marquárdt, 1990; Parsons, 1984

Severe reduction in speech intelligibility:
  Crary, 1984; Marquardt and Sussman, 1991; Velleman, Strand, Pollock and Hall, 1992

Unsteady pitch and increased segmental duration:
  McClumpha and Logue, 1972

Monotone and slow rate:
  Aram and Glasson, 1979; Edwards, 1973; Guyette and Diedrich, 1983; McClumpha and Logue, 1972; Yoss and Darley, 1974; Rosenbek and Wertz, 1972; Shriberg, 1993

Acoustic measures of fundamental frequency and duration/no consistent group patterns:
  Hall, Jordan and Robin, 1993

Speech Perception Characteristics

Deficits in auditory perception:
  Robin, Hall and Jordan, 1986

Deficits in auditory discrimination:
  Snow, Marquardt and Davis, 1993

Deficits in perception and production of rhyme:
  Marion, Sussman and Marquardt, 1993

Language Characteristics

Age-appropriate receptive language abilities:
  Aram and Glasson, 1979

Expressive skills significantly less developed than receptive skills:
  Riley, 1984; Snyder, Marquardt and Peterson, 1977

Errors in both syntax and morphology:
  Ekelman and Aram, 1983

Deficits in concept comprehension:
  Hall, Hardy and LaVelle, 1990

Cognitive Characteristics

Significantly lower performance than verbal scores on intelligence testing:
  Ferry, Hall and Hicks, 1975; Gubbay, Ellis, Walton and Court, 1965

Gender Characteristics

Three to one/males to females: Hall *et al.*, 1993

Praxis Characteristics

Poor non-speech praxis abilities:
  Rosenbek and Wertz, 1972; Smartt, LaLance, Gray and Hibbett, 1976; Yoss and Darley, 1974

Normal praxis abilities:
  Aram and Horwitz, 1983

Development milestone delays:
  Palmer, Wurth and Kinchloe, 1964

General clumsy motor development for self-help skills:
  Crary, 1984; Gubbay *et al.*, 1965; Hall *et al.*, 1993; Walton, Ellis and Court, 1962; Yoss and Darley, 1974

Neurological Characteristics

Failure to identify specific neuroanatomical abnormalities:
  Darwish, Pearce, Gaines and Harasym, 1982; Denays, Tondeur, Foulon, Verstraeten, Ham, Piepsz and Noel, 1989; Horwitz, 1984

Consistent neurological and EEG findings:
  Denays *et al.*, 1989; Hall *et al.*, 1993; Horwitz, 1984; Rosenbek and Wertz, 1972; Yoss and Darley, 1974

Source: B. L. Davis, K. J. Jakielski, and T. P. Marquardt, "Developmental Apraxia of Speech: Determiners of Differential Diagnosis," *Clinical Linguistics and Phonetics, 12* (1998): 27. Reprinted with permission.

The second reason for the controversy surrounding childhood apraxia of speech stems from concerns about applying the label *apraxia* because, unlike the adult form of apraxia, it is often not possible to document specific neurological damage that might have led to the problem. This latter question is another reason that CAS is often included with Speech Sound Disorders of Unknown Origin (see next section). However, in some cases a potential causal agent can be identified. Thus, CAS may not clearly fit into either the organic or unknown group. As such, it seems appropriate to discuss it separately here.

In 2002, in an effort to resolve some of the controversy, the American Speech-Language-Hearing Association (ASHA) established an ad hoc committee on CAS. The committee reviewed the extensive and somewhat confusing literature in this area and in 2007 presented their findings. After considerable feedback, a position statement and the committee's technical report were adopted by ASHA's legislative council (ASHA, 2007a, 2007b). You may refer to the ASHA website, where both documents can be obtained for more detailed study. The ASHA position statement defines CAS as follows:

> *Childhood apraxia of speech (CAS)* is a neurological childhood (pediatric) speech sound disorder in which the precision and consistency of movements underlying speech are impaired in the absence of neuromuscular deficits (e.g., abnormal reflexes, abnormal tone). CAS may occur as a result of known neurological impairment, in association with complex neurobehavioral disorders of known or unknown origin, or as an idiopathic neurogenic speech sound disorder. The core impairment in planning and/or programming spatiotemporal parameters of movement sequences results in errors in speech sound production and prosody. (2007a, pp. 1–2)

Note that the definition limits CAS to problems with speech; the coexisting but separate difficulties that children with CAS may demonstrate with nonspeech oral movements are thought to indicate the comorbidity of either an underlying neuromuscular problem (i.e., dysarthria) or oral apraxia.

The ASHA definition also emphasizes that although CAS is seen as a neurological problem, it may arise in more than one way. It may be a reflection of a known neurological condition such as cerebral palsy. It may also be comorbid with "known neurobehavioral disorders" such as autism, Fragile X syndrome, or Rhett syndrome. In many cases, however, the origin of CAS is unknown (idiopathic).

The position statement has not solved all of the issues with CAS. It states very clearly that "at present, there is no validated list of diagnostic features of CAS that differentiates this symptom complex from other types of childhood speech sound disorders" (ASHA, 2007a, p. 2). That is, experts still don't fully know what it is that makes CAS distinct from other disorders. However, as the definition indicates, the primary problem appears to be one of "...planning and/or programming..." for speech. The position statement then mentions an emerging consensus about three specific speech production features that may be unique to CAS. The first is inconsistent errors on vowels and consonants; in this case, the term *inconsistent* specifically refers to multiple attempts at the same word resulting in different productions. Thus, a child with CAS who attempts the word *music* several times might produce them as /muzu/, /ugɪ/, and /mɪzu/. A second emerging feature of CAS is difficulty with prosody, particularly as it relates to the use of phrasal or lexical stress. Shriberg, Aram, and Kwiatkowski (1997b), for example, noted a tendency toward excessive and equal stress in two-syllable words. To continue with our example, production of the word *music* by a child with CAS may be perceived as MUSIC instead the normal MUsic (equal stress on both syllables rather than just the first). One study suggested that the difference between the syllables may be present but it may not be perceptible to listeners (Munson, Bjorum, and Windsor, 2003). The third emerging feature of CAS cited in the position statement (which may be difficult to see in most clinical situations) is lengthened and disrupted transitions between syllables and sounds. A study by Maasen, Nijland, and van der Meulen (2001), for example, showed stronger "anticipatory coarticulation" in children with CAS compared to typically speaking children.

These emerging characteristics raise the question of whether childhood apraxia of speech should be described as a purely motor speech disorder. Marquardt, Jacks, and Davis (2004) note that the inconsistency observed in CAS just as easily may be a product of an imprecise underlying phonological representation rather than a pure speech motor programming problem. As well, problems with the prosody of speech (i.e., excessive and equal stress) may indicate some lack of detail in the underlying representation about the hierarchical organization of speech. When combined with reports that children with CAS exhibit difficulty with reading and spelling (Gillon and Moriarty, 2007), it points to CAS being the result of a combination of representational and motor speech difficulties (McNeill, 2007). Such a conclusion remains speculative at this point.

An important related question is the prevalence of CAS given that there appears to have been an increase in the use of this diagnostic label in recent years. According to the ASHA Technical Report, this increase may be largely because of confusion over the exact characteristics of CAS (ASHA, 2007b). Unfortunately, there have been no systematic population studies (ASHA, 2007b), but one recent estimate, based on clinical referral data, suggests a prevalence of one to two cases per 1,000 children (Shriberg, Aram, and Kwiatkowski, 1997a). If the emerging features are confirmed by additional research, clinicians may soon be able to obtain a more precise estimate of the prevalence of CAS.

Chapter 7 presents some suggestions for assessment and treatment of CAS.

SPEECH SOUND DISORDERS OF UNKNOWN ORIGIN

The second and largest group of children with speech sound disorders is one that has puzzled investigators for many years. It includes those for whom there is no obvious cause. This has long raised the question: If we don't know how the problem arose in the first place, how do we help these children? Lacking clear answers, speech-language pathologists have for many years tended to do two things. First, we have often assumed this is a single group, and second, we have tended to treat them all the same way. Until about the 1970s, most SLPs referred to these children as having *functional articulation disorders* (a term still used by some today). The word *functional* implies that these children have some sort of learning difficulty. And in this context, the word *articulation* implies that the problem is with learning to physically produce individual speech sounds. So, for many years these children received what is now called *traditional articulation therapy* (sometimes also called *phonetic therapy*), which is a motor skill–oriented approach to therapy. This approach will be described in a later chapter.

In the 1970s, speech-language pathology began to be influenced by developments in the field of linguistics, particularly those brought forth by the publication of *The Sound Pattern of English* (Chomsky and Hallé, 1968), *A Dissertation on Natural Phonology* (Stampe, 1979), and *Phonological Disability in Children* (Ingram, 1976). These publications, combined with a growing interest in disorders of language (independent of difficulties with speech), forced SLPs to consider that in addition to learning how to physically produce speech sounds, children also have to learn how the sounds of their language are organized (i.e., they had to learn the phonology of the language). These publications and the subsequent research they spawned also made SLPs realize that there were patterns among what had always seemed like unrelated collections of individual errors. Previously, if a child said [wit] for *with,* [pan] for *fan,* and [too] for *Sue,* the diagnosis would have been simply that they had not learned to physically produce /θ/, /f/, and /s/. Therapy would focus on teaching the child to perceive and produce each of those sounds one by one. However, the new insights from linguistics made SLPs consider that these three errors might be related in some way. All of the intended sounds represent fricative targets being replaced by stop consonants. The work of Chomsky and Hallé suggested that in this case the child may be having troubling learning the *continuant* feature, which all fricatives share. Stampe took a different perspective and suggested that the child might have an immature speech production or perception system, and thus was temporarily unable to either perceive or produce fricatives. To get around this temporary limitation, Stampe suggested that the child was simplifying all fricatives to stops (a pattern known as *stopping*). As the child's perception or production systems matured, he or she would no longer find it necessary to simplify and would suppress the pattern (i.e., the child would, in this case, "stop stopping"). Ingram's book was perhaps the first to attempt to translate these developments in linguistic theory for the practicing clinician by speaking of "explicitly principled therapy." The net result was that the field suddenly began referring to these children as having *developmental phonological disorders* or simply *phonological disorders.* The emphasis had changed from articulation to phonology.

This change in labels was also accompanied by changes in the approach to assessment and treatment. Many clinicians began to switch from teaching about the physical aspects of production to teaching children how using different sounds results in changes in meaning. This approach (also to be described in a later chapter) is called variously *contrast therapy, phonological therapy,* or *phonemic therapy.* Whatever it was called, many SLPs began to report that these children were progressing through therapy much more quickly than before with a sound-by-sound approach. Researchers began to validate this observation empirically. Klein (1996), for example, retrospectively compared 19 children who had received traditional articulation therapy with 17 children who had received phonological therapy. The two groups had been treated at different times by different clinicians, but within each group the therapy had been relatively controlled within a single university clinic. Klein reported that the children in the phonological therapy group spent significantly fewer months in therapy (13.5 vs. 22.3 months), were significantly less severely involved at their last treatment session, and were significantly more likely to have been dismissed from therapy with normal speech (17/17 vs. 2/19).

Unfortunately, this change in treatment approach was not universally successful. Even though outcomes tend to be better for many of these children, they do not all benefit equally. Some actually respond better to traditional articulation therapy, and some don't respond well to either approach. It is still not completely clear how to determine which child will respond best to which form of intervention.

In an attempt to more fully understand this group, researchers have examined a whole variety of variables to see whether these children differ in some more specific way from children who were developing speech normally or from those with organically based problems. To date, no consensus has emerged. As quickly as one study reports some unique difference, another study asks the same question and reveals contradictory results. For example, Dworkin (1978) reported that children with "functional articulation disorders" had lower tongue strength and slower diadochokinetic rates than typically speaking children. However, a follow-up study by Dworkin and Culatta (1985) revealed no such differences. Despite the lack of a consensus on the problem these children have, researchers have identified a whole range of factors that appear to be at least related to speech sound disorders. Later in this chapter we will discuss some of those factors. Relative to classification, however, the failure to identify any single factor that is unique to this group has led many to conclude that this may not be a single group. Perhaps there are subgroups. Several groups of investigators have tried to sort out what the subgroups might be.

One possible approach suggested in the literature is to subdivide the group based on severity. Perhaps children with milder problems will respond better to particular treatments and those with more severe problems will respond better to other treatments. There are at least three problems with such an approach. First, although it is certainly true that children with speech sound disorders can be found anywhere along the continuum of severity (e.g., mild, moderate, or severe), there are no gold standards for determining severity of involvement in this population (Flipsen, Hammer, and Yost, 2005). Drawing the lines between the groups is therefore problematic. Second, if subgroups actually exist based on some other dimension, creating subgroups based on severity would only result in somewhat smaller but still heterogeneous groups. Third, and perhaps most important, "there seems to be no evidence that severity measures discriminate between subgroups of children with speech disorder in terms of the type of intervention indicated, or outcome" (Dodd, 2005, p. 5).

At least three other perspectives (etiological, psycholinguistic, symptomological) have begun to show potential for defining subgroups of children with speech sound disorders of unknown origin. The following sections describe these perspectives. It is important to note that no strong consensus has yet been reached about the best way to subdivide this population. What follows are very much three "works in progress."

Classification by Possible Etiology

With each of the organically based subgroups, the cause was obvious. Shriberg (1982) argued that, in the case of speech sound disorders of unknown origin, the cause may simply be much more difficult to find. Despite the added difficulty, however, isolating the specific causes offers the possibility of both a better understanding of the nature of the problem and a better match between the child's problem and the chosen treatment approach.

The search for not so obvious causes is complicated by the fact that in many cases what originally caused the problem (a *distal cause*) may have led to other problems (a *proximal cause*) that may now be maintaining the disorder (the distal cause may or may not still be operating). To illustrate, consider the child born with a significant hearing loss. The hearing loss results in an inability to hear all of the fine details of speech. This then may lead to poorly developed or distorted long-term storage of the sound system (what linguists call a poorly developed or distorted *underlying representation*). This may contribute to inaccurate production; it would be difficult to accurately produce something if you don't have an accurate sense of what the target is supposed to sound like. The hearing loss led to the problem originally and thus is the *distal cause* of the problem, but the poorly developed or distorted underlying representations may be the maintaining or *proximal cause* of the problem.

An early component of the search for etiological subgroups involved the identification of *causal correlates* or factors that appeared very often in the case histories of these children (Shriberg and Kwiatkowski, 1994). This analysis yielded several candidates for possible subgroups. However, this approach proved to be insufficient, as detailed case history information is not always available. Parents, who are often the primary source of case history information, may also not have very reliable memories about their children's histories (Majnemer and Rosenblatt, 1994). Complicating matters even further is that many children present with more than one of the causal correlates. This led Shriberg and his team to search for *diagnostic markers,* or speech characteristics, that are unique to each of the possible subgroups. Such markers are thought to offer insight into the perceptual, cognitive, or speech processing mechanisms involved. These processing mechanisms then serve as confirmatory evidence for the subgroups by suggesting theoretical pathways from a distal cause to a particular subgroup. The diagnostic markers may also be ultimately useful clinically. They may, for example, serve as potential treatment targets or at least help to identify such targets. An understanding of both the diagnostic markers and the processing mechanisms leading to those markers might also help identify the best approach to treating those particular targets (Flipsen, 2002b).

Shriberg and colleagues have postulated seven "putative" (i.e., potential and somewhat supported) subgroups (Shriberg, Lewis, Tomblin, McSweeny, Karlsson, and Scheer, 2005), which are highlighted in Table 4.5. The first five of the subgroups are classed as forms of Speech Delay. In such cases these children present with speech that is significantly behind developmental expectations during the preschool years. These children then typically qualify for and receive therapy. The distal cause for all five subgroups is currently thought to be some form of genetic difference (some may also include the influence of environmental factors). Several recent studies have identified gene loci that appear to be associated with speech sound disorders (e.g., Lewis et al., 2006; McDermot et al., 2005; Shriberg, Ballard, Tomblin, Duffy, Odell, and Williams, 2006). For each subgroup, however, the specific genetic difference (not definitively identified yet) is thought to lead to a different processing mechanism and thus to different diagnostic markers.

Evidence supporting the validity of Shriberg's etiological subgroups is starting to accumulate. The largest subgroup, Speech Delay–Genetic (SD–GEN), includes approximately 56 percent of these children who have one or more family members who have or have had speech or language problems. A particularly high proportion of omission errors especially on later developing consonants (Shriberg et al., 2005) is suggested as the diagnostic marker for this group; this suggests that they may be having difficulty identifying the phonemic details of the language (a cognitive-linguistic problem). Lewis, Freebairn, Hansen, Miscimarra, Iyengar, and Taylor (2007) reported findings that support a unique cognitive-linguistic proximal cause for this subgroup. In that study, parents of children with speech sound disorders, who themselves had a history of therapy for speech sound disorders, performed significantly less well compared to parents without such histories on some standardized measures of spoken language and spelling.

■ **TABLE 4.5**   Shriberg's Seven Putative Subtypes of Speech Sound Disorders of Unknown Origin

Group	Abbreviation	Prevalence[1]	Distal Cause	Proximal Cause (Processing Mechanism)	Diagnostic Markers
Speech Delay–Genetic	SD–GEN	56%	Genetic (polygenic) / environmental	Cognitive-Linguistic Processing	> deletion errors
Speech Delay–Otitis Media with Effusion	SD–OME	30%	Genetic (polygenic) / environmental	Auditory-Perceptual Processing	> backing errors; I–S gap[2]
Speech Delay–Developmental Psychosocial Involvement	SD–DPI	12%	Genetic (polygenic) / environmental	Affective-Temperamental Deficit	> severity?
Speech Delay–Apraxia of Speech	SD–AOS	???	Genetic (monogenic? or oligogenic?)	Speech-Motor Control	Lexical stress ratio; > coefficient of variation ratio
Speech Delay–Dysarthria	SD–DYS	???	Genetic (monogenic? or oligogenic?)	Speech-Motor Control	???
Speech Errors–Sibilants	SE–/s/	???	Environmental	Phonological Attunement	> first spectral moment for /s/
Speech Errors–Rhotics	SE–/r/	???	Environmental	Phonological Attunement	< F3–F2

[1]Percentage of those children in the population who have speech sound disorders of unknown origin.
[2]I–S = Intelligibility–Speech Gap (intelligibility far lower than predicted by speech sound accuracy).

A second subgroup, Speech Delay–Otitis Media with Effusion (SD–OME), includes approximately 30 percent of these children who have histories of early and frequent episodes of OME. At least two specific diagnostic markers have been proposed. Shriberg, Flipsen, Kwiatkowski, and McSweeny (2003) identified the *intelligibility-speech gap*. The conversational speech of these children was consistently less understandable than children without such histories. However, looking only at the portions of speech that could be understood, the accuracy of their consonant production was better than seen in some of the other subgroups. In other words, their speech was less well understood than would be expected, given the accuracy of their consonant production. Shriberg, Kent, Karlsson, McSweeny, Nadler, and Brown (2003) proposed a second diagnostic marker involving a higher frequency of backing errors (a very atypical pattern of using posterior sounds such as velar or palatal sounds in place of more anterior sounds such as alveolars). Like the SD–GEN subgroup, these two markers suggest difficulty extracting relevant phonemic details from the input language. In the case of SD–OME, the mechanism is thought to be intermittent hearing loss (Shriberg, Friel-Patti, Flipsen, and Brown, 2000).

A third possible subgroup, Speech Delay–Psychosocial Involvement (SD–DPI), is thought to include up to 12 percent of this population. Although the speech of this group has been characterized as more severely delayed than some of the other subgroups, a more specific diagnostic marker has yet to be identified. Hauner, Shriberg, Kwiatkowski, and Allen (2005) suggested that these children present with either (1) "approach-related negative affect" (i.e., described as aggressive, angry, or manipulative/control seeking) or (2) "withdrawal-related negative affect" (socially withdrawn, shy/fearful, or extremely taciturn). Thus, it is thought that these children may have temperaments that make it more difficult for them to obtain the feedback they need to develop and/or normalize their speech skills. These children may also be easily frustrated by their inability to communicate effectively and/or less likely to persist in their communication attempts.

Two other subgroups proposed by Shriberg include those with motor speech involvement. As noted earlier in the discussion of CAS, there is some justification for including at least those children with an idiopathic form of CAS in the population of speech sound disorders of unknown origin (referred to in Table 4.5 as SD–AOS). Additional details on CAS can be found in the previous section. The other subgroup of the speech delay type includes those children with subtle or less obvious forms of dysarthria (SD–DYS). As indicated in Table 4.5, it is not yet clear which task(s) or speech behavior(s) would qualify as viable diagnostic markers for this subgroup.

The last two subgroups proposed by Shriberg (Speech Errors–/s/ and Speech Errors–/r/) are currently thought to reflect an environmental distal cause. Shriberg and associates (2005) noted that these children are not typically identified as requiring treatment for speech sound problems as preschoolers. Rather, they may have a "disposition to respond to the environmental press for mastery of speech sounds in the ambient language" (p. 838). In other words, they may be so motivated to communicate that they attempt to master some aspects of speech before they are fully ready to do so. They may then adopt a production pattern that is less than optimal but that is retained well into the school years. It should be noted that speech errors in this case are not necessarily the same as "residual errors," which reflect distortion errors observed in adolescents and adults. As their name implies, residual errors are leftover errors from the preschool period that do not self-correct and may be resistant to treatment. But these residual errors come from one of two different sources. They may be remnants of either Speech Errors (RE–SE) or one of the five subgroups of Speech Delay (RE–SD). Although listeners cannot usually hear the difference between them, residual errors from these two sources have been shown to be acoustically distinct from each other (Karlsson, Shriberg, Flipsen, and McSweeny, 2002; Shriberg, Flipsen, Karlsson, and McSweeny, 2001).

Classification by Psycholinguistic Deficit

A second possible perspective that might be used to subdivide children with speech sound disorders of unknown origin into subgroups is to focus on the current underlying difficulty these children might be having with processing speech in the brain. Stackhouse and Wells (1997) argue that an etiological (what they term a "medical") approach to identifying the problem a particular child is having is limited both because causes are often not apparent and because existing etiological schemes don't always point directly to specific treatment options. On the other hand, they argue that a focus on error patterns (what they term a "linguistic" approach) provides a description only of the output behavior and fails to explain why certain speech behaviors are occurring (i.e., it fails to account for even what we have here called the proximal cause). The better solution, according to Stackhouse and Wells, is to apply a psycholinguistic model. Psycholinguistic models (discussed briefly in Chapter 3) have been used for many years in the field of speech-language pathology (see Baker, Croot, McLeod, and Paul, 2001, for a review). Stackhouse and Wells provide a specific model for examining psycholinguistic processing in children with speech sound disorders (see Figure 4.1).

Note the term *phonological* that is used in Figure 4.1. Stackhouse and Wells (1997) point out that it is "important to distinguish a *phonological problem*—a term used to describe children's speech output difficulties in a linguistic sense—from a *phonological processing problem*—a psycholinguistic term used to refer to the specific underlying cognitive deficits that may give rise to speech and/or literacy difficulties" (p. 8). Pascoe, Stackhouse, and Wells (2005) presented a detailed case study of the application of this model.

Stackhouse and Wells (1997) did not necessarily develop their model with the specific intention of identifying subgroups. However, because their approach provides for the creation of a profile of the difficulty each child may be experiencing, using it to identify

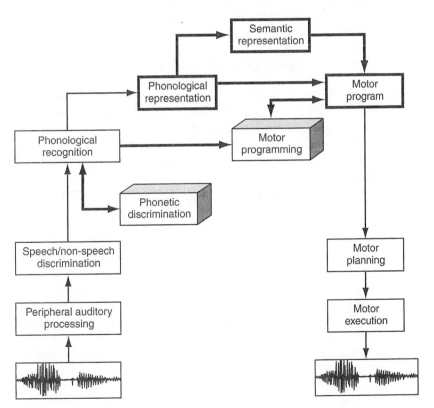

■ FIGURE 4.1 Speech processing model by Stackhouse and Wells (1997).

Note: The broad arrows and shaded boxes represent processes hypothesized to occur offline.

Source: From *Children's Speech and Literacy Difficulties: A Psycholinguistic Framework* (p. 350) by J. Stackhouse and B. Wells, 1997. Copyright John Wiley & Sons Limited. Reproduced with permission.

subgroups seems at least plausible. One might, for example, evaluate large groups of children with speech sound disorders of unknown origin to determine if certain profiles are more common than others. Stackhouse (2000) used this approach in a longitudinal study to suggest how different profiles might help differentiate children with speech sound disorders who have later literacy problems from those who learn to read normally.

Classification by Symptomatology

Barbara Dodd and her colleagues take the view that neither of the preceding two approaches is adequate for classification of speech sound disorders of unknown origin. Dodd, Holm, Crosbie, and McCormack (2005) note that "there is as yet no theoretically adequate or clinically relevant explanation of disordered speech . . . current models of the speech-processing chain . . . fail to disentangle causal, co-morbid, and consequent difficulties" (p. 44). Dodd and her colleagues argue that "surface error patterns" (i.e., symptoms) provide the best perspective on classification and that such patterns do in fact explain the nature of the disorder. They have suggested four possible subgroups. A recently published test, the *Diagnostic Evaluation of Articulation and Phonology (DEAP)* (Dodd, Hua, Crosbie, Holm, and Ozanne, 2006) was specifically developed to allow clinicians to classify children using this system of subgroups.

The first subgroup proposed by Dodd is *articulation disorder* in which the child produces consistent substitution or distortion errors on a limited number of phonemes (often /s/ or /r/). Errors don't change whether the production is spontaneous or imitated. In a cohort study of 320 children with speech sound disorders, Broomfield and Dodd (2004) classified 40 (12.5 percent) children into this subgroup.

The second and largest of Dodd's subgroups, *phonological delay* includes children whose errors can be described using phonological process labels that are also seen in much younger typically developing children (i.e., developmental patterns). Broomfield and Dodd (2004) classified 184/320 (57.5 percent) children into this subgroup.

Dodd's third subgroup, *consistent phonological disorder*, includes children who produce developmental patterns but also produce nondevelopmental patterns (i.e., those not usually produced by typically developing children). In this case, the nondevelopmental patterns are produced consistently. Broomfield and Dodd (2004) classified 66/320 (20.6 percent) children into this subgroup.

Dodd's final and smallest subgroup, *inconsistent phonological disorder*, includes children who produce nondevelopmental error patterns but do so inconsistently. In this case, inconsistency refers to variations in output on repeated productions of the same words. Interestingly this happens to also be one of the "emerging features" discussed earlier with reference to CAS. Broomfield and Dodd (2004) classified 30/320 (9.4 percent) children into this subgroup.

Dodd's efforts have included attempts to empirically validate the categories. Such validation is being sought by demonstrating that the children in different groups respond differentially to different treatment approaches. For example, Dodd and Bradford (2000) presented case study data on three children: A child with a consistent phonological disorder received the most benefit from a phonological contrast approach, whereas two children with inconsistent phonological disorders initially responded most quickly to a core vocabulary approach. Once these latter children's errors became more consistent, one of them responded more quickly to phonological contrast therapy. These same associations between subgroup membership and response to therapy were also observed in a follow-up group study including a total of 18 children (Crosbie, Holm, and Dodd, 2005).

SUMMARY OF CLASSIFICATION

As comprehensive as the preceding discussion is, it only represents some current best guesses as to how to classify children with speech sound disorders. Other perspectives are also possible. Clearly, considerable work remains. For the organically based disorders, clinicians know a great deal about how to assess and treat these children. As mentioned previously, specialized texts are available. Considerable progress has also been made in understanding the nature of the problem where the origin is currently unknown, but clinicians do not yet have a clear consensus about the exact nature of this group. Lacking such a consensus, speech-language pathologists are left to choose from a number of available options for the assessment and intervention for these children. These options are outlined in subsequent chapters.

FACTORS RELATED TO SPEECH SOUND DISORDERS

In the preceding pages we have reviewed attempts that have been made to group various factors related to speech sound disorders of unknown origin into groups or classifications. The effort to classify origins is moving the field ahead in terms of how to view disorders of unknown etiology. However, no single factor that might describe this group of clients has emerged. It appears that some factors examined to date may be associated with at least some of these children. An appreciation of these factors is important, given that the question of subgroups is still not fully resolved. Perhaps more important, clients, families, and clinicians are all interested in these factors, as they may offer insight into the nature of the problem for specific children.

Several approaches have been taken to examining related factors. One of the more common approaches has been the use of correlational studies. Such studies explore whether speech sound production and selected variables covary or coexist within individuals. Stated more simply, they seek to determine whether one variable (such as status of speech sound production skill) is related to another variable (such as intelligence). A high correlation between two variables implies that such variables are related to each other. For example, a high correlation between a measure of intelligence and the acquisition of speech sounds would indicate that a high number of correct articulatory responses co-occur with a high score on a measure of intelligence, and a low number of correct articulatory responses co-occur with a low score on a measure of intelligence. A low correlation, on the other hand, would indicate that the score obtained on an articulatory measure and the score on an intelligence measure do not covary and are not systematically related to each other. When a correlation is high, the status of one variable can sometimes be predicted from knowledge of the status of the second variable. This does not mean, however, that a causal relationship exists between the two; it simply means that they are related to each other. The frequently cited warning, "Correlation does not imply causation," speaks to precisely this issue. Correlational studies are, however, useful for purposes of identifying topics worthy of further study.

In correlational studies, investigators typically have looked at a single variable (for example, speech sound discrimination) as it relates to articulatory status. A second approach to examining related factors has been the use of multivariate analysis techniques to look at the relationship between speech sound status and several variables simultaneously within individuals.

A third approach used for examining potential factors involves comparisons between normal children and children with speech sound disorders on a variable of interest, for example, reading performance. When reviewing studies of this type, several points should be kept in mind. First, as stated earlier, a statistically significant difference between the groups on a particular variable (for example, language comprehension) does not imply a causal relationship. Other variables may account for the differences found between the groups. For example, if children with speech sound disorders were found to have poorer reading skills than a normal control group, differences in reading performance may be related to something other than poor articulation (e.g., phonological awareness). Such studies, however, may point to areas that are worthy of further exploration in terms of how they relate to phonological performance. Second, statistical significance does not imply clinical/practical significance for two reasons: (1) group trends frequently do not reflect individual performance and (2) relatively small quantitative differences resulting in statistically significant differences may have limited clinical utility. In a study reported by Dubois and Bernthal (1978), a small but statistically significant difference was found between two types of speech sound measures (spontaneous picture naming and a delayed imitation sentence production), and yet the numerical difference in average performance, based on a 20-item task, was less than 2 items. Because of the small numerical difference, the clinical or practical significance of such group findings might be questioned.

A fourth approach used to examine related factors is to present descriptive profiles of children who evidence speech sound disorders and trace their history over time. A comprehensive investigation of speech-language, prosody, and voice characteristics of children with speech sound disorders was reported by Shriberg and Kwiatkowski (1994). None of the factors studied were good predictors for short- or long-term normalization.

Winitz (1969) has suggested that some variables that have been studied in relation to speech sound disorders may best be viewed as macrovariables (variables formed from several other variables). The variable of age, for example, may be comprised of such components as physical maturation, motor coordination, cognition, and linguistic maturity. As Winitz pointed out, although a macrovariable may be found to correlate with speech sound production skill, the individual components accounting for the correlation may be difficult to identify.

At the present time, the largest group of identified causal factors are in the area of structure and function of the speech and hearing mechanism. These will be discussed first. Next, we will discuss cognitive-linguistic factors, and in the final section we will discuss psychosocial factors.

STRUCTURE AND FUNCTION OF THE SPEECH AND HEARING MECHANISM

An obvious consideration when evaluating an individual's phonologic status relates to the potential for problems that may be manifested in the structure and function of the speech and hearing mechanisms. Such problems may require medically related interventions such as surgical management for a child with cleft palate in order for the child to achieve velopharyngeal closure for production of stops, fricatives, and affricates.

Otitis Media (OME)

It has long been supposed that frequent episodes of middle ear disease, which are accompanied by a buildup of liquid in the middle ear space (also called *otitis media with effusion*, or *OME*), may result in a delay in speech sound development. This is, of course, the basis for Shriberg's SD–OME subgroup of speech sound disorders of unknown origin discussed previously. The assumption is that the accumulating liquid blocks the transmission of sound, resulting in a mild to moderate hearing loss. Although the condition invariably resolves and hearing usually returns to normal, frequent episodes may result in a history of inconsistent auditory input. Unfortunately, the research results to confirm these assumptions has been quite mixed. Shriberg, Flipsen, and colleagues (2000) identified 27 separate studies conducted on this question. Of the 27 studies, 17 (63 percent) suggested no impact, while 21 (78 percent) suggested some significant impact. (Some studies included comparisons using multiple measurement approaches; both impacts and no impacts were reported in some studies.)

Several reasons might account for this unclear picture. First, the majority of children experience at least one episode of OME during the preschool years (Adams and Benson, 1991). Assuming an average duration of 29 days per episode (Teele, Klein, Rosner, and the Greater Boston Otitis Media Study Group, 1984), a single episode would be unlikely to lead to a long-standing problem with the production of speech sounds. Some children, however, seem predisposed to multiple episodes of OME. Although comparisons were usually made between children with "frequent" OME and those with few or no episodes, the studies in this area differed widely as to their definition of the term *frequent*.

A second factor in the mixed findings for OME is that the studies differed in the reliability of documenting actual episodes of OME. Some investigators relied solely on parent report, while others evaluated available medical records. Even for studies using medical records, however, some physicians made their diagnosis by visualizing the tympanic membrane, while others used tympanometry (even within the same study). Another complication to identifying OME is reports from longitudinal studies such as those by Marchant and associates (1984) of "silent otitis," or episodes in which the child displays no actual symptoms. Thus, some children in the so-called control groups in some studies may have actually had OME that was not identified.

A third complication in the OME research is that few studies document or report the hearing status of the children during OME episodes. Although a temporary conductive hearing loss is often present during episodes of OME, the extent of the loss can vary widely across children. The timing of any hearing loss may also be crucial. Hearing loss occurring between 12 and 18 months of age may be especially troublesome for speech sound development (Shriberg, Friel-Patti, Flipsen, and Brown, 2000).

A fourth factor is access to medical care. Prompt medical treatment of OME may prevent significant accumulation of liquid in the middle ear space and thus eliminate the resulting hearing loss. If the children in the studies did not all have equal access to such treatment, or if the treatment was not applied consistently, it should not be surprising that study outcomes varied widely.

A final factor that might account for some of the mixed findings in the OME studies is variation in socioeconomic status (SES) of the children both within and across studies. Socioeconomic status will be discussed in more detail below, but children from low SES backgrounds appear to be at higher risk for speech sound disorders because of either poorer-quality language stimulation and/or poorer access to health care.

Clearly, all of the above factors interact, making the question of whether OME can impact speech sound acquisition a very difficult one to answer. One proposal has been to design better studies where children are recruited in the first year of life and monitored carefully over time. Roberts, Rosenfeld, and Zeisel (2004) surveyed 14 such prospective studies using a statistical technique known as *meta-analysis* and concluded that there were "no to very small associations of OM to speech and language development in most children" (p. 247). Roberts and colleagues did note that such a conclusion assumes an optimal learning environment, which may not always be present. Thus, particular children may be at greater risk for delayed speech development from OME. Findings from a study by Shriberg, Flipsen, and colleagues (2000) support such a conclusion. Using two different groups, these authors reported that having frequent OME resulted in no increased risk of delayed speech in a group of children from a university-affiliated, general pediatric clinic group but a significantly increased risk of approximately 4.6 times for a group of Native American children living on a reservation. Children in the latter group were from a lower SES background and had poorer access to good-quality medical care.

Speech Sound Perception

Speech-language pathologists have long been interested in a possible relationship between the perception (often referred to as *discrimination*) and production of speech sounds in individuals with normal auditory acuity. In the early days of the profession, many clinicians assumed that a major reason children produced sounds in error was because they didn't properly discriminate one sound from another. Phonemic perception is a form of auditory perception in which the listener and/or speaker distinguishes the sound contrasts used in a language. Linguistic or phonemic perception also includes the storing and accessing of sounds for the recognition of words that are heard. From a clinical perspective, this skill includes the ability to detect differences between sounds in the language and differences between correct and incorrect productions. Clinicians are interested in determining whether or not production errors are related to errors in perception of speech sounds. Numerous investigations have been conducted to ascertain the relationship between production and perception in children with normal phonologic development and children with delayed phonologic development.

As was stated in the discussion of normal acquisition (see Chapter 3), some scholars view phonemic perception as essentially completed by the time the normally developing child has acquired the first 50 words. If this assumption is correct, it follows that the child's speech sound production errors can be ascribed primarily to difficulties in motor (articulatory) control and/or phonologic (linguistic) factors, rather than perception. If, however, the acquisition and development of speech sound perception continues into the preschool and even the early school years, or if some children with phonological delays also are delayed in the development of speech sound perception, some production errors may be the result of a mismatch between the adult form of the word and the child's perception and underlying representation (storage) of the word. In other words, some children's production errors may be related to phonemic perception. Finally, many treatment programs include auditory perceptual tasks (e.g., discrimination, auditory bombardment) on the assumption that such tasks help the child to learn the adult sound system.

Before discussing studies concerning the relationship between production and perception, it is useful to recall some of the previously reviewed data on auditory perception in normal infants and young children. In Chapter 3, evidence was presented that infants can perceive many contrasts used in the phonology of their language at the time they begin to speak. Indeed, experiments have shown that infants under 1 year of age are able to discriminate between many speech sounds (Eimas, Siqueland, Jusczyk, and Vigorito, 1971; Butterfield and Cairns, 1974; Jusczyk and Luce, 2002). Apparently, within the first few months of life, infants perceive differences in the acoustic signal as categorical differences similar to those serving as phonemic contrasts in adult languages. Speech sound perception experiments also suggest that as children begin to speak words, they do not perceive all of the relevant phonologic contrasts. This finding may be explained in part by the fact that infant perception tasks typically require only that the participant note changes in the acoustic signal, whereas linguistic or phonemic perception involves an active attention to contrasting speech sounds and sequences in order to identify, store, recognize and retrieve distinct lexical items. The skills required for nonlinguistic discrimination (same-different distinctions) tested in investigations of infant perception are very different from those required to distinguish and store lexical items.

Perceptual discrimination experiments with preschoolers, beginning with children at approximately age 2, have shown that young children can make most of the phonologic distinctions in English. Barton (1976), who attempted to determine whether normal 2-year-olds had full or partial linguistic perception, reported that although his participants were unable to make all of the perceptions required on the experimental tasks, they were able to perceive sounds they were not producing. He concluded that their perception was more advanced than their production and suggested that they may have had full or nearly full perception at this early age. He also pointed out that word familiarity influenced the children's performance on perceptual tasks: Children made more errors on the perception of new or unfamiliar words than on words they knew well, a finding that has been reported by other investigators.

Perceptual errors may result from a partially correct internal representation that becomes more accurate with increased exposure to the adult speech models. If a child fails to notice the discrepancy between his or her initial internal representation and the adult form, a perceptually based production error may be the result.

The study of young children's perceptual skills is of interest to both clinicians and researchers. The extent to which the findings based on children with normal perceptual and production skills are applicable to the phonologically delayed population is unclear, since it is not certain that inferences can be drawn from normal to phonologically delayed speakers. Locke (1980a) suggested that a difference may exist between the role of perception in the acquisition of phonologic errors and its role in the maintenance of a speech sound disorder.

Clinical research on speech sound perception and its relationship to speech sound disorders has sought to determine (1) if a relationship exists, (2) the relationship between general and phoneme-specific measures of discrimination and production as well as that between external and internal discrimination, and (3) the relationship between perceptual training and production.

Relationship between Speech Sound Disorders and Speech Sound Discrimination

The possibility of a relationship between speech sound disorders and speech sound (auditory) perception was first investigated in the 1930s. This early perceptual research, referred to as *speech sound discrimination research*, relied primarily on general measures of speech sound discrimination (tests measuring many sound contrasts), which required the participant to judge whether word or nonsense pairs verbally presented by the examiner were the same or different. In such tests, there was generally no attempt to compare the specific phoneme production errors with the specific perception errors the participant might have made.

Travis and Rasmus (1931) found that on a discrimination test of 366 paired nonsense-syllable items, normal participants performed significantly better than participants with mild speech sound disorders. Other researchers comparing the discrimination skills of normal speakers and speakers with speech sound errors (Kronvall and Diehl, 1954; Clark, 1959) reported similar findings; that is, normal speakers had significantly better skills, and several investigators found a positive correlation between performance on an articulation test and performance on a test of speech sound discrimination (Reid, 1947a; Carrell and Pendergast, 1954).

A number of studies, however, found no relationship between discrimination and speech sound productions. In a study similar to that of Travis and Rasmus, Hall (1938) reported no significant differences in discrimination skill between normal speakers and two groups of speakers with mild and severe speech sound disorders. Hansen (1944), who studied discrimination and articulation in a college-age population, also reported little relationship between the two variables; likewise, Mase (1946), Prins (1962b), Garrett (1969), and Veatch (1970) found no significant differences in speech sound discrimination skills between children with speech sound disorders and normal speakers.

Sherman and Geith (1967) suggested that one reason for the equivocal findings may have been that experimental groups were chosen on the basis of articulatory proficiency rather than speech sound discrimination performance, and consequently etiologies associated with articulatory-impaired students may not have been limited to individuals with poor speech sound discrimination skills. To control for perceptual skill, Sherman and Geith administered a 50-item speech sound discrimination test to 529 kindergarten children and then selected from this group 18 children with high discrimination scores and 18 with low scores. These two groups were given a 176-item picture-articulation test. The authors reported that children with high speech sound discrimination scores obtained significantly higher articulation scores than the group with lower discrimination scores. They concluded that poor speech sound discrimination skill may be causally related to poor articulation performance.

Schwartz and Goldman (1974) investigated the possible effects on performance by young children of the type of discrimination task required and found that their participants consistently made more errors when stimulus words were presented in a paired-comparison context (goat and coat; coat and boat) than when target words were included in carrier phrase and sentence contexts (as in "The man brought a coat"). They also found that when background noise was present during stimulus presentation, performance was poorer, particularly for the paired-comparison words. The authors urged speech-language pathologists to test discrimination with tasks that are meaningful and familiar to children, and under the kind of listening conditions the child is likely to encounter in his or her environment.

After reviewing the early articulation and discrimination literature, Weiner (1967) attributed variations in findings to the fact that (1) different types of discrimination tasks were used, (2) participants of different age levels were used, and (3) participants reflected varying degrees of articulatory defectiveness from one study to another. He further concluded that speech sound discrimination is a developmental skill, which ceilings at about 8 years, and that a positive relationship exists between auditory discrimination problems and more severe articulation difficulties at age levels below 9 years. After reviewing the studies on the relationship between auditory discrimination and articulation performance, Winitz (1984) identified a number of factors that may account for the absence of consistent reports of a positive relationship between articulatory performance and speech sound discrimination measures: (1) a lack of relevance of the discrimination test items, (2) a lack of consideration of the child's specific speech sound errors, and (3) a lack of consideration of phonetic context in which the production error occurs.

Relationship between General and Phoneme-Specific Measures; External and Internal Monitoring

In most of the investigations cited above, discrimination was tested through general speech sound discrimination measures—that is, tasks comprised of items sampling a wide variety of sound contrasts (e.g., *s*un-*b*un, *k*ey-*t*ea, *sh*oe-*z*oo) and designed to examine the participant's overall capacity to distinguish among a large number of speech sounds in a variety of phonetic contexts. Locke (1980a) pointed out that in testing speech sound perception of clients with speech sound disorders, the critical issue is the clients' ability to discriminate the sound or segments that they misarticulate. Although clients may not have a general problem with speech sound discrimination, they may have phoneme-specific perceptual difficulties on sounds they misarticulate. Perceptual testing should involve stimuli that focus on the children's specific production errors.

Locke (1980a) recommended going a step further, urging that measures of sound perception should not only be phoneme specific but also context specific. He argued that perceptual tasks should reflect the child's production errors and reflect those phonetic environments (words) in which error productions occur and include both the error productions and the target productions.

Locke studied children's ability to discriminate sounds they produced in error when those sounds were reproduced and contrasted with the correct sound by the adult examiner. Specifically, 131 children were tested on a perceptual task in which the examiner produced imitations of the participant's error productions, and the participants were then required to judge whether the examiner's productions were correct productions of the target word. Locke reported that 70 percent of the children correctly perceived the correct and incorrect forms of the target words, thus indicating that many children could correctly discriminate sounds made by an adult, that they produced in error. About one-third of the contrasts misproduced were also misperceived, but the misperceptions were not evenly distributed across all misproductions. Although the substitution of one voiceless fricative for another accounted for 49 percent of the production errors, these contrasts accounted for 89 percent of the misperceptions.

In a study of 14 2-year-old children, Eilers and Oller (1976) found some perceptual confusions in word and nonsense pairs where production of one segment was substituted for another. Yet other common production errors were discriminated by most of their participants. They concluded that some production errors may be related to perceptual difficulties and others to motor constraints.

Strange and Broen (1980) compared 21 children between the ages of 2 and 11 on their production and perception of word-initial /w/, /r/, and /l/. They concluded from their data that both perception and production of phonemic contrasts develop gradually and that perception of a contrast usually preceded its production.

Velleman (1983) collected data from children ages 3 to 5 on a production task that included naming of pictures and objects in a play situation and the imitation of nonsense syllables. She then tested the children's perception of /s/ and /θ/—/s/ because it is easy to perceive and /θ/ because it is not "acoustically salient" and is thus relatively difficult to perceive—and computed a correlation between the two tasks. The data confirmed her hypothesis that some frequently occurring production errors in children's speech are easier to perceive than others. Since contrasts involving /s/ were relatively easily perceived, Velleman inferred that the late acquisition of /s/ could be ascribed to motor constraints. In contrast, the /θ/ versus /f/ contrast is a difficult distinction to make and, as she predicted, only children with high perception scores (over 80 percent) obtained high production scores on these phonemes. More errors were made on both perception and production in the case of /s/, and there was no significant correlation between the two measures.

In summary, some speech sound contrasts remain difficult to discriminate as late as 3 years or older, even in normal developing children. There does not, however, appear to be a correlation between many of the production errors seen in children and measures of speech sound perception. This finding suggests that while perception might be a factor in some misarticulations, this factor cannot account for others.

An additional testing variable frequently considered in phoneme-specific discrimination testing is the source of the speech production that the participant is required to judge. When the task involves discrimination of a stimulus presented from an external source, such as speech productions from another person or recorded stimuli, it is termed *external discrimination*, or monitoring. External discrimination can also include *external self-discrimination*, of which listening to and making judgments of tape-recorded samples of one's own speech is an example.

When the discrimination or perceptual task involves a judgment of one's own ongoing speech sound productions, it is called *internal discrimination*, or internal monitoring. During internal discrimination, the speaker has available both air- and bone-conducted auditory cues.

Studies of speech sound discrimination skills of young children with delayed speech sound development have indicated that children frequently were able to make external judgments of sound contrasts involving their error sounds (Locke and Kutz, 1975; Chaney and Menyuk, 1975). In a study employing phoneme-specific discrimination tasks, Aungst and Frick (1964) utilized the *Deep Test of Articulation* (McDonald, 1964b), in which the /r/ was tested in 58 productions, to study the relationship between /r/ production and four measures of speech sound discrimination. Three of the discrimination tasks were designed by the investigators to assess participants' discrimination of their own /r/ productions as they occurred in a set of 30 words. These discrimination tasks required each participant to (1) make an immediate right-wrong judgment of his or her /r/ production after speaking each word, (2) make right-wrong judgments of his or her /r/ productions after such productions had been audio recorded and played back, and (3) make same-different judgments of his or her /r/ productions as they followed the examiner's correct productions presented via audio tape recording. The fourth discrimination task was the *Templin Test of Auditory Discrimination* (Templin, 1957), a general test of external discrimination. The participants were children, 8 years or older, who made errors only on /r/. The authors reported high correlations among their three discrimination tasks but low correlations between each of those tests and the Templin general discrimination measure. Moderate correlation coefficients of .69, .66, and .59 were obtained between each of the three phoneme-specific discrimination tasks and scores on the *Deep Test of Articulation* for /f/. In contrast, the Templin discrimination test scores did not correlate well with the articulation measure. These findings indicate some relationship between performance on the *Deep Test of Articulation* and the phoneme-specific discrimination measures but not between the *Deep Test of Articulation* and the general test of discrimination.

Lapko and Bankson (1975) also compared external and internal monitoring with consistency of articulation, as measured by the *Deep Test of Articulation*, in a group of 25 kindergarten and first-grade children exhibiting misarticulations of /s/. All measures were phoneme-specific to /s/. They reported a significant correlation (r = .55) between the child's ability to discriminate his or her own productions of /s/ and the consistency of misarticulation of /s/. In other words, those participants with the higher number of correct productions on the *Deep Test of Articulation* also had higher scores on the measure of internal discrimination. A significant correlation was not obtained between external monitoring tasks and articulation consistency as measured on the *Deep Test of Articulation*.

Wolfe and Irwin (1973) and Stelcik (1972) provided further evidence of a positive correlation between articulatory skill and self-monitoring (internal monitoring) of error sounds. But the results of other investigations (Woolf and Pilberg, 1971; Shelton, Johnson, and Arndt, 1977) have indicated that the findings in such studies may be influenced by factors such as the consistency of misarticulation, type of discrimination task used to test internal monitoring, and nature of the stimulus items.

Hoffman, Stager, and Daniloff (1983) suggested that current phoneme-specific, external discrimination tasks may not be sensitive to allophonic variations that might be perceived by misarticulating children. For example, the prevocalic voicing contrast that a misarticulating child perceives and produces may not be within the perceptual boundary of an adult phoneme and, consequently, not perceived by the adult; what the child may perceive as a contrast between adult allophones of /z/ may not be perceived by the adult listener because both allophones are within the adult's perceptual boundary of /z/. Such sound variations may be used by some children to contrast forms that are not used in a contrastive manner by adults. It would follow that an adult examiner would evaluate such contrasts as a mismatch between the child's production and the adult standard. These authors have suggested that "meaningful subgroups of misarticulating children may be found to manipulate subphonemic, that is allophonic, acoustic cues in nonstandard manners and thus lead to their identification as misarticulations" (p. 214).

Discrimination Improvement and Articulatory Productions

The influence of discrimination training on production has also been considered by investigators. Historically, clinicians routinely conducted some type of discrimination training, or "ear training," as a precursor to production training; however, that is no longer the case. Investigators have attempted to determine whether or not a functional relationship exists between speech sound production and discrimination and more specifically, whether discrimination training affects production.

Sonderman (1971) reported an investigation designed to assess (1) the effect of speech sound discrimination training on articulation skills and (2) the effect of articulation training on speech sound discrimination skill. Holland's speech sound discrimination program (1967) and the S-Pack (Mowrer, Baker, and Schutz, 1968) were administered in alternate sequence to two matched groups of 10 children between 6 and 8 years old, all of whom produced frontal lisps. Four measures were administered to obtain pre-training and post-training profiles for each child: (1) the Wepman Test of Auditory Discrimination (a general test of external monitoring skills), (2) a /s/ specific discrimination test, (3) an examiner-designed general articulation test, and (4) the criterion test from the S-Pack (a deep test of the /s/). Improvement in both discrimination and articulation scores was obtained from both discrimination training and articulation training, regardless of the sequence in which the two types of training were conducted. Articulatory improvement did not necessarily mean that speech sound errors were corrected. Rather, shifts from one type of error to another (e.g., omission to substitution; substitution to distortion) were regarded as evidence of improvement.

Williams and McReynolds (1975) explored the same question that Sonderman did. Two participants were first given production training followed by a discrimination probe, then discrimination training followed by a production probe. Two additional participants received the discrimination training first and the production training second. The probe measures, administered to determine if changes occurred in one modality after training in the other, indicated that production training was effective in changing both production and discrimination; in contrast to Sonderman (1971), however, Williams and McReynolds (1975) found that discrimination training was effective in changing only discrimination and did not generalize to production.

Shelton and colleagues (1977) explored the influence of articulation training on discrimination performance. One group of participants received production training on the /r/

and a second group on the /s/, and pre- and post-discrimination probes, consisting of 40 items specifically related to the error sound, were administered. Results indicated that both groups of participants improved in articulation performance, but no improvement was noted in discrimination performance. The authors suggested that the variance between their results and those of other investigators presumably could be accounted for by one or more unidentified participant or procedural variables.

Rvachew (1994) studied the influence of various types of speech perception training that were administered concurrently with traditional speech sound training. Twenty-seven (27) preschoolers with phonologic impairment who misarticulated /s/ were randomly assigned to three groups each of which received one of the following types of discrimination training: (1) listening to a variety of correctly and incorrectly produced versions of the word *shoe*; (2) listening to the words *shoe* and *moo*; and (3) listening to the words *cat* and *Pete*. Following six weekly treatment sessions, children who received types 1 and 2 training demonstrated superior ability to articulate the target sound in comparison to those who received type 3 training. Based on her data, Rvachew (1994) suggested that "speech perception training should probably be provided concurrently with speech production training" (p. 355). A later report of Rvachew, Rafaat, and Martin (1999) further supported this conclusion. Through two complementary studies, these researchers explored the relationship of stimulability, speech perception ability, and phonological learning. In the first study, participants were treated individually using a cycles approach as prescribed by Hodson (1989). They reported that children who were stimulable for a target sound and who demonstrated good pre-treatment perceptual ability for that sound made more progress in therapy than those who were stimulable for the target sound but had poor speech sound perception for that sound. Children who were not stimulable did not make progress regardless of their perceptual skills. A second study included both individual and group instruction for the participants. Lessons involved phonetically based production activities, and a computer-based program of perceptual training (SAILS, 1995). Results from the second study indicated that all children, regardless of pre-treatment stimulability and /or speech perception skills made progress in production. The authors concluded that "despite the independence of stimulability and speech perception ability before training, there is reason to believe that speech perception training may facilitate the acquisition of stimulability if both production and perception training are provided concurrently to children who demonstrate unstimulability and poor speech perception for the target sound" (p. 40).

The findings reported by Rvachew and colleagues suggest that for children with poor speech sound perception of a target sound, including perceptual training along with production training produces positive clinical outcomes in terms of sound acquisition. This conclusion is supported by findings of a third related study (Rvachew, Nowak, and Cloutier, 2004). In this case, the SAILS perception training program was combined with phonological awareness training (letter recognition, sound-symbol association, onset identification) and compared to a computer-based program for vocabulary development. The two approaches were used concurrently with speech production training. Half of the 34 preschool children were randomly assigned to each group. Findings again showed significantly superior outcomes for the children who received the perception training. Interestingly, the two groups did not differ on phonological awareness outcomes.

Self-Monitoring

Other groups of investigators (Koegel, Koegel, and Ingham, 1986; Koegel, Koegel, Van Voy, and Ingham, 1988) have looked at a related topic and examined the relationship between self-monitoring skills and response generalization into the natural environment. School-age children were provided specific training in self-monitoring of the speech productions. These investigators reported that generalization of correct articulatory responses of the target sounds did not occur until a self-monitoring task was initiated in the treatment program. They concluded that such self-monitoring was required for generalization of the target sounds in the natural environment to occur.

An effort was made by Gray and Shelton (1992) to replicate these findings. They employed self-monitoring procedures, which differed slightly from those employed in the studies by Koegel and colleagues (1986, 1988) with eight elementary school children. Results of their study did not replicate the positive treatment effects reported by Koegel and colleagues (1986, 1988). The authors indicated that different, participant, treatment, and environmental variables may have accounted for different outcomes.

Summary

A relationship appears to exist between speech sound perception and production in some children with impaired phonology although the precise nature of the relationship has not been determined. The suggestion of Lof and Synan (1997) that perceptual testing should focus on speech sounds that a child misarticulates is well supported by research data. Self-monitoring of error productions would appear to be an important skill for normal articulation, but instruments to assess such a skill are lacking. Further data are needed to better understand the relationship between discrimination errors and speech sound disorders. Although the efficacy of speech sound discrimination training as a predecessor to production training has often been questioned, when perceptual deficiencies are present, perceptual training prior to or concurrent with direct instruction would seem appropriate.

Minor Structural Variations of the Speech Mechanism

Speech clinicians, as part of an oral-mechanism examination, are required to make judgments about the structure and/or function of the lips, teeth, tongue, and palate. These oral structures can vary significantly, even among normal speakers. Investigators have attempted to identify relationships between speech sound disorders and structural variations of the oral mechanism.

Major variations were discussed previously under organically based disorders. The following sections highlight lesser variations and their potential impact on speech sound production. Although a strict cause-effect relationship has not been established, such variations may contribute to the difficulty that some children experience.

Lips

Approximation of the lips is required for the formation of the bilabial phonemes /b/, /p/, and /m/; lip rounding is required for various vowels and the consonants /w/ and /hw/. An impairment that would inhibit lip approximation or rounding might result in misarticulation of these sounds. Fairbanks and Green (1950) examined various dimensions of the lips in 30 adult speakers with superior consonant production and 30 with inferior consonant production and reported no differences on various lip measurements between the two groups.

Certain deformities of the lips such as the enlarged lips in Ackerman syndrome (Ackerman, Ackerman, and Ackerman, 1973) or congenital double lips (Eski, Nisanci, Aktas, and Sengezer, 2007) may interfere with speech production but does not in every case. These findings suggest that only major deviations in lip structure or function are likely to impact speech sound production.

Teeth

Several English consonants require intact dentition for correct production. Labiodental phonemes (/f/ and /v/) require contact between the teeth and lower lip for their production, and linguadental phonemes require interdental tongue placement for /ð/ and /θ/ productions. The tongue tip alveolars (/s/, /z/) require that the airstream pass over the cutting edge of the incisors.

Researchers investigating the relationship between deviant dentition and consonant production have examined the presence or absence of teeth, position of teeth, and dental occlusion. *Occlusion* refers to the alignment of the first molar teeth when the jaws are closed, and *malocclusion* refers to the imperfect or irregular position of the teeth when jaws are closed. Lay terms to describe different types of occlusion include open bite and overbite. Examples of different types of occlusion may be seen in Figure 4.2.

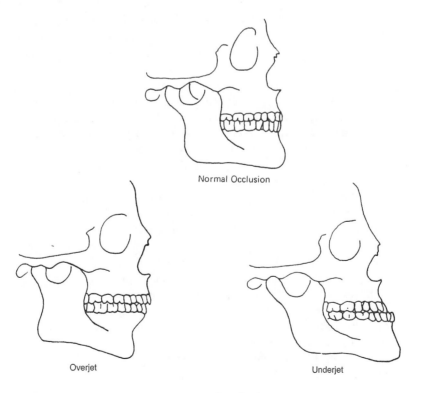

Normal Occlusion

Overjet

Underjet

■ **FIGURE 4.2**   Examples of types of occlusions.

Bernstein (1954) identified malocclusions in children with normal and defective speech but did not find a higher incidence of malocclusion in children with speech sound problems than in children with normal skills. He found that speech sound errors were generally not related to malocclusion, except in the case of the open bite (the teeth do not come together from the first or second molar on one side to the same tooth on the opposite side). Fairbanks and Lintner (1951) examined molar occlusion, occlusion of the anterior teeth, and anterior spaces in 60 adults, 30 of whom were judged to have superior speech sound skills and 30 with inferior skills. They found that neutrocclusion (normal jaw relationship with a slight malocclusion in the anterior segments) tended to predominate in the group of superior speakers, and distocclusion (malocclusion with retrusion of the mandible) and mesiocclusion (malocclusion with protrusion of the mandible) tended to occur more often in the group of speakers with production errors. When data on the participants were divided according to (1) no marked dental deviation and (2) one or more marked dental deviations, the authors found that marked dental deviations occurred significantly more frequently in the inferior speakers than in the superior ones. Open bite was present in the inferior speaking group but not in the superior speaking group. Laine, Jaroma, and Linnasalo (1987) conducted a study of speech errors and incisor teeth issues in 451 college-age students in Finland. They reported significantly larger amounts of horizontal overjet or vertical overbite in participants with "audibly clear" /s/ distortions compared to their peers with no speech errors.

Although speakers with normal articulatory skills tend to have a lower incidence of malocclusion than speakers with articulatory errors, malocclusion itself does not preclude normal production. Subtelny, Mestre, and Subtelny (1964) found malocclusion to coexist with both normal and defective speech. They also noted that during /s/ production, normal speakers with malocclusion (distocclusion) tended to position the tongue tip slightly to the rear of the lower incisors (i.e., what some have called a tongue-tip down /s/) when compared to normal speakers with normal occlusion.

Starr (1972) reported several clinical observations concerning dental arch relationships and speech production skills. He stated that a speech sound problem is highly probable in individuals with a short or narrow maxillary (upper) arch and a normal mandibular (lower) arch. The consonants likely to be affected by such conditions are /s, z, ʃ, tʃ, f, v, t, and d/. He further noted that rotated teeth and supernumerary (extra) teeth do not generally present significant speech problems.

Another area of interest to investigators has been the influence of missing teeth on speech sound skill. Bankson and Byrne (1962) examined the influence of missing teeth in kindergarten and first-grade children on the production of /s/, /ʃ/, and /f/ in the word-initial, medial, and final positions, and /z/ in the word-medial position. Initially, participants were identified either as children who had correct articulation with their teeth intact or as children who had incorrect articulation with their teeth intact. After four months, articulation skills were reassessed and the number of missing central or lateral incisors tabulated. A significant relationship was found between presence or absence of teeth and correct production of /s/, but not of /f/, /ʃ/, or /z/. However, some children maintained correct production of /s/ despite the loss of incisors.

Snow (1961) examined the influence of missing teeth on consonant production in first-grade children. Participants were divided into two groups: those with normal incisors and those with missing or grossly abnormal incisor teeth. The consonants examined were /f/, /v/, /θ/, /ð/, /s/, and /z/. Although Snow found that a significantly larger proportion of children with dental deviations misarticulated consonants, she also found that three-quarters of the children with defective dentition did not misarticulate these sounds. In contrast to Bankson and Byrne, who noted significant differences only for /s/, Snow found significant differences for all phonemes. Snow suggested that although dental status may be a crucial factor in sound productions for some children, it does not appear to be significant for most. This conclusion is supported by Gable, Kummer, Lee, Creaghead, and Moore (1995), who examined 26 children whose incisor teeth had to be extracted before age 5 years. At age 8 to 10 years, the speech sound production skills of these children were not significantly different from that of an age-matched group of children without the premature extractions. However, Pahkala, Laine, and Lammi (1991) reported that earlier appearance of the permanent teeth was associated with a decreased occurrence of speech sound disorders in a group of children acquiring Finnish.

Tongue

The tongue is generally considered the most important articulator for speech production. Tongue movements during speech production include tip elevation, grooving, and protrusion. The tongue is relatively short at birth, growing longer and thinner at the tip with age.

Ankyloglossia, or *tongue-tie,* are terms used to describe a restricted lingual frenum (sometimes called the *frenulum*). At one time, it was commonly assumed that an infant or child with ankyloglossia should have his or her frenum clipped to allow greater freedom of tongue movement and better articulation of tongue tip sounds, and frenectomies (clipping of the frenum of the tongue) were performed relatively frequently. However, McEnery and Gaines (1941) examined 1,000 patients with speech disorders and identified only 4 individuals with abnormally short frenums. Their most extreme case of a short frenum was a 10-year-old boy, whose only error was a /w/ for /r/ substitution; the error was corrected following speech instruction. The authors recommended against surgery for ankyloglossia because of the possibility of hemorrhages, infections, and scar tissue.

Fletcher and Meldrum (1968) examined the relationship between length of the lingual frenum and articulation. They compared two groups of sixth-grade students, 20 with limited lingual movement and 20 with greater lingual movement, and reported that participants with restricted lingual movement scored within normal limits on a measure of articulation but tended to have more articulation errors than the group with greater lingual movement. The possibility of some relationship between frenum length and speech sound problems is supported by a more recent study that examined 200 children age 6 to 12 years. Ruffoli and colleagues (2005) classified the severity of ankyloglossia based on frenum length and reported "a relationship between the presence of speech anomalies and a decreased mobility of the tongue, but only for those subjects who frenulum length resulted in moderate or severe levels of ankyloglossia" (p. 174).

Clipping of the frenum does still occur, which raises the question as to whether it makes a difference. Messner and Lalakea (2002) reported results from a group of children age 1 to 12 years who underwent such procedures. Formal speech evaluations by speech-language pathologists indicated that 9 of 11 (82 percent) of the children with pre-operative speech errors had improved their speech. A similar study by Heller, Gabbay, O'Hara,

Heller, and Bradley (2005) reported improvement in 10 of 11 (91 percent) cases. These findings suggest that frenum clipping may make a difference.

Although too large a tongue (*macroglossia*) or too small a tongue (*microglossia*) might be expected to affect speech sound skills, there appears to be little relationship between the two. However, these variables have not been adequately investigated. The tongue is a muscular structure capable of considerable change in length and width and thus, regardless of size, is generally capable of the mobility necessary for correct sound productions.

One area where the question of the relationship between tongue size and speech sound production skill has been indirectly studied is in some attempts to improve the speech of individuals with Down syndrome. Recall that these individuals have *relative macroglossia* or normal-sized tongues in a small oral cavity. For some time it was assumed that if tongue size is critical to the speech of these individuals, perhaps reducing tongue size might improve their speech. Partial glossectomies (i.e., removal of part of the tongue) were performed on a small number of individuals with Down syndrome during the late 1970s and early 1980s. Objective analysis, however, suggested that such procedures do not result in any significant improvement in speech intelligibility (Klaiman, Witzel, Margar-Bacal, and Munro, 1988; Margar-Bacal, Witzel, and Munro, 1987; Parsons, Iacono, and Rozner, 1987). Klaiman and associates did report that speech was judged to be more visually acceptable following a glossectomy. These procedures are still performed on occasion, although usually the goal is to improve a compromised airway, which can be a problem in some individuals with Down syndrome. The question of the effect of macroglossia on speech sound production remains an open one.

Hard Palate

The relationship between speech sound disorders and variations in hard palate dimensions has received limited attention. Fairbanks and Lintner (1951) measured the hard palates of a group of young adults with superior consonant articulation and a group with inferior consonant articulation. They reported no significant differences in cuspid width, molar width, palatal height, and maximum mouth opening. Removal of any part of the maxilla, if not restored surgically or prosthetically, may create a serious problem for the speaker.

Oral Sensory Function

Oral sensory and kinesthetic feedback play a role in the development and ongoing monitoring of articulatory gestures, and thus the relationship between oral sensory function and speech sound productions has been of interest. Some treatment approaches include the practice of calling the client's attention to sensory cues. Bordon (1984) indicated the need for awareness of *kinesthesis* (sense of movement and position) during therapy. Almost any phonetic placement technique used to teach speech sounds usually includes a description of articulatory contacts and movements necessary for the production of the target speech sound.

The investigation of *somesthesis* (sense of movement, position, touch, and awareness of muscle tension) has focused on (1) temporary sensory deprivation during oral sensory anesthetization (nerve block anesthesia) to determine the effect of sensory deprivation on speech production and (2) assessment of oral sensory perception such as two-point discrimination or oral form discrimination to see if such sensory perception was related to articulatory skill. Considerable research into oral sensory functioning was conducted in the 1960s using a variety of methods to assess oral tactile sensitivity in order to understand if a relationship existed between these sensory tasks and articulation performance. Later research examined articulation of individuals during periods of temporary sensory deprivation, sometimes referred to as *oral blockade*.

Netsell (1986) has suggested that it is likely that adults are not consciously aware of specific speech movements during running speech. He also speculated that children may not be aware of articulatory movements during the acquisition period. If Netsell is correct, the clinician who attempts to utilize somesthetic senses in monitoring running speech may be asking the client to respond to information that is not available at a conscious level without instruction.

Oral Tactile Sensitivity

Early investigators of oral sensory function attempted to explore the sensitivity or threshold of awareness of oral structures to various stimuli. Ringel and Ewanowski (1965) studied oral tactile sensitivity utilizing an esthesiometer, a device used in the measurement of two-point discrimination. They examined discrimination sensitivity of various structures in a normal population and found that the maximal to minimal awareness hierarchy for two-point stimulation (awareness of two points rather than one) was tongue tip, finger tip, lip, soft palate, alveolar ridge, and that the midline of structures tended to be more sensitive than the lateral edges.

Fucci and associates (Arnst and Fucci, 1975; Fucci, 1972) measured the threshold of vibrotactile stimulation of structures in the oral cavity in both normal and speech-disordered individuals. These investigators found that participants with misarticulations tended to have poorer oral sensory abilities than normal speaking participants.

Oral Form Recognition

Oral sensory function has also been investigated extensively through form recognition tasks. Ringel, Burk, and Scott (1970) speculated that form identification (*oral stereognosis*) may provide information on nervous system integrity since the recognition of forms placed in the mouth was assumed to require integrity of peripheral receptors for touch and kinesthesis as well as central integrating processes. Most form recognition tasks require the participant to match forms placed in the oral cavity with drawings of the forms, or to make same-different judgments. Participants tend to improve on such tasks until adolescence when they ceiling-out (i.e., achieve maximum performance possible). Stimuli for such testing are typically small, plastic, three-dimensional forms of varying degrees of similarity, such as triangles, rectangles, ovals, and circles.

Investigators who have studied the relationship between oral form recognition and articulation performance have reported inconsistent results. Arndt, Elbert, and Shelton (1970) did not find a significant relationship between oral form recognition and articulation performance in a third-grade population. But Ringel, House, Burk, Dolinsky, and Scott (1970) reported significant differences on an oral form-matching task between normal-speaking elementary school children and children with articulation errors. Speirs and Maktabi

(1990) reported similar findings. Ringel and associates analyzed their data in greater detail and noted that children with severe misarticulations made more form-recognition errors than children with mild articulation problems. However, a study by Hetrick and Sommers (1988) failed to find differences related to severity of errors.

Some researchers have investigated the relationship between production of specific phonemes and oral sensory function. McNutt (1977) found that children who misarticulated /r/ did not perform as well as the normal speakers on oral form perception tasks; there were, however, no significant differences between the normal speakers and the children who misarticulated /s/.

Bishop, Ringel, and House (1973) compared oral form-recognition skills of deaf high school students who were orally trained (taught to use speech), and those who were taught to use sign language. The authors noted skill differences that favored the orally trained students and postulated that "while a failure in oroperceptual functioning may lead to [speech sound] disorders ..., a failure to use the oral mechanism for speech activities, even in persons with normal orosensory capabilities, may result in poor performance on oroperceptual tasks" (p. 257).

Locke (1968) examined the relationship between articulation skills and oral form-recognition scores from a different perspective. Rather than comparing the performance of normal-speaking children with those of children who demonstrated speech sound errors, he compared the performance on an articulation learning task of 10 normal children with high form-recognition scores with that of 10 normal children with low form-recognition scores. Each participant was required to imitate three German sounds heard on a tape recording of a native German speaker. Locke found that the group with high form-perception scores obtained significantly better production scores on two of the three consonant sounds than the group with low form-identification scores.

McDonald and Aungst (1970) pointed out that an individual can have good articulation skills despite poor oral form-recognition scores. They cited the case of a 21-year-old neurologically impaired male who articulated normally yet demonstrated difficulty in oral form identification and in two-point discrimination on the tongue.

Oral Anesthetization

The relationship between speech sound productions and oral sensory functions has also been examined through sensory deprivation. To study the role of oral sensation during speech, researchers have induced temporary states of oral sensory deprivation through the use of oral nerve-block and topical anesthetization (similar to what occurs prior to dental work). Then they have compared speech under normal conditions with speech under anesthetization on a variety of dimensions, such as overall intelligibility, vowel and consonant articulation, rate, phoneme duration, and physiological and acoustic characteristics.

Gammon, Smith, Daniloff, and Kim (1971) examined the articulation skills of eight adult participants reading 30 sentences under four conditions: (1) normal, (2) with masking noise present, (3) nerve-block anesthesia, and (4) nerve-block anesthesia with masking noise. They noted few vowel distortions under any of the conditions and a 20 percent rate of consonant misarticulation (especially fricatives and affricates) under anesthesia and under anesthesia with noise. Scott and Ringel (1971) studied the articulation of two adult males producing lists of 24 bisyllabic words under normal and anesthetized conditions. They noted that articulatory changes caused by sensory deprivation were largely non-phonemic in nature and included loss of retroflexion and lip-rounding gestures, less tight fricative constrictions, and retracted points of articulation contacts.

Prosek and House (1975) studied four adult speakers reading 20 bisyllabic words in isolation and in sentences under normal and anesthetized conditions. Although intelligibility was maintained in the anesthetized condition, speech rate was slowed and minor imprecisions of articulation were noted. The authors reported that, when anesthetized, speakers produced consonants with slightly greater intraoral air pressure and longer duration than under the normal nonanesthetized condition.

In summary, studies involving anesthetization found that speech remained intelligible although participants did not speak as accurately under this condition as they did under normal conditions. However, the participants in these studies were adult speakers with normal articulation skills prior to the sensory deprivation. It is unclear if reduced oral sensory feedback might interfere with the acquisition of speech or affect remediation.

Oral Sensory Function and Speech Sound Learning

Jordan, Hardy, and Morris (1978) studied the influence of tactile sensation as a feedback mechanism in speech sound learning. Their participants were first-grade boys, nine with good articulation skills and nine with poor articulation skills. Participants were fitted with palatal plates equipped with touch-sensitive electrodes and taught to replicate four positions of linguapalatal contact, with and without topical anesthesia. Children with poor articulation performed less well on tasks of precise tongue placement than children with good articulation. Participants with poor articulation were able to improve their initially poor performance when given specific training on the tongue placement tasks.

Wilhelm (1971) and Shelton, Willis, Johnson, and Arndt (1973) used oral form-recognition materials to teach form recognition to misarticulating children and reported inconsistent results. Wilhelm reported articulation improved as oral form recognition improved. Shelton and colleagues reported results that did not support that finding. Ruscello (1972) reported that form-recognition scores improved in children undergoing treatment for articulation.

Summary

The role of normal oral sensory function or somesthetic feedback in the development and maintenance of speech production is complex. Despite efforts to identify the relationship between oral sensory status and articulatory performance, conclusive findings are lacking. A review of the literature, however, has revealed the following:

1. Oral form recognition improves with age through adolescence.
2. The role of oral sensory feedback in the acquisition of phonology is unclear.
3. Individuals with poor articulation tend to achieve slightly lower scores on form-perception tasks than their normal-speaking peers. However, some individuals with poor form-identification skills have good articulation.
4. During anesthesia, intelligibility is generally maintained but articulation tends to be less accurate.

5. Although some individuals with speech sound disorders may also have oral sensory deficits the neurological mechanisms underlying the use of sensory information during experimental conditions may differ from those operating in normal running speech.

6. Information concerning oral sensory function has not been shown to have clinical applicability.

7. It is important to distinguish between the effects of sensory deprivation in individuals who have already developed good speech skills and the effects in individuals with speech sound disorders.

8. The effects of long-term sensory deprivation have yet to be explored.

MOTOR ABILITIES

Because speech is a motor act, researchers have explored the relationship between speech sound production and motor skills, investigating performance on gross motor tasks as well as oral and facial motor tasks.

General Motor Skills

Studies focusing on the relationship between general or gross motor skills and articulatory abilities have yielded inconsistent and inconclusive results. It may be concluded, however, that individuals with speech sound problems do not have significant retardation in general motor development.

Oral-Facial Motor Skills

Speech is a dynamic process that requires the precise coordination of the oral musculature. During ongoing speech production, fine muscle movements of the lips, tongue, palate, and jaw constantly alter the dimensions of the oral cavity. An assessment of the client's oral motor skills is typically a part of a speech mechanism examination. Tests of diadochokinetic rate or maximum repetition rate (rapid repetition of syllables) have been used frequently to evaluate oral motor skills. Diadochokinetic rate is established either with a *count by time* procedure, in which the examiner counts the number of syllables spoken in a given interval of time, or a *time by count* measurement, in which the examiner notes the time required to produce a designated number of syllables. The advantage of the time by count measurement is that few operations are required since the examiner need only listen to the syllable count and turn off the timing device when the requisite number of syllables is produced. Performance is then sometimes compared to normative data. The syllables most frequently used to assess diadochokinetic rates are /pʌ/, /tʌ/, and /kʌ/ in isolation, syllable repetition, and the sequences /pʌtʌ/, /tʌkʌ/, /pʌkʌ/, /pʌtʌkʌ/. There is evidence that diadochokinetic rates improve with age. Fletcher (1972) examined diadochokinetic rates in normal children ages 6 to 13 years using a count by time procedure. He reported that children increased the number of syllables produced in a given unit of time at each successive age from 7 to 13 years. Data reported by Canning and Rose (1974) indicated that adult values for maximum repetition rates were reached by 9- to 10-year-olds, whereas Fletcher's data show a convergence after age 15.

McNutt (1977) and Dworkin (1978) examined diadochokinetic rates of children with specific misarticulations and of their normal-speaking peers. McNutt examined the rate of alternating syllable productions (e.g., /dʌgə/) in children with normal articulation, children with /s/ misarticulation, and children with /r/ misarticulation. Both groups of children with misarticulations were noted to be slower than normal speakers in syllable production rates. Dworkin examined lingual diadochokinetic rates for the syllables /t ʌ/, /d ʌ/, /k ʌ/, and /g ʌ/, in normal speakers and frontal lisping speakers aged 7 to 12 years. The mean rate of utterances of the syllables tested was significantly lower in participants in the group with speech sound errors.

Some researchers have questioned the usefulness of rapid syllable repetition tasks and their relationship to articulation skills because the movements of articulation are produced by the simultaneous contraction of different groups of muscles rather than the alternating contraction of opposed muscles (McDonald, 1964a). The idea of a different pattern of organization of the muscle movements for diadochokinetic (DDK) tasks is supported by at least two studies of speech kinematics or movement patterns (Adams, Weismer, and Kent, 1993; Smith, Goffman, Zelaznik, Ying, and McGillem, 1995). Findings from these studies suggest that speakers modify the way they move their articulators at fast rates compared to normal rate. This suggests that fast rate productions are qualitatively different from normal rate productions. This makes it difficult to know how meaningful problems observed at fast rates really are.

Winitz (1969) also pointed out that because normal speakers have a history of success with speech sounds, they may have an advantage over speakers with misarticulations on diadochokinetic tasks. Tiffany (1980) pointed out that little is known about the significance of scores obtained on DDK tasks and thus "such measures appear to lack a substantial theoretical base" (p. 895). The one exception to this generality relates to those children that might be considered to evidence childhood apraxia of speech (discussed elsewhere in this chapter). Poor performance in diadochokinetic tasks is often reflective of syllable sequencing problems evident in this population. Another exception would be clients with a history of unusual or delayed oral-motor development, which may be evidenced in sucking, feeding, and swallowing in addition to delayed speech sound development. These children may evidence problems with muscle tone and movement of the oral structures, including independent movement of the tongue and/or lips from the jaw. It would appear that slow or weak oral-motor development may be a contributing factor to the presence of a speech sound disorder.

Although difficult to measure in most clinical settings, another perspective on possible motor deficits in speech sound disorders has involved the measurement of tongue strength. Dworkin and Culatta (1985) found no significant difference in the maximum amount of tongue force that could be exerted by children with speech sound disorders compared to children without any speech difficulties. Dworkin (1978) showed differences specific to children who were producing /s/ errors. A study by Bradford, Murdoch, Thompson, and Stokes (1997) revealed reduced tongue strength in children diagnosed with childhood apraxia of speech (CAS) compared to children with inconsistent phonological disorder and normal-speaking children. However, Robin, Somodi, and Luschei (1991) failed to find such a difference for the children with CAS in their study.

Like diadochokinetic rates, the value of measuring maximum tongue strength has been questioned. It has been suggested that people likely use only about 20 percent of their tongue strength capability during speech (Forrest, 2002; Kent, Kent, and Rosenbek, 1987). An alternative to measuring maximum tongue strength was conducted by Speirs and Maktabi (1990), who measured fine tongue control by asking their participants to maintain a low level of target pressure for short periods. The children with speech sound disorders showed significantly less stability (i.e., poorer fine control) than children without speech errors. In the previously mentioned study by Robin and colleagues (1991), although there was no difference in maximum strength, the children with CAS were significantly poorer at maintaining tongue pressure at 50 percent of maximum compared to normal-speaking children. Such findings lend some support to the idea that some children with speech sound disorders may have subtle motor deficiencies or delays.

Summary

Individuals with speech sound problems have not been shown to exhibit significantly depressed motor coordination on tasks of general motor performance. The relationship between oral-motor skills and articulation skills in speech sound disorders of unknown origin remains uncertain. Although such individuals have been found to perform more poorly on diadochokinetic tasks than their normal-speaking peers, these results cannot be accurately interpreted until the relationship between diadochokinetic tasks and the ability to articulate sounds in context is clarified.

Findings of tongue strength studies suggest that although overall strength may not be a problem for children with speech sound disorders, a more important issue may be fine tongue control or stability. It is not yet clear whether such findings represent children with speech sound disorders in general or if they are limited to only subgroups of this population such as those with abnormal tone or those with CAS.

ORAL MYOFUNCTIONAL DISORDERS/TONGUE THRUST

Oral myofunctional disorders (OMD) are observed by speech-language pathologists and include such phenomena as tongue thrusting, unusual oral movements, finger sucking, lip insufficiencies, and dental and oral structure deficiencies. The concern of speech-language pathologists relates to speech differences and disorders that may be related to such oral variations. Since tongue thrusting is the oral myofunctional disorder most commonly encountered by speech-language pathologists, in this section we will focus on this phenomena.

Tongue thrust has been defined as frontal or lateral tongue thrust or strong contact of the tongue with the teeth during swallowing, as well as inadequate lip closure or incorrect tongue rest posture (Neiva and Wertzner, 1996). Proffit (1986) pointed out that tongue thrust is something of a misnomer since it implies that the tongue is thrust forward forcefully, when in reality such individuals do not seem to use more tongue force against the teeth than nonthrusters. Rather, *tongue thrust swallow* implies a directionality of tongue activity in swallowing. Other terms sometimes used to describe these behaviors include *reverse swallow, deviant swallow*, and *infantile swallow*. These terms should be avoided because of their inherent faulty implications (Mason, 1988). The most salient features of a tongue thrust swallow pattern, according to Mason and Proffit (1974), include one or more of these conditions:

1. During the initiation of a swallow, a forward gesture of the tongue between the anterior teeth so that the tongue tip contacts the lower lip;
2. During speech activities, fronting of the tongue between or against the anterior teeth with the mandible hinged open (in phonetic contexts not intended for such placements); and
3. At rest, the tongue carried forward in the oral cavity with the mandible hinged slightly open and the tongue tip against or between the anterior teeth. (p. 116)

Everyone starts out life as a tongue thruster because at birth the tongue fills the oral cavity, making tongue fronting obligatory. Sometime later, the anterior tongue-gums/teeth seal during swallowing is replaced with a superior tongue-palate seal. There is some debate about when most children make this change. Hanson (1988b) suggested that this happens by age 5 years. A review of published studies by Lebrun (1985), however, concluded that "tongue thrust swallowing is the rule rather than the exception in children under 10 years of age" (p. 307).

Tongue thrust during swallow and/or tongue fronting at rest can usually be identified by visual inspection. Mason (1988) has pointed out that two types of tongue fronting should be differentiated. The first is described as a *habit* and is seen in the absence of any morphological structural delimiting factors. The second is *obligatory* and may involve factors such as airway obstruction or enlarged tonsils with tongue thrusting being a necessary adaptation to maintain the size of the airway to pass food during swallow. Oral myofunctional therapy for obligatory tongue fronting has been questioned by Shelton (1989) because of the poor prognosis for change.

Wadsworth, Maul, and Stevens (1998) indicated that tongue thrust swallow frequently co-occurred with resting forward-tongue posture (63 percent), open bite (86 percent), overjet (57 percent), abnormal palatal contour (60 percent), and open mouth posture (39 percent). Marshall (1992) indicated that some children who tongue thrust are described as having a tongue that is "too big." However, she indicated that low muscle tone (flaccidity) of the tongue is often the real problem. She also attributes tongue thrusting to tongue instability, jaw instability, allergies, and poor sensory awareness.

Hanson (1988a) suggested that a better description for these tongue position and movement behaviors would be "oral muscle pattern disorders." Orthodontists and speech-language pathologists have been interested in tongue thrusting and a forward tongue resting posture because of the perception that tongue function can cause certain types of (1) malocclusion problems, (2) altered patterns of facial development, and (3) speech sound problems. The type of speech sound disorder associated with tongue thrust and malocclusion is a frontal lisp characterized by anterior tongue placement for /s/ and /z/. The number of lisps is higher in children who evidence tongue thrusting than for children who do not evidence such behavior. Sometimes tongue thrust is also associated with anterior placement of /ʃ/, /tʃ/, /dʒ/, /ʒ/, /t/, /d/, /l/, and /n/.

Impact of Tongue Thrust on Dentition

The current view is that the resting posture of the tongue affects the position of the teeth and jaws more than does the tongue function during swallowing (tongue thrust) or speaking

(Proffit, 1986). Tongue thrusting may play a role in maintaining or influencing an abnormal dental pattern when an anterior resting tongue position is present. If the position of the tongue is forward (forward resting position) and between the anterior teeth at rest, this condition can impede normal teeth eruption and can result in an anterior open bite. However, tongue thrusting patients, in the absence of an anterior tongue resting position, are not thought to develop malocclusions. The pressure or force on dentition associated with tongue thrust during speaking and swallowing are of short duration and do not exert enough force on the dentition to cause problems of dental occlusion. Mason (1988) pointed out that individuals who exhibit a tongue thrust pattern and forward tongue posture create morphological conditions that can potentially lead to dental occlusion problems and would be much more likely to develop a malocclusion than when only a tongue thrust is present.

Tongue Thrust and Presence of Speech Sound Errors

Investigators have reported that speech sound errors, primarily sibilant distortions, occur more frequently in children who evidence tongue thrust than in those who do not. Fletcher, Casteel, and Bradley (1961) studied 1,615 school children ages 6 to 18 and found that children who demonstrated a tongue thrust swallow pattern were more likely to have associated sibilant distortions than children who did not. They also reported that participants with normal swallow patterns demonstrated a significant decrease in sibilant distortion with age, whereas tongue thrusters did not.

Palmer (1962) found that clients referred for marked tongue thrusting nearly always demonstrated a sibilant "difference" but that the difference was perceived as only a slight lisp. He reported that such differences also occurred on /t/, /d/, and /n/.

Jann, Ward, and Jann (1964) examined the relationship among speech defects, tongue thrusting, and malocclusion in children in the early primary grades and reported a high incidence of /s/, /z/, and /l/ variations in children with tongue thrust swallow patterns.

Wadsworth and colleagues (1998) reported that of 200 children from grades kindergarten through 6 who were enrolled in speech therapy, 77 percent of children with a defective /s/ evidenced abnormal rest tongue position and 76 percent exhibited a tongue thrust swallow.

Subtelny and colleagues (1964) used radiographic techniques to examine the relationship between normal and abnormal oral morphology and /s/ production. Their participants, 81 adolescents and adults, were divided into three groups: (1) normal speakers with normal occlusion, (2) normal speakers with severe malocclusion, and (3) abnormal speakers with severe malocclusion. In contrast to earlier investigators, these authors found that the incidence of tongue thrusting and malocclusion in normal speakers was comparable to that in abnormal speakers. This finding is consistent with the reported developmental decrease in the reverse swallow pattern. By contrast, Khinda and Grewal (1999) examined the relationship among tongue thrusting, anterior open bite, and speech sound disorders. In a group of children with tongue thrust and normal occlusion, 30 percent demonstrated speech sound disorders compared to 95 percent of children with tongue thrusting combined with an anterior open bite. Thus, significantly more speech sound disorders were associated with the combination of tongue thrust and anterior open bite.

Treatment Issues

Hanson (1994), in a review of the 15 studies that examined the effectiveness of tongue thrust therapy, reported that 14 of the investigators indicated that swallowing and resting patterns were altered successfully. Most studies reviewed patients at least one year following the completion of treatment. Only one study of five participants (Subtelny, 1970) found therapy to be ineffective in correcting the disorders.

Other support for tongue thrust intervention has often come from clinical reports by clinicians who conduct oral myofunctional therapy. For example, Hilton (1984) stated, "In my experience, many tongue-fronting children who begin speech articulation therapy without having had the early sensorimotor and stretching activities of myotherapy ... begin with an unnecessary handicap.... I provide every tongue-fronting speech articulation case these initial oral awareness, control, and flexibility exercises prior to initiation of the place-feature oriented therapy" (p. 51). Umberger and Johnston (1997) agreed that combined speech therapy and oral myofunctional therapy provides the best opportunity for improved speech accompanying reduced tongue thrusting.

The official statement adopted by the American Speech-Language-Hearing Association (ASHA) Legislative Council (ASHA, 1991) on the role of the speech-language pathologist in assessment and management of oral myofunctional disorders includes the statement: "Investigation, assessment, and treatment of oral myofunctional disorders are within the purview of speech-language pathology" (p. 7).

1991 Position Statement

According to American Speech-Language-Hearing Association:

1. Oral myofunctional phenomena, including abnormal fronting (tongue thrust) of the tongue at rest and during swallowing, lip incompetency, and sucking habits, can be identified reliably. These conditions co-occur with speech misarticulations in some patients.
2. Tongue fronting may reflect learned behaviors, physical variables, or both.
3. Published research indicates that oral myofunctional therapy is effective in modifying disorders of tongue and lip posture and movement.
4. Investigation, assessment, and treatment of oral myofunctional disorders are within the purview of speech-language pathology.
5. The speech-language pathologist who desires to perform oral myofunctional services must have the required knowledge and skills to provide a high quality of treatment. The provision of oral myofunctional therapy remains an option of individual speech-language pathologists whose interests and training qualify them.
6. Evaluation and treatment should be interdisciplinary and tailored to the individual. The speech-language pathologist performing oral myofunctional therapy should collaborate with an orthodontist, pediatric dentist, or other dentists, and with medical specialists such as an otolaryngologist, pediatrician, or allergist, as needed.
7. Appropriate goals of oral myofunctional therapy should include the retraining of labial and lingual resting and functional patterns (including speech). The speech-language pathologist's statements of treatment goals should avoid predictions of treatment outcome based on tooth position or dental occlusal changes.

8. Basic and applied research is needed on the nature and evaluation of oral myofunctions and the treatment of oral myofunctional disorders. (p. 7)

The ad hoc committee report (ASHA, 1989) on the labial-lingual posturing function developed the above statement based on the following concepts relative to oral myofunctional phenomena as they relate to communication disorders:

1. All infants exhibit a tongue thrust swallow as a normal performance.
2. This pattern changes with growth and maturation to the extent that many different swallow patterns can be identified from infancy to adulthood.
3. At some time in development, a tongue protrusion swallow is no longer the norm and can be considered undesirable or as a contributing and maintaining factor in malocclusion, lisping, or both.
4. A related condition that has a stronger link to malocclusion is a forward resting posture of the tongue. . . . This is consistent with orthodontic theory and research that long-acting forces against the teeth result in tooth movement whereas short-acting (intermittent) forces are not as likely to cause tooth movement.
5. There is descriptive evidence that during the course of oral myofunctional therapy some individuals have corrected or controlled a tongue thrust swallow and an anterior resting posture.
6. Diagnostic attention should be directed toward determining whether a tongue thrust swallow and a forward tongue resting posture coexist in a given patient. When these conditions coexist, a greater link to malocclusion would be expected than from a tongue thrust swallow alone. However, there is insufficient evidence to show that a forward tongue posture and tongue thrust swallow are more detrimental than a tongue forward resting posture alone. There is also some evidence that a tongue forward resting posture or tongue thrust swallow and lisping coexist in some persons. Correction of tongue function or posture may facilitate correction of the lisp or the interdentalization of the /t/, /d/, /n/, and /l/ phonemes.
7. In normal development, slight separation of the lips at rest ("lip incompetence") is normal in children. With growth, the lips typically achieve contact at rest in the teenage years. Some individuals, however, persist in a lips-apart posture after development has advanced sufficiently to permit lip closure. Such individuals may be candidates for treatment.
8. There is some evidence that lip exercises can be successful in facilitating a closed-lip posture.
9. Sucking habits (e.g., finger, thumb, tongue, lips) can influence dental development. When tongue thrusting and thumb sucking coexist with dental problems, developmental correction of the tongue thrust would not be expected until the thumb, finger, or sucking habit ceases.
10. Other variables besides learning influence tongue posture. They include posterior airway obstruction, which may involve tonsils, adenoids, nasal blockage, high posterior tongue position with a short mandibular ramus, or a long soft palate. Many morphologic features or combinations of features can reduce oral isthmus size and obligate the tongue to rest forward. Diagnostic procedures should distinguish such patients from those with other forward tongue postures or functions. The obligatory tongue forward posture group would seem unlikely candidates for myofunctional therapy in the absence of medical treatment. Any indicated remedial medical procedures are usually carried out prior to consideration of myofunctional therapy.

Summary

1. Existing data support the idea that abnormal labial-lingual posturing function can be identified, including abnormal fronting (tongue thrust) of the tongue at rest and during swallowing, lip incompetency, and sucking habits.
2. A forward tongue resting posture has the potential, with or without a tongue thrust swallow, to be associated with malocclusions.
3. There is some evidence that an anterior tongue resting posture or a tongue thrust swallow and speech production errors coexist in some persons.
4. Oral myofunctional therapy can be effective in modifying disorders of tongue and lip posture and movement.
5. Assessment and treatment of oral myofunctional disorders that may include some nonspeech remediation are within the purview of speech-language pathology but should involve interdisciplinary collaboration.
6. Research is needed on the nature and evaluation of oral myofunctions and the treatment of such disorders.

COGNITIVE-LINGUISTIC FACTORS

A second category of variables that have been studied relative to a possible relationship to speech sound disorders is that of cognitive-linguistic factors. Historically, the field of communication sciences and disorders has been interested in the relationship between intelligence and the presence of speech sound disorders. In more recent years, investigators have sought to describe the relationship between disordered phonology and additional aspects of cognitive-linguistic functioning. This not only is useful in determining the type of instructional/intervention program that may be most efficacious for the child's overall language development but it also helps to provide a better understanding of interrelationships of various components of language behavior.

Intelligence

The relationship between intelligence (as measured by IQ tests) and speech sound disorders has been a subject of interest for many years, and of several investigations. In a study of elementary and junior high school students, Reid (1947a, 1947b) reported that articulation proficiency could not be predicted from intelligence scores when the IQ was 70 or above. Winitz (1959a, 1959b), in his investigation of 150 children, reported similarly low positive correlations between scores obtained on the *Wechsler Intelligence Scale for Children* and the *Templin-Darley Articulation Screening Test*. Thus, in terms of the relationship between intelligence and articulation in children of normal intelligence, data have indicated that one is not a good predictor of the other.

A second perspective on the relationship between intelligence and phonology may be gleaned from studies of the phonological status of developmentally delayed individuals. Prior to 1970, a number of studies were conducted to explore the prevalence of speech sound disorders in developmentally delayed individuals. Typical of these studies are those of Wilson (1966), Schlanger (1953), and Schlanger and Gottsleben (1957). Wilson used the

Hejina Articulation Test in his study of 777 children with cognitive impairments (what we used to call *mental retardation*) whose chronological ages ranged from 6 to 16 years. He reported that 53.4 percent of the children evidenced speech sound disorders. Errors of substitution, omission, and distortion tended to decrease as the mental ages of the children increased. Wilson (1966) concluded that "there is a high incidence of articulatory deviation in an educable mentally retarded population, and the incidence and degree of severity is closely related to mental-age levels" (p. 432). Wilson's findings also indicated that articulatory skills, which continue to improve until approximately age 8 in the normal population, continue to show improvement well beyond that age in the cognitively impaired population.

Schlanger (1953) and Schlanger and Gottsleben (1957) reported similar findings to Wilson in their studies of speech production in individuals with cognitive impairment. Schlanger investigated 74 children in a residential school; the children's mean chronological age (C.A.) was 12;1, and their mean mental age (M.A.) was 6;8. Of the 74 children, 56.7 percent were found to have speech sound disorders. In their study of 400 randomly selected residents at a training school with a C.A. mean of 28;9 and a M.A. of 7;8, Schlanger and Gottsleben reported that 78 percent presented speech delays ranging from slight to severe. Individuals with Down syndrome (DS) or whose etiologies were based on central nervous system impairment demonstrated the most pronounced speech delay.

As noted previously in our discussion of classification and genetic syndromes, the developmental pattern for speech sounds in persons with cognitive impairments are generally similar to that of younger typically developing children (Bleile, 1982; Smith and Stoel-Gammon, 1983; Sommers, Reinhart, and Sistrunk, 1988). However, Kumin, Council, and Goodman (1994) reported a great deal of variability in the age at which sounds emerge in the speech of children with DS. They also stated that these children do "not appear to follow the same order as the norms for acquisition for typically developing children" (p. 300), and also that emergence of some sounds were as much as five years later than the age in which normally developing children acquire a sound.

Shriberg and Widder (1990) indicated that findings from nearly four decades of speech research in cognitive impairment can be summarized as follows:

1. Persons with cognitive impairments are likely to have speech sound errors.
2. The most frequent type of error is likely to be deletions of consonants.
3. Errors are likely to be inconsistent.
4. The pattern of errors is likely to be similar to that of very young children or children with speech sound disorders of unknown origin.

Several investigators have explored the speech patterns of individuals with DS, a genetically controlled subset of individuals with cognitive impairment. Sommers and colleagues (1988) reported that among the speech sound errors evidenced by children with DS, ages 13 to 22 years, some were phonemes frequently seen in error in 5- and 6-year-olds of normal intelligence (i.e., /r/, /r/ clusters, /s/, /s/ clusters, /z/, /θ/, and /v/). The authors indicated that these errors would appear to support the assertion that the phonological development of children with DS follows the same general pattern as that of normal children. However, they also reported that DS children evidenced errors not typically seen in normal 5- and 6-year-olds (e.g., deletion of alveolar stops and nasals). They further reported that imitative and spontaneous single-word picture-naming responses of their participants failed to identify many of the omission errors found in connected speech samples of their participants.

Rosin, Swift, Bless, and Vetter (1988) studied the articulation of children with Down syndrome as part of a study of overall communication profiles in this population. They compared a group of 10 DS male participants (C.A. = 14;7 years) with a control group of individuals with other forms of cognitive impairment and two control groups of individuals with normal intelligence representing two age levels (C.A. 6;1, 15;5). They reported that as M.A. increased across participants, intelligibility on a language sample increased. The DS group was also significantly different from the group of individuals with other forms of cognitive impairment and the younger age normal group (the older group was not compared) in terms of the percent of consonants correctly articulated on the *Goldman-Fristoe Test of Articulation.*

In addition to the speech measures mentioned above, Rosin and colleagues (1988) also included other language measures, an oral motor evaluation, and aerodynamic measures in their assessment. They reported that the DS group had difficulty with production measures as demands for sequencing increased (e.g., consonant-vowel repetitions, length of words). The DS group needed a significant amount of cueing in order to articulate the target /pataka/, and had more variable intraoral pressure when producing /papapaps/. The mean length of utterance of the DS group was also significantly shorter than the mentally retarded and normal groups. The authors indicated that these findings are in accord with observations of others and suggested that sequencing underlies both oral motor control and language problems evidenced in DS participants.

Summary

Investigators concur that there is a low positive correlation between intelligence and speech sound production skill within the range of normal intelligence. Thus, it can be inferred that intellectual functioning is of limited importance as a contributing factor to articulatory skill, and can be viewed as a poor predictor of articulation. On the other hand, a much higher correlation has been found between intelligence and articulation in the cognitively impaired population. The articulatory skills in a subgroup of individuals cognitive impairment (those with DS) reflect error patterns similar to those seen in young normally developing children; however, they also evidence errors that are considered different or unusual when compared to normal developing children.

Language Development

Because phonology is one component of a child's developing linguistic system, there has been an interest in the relationship between phonologic development and development of other aspects of language (i.e., morphology/syntax, semantics, pragmatics). Of particular interest to speech-language pathologists has been the extent to which there is a co-existence (or comorbidity) of speech sound disorders and language disorders.

How common it is for two conditions to co-occur depends on how the question is framed. One might ask: How common is it in the population for a person to have both disorders? This results in a very small number, which may hide the significance of the problem. Speech-language pathologists don't usually deal with the whole population; they deal with whoever is referred to them. A clinically more meaningful question is: When we are dealing with an individual who has one disorder, how likely is it that this person will also have a second disorder at the same time? Answering that question will depend on which disorder is used in the denominator for the calculation (also called the *index disorder*). One might ask: What percentage of individuals with speech sound disorders also have a language disorder? Or What percentage of individuals with a language disorder also have a speech sound disorder? Shriberg and Austin (1998) reviewed the existing literature in this area and their findings are summarized in Table 4.6. For our discussion here, the more interesting values are those using speech as the index disorder. Using the data in Table 4.6 and some additional

■ **TABLE 4.6** Estimates of the Comorbidity of Speech and Language Disorders

			Comorbidity Estimates by Index Disorder	
Study	**n**	**Mean Age***	**Speech Index**	**Language Index**
Paul (1993)	37	3[b]		37%
Whitehurst et al. (1991)	22	3		35
Connell, Elbert, and Dinnsen (1991)	23	4	43%	
Shriberg, Kwiatkowski, Best, Hengst, and Terselic-Weber (1986)	33	4	60	
Shriberg and Kwiatkowski (1994)	64	4	66	
Bishop and Edmundson (1987)	66	4[c]		74
Paul (1993)	37	4[b]		16
Tallal, Ross, and Curtiss (1989)	76	4		60
Bishop and Edmundson (1987)	67	4.5[c]		55
Shriberg et al. (1986)	38	5	50	
Bishop and Edmundson (1987)	68	5[c]		34
Tomblin (1996a)	862	5		25
Paul and Shriberg (1982)	30	6	66	
Shriberg and Kwiatkowski (1982)	43	6	77	
Schery (1985)	718	7	75[d]	75[d]
St. Louis, Ruscello, Grafton, and Hershman (1994)	20	7[e]	45	
St. Louis et al. (1994)	20	7[e]		65
Ruscello, St. Louis, and Mason (1991)	24	12.5	54[f]	
Ruscello et al. (1991)	24	12.5	21[g]	

[a]Ages rounded up at .5, unless mean age was provided within narrow age range.
[b, c]Same children followed longitudinally.
[d]No index disorder in this survey.
[e]Estimated.
[f]Classified as having delayed articulation.
[g]Classified as having residual errors.

Source: L. D. Shriberg and D. Austin, "Comorbidity of Speech-Language Disorder: Implications for a Phenotype Marker for Speech Delay" in R. Paul (Ed.), *Exploring the Speech-Language Connection* (Baltimore: Paul H. Brookes Publishing Co., Inc., 1998), p. 91. Reprinted by permission.

data they generated themselves, Shriberg and Austin concluded that up to approximately 60 percent of preschool children with speech sound disorders also have some type of language disorder. Shriberg and Austin also concluded that if we limit our discussion to coexisting *receptive language disorders*, the corresponding figure drops to 20 percent. Shriberg and Austin summarized this literature to say that there is some support for the idea that children who have more severe speech sound disorders may also be more likely to have coexisting expressive language disorders.

Some investigators have attempted to further study and explain the interaction between phonology and other aspects of language, especially syntax. A common perception is that language is organized "from the top down"—in other words, a speaker goes from pragmatic intent, to semantic coding, to syntactic structure, to phonologic productions. Thus, higher-level linguistic formulations may ultimately be reflected in a child's phonologic productions. If this theory is accurate, it might be expected that the more complex the syntax, the more likely a child is to evidence linguistic breakdown, which may then be evidenced in phonologic productions. Schmauch, Panagos, and Klich (1978) conducted a study in which 5-year-old children with phonologic and language problems were required to produce certain nouns (drawn from phonologic inventories) in three syntactic contexts—that is, an isolated noun phrase (the simplest context), a declarative sentence, and a passive sentence (the most complex context). These investigators reported a 17 percent increase in speech sound errors between the noun phrase and each of the sentence contexts. They also reported that later developing consonants were those most influenced by syntactical complexity and that error productions reflected quantitative rather than qualitative changes.

A follow-up study of the top-down notion was conducted by Panagos, Quine, and Klich (1979). In this study, 5-year-old children were required to produce 15 target consonants in noun phrases, declarative sentences, and passive sentences; consonants appeared in the initial and final word-positions of one- and two-syllable words. Syntax was again found to significantly influence speech sound accuracy, as did number of syllables in target words. Word position did not influence accuracy. The authors further reported that two sources of complexity—phonologic (including difficulty with later developing consonants as well as specific contexts) and syntactic—combined additively to increase the number of speech sound errors. From the easiest context (final word position of one-syllable words in noun phrases) to the hardest (final word position of two-syllable word in passive sentences), there was a 36 percent increase in speech sound errors. The effects of grammatical complexity were cumulative.

A second perspective on the language-phonology relationship suggests that linguistic influences operate "from the bottom up." In this view, language expression is regulated by feedback (internal and external) from phonologic performance. Feedback from phonologic performance is needed to maintain syntactic processing and accuracy, especially when errors occur and must be corrected.

Panagos and Prelock (1982) conducted a study to test the hypothesis that phonologic structure influences children's syntactic processing. Ten children with language disorders were required to produce sentences containing words with varying syllable complexity—that is, *simple*: "The (CV) kid (CVC) pushed (CVCC) the (CV) car (CVC) in (VC) the (CV) room (CVC)," and *complex*: "The (CV) chocolate (CVCVCVC) is (VC) in (VC) the (CV) napkin (CVCCVC)." In addition, sentence complexity was varied from unembedded ("The girl washed the doll in the tub") to right embedded ("The cook washed the pot the boy dropped") to center embedded ("The lady the uncle liked sewed the coat"). The results of the study supported the hypothesis. When participants repeated sentences containing words of greater syllable complexity, they made 27 percent more syntactic errors. In addition to this bottom-up influence, Panagos and Prelock (1982) also reported that syntactic complexity further compounded production difficulties. From the unembedded to the center embedded, there was a 57 percent increase in phonologic errors.

These findings support the view that a simultaneous top-down bottom-up relationship exists between language and phonology. Another way of expressing this concept is to consider that children with disordered language-phonology have a limited encoding capacity; and the more this capacity is strained at one level or another, the greater the probability of delay in one component or more of language. It should be pointed out that the investigators who have examined the affect of complexity on the language-phonology relationship have typically employed elicited imitation tasks, and thus complexity of utterances was controlled by the investigators. It can be argued that with this type of performance task, structural simplifications are the expected outcomes. Elicited imitation tasks do not reflect the conditions present when a child is engaged in conversation, and thus we cannot assume that constraints of the nature demonstrated by Panagos and Prelock (1982) can predict behavior in a conversational context (Paul and Shriberg, 1984).

In an investigation by Paul and Shriberg (1982) designed to study phonologic productions as they relate to particular morphophonemic structures, continuous speech samples were obtained from 30 children with speech delays. They reported that certain of their participants were able to produce complex morphosyntactic contexts spontaneously, which did not result in phonologic simplifications. In other words, some of their participants were able to maintain a similar level of phonologic production in spite of producing more complex syntactic targets. They (Paul and Shriberg, 1984) suggested that children may "do things other than phonologic simplification in an attempt to control complexity in spontaneous speech" (p. 319). They summarized by indicating that some children with speech delays are sometimes able to allocate their limited linguistic resources to realize phonologic targets consistent with their linguistic knowledge in the context of free speech, even though at other times they may use avoidance strategies or other means of reducing the encoding load.

The simultaneous top-down bottom-up relationship between phonology and other aspects of language is reflected in the concept of a snyergistic view of language (Schwartz, Leonard, Folger, and Wilcox, 1980; Shriner et al., 1969). This perspective assumes a complex interaction and interdependency of various aspects of linguistic behaviors including language and phonology.

Several investigators have studied whether intervention focused on one aspect of the linguistic domain (e.g., morphosyntax) facilitates gains in an untreated domain (e.g., phonology). Matheny and Panagos (1978) looked at the effects of syntactic programming on phonologic improvement and the effects of phonologic programming on syntactic improvement in school-age children. Each group made the greatest gains in the treated domain as compared to a control group, but also made improvements in the untreated domain. Similar findings were reported by Wilcox and Morris (1995). They reported that children with phonological and language impairments who participated in a preschool language-focused program made gains not only in language but also in phonology, based on comparison to a control group. Hoffman, Norris, and Monjure (1990), in a study based on two siblings from a set of triplets, also found that a narrative intervention program facilitated gains in both language and phonology for one brother, while gains in phonology only were achieved by the brother who only received phonologic instruction.

One of the more comprehensive studies of cross-domain improvement between language (morphosyntax) and phonology was reported by Tyler and colleagues (2002). They compared treatment outcomes for three groups of children, all of whom evidenced both phonologic and morphosyntactic disorders: (1) Group 1 received morphosyntactic instruction for a 12-week block, followed by 12 weeks in phonology; (2) Group 2 reversed the order of the 12-week blocks; and (3) Group 3 served as a control group. These investigators reported that in comparison to the control group, both interventions were effective; however, only morphosyntactic instruction led to cross-domain improvement (i.e., language therapy improved phonology but not the reverse).

These findings have not been supported in all investigations of cross-domain improvements.

Tyler and Watterson (1991) reported that participants with a severe overall language and phonological disorder made improvements in language when presented with language therapy; however, gains were not made in phonology (they actually reported a tendency for performance to become slightly worse). On the other hand, participants with mild-moderate but unequal impairments in phonology and language improved in both areas when presented with phonologic therapy. The authors suggested that a language-based intervention program may not result in improvement in phonologic as well as other language skills for children whose disorders are severe and comparable in each domain. However, children with less severe problems in one or both domains may benefit from therapy with either a language or phonology focus.

Fey, Cleave, Ravida, Long, Dejmal, and Easton (1994) conducted an experimental treatment program with 26 participants, ages 44 to 70 months, with impairments in both grammar and phonology. Eighteen children received language intervention (grammar facilitation) in accord with one or another of two designated teaching approaches and eight children served as controls. Results indicated that despite a strong effect for intervention on the children's grammatical output, there were no direct effects on the participants' speech sound productions. The authors indicated that trying to improve intelligibility by focusing on grammar is not defensible for children in the age and severity range of their participants. They further indicated that for most children who have impairments in both speech and language, intervention will need to be focused on both areas. While this study only examined one form of language intervention that anticipated phonologic effects, these data provide strong evidence that in children ages 4 to 6, treatment approaches should address phonologic problems directly if changes in phonologic performance are to be expected.

Tyler and colleagues (2002) have indicated that differences in findings between their study and that of the Fey and colleagues (1994) study may be due to differences in goal selection, intervention techniques, or measures used to determine changes in phonology. Further clinical studies are needed to clarify the synergistic relationship between language and phonology, including cross-domain improvements. The influence of age, nature and severity of both language and speech sound disorders, treatment approaches employed, and measures used to ascertain progress all need further study.

Summary

Research has shown that up to 60 percent of younger children with speech sound disorders are likely to also have language delay. It is a much smaller proportion (perhaps up to 20 percent) if we consider only receptive language problems. Language and phonology may be related in what has been termed a synergistic relationship. Investigators face the challenge of further defining the intricacies of the relationship between phonology and other linguistic behaviors in terms of both development and clinical management of disorders. It appears that for children with language impairment and moderate to severe phonologic delay, direct phonologic intervention may be required in order to impact phonology. Further research in cross-domain generalization is needed to guide clinical practice in this area.

Academic Performance

The relationship between speech sound disorders and academic performance is of interest to clinicians working with school-age children since oral language skills are fundamental to the development of many literacy related academic skills such as reading and spelling. Because the use of sounds in symbolic lexical units is a task common to learning to speak, read, and write, researchers for many years have studied the co-occurrence of reading and speech sound disorders, and have discussed possible common factors underlying the acquisition of literacy and other language-related skills.

Hall (1938) compared 21 children with speech sound disorders of unknown origin with a normal control group on the *Gates Silent Reading Test* and the *Iowa Silent Reading Test* and reported no significant differences in silent reading achievement between the two groups. Everhart (1953) also used the *Gates Silent Reading Test* and reported no significant relationship between speech sound disorders and reading ability, although boys with normal articulation tended to obtain higher reading scores than the overall group of children with speech sound disorders.

The relationship between reading readiness and speech sound disorders was studied by Fitzsimons (1958) and Weaver, Furbee, and Everhart (1960). Fitzsimons used the *Metropolitan Reading Readiness Test* to determine the status of reading readiness and reported that below grade-level scores were more frequent among children with speech sound disorders than among those with normally developing articulation. Weaver and colleagues (1960) reported a significant relationship between articulatory performance and reading readiness as well as between articulatory performance and reading scores.

Flynn and Byrne (1970) took a different approach to this question. They compared articulatory performance of 52 advanced and 42 delayed third-grade readers on the *Templin-Darley Tests of Articulation*. Those who scored 4.2 or higher on the *Iowa Test of Basic Skills* were classified as advanced readers; those who scored 2.2 or lower were classified as delayed readers. The authors reported no significant difference between the two groups in articulation test scores.

Lewis and Freebairn-Far (1991) conducted a cross-sectional study designed to examine the performance of individuals with a history of a preschool speech sound disorder on measures of phonology, reading, and spelling. Groups of participants included at least 17 individuals from each of the following categories: preschool, school age, adolescence, and adulthood. Normal comparison groups at each age level were also tested. Significant differences between the disordered and normal groups were reported on the reading and spelling measures for the school-age group, and on the reading measure for the adult group. Although the reading and spelling measures for the adolescent group and the spelling measure for the adult group did not reach significance, the trend was for the individuals with histories of disorders to perform more poorly than normals. Data also indicated that participants who evidenced a speech sound disorder accompanied by additional language problems performed more poorly on measures of reading and spelling than participants with speech sound disorders only. The authors indicated that children evidencing phonologic impairment are at risk for reading and spelling problems in school and may have special educational needs.

Felsenfeld, McGue, and Broen (1995) conducted a comparison study of the children of 24 adults with a documented history of a phonologic-language disorder that persisted from childhood until at least grade 11 (proband group), and 28 adults who were known to have had normal abilities as children (control group). Included among the comparison variables were several categorized under "educational performance." Results revealed that 28 percent of the children of the proband group repeated at least one grade, compared to 0 percent from the control group. Likewise, 22 percent of the proband children compared to 4 percent of the controls had received academic tutoring. Speech treatment had been received by 33 percent of the proband group and 0 percent of the control group. They also reported that half of the school-age children who were receiving speech treatment were also either participating in remedial academic services and/or had repeated a grade.

Although interest has traditionally focused on the co-occurrence of reading-spelling and speech sound disorders in children, more recently there has also been interest in children's ability to process phonology as part of various reading tasks. More specifically, some students with reading disabilities may lack awareness of individual sounds, have difficulty dividing words into sounds, and recalling sound-symbol relationships (phonologic awareness). Catts (1986) found that children with reading disabilities may have problems with these linguistically oriented tasks and yet not reflect phonologic impairment.

Investigators have attempted to apply phonologic concepts to aid in the understanding of reading and spelling disorders. This activity is based on the assumption that acquisition of speaking, reading, and writing skills involves the analysis of sounds in lexical units, which may be related to underlying cognitive-linguistic processes. In particular, the concepts of phonologic processes and underlying internal knowledge of the sound system have been employed to aid in understanding the development of spelling and reading skills (Hoffman and Norris, 1989).

Liberman and Shankweiler (1985), in a discussion of the phonologic basis of literacy, indicated that reading success was related to the degree to which children were aware of "underlying phonologic structure" and that poor readers often were unable to segment words into their phonologic constituents. They suggested that a relationship exists between children's readiness for reading and spelling and their metalinguistic awareness of the internal structure of words. O'Conner and Jenkins (1999) reported that performance on phonological awareness tasks (e.g., initial sound identification, rhyme production, phoneme segmentation) in kindergarten predicted differences in reading achievement at the end of first grade, and was reliable in identifying children who would later be diagnosed as having a reading disability.

Catts (1991) suggested that speech-language pathologists working in school systems should seek to develop programs designed to facilitate "phonologic awareness" in children, particularly those at risk for reading disabilities. Catts suggested that "phonologic awareness" activities might include activities designed to increase awareness of syllables, phonemes, manner of phoneme production, and sound positions in words. Activities to accomplish these goals could include sound play, rhyming, alliteration, and segmentation tasks. This topic, including how it relates to speech sound disorders, is discussed in greater detail in Chapter 9.

Hoffman and Norris (1989) analyzed spelling errors of 45 elementary school children for evidence of phonologic process patterns. They reported that many of the spelling errors involved both syllable reduction and feature changes similar to the sound simplifications seen in the speech of young children with normal speech development. They further indicated that even though children had acquired normal speech, they exhibited spelling errors similar to those seen in the speech simplifications of younger children. Hoffman (1990) related specific types of developmental spelling patterns to stages of normal phonologic acquisition. For example, "precommunicative spellings" (seemingly random selection of letters of the alphabet to represent words) were described as parallel to the random sound productions of babbling. "Semiphonetic spellings" (letters used to represent sounds, but only some of the sounds are represented, e.g., *E* for *eagle*) were described as parallel to the stage where children delete syllables or segments and substitute sound classes for one another. Hoffman also indicated that because the speech-language pathologist is the school-based professional who has the most detailed knowledge of sound perception and production, phonologic organization, stages of acquisition, and methods of phonologic description, he or she is in a good position to serve as a resource to teachers regarding the application of phonologic concepts to the understanding of spelling errors. Chapter 9 focuses on phonological awareness and its relationship to literacy and the role of the speech-language pathologist in literacy.

Summary

Research investigations that have focused on the co-occurrence of speech sound disorders and literacy impairments indicate a possible relationship between these disorders in some children. Data indicate that young children with severe speech sound and/or other language disorders are at risk for academic problems, and there may be a familial propensity for such difficulties. The role of "phonologic awareness" in the development of reading and spelling skills has been the focus of a lot of study in the last decade. It appears that there is a relationship between phonological awareness and later literacy skills and that children with speech sound disorders are at risk for problems in both areas. Parallels have been made between the use of phonologic processes and stages in the acquisition of oral language and acquisition of reading and spelling skills. It has been suggested that speech-language pathologists are in a unique position to offer assistance to the classroom teacher in their efforts to assist children at risk for reading and/or spelling problems.

PSYCHOSOCIAL FACTORS

Psychosocial factors represent a third cluster of variables that have long fascinated clinicians in terms of their potential relationship to phonology. Age, gender, family history, and socioeconomic status have been studied in an effort to better understand factors that may precipitate or otherwise be associated with phonologic impairment.

Age

The literature on speech sound acquisition was reviewed in Chapter 3. Investigations have revealed that children's articulatory and phonologic skills continue to improve until approximately 8 years of age, by which time the normal child has acquired most aspects of the adult sound system. In fact, it appears that by age 4 normally developing children have articulation skills that closely resemble that of adults.

Speech-language pathologists use normative information concerning phonologic development as a guide in case selection and for determining treatment goals. Clinicians should keep in mind that the order in which sounds are incorporated into speech varies from child to child and does not necessarily follow a specific sequence. There is no indication that one sound is dependent on any other for its development.

Speech-language pathologists have shown a particular interest in the effect of maturation on children identified as having speech sound disorders. Roe and Milisen (1942) sampled 1,989 children in grades 1 through 6 who had never received any formal speech therapy. They found that the children's mean number of articulation errors decreased between grades 1 and 2, grades 2 and 3, and grades 3 and 4. In contrast, the difference in the mean number of errors between grades 4 and 5 and grades 5 and 6 was not significant. The authors concluded that maturation was responsible for improvement in articulation performance between grades 1 and 4 but was not an appreciable factor in articulation improvement in grades 5 and 6.

Sayler (1949) assessed articulation in 1,998 students in grades 7 through 12 as they read sentences orally. His findings indicated a slight decrease in the mean number of articulation errors at each subsequent grade level, but because the improvement in speech sound productions was so small, he concluded that maturation does not appear to be an appreciable factor in improvement in the middle school and secondary grades. Children in upper elementary and secondary grades appear to be more consistent in their phonologic patterns than children in the lower elementary grades.

Factors that relate to normal phonologic variations during the school years include refinement of the timing of sequential articulatory gestures, the influence of reading and spelling, and peer influence (Chapter 3 of this book). These factors, however, would result in, at most, only minor phonologic variations within this age group.

Summary

Acquisition by a child of the adult speech sound system has been shown to be related to maturation. There is a direct correlation between improvement in articulation skills and age through approximately age 8, when phonologic mastering is essentially complete in normally developing, children. Maturation generally is not a factor in speech sound acquisition after age 9 in normally developing children.

Gender

Child development specialists have long been interested in contrasts between males and females in phonologic acquisition, and, likewise, speech-language pathologists have investigated the relationship between gender and articulation status. Research in this area has focused on (1) a comparison of phoneme acquisition in males and females and (2) a comparison of the incidence of speech sound disorders in males and females.

Dawson (1929) examined the articulatory skills of 200 children from grades 1 through 12 on six measures of articulation. He reported that until approximately age 12, girls were slightly superior to boys in their articulatory skills. Templin (1963) reported similar findings: "In articulation development, girls consistently are found to be slightly accelerated . . . in all instances the differences are relatively small and often are not statistically significant" (p. 13).

Smit, Hand, Freilinger, Bernthal, and Bird (1990) conducted a large-scale normative study of phonologic development in children ages 3 through 9 from Iowa and Nebraska. They reported that the Iowa-Nebraska girls appeared to acquire sounds at somewhat earlier ages than boys through age 6. The differences reached statistical significance only at age 6 and younger and not in every preschool age group. Kenney and Prather (1986), who elicited multiple productions of frequent error sounds, reported significant differences favoring girls in the age range 3 through 5.

Speech surveys conducted by Hall (1938), Mills and Streit (1942), Morley (1952), Everhart (1960), and Hull, Mielke, Timmons, and Willeford (1971) indicated that the incidence of speech sound disorder was higher in males than females, regardless of the age group studied. Smit and colleagues (1990) stated that "it is a well-known fact that boys are at much greater risk than girls for delayed speech, and this propensity continues to be reported" (p. 790).

Summary

The sex of a child does not appear to be a significant factor in phonologic acquisition. It should be recognized, however, that at certain ages females tend to be slightly ahead of males in phonologic acquisition. Many current tests of speech sound acquisition include separate normative data for males and females. Sex as a factor is also reflected in the fact that significantly more male than female children are identified as having speech sound disorders.

Family Background

Researchers have been interested in the influence of family background, both environmental and biological, and how it may affect a child's speech and language development. In the following paragraphs we will review literature related to family background and phonology organized around three topics: (1) socioeconomic status, (2) family transmission, and (3) sibling influences.

Socioeconomic Status

The socioeconomic status of a child's family, as measured by parents' educational background, parental occupation, income, and location of family residence, is a significant part of the child's environment. Since some behavioral deficiencies occur more frequently in lower socioeconomic environments, socioeconomic status has been of interest to speech-language clinicians as a possible factor in language development.

Everhart (1953, 1956) explored the variable of parental occupational status in an investigation of the relationship between articulation and other developmental factors in children. In speech surveys of children in grades 1 through 6, those classified as having speech sound disorders were compared to children with normal speech development with respect to parental occupation. No significant differences were found, and Everhart concluded that the occurrence of speech sound disorders in children was not related to parental occupation.

Templin (1957) analyzed developmental language data from children ages 3 to 8 years in terms of parental occupation and reached a somewhat different conclusion. She used the *Minnesota Scale for Parental Occupations* to categorize parental occupation. At each age level, children whose parents were in the upper occupational group had fewer misarticulations than the children in the lower occupational group. In particular, 4-, 4 1/2-, and 7-year-old children whose parents were in the lower occupational group had significantly more articulation errors than those whose parents were in the upper group. Templin concluded that parental occupation seemed to be a factor in children's articulation skill until about age 4 but that parental occupation no longer seemed to influence articulation development by the time children were 8 years old.

Weaver and colleagues (1960) also investigated the relationship between parental occupation and articulation proficiency in 592 first-grade children and found that a greater number of children with normal articulation skills came from homes in the upper occupational group, whereas more children with articulation errors came from homes in the lower occupational group. The poorest articulation proficiency, as judged by number of articulation errors, was found among children from the two lowest occupational classes.

Prins (1962a) found no significant correlation between articulation and socioeconomic level for 92 articulatory defective children between the ages of 2 and 6 years. Likewise, Smit and colleagues (1990) in the Iowa-Nebraska normative study reported that socioeconomic level did not have a significant relationship to articulatory performance. After an extensive review of the literature on the relationship between articulation and socioeconomic status, Winitz (1969) concluded that "more misarticulating children and more articulatory errors are found in the lower socioeconomic groups than in the upper socioeconomic groups. However, when a correlational index is used, the relationship is low or nonsignificant" (p. 147).

These findings overall suggest that speech sound disorders are not that strongly associated with low SES (i.e., growing up in a low SES household does not guarantee a problem with speech sounds). However, when combined with other factors, low SES may interact to result in a speech sound disorder. Recall our previous discussion of how children with frequent otitis media who also grow up in low SES households are at significantly increased risk of developing a speech sound problem.

Familial Tendencies

It is not uncommon for speech-language pathologists to observe a family history of developmental speech and language disorders. While information of this nature is often noted in diagnostic reports, until the 1980s few systematic attempts were made to study speech sound disorders as they related to family history. Neils and Aram (1986) obtained reports from the parents of 74 preschool language-disordered children and indicated that 46 percent reported that other family members had histories of speech and language disorders. Of this group, 55 percent were reported to have speech sound disorders, the most prevalent type of familial disorder reported. Shriberg and Kwiatkowski (1994) reported data from 62 children, ages 3 to 6 years with developmental phonologic disorders. They found that 39 percent of the children had one member of the family with the same speech problem, while an additional 17 percent (total = 56 percent) had more than one family member with the same speech problem.

Two twin studies have been reported that contribute to our understanding of familial influences, including genetic factors that may relate to speech sound disorders. Matheny and Bruggeman (1973) studied 101 same-sex twin sets, 22 opposite-sex twin sets, and 94 siblings between the ages of 3 and 8 years. An articulation screening test was administered to each child. Monozygotic twins' articulation screening correlated more closely with each other than did dizygotic twins' scores. The authors concluded that there is a strong hereditary influence on articulation status. In addition, sex differences were found to favor females. Locke and Mather (1987) examined speech sound productions in 13 monozygotic and 13 dizygotic twin sets. They reported more phonetic concordance in the monozygotic than the dizygotic twins (i.e., the identical twins were more similar in their errors patterns than the fraternal twins).

Lewis, Ekelman, and Aram (1989) examined the familial basis of speech sound disorders by comparing sibling articulation status for a group of children identified as evidencing a severe speech sound disorder, and a group who reflected normal speech development. Assessment measures included the *Natural Process Analysis*, repetition of 50 multisyllabic words, and the *Screening Test for Developmental Verbal Apraxia*. In addition, language, gross- and fine-motor skills, and reading were assessed. Family histories of communication disorders and/or learning disabilities were noted. Results revealed that the siblings of the children with communication disorders performed more poorly than control siblings on phonology and reading measures. Disordered participants' phonologic skills correlated positively with those of their siblings, whereas controls' scores did not. Families of children with disorders reported significantly more members with speech and language disorders and dyslexia than did families of controls. Sex differences were reflected in the incidence but not in the severity or type of disorder present. The authors concluded that their findings suggested a familial basis for at least some forms of severe speech sound disorders.

One of the most interesting studies of the familial basis of phonologic impairments was conducted by Felsenfeld and colleagues (1995). These investigators utilized speech and academic development data involving 400 normally developing children that were gathered between 1960 and 1972 by Templin and Glaman (1976). From this sample, two follow-up groups were identified consisting of 24 adults with a history of a moderate phonologic-language disorder as children, and a control group of 28 adults with a documented history of normal articulation development. They reported that the children of the "disordered" participants performed significantly more poorly on all tests of articulation and expressive language functioning and were significantly more likely to have received articulation treatment than were the children of the control participants. There was, however, no evidence that specific misarticulations or phonologic processes could be identified with the "disorders" families.

Recall also the previously mentioned study by Lewis and colleagues (2007) comparing parents of children with speech sound disorders who themselves had histories of speech sound disorders against parents of similar children without such histories. The parents with histories of speech sound disorders themselves performed significantly poorer on standardized tests of spoken language and spelling.

It may be inferred from these studies that genetic or biological inheritance factors may precipitate the speech sound disorder, yet it is often difficult to separate environmental from genetic/biological influences. A study that examined environmental influences was reported by Parlour and Broen (1991). Their research was predicated on the possibility that individuals who themselves experienced significant speech and language disorders as children are likely to become adults who will provide a less than optimal cultural or linguistic milieu for their own families.

Parlour and Broen (1991) collected follow-up family data of adults with and without a childhood history of delayed phonologic development. Both groups of participants were originally part of the large normative study that was conducted by Mildred Templin (1968) 28 years earlier. The group who had displayed a moderate to moderately severe speech sound disorder in early elementary school was comprised of 24 individuals. The control group was comprised of 28 adults who had evidenced average or better articulation during the same time period. Two environmental measures, the *Preschool HOME Scale* and the *Modified Templin Child-Rearing Questionnaire,* were employed to ascertain qualitative aspects of a child's environment including physical, emotional, and cognitive support available to preschool children, and child-rearing practices. These two measures included direct observation of the examiner, parental reports, and parental responses to a written questionnaire.

The two groups performed in a generally comparable manner for all of the environmental domains sampled, with one exception, acceptance, which assessed disciplinary practices. Parlour and Broen (1991) reported that families with a history of speech sound disorders were more reliant on physical punishment than were control families. In terms of future research efforts, the authors suggested that although differences were generally not significant between the groups, the disordered group received lower mean scores than controls on each of the Home subscales, suggesting that some subtle differences may have been present, particularly for domains involving the use of punishment, learning, and language stimulation.

Sibling Influences

Another factor of interest to investigators of phonologic acquisition has been sibling number and birth order. Since the amount of time that parents can spend with each child decreases with each child added to a family, some clinicians have questioned whether sibling status is related to articulatory development. Koch (1956) studied the relationships between certain speech and voice characteristics in young children and siblings in two-child families. In this study, 384 children between 5 and 6 years old were divided into 24 subgroups matched individual by individual on the basis of age, socioeconomic class, and residence. Data on speech and voice characteristics consisted of teachers' ratings. Koch reported that firstborn children had better articulation than secondborn, and the wider the age difference between a child and his or her sibling, the better the child's articulation.

Likewise, Davis (1937) reported that children without siblings demonstrated superior articulatory performance to children with siblings and to twins. On the other hand, Wellman, Case, Mengert, and Bradbury (1931) did not find a significant relationship between the number of siblings and level of articulation skill for 3-year-olds.

Twins have been reported to present unique patterns of speech sound acquisition (Perkins, 1977; Powers, 1971; Winitz, 1969). From birth, twins receive speech stimulation not only from others within their environment but also from each other. Powers (1971) indicated that the "emotional ties of twins, too, are likely to be closer than those of singled siblings, which further augments their interdependence in speech" (p. 868). It is not uncommon for twins to reflect common phonologic patterns and use similar phonologic processes. Schwartz and colleagues (1980) reported, however, that in the very early stages of phonologic acquisition (the first 50 words), similarities in phonemes used, including phonologic patterns and lexical items, were not present. Unique patterns of speech occasionally found in twins 2 years and older that have little resemblance to adult models and have meaning only to the twins are termed *idioglossia*.

Summary

Little relationship exists between socioeconomic status and speech sound disorders based on available reports. Although greater numbers of misarticulating children tend to be found in lower socioeconomic groups (especially children under 4 years), socioeconomic status by itself does not appear to contribute significantly to the presence of a speech sound disorder.

Studies of phonologic development in twins, as well as in families with a history of phonologic impairment, suggest some sort of familial propensity toward the presence of such a disorder. Investigations examining phonologic status and sibling relationships are limited, but findings have been fairly consistent. Firstborn and only children exhibit better articulation performance than children with older siblings or twins. The age span between siblings also appears to affect phonologic proficiency, with better articulation associated with wider age differences. One can speculate that the firstborn or only child receives better speech models and greater stimulation than the child who has older siblings. The possibility also exists that older siblings produce "normal" developmental phonologic errors and, thus at points in time present imperfect speech models to younger siblings. Unique patterns of sound productions have been reported in twins; reasons for these patterns are speculative and tend to focus on the stimulation each twin receives from the other. Unique speech patterns have, however, been reported, even in very young twins.

Personality

The relationship between personality characteristics and phonologic behavior has been investigated to determine if particular personality patterns are likely to be associated with speech sound disorders. Researchers have examined not only the child's personality traits but also those of the child's parents, using various assessment tools.

Bloch and Goodstein (1971) concluded, in a review of the literature, that personality traits and emotional adjustment of individuals with speech sound disorders have shown contradictory findings and attributed this to two major problems with the investigations: (1)

the criteria for defining articulatory impairment has varied from one study to the next and (2) the tools or instruments used to assess personality and adjustment have varied in their validity and reliability.

In a causal-correlates profile based on 178 children with developmental phonologic disorders, Shriberg and Kwiatkowski (1994) presented data on psychosocial inputs (parental behaviors) and psychosocial behaviors (child characteristics) that were descriptive of this population. Twenty-seven (27) percent of the parents were judged to be either somewhat or considerably ineffective in terms of behavioral management, and 17 percent were either somewhat or considerably overconcerned about their child's problem. An even smaller percentage of parents indicated that it was their perception that their child had difficulty with initial acceptance by peers. Over half the children (51 percent) were described as somewhat too sensitive (easily hurt feelings), and an additional 14 percent were described as overly sensitive (very easily hurt feelings). They reported that their descriptive data indicated that "a significant number of children with developmental phonologic disorders experience psychosocial difficulties" (p. 115). They indicated, however, that one cannot be completely certain that sampling biases did not inflate the magnitudes of the findings, or whether the participants would differ significantly from data in a nonspeech-delayed group.

Summary

While certain personality characteristics have been linked to some children with developmental phonologic impairments, no clear picture of personality variance from normals has emerged in this population. Likewise, certain parental/home variables have been associated with this population, but the strength of that association is unclear. Further studies involving normal–disordered child comparisons are necessary before a definitive statement regarding this causal-correlate can be made.

CONCLUSION

The field has made great strides in understanding children with speech sound disorders. For many of these children, the cause of the problem is known, and specific approaches to assessment and intervention are being developed. In other cases, however, the origin of the problem is not known. This latter group of children does not consistently respond to the same intervention approaches, suggesting that there may be subgroups. Several research teams are attempting to unravel possible subgroups.

A great deal has been discovered that can assist the speech-language pathologist in assessing phonologic status, planning remediation programs, and counseling clients and their parents. Yet, many questions remain unanswered. One truth that emerges from the literature, however, is the absence of any one-to-one correspondence between the presence of a particular factor and the precise nature of most individuals' phonologic status. Prediction of cause-effect relationships represents a scientific ideal, but determination of such relationships in the realm of human behavior, including communication disorders, is often difficult.

■ **QUESTIONS FOR CHAPTER 4**

1. What is meant by an "organically based" speech sound disorder? Cite some examples.

2. Briefly outline the three ways investigators have tried to identify subgroups of speech sound disorders of unknown origin.

3. Cite specific examples wherein knowledge of etiology is highly important, if not essential, to developing an effective and efficient intervention program.

4. What is the relationship of speech sound perception and speech sound errors?

5. What is the relationship between phonological disorders and morphosyntactic language impairments?

6. What is the relationship of phonological delay, phonological awareness, and a child's acquisition of literacy?

7. Explain why "correlation does not imply causation."

8. How is each of the following factors related to clinical phonology and speech production?

   a. Otitis media

   b. Tongue thrusting

   c. Missing teeth

   d. Apraxia

   e. Cognitive impairment

   f. Severe language impairment

   g. Poor literacy skills

   h. Lower socioeconomic status

   i. Dental braces

   j. Significant hearing loss

   k. Family history of phonological difficulties

   l. Removal of part of the tongue

Phonological Assessment Procedures

NICHOLAS W. BANKSON
James Madison University

JOHN E. BERNTHAL
University of Nebraska–Lincoln

PETER FLIPSEN JR.
Idaho State University

PHONOLOGICAL SAMPLING

One of the unique contributions of the field of speech-language pathology to the assessment of verbal behavior is the development of *phonological assessment* instruments. For several decades, phonological/articulation assessment procedures have remained almost the exclusive domain of speech-language clinicians, although linguists, child development specialists, psychologists, pediatricians, and special educators also use such tools.

Evaluation of an individual's phonological status typically involves description of his or her speech sound production system and comparing this system to the adult standard of the speaker's linguistic community *(relational analysis)* in order to determine which sounds are produced correctly. For speakers with limited phonological repertoires, the speech sound system is often described independent of the adult standard *(independent analysis),* in which case the examiner simply wants to know what speech sounds are produced, regardless of whether they are used correctly or not. Phonological assessment is often done in the context of a communication evaluation that also includes assessment of voice quality, resonance, fluency, syntax, semantics, pragmatics, discourse, and prosodic aspects of language. Additional related measures such as hearing testing and an oral mechanism examination are usually included in a comprehensive communication evaluation/assessment. Although some clinicians have differentiated between phonological delay (children whose speech sound errors are similar to those found in younger normally developing children) and phonological disorders (children whose speech sound errors differ from normal developing children), we will not differentiate between the two here. In reality, most children with multiple misarticulations will have errors that fall into both categories.

Phonological assessment is used to describe the phonological status of an individual and:

1. Determine whether his or her speech sound system is sufficiently different from normal development to warrant intervention.
2. Determine treatment direction, including target behaviors and strategies to be used in the management of the client.
3. Make prognostic statements relative to phonological change with or without intervention/therapy.
4. Monitor change in phonological performance across time.
5. Identify factors that may be related to the presence or maintenance of a phonological disability/delay.

In addition, the speech-language pathologist (SLP) may be called on to identify and describe dialectal variations of Standard American English. The need to describe such differences usually follows a request or inquiry for accent reduction by individuals who speak a regional or cultural dialect or for whom English is a second language. In the case of a client referred for a phonologic evaluation whose speech reflects dialectal differences, the speech-language pathologist must be able to differentiate which phonological characteristics reflect dialect differences and which reflect a speech disorder.

The primary purposes of a phonological assessment are to determine whether an individual needs phonological instruction, and if so, the direction of such treatment. To make these determinations, the clinician engages in a multistep process that involves sampling the client's speech through a variety of procedures, analyzing the data gathered, interpreting the data that have been analyzed, and then making clinical recommendations. In this chapter, we will discuss various sampling and testing procedures and discuss factors and issues that should be taken into consideration when analyzing and interpreting speech sound samples. This chapter will focus on impairments rather than accent/dialect reduction since the latter will be discussed in detail in Chapter 8. At the end of this chapter, you will find a case history of a child to whom procedures discussed in this chapter are applied.

SCREENING FOR PHONOLOGICAL DISORDERS

A complete phonological assessment, including analysis and interpretation of results, is not something that can be done quickly. Because of this time expenditure, clinicians will often do a screening to determine if a more comprehensive phonological assessment is warranted. Screening procedures are not designed to determine the need or direction of therapy, but rather to identify individuals who merit further evaluation from those for whom further assessment is not indicated. Screening might include (1) screening children at a preschool or "kindergarten roundup" to determine whether they have age-appropriate phonological skills; (2) screening children in grade 3 (by which time maturation should have resolved most developmental errors); (3) screening individuals preparing for occupations, such as broadcast journalism, that require specific speech performance standards; and (4) screening the phonological status of clients referred for a suspected communication impairment.

In screening, individuals are not identified as candidates for therapy, but rather are simply identified as needing further assessment. Additional testing is often required before statements about the presence or absence of a phonological disorder can be made, and it is certainly required for determining the direction for treatment. Instruments used for screening consist of a limited sampling of speech sound productions, which can usually be administered in five minutes or less. Screening measures can be categorized as informal or formal. Informal measures are often used when people wish to develop their own screening tools in order to meet their particular needs. Formal measures are often employed when users desire established norms or testing methodologies that are more uniform.

Informal Screening Measures

Informal screening measures are usually devised by the examiner and are tailored to the population being screened. Although informal procedures can be easily and economically devised, they do not include standardized administration procedures or normative data, which are characteristics of formal screening measures. An example of an informal screening procedure that could be used with a group of kindergarten children would be where the examiner asks each child the following:

1. State your name and address.
2. Count to ten; name the days of the week.
3. Tell about a television show.

If the subjects are adults, the examiner might ask them to do one or all of the following:

1. Read sentences designed to elicit several productions of frequently misarticulated sounds, such as /s/, /r/, /l/, and /θ/. For example, "I saw Sally at her seaside house; Rob ran around the orange car."
2. Read a passage with a representative sample of English speech sounds, such as the "Grandfather Passage."

   Grandfather Passage. You wish to know all about my grandfather. Well, he is nearly 93 years old, yet he still thinks as swiftly as ever. He dresses himself in an old black frock coat, usually several buttons missing. A long beard clings to his chin, giving those who observe him a pronounced feeling of the utmost respect. When he speaks, his voice is just a bit cracked and quivers a bit. Twice each day he plays skillfully and with zest upon a small organ. Except in winter when the snow or ice prevents, he slowly takes a short walk in the open air each day. We have often urged him to walk more and smoke less, but he always answers, "Banana oil." Grandfather likes to be modern in his language.

3. Engage in an informal conversation about topics of interest such as a recent vacation or a current event.

Criteria for failure of informal screening are determined by the examiner. An often-used rule of thumb is "If in doubt, refer for further testing." In other words, an examiner who suspects that the client's speech sound system is not appropriate for his or her age and/or linguistic community should be referred for a more complete assessment. The examiner may also choose to determine or establish performance standards on the screening instrument that will help identify those referred for further testing. Those individuals with the greatest need for additional testing and probable intervention will usually be obvious to the examiner from even a small sample of their speech and language.

Formal Screening Measures

Formal screening measures include published elicitation procedures for which normative data and/or cut-off scores are often available. These formal measures are usually one of three types: (1) tests designed solely for screening phonology, (2) tests that are related or part of a more comprehensive phonological assessment, and (3) tests that screen phonology as well as other aspects of language. Tests designed explicitly for screening phonology are often used when screening phonology is the primary goal. Those instruments that combine phonological screening with other aspects of language screening are most commonly used for more general communication disorders screening, wherein information on phonology is just part of the communication behavior that is of interest.

The following is a formal phonology screening test that is not part of a larger phonology test or a more comprehensive communication screening.

Denver Articulation Screening Exam (DASE) (Drumwright, 1971)

The DASE is a 5-minute test to detect articulation disorders in children $2\frac{1}{2}$ to 7 years. It consists of 22 pictures that the testee is required to produce following the tester's model. The author indicates that this test is especially useful with children who are shy or immature, or who have a short attention span. The examiner is asked to judge intelligibility on a 4-point scale, with 1 being "easy to understand" and 4 being "can't evaluate." Children are ranked "normal to abnormal," depending on composite articulation and intelligibility scores.

The following is an example of a formal screening measure that is part of a more comprehensive assessment of phonology.

Diagnostic Screen (Dodd, Hua, Crosbie, Holm, and Ozanne, 2006)

The *Diagnostic Screen* is related to *The Diagnostic Evaluation of Articulation and Phonology (DEAP)* instrument. The screening portion includes 22 pictures that are imitated following examiner production, requires 5 minutes to administer, and provides an indication of whether further assessment may be appropriate. The authors indicate that the screening test is especially useful with children who are shy or immature, or who have a short attention span.

The following tests include screening of phonology as part of an overall speech and language screening.

Fluharty Preschool Speech and Language Screening Test–Second Edition (Fluharty, 2000)

This test was designed for children, ages 3 through 6 years. The articulation portion of the test uses 15 pictured objects to elicit 30 target sounds. Some stimulus items are designed to assess two sounds. Standard scores and percentiles for the subtests are included.

Speech-Ease Screening Inventory (K–1) (Pigott, Barry, Hughes, Eastin, Titus, Stensil, Metcalf, and Porter, 1985)

This test was designed for kindergartners and first-graders. The overall test takes 7 to 10 minutes to administer, with the articulation section being comprised of 12 items. Through sentence completion items, 14 phonemes and three blends are assessed. Cut-off scores for phoneme error counts indicative of the need for further testing are provided.

Preschool Language Scale (Zimmerman, Steiner, and Pond, 1992)

This test was designed for children, ages 1 through 7. The "articulation screener" portion of the test consists of 37 items that test 18 speech sounds plus one consonant cluster. Performance levels expected for children are provided.

Summary

Screening procedures are not designed to determine the need or direction of treatment. Rather, their purpose is to identify individuals for further testing. The criteria for failure on informal screening tests are often left up to the examiner. When available, standard scores and percentile ranks aid the examiner in establishing such criteria. It is not uncommon for a score one standard deviation below the mean to be used as a cut-off score. For some instruments, cut-off scores or age expectation scores are provided.

COMPREHENSIVE PHONOLOGICAL ASSESSMENT: ASSESSMENT BATTERY

Sampling procedures involved in phonological assessment are more in-depth and detailed than those described for screening. When doing a phonological analysis, the clinician usually employs several assessment instruments and sampling procedures since no one sampling procedure or test provides all a clinician needs to know when making case selection decisions and determining the direction that an intervention program should take. A phonological evaluation typically involves phonological productions in speech samples of varying lengths (e.g., syllables, words, phrases), phonetic contexts, and in response to various elicitation procedures (e.g., picture naming, imitation, conversation). This collection of samples is often referred to as an *assessment battery*.

As already stated, the two major purposes of a phonological assessment are to determine the need for and direction of treatment. It is to these purposes that most of the writings, research, and testing materials on phonological disorders have been addressed. In the following pages, components of a phonological evaluation battery, with an emphasis on procedures for obtaining phonological samples, are presented. Following this, analysis and interpretation of data collected through sampling procedures are discussed. Throughout this chapter, an attempt is made to synthesize the available literature and make suggestions based on the authors' clinical experience.

Phonological Samples Included in the Test Battery

Connected/Conversational Speech Sampling

Rationale.   All phonological evaluations should include a sample of connected speech. Since the ultimate objective of phonological treatment is correct production of sounds in spontaneous conversation, it is important that the examiner observe sound productions in as "natural" a speaking context as possible. Such samples allow one to transcribe phoneme productions in a variety of phonetic contexts, to observe error patterns, and to judge the severity of the problem and the intelligibility of the speaker in continuous discourse. Sounds produced in connected speech may also be studied in relation to other factors such as speech rate, intonation, stress, and syllable structure. In addition, connected speech samples allow for multiple productions of sounds across lexical items.

Because spontaneous connected speech samples are the most valid or representative sample of phonological performance, some clinicians suggest that phonological analyses should be exclusively based on this type of sample (Shriberg and Kwiatkowski, 1980; Stoel-Gammon and Dunn, 1985; Morrison and Shriberg, 1992). Connected speech samples have the advantage of allowing the examiner to transcribe sound productions within the context of the child's own vocabulary and in running speech, which includes his natural prosodic patterns. In addition, these samples can be used for other types of language analysis. Sometimes, however, there are practical problems associated with relying solely on such samples. Many individuals with severe phonological problems may be almost unintelligible, and it may be impossible or very difficult to reliably determine and/or transcribe what they are attempting to say in conversational speech. Some children may be reluctant to engage in conversational dialogue with an adult they do not know. It may also be an almost impossible task to obtain a spontaneous speech corpus that contains a representative sample of English phonemes.

Ingram (1989a) suggested that difficulty in obtaining a "cross-section of the sounds in English" (representative sample) may not be a critical issue. He argued that if a spontaneous sample is of "sufficient size," the child's preference for sounds is revealed. Sounds missing from the sample may reflect a "selective avoidance" by the child; that is, the child chooses not to produce them. However, the absence of specific sounds in a child's spontaneous speech may reflect an infrequent occurrence of those sounds in English rather than selective avoidance; and even if the inference of selective avoidance is valid, clinicians may want the benefit of information about other productions. In summary, although connected speech samples are an essential part of an assessment battery, most clinicians do not rely on this type sample exclusively.

Elicitation Procedures.   The customary and preferred method for obtaining a sample of connected speech is to engage a client in spontaneous conversation. The clinician may talk with the client about such things as his or her family, television shows, or places the client has visited. The samples should be recorded so that the clinician can play them back as often as required to accurately transcribe the client's utterances. Clinicians should make notes about topics covered and errors noted to facilitate later transcription.

Some clinicians have the client read a passage orally as an alternative method for obtaining a connected sample of speech. Although this procedure provides a sample of connected speech, it has been demonstrated that usually fewer errors occur in a reading sample obtained in this manner than in a corpus of conversational speech (Wright, Shelton, and Arndt, 1969). Moreover, clinicians frequently test children who have not yet learned to read, in which case this procedure is obviously not a viable option.

Some speech sound tests specify procedures for obtaining a sample of connected speech. For example, in the "Sounds-in-Sentences" subtest of the *Goldman-Fristoe Test of Articulation* (Goldman and Fristoe, 2000), the client listens to a story while viewing accompanying pictures and is then asked to repeat the story. Such a delayed imitation task is designed to elicit particular sounds in certain phonetic contexts.

A more spontaneous method than either the immediate or delayed imitation technique is for the client to tell a story about a series of pictures selected to elicit target words and sounds. Dubois and Bernthal (1978) compared productions in the same word stimuli elicited through a picture-naming task, a delayed imitation task, and a storytelling task. They reported that the greatest number of errors were found on the storytelling task and the smallest number on the picture-naming task. These findings were not surprising, since the task of naming single words requires different skills than the sequencing of words in phrases and sentences. Although the differences between the methods were statistically significant, the authors interpreted the differences as clinically nonsignificant. They did, however, report that some individuals varied from group trends in their production of certain sounds, depending on the task; for example, some children made significantly more errors on the delayed imitation task than on the picture-naming task.

Summary.   A connected speech sample is a crucial part of any phonological assessment battery because it allows (1) assessment of overall intelligibility and severity, (2) determination of speech sound usage in its natural form, and (3) a database from which to judge the accuracy of individual sounds, patterns of errors, and consistency of misarticulations. The preferred method for obtaining connected speech samples is to engage the client in spontaneous conversation. If, for some reason, this cannot be accomplished, alternate procedures that can be used include (1) conversational responses elicited via picture stimuli or toys, (2) utilization of a reading passage, and (3) telling a story following the clinician's model (delayed imitation).

Single-Word/Citation Form Sampling

Rationale.   From the standpoint of widespread usage, analyzing phoneme productions in a corpus of single-word productions (usually elicited by having an examinee name pictures) has been a common method for assessing speech sounds. Single words provide a discrete, identifiable unit of production that examiners can usually readily transcribe. Since transcribers often are interested in observing the production of only one or perhaps two segments per word, they are thus able to transcribe and analyze single-word samples more quickly than multiple or connected word samples. Even though a test may prescribe the scoring of only one or two sounds, we would recommend that the tester transcribe the entire word, including vowels. The efficiency of analyzing sound productions from single-word productions has resulted in widespread usage of such stimuli. As suggested earlier, this type of sampling provides data that are supplemental to information obtained from the connected speech sample.

When sampling single words, it is typical for only one or two consonants to be targeted and scored in a word. Sound positions include sounds in the *initial* position (sound at the beginning of a word, e.g., /b/ in /bot/), *final* position (sound at the end of a word, e.g., /t/ in /ræbɪt/), and *medial* position (all sounds between the initial and final sounds, e.g., /ɔ/, /k/, and /ɪ/ in /wɔkɪŋ/).

In some instances, the prefixes *pre-, inter-,* and *post-* are each combined with the term *vocalic* to describe the location of a consonant sound within syllables. *Prevocalic* position refers to consonants that precede a vowel (CV) and therefore initiate the syllable (e.g., *s*oap, *c*at). *Postvocalic* position refers to consonants that follow the vowel (VC) and therefore terminate the syllable (e.g., soa*p*, ca*t*). *Intervocalic* position involves a consonant that is embedded (VCV) between two vowels (e.g., ca*m*el, ea*g*er). A singleton consonant in the initial position of a word is prevocalic. Likewise, a singleton sound in word-final position is postvocalic. A consonant in the intervocalic position serves the dual function of ending the preceding syllable and initiating the following syllable. Ingram (1981) suggested that when one consonant occurs between two vowel nuclei, such "ambisyllabic" consonants may be viewed as being shared by both syllables. The intervocalic consonant would be in the word-medial position, since *medial* refers to somewhere between the first and the last sounds of the word. A medial consonant may stand next to another consonant and serve to initiate (release) or terminate (arrest) a syllable, and therefore is not necessarily intervocalic. Thus, references to initial, medial, and final positions refer to location of consonants in a word, whereas the terms *prevocalic, intervocalic, postvocalic, releasor, arrestor, onset,* and *code* refer to consonant position relative to syllables.

Speech sound productions are influenced by the complexity of the syllables and words in which they are produced. We know that the number and juxtaposition of phonemes make some syllables more difficult to produce than others. For example, a syllable such as /go/ is easier to produce than /grop/. The first syllable shapes to develop are generally CV, VC, and CVCV, which constitute the simplest syllable shapes.

One of the key issues in assessment concerns the correlation between phonological productions that occur in citation form (single words) and those that occur in connected speech. Research findings support a positive correlation between responses obtained from naming pictures and speech sound productions in spontaneous speaking situations. It should be noted, however, that in some clients, differences are frequently observed between these two types of measures. Clinicians need to be aware that sound productions in single words may not accurately reflect the same sounds produced in a spontaneous speech context.

Morrison and Shriberg (1992) reviewed 40 years of studies that were designed to compare citation-form testing (single-word testing) with continuous-speech sampling. They reported that, in general, more errors occur in spontaneous connected speech as compared to production of single words, although there were instances in which speech sound errors were more frequent in word naming. However, in their own research they reported that children produced sounds more accurately in connected speech than they did in citation-form testing.

Single-word testing does not provide the tester an opportunity to evaluate the effect of context on speech sound productions (coarticulation). As discussed in Chapter 1, coarticulatory effects transcend phonetic, syllabic, and lexical (word) boundaries. Gallagher and Shriner (1975) reported that children's /s/ productions were affected by position in CCV consonant clusters. Curtis and Hardy (1959) reported that /r/ was more likely to be produced correctly in consonant clusters than in single phoneme productions. Hoffman, Schuckers, and Ratusnik (1977) reported that /r/ was influenced by factors such as lexical constraints (within vs. across word boundaries) and phonetic contexts. For example, when /r/ was embedded in nonlexically constrained contexts (e.g., "The sick *rat* dies"), production was facilitated in the environment of /s/ as compared to /m/, /p/, and /t/. Variations in consonant production when sounds are elicited in consonant-plus-vowel contexts rather than in consonant clusters are widely recognized.

Despite reservations concerning some of the inferences that can be made about conversational speech on the basis of single-word samples, most clinicians value and include single-word productions in the assessment battery. Single-word tests, which can provide the clinician with information concerning phonetic skills, typically include all consonant phonemes in a language, and can provide phonological data in a relatively short time. In addition, for unintelligible clients, the tester has the advantage of knowing the productions the client has attempted to say. Because of the variations and because of the different kinds of data each sample provides in productions of single words versus connected speech, we recommend that both should be included in the assessment battery.

Elicitation Procedures.   The customary way to elicit single-word productions is through the administration of a single-word articulation test (generally called a *speech sound inventory*), where a client names single words in response to picture stimuli. Single words may also be obtained by having a child name toys or objects. For young children, the clinician may simply wish to transcribe single-word productions the child produced spontaneously. Since picture-naming tests are the typical method for sampling single words, the following discussion will focus on this type of sampling procedure.

Speech sound inventories typically sample consonants, consonant clusters, and occasionally vowels and diphthongs. Consonants are often assessed in the initial, medial, and final positions of words—for example, /s/ in *s*aw, pen*c*il, hou*s*e; /ʃ/ in *s*hoe, sta*t*ion, fi*s*h, or in word-initial and final positions. Some instruments elicit sounds only in the initial and final positions (see Figure 5.1). The specific sounds included in inventories vary from test to test but almost always include those sounds that have a high frequency of error in children's speech. Studies have shown the following as the most frequently misarticulated sounds: /s, z, θ, ð, ʃ, ʒ, tʃ, dʒ, v, r, hw/. With the exception of the /hw/ (a phoneme that is often collapsed with /w/ in English), these sounds are among those items usually included in single-word tests.

As stated previously, speech sound inventories have traditionally placed little emphasis on the assessment of vowels. Undoubtedly this is a reflection of the fact that most preschool and school-age children with phonological disorders have problems primarily with consonants and that vowels are typically mastered at a relatively early age. As speech pathologists are increasingly involved in early intervention programs for children at risk for communication impairments, vowel productions have, however, been increasingly scrutinized. Although some speech sound tests do target vowels, the examiner is encouraged to transcribe vowel productions even though a test is designed to examine only consonants.

Consonant Inventory

Circle the I or F to indicate an error on an initial or final consonant or consonant cluster

# Target Word / Phonetic Transcription	Word Correct	Transcription of Child's Production	Modeled	p	b	m	w	f	v	θ	ð	t	d	s	z	n	l	ʃ	tʃ	dʒ	j	r	k	g	h	ɚ	clusters	Notes
1. cat kæt	☐	_____	☐									F											I					
2. gate get	☐	_____	☐									F												I				
3. cup kʌp	☐	_____	☐	F																			I					
4. candy kændi	☐	_____	☐																				I					
5. dog dɔg	☐	_____	☐										I											F				
6. bed bɛd	☐	_____	☐		I								F															
7. boat bot	☐	_____	☐		I							F																
8. goat got	☐	_____	☐									F												I				
9. gun gʌn	☐	_____	☐													F								I				
10. cow kau	☐	_____	☐																				I					
11. crab kræb	☐	_____	☐		F																						I	
12. coat kot	☐	_____	☐									F											I					
13. wagon wægən	☐	_____	☐				I																	F				
14. cake kek	☐	_____	☐																				I/F					
15. knife naɪf	☐	_____	☐					F								I												
16. hat hæt	☐	_____	☐									F													I			
17. rabbit ræbɪt	☐	_____	☐									F										I						
18. balloon bəlun	☐	_____	☐		I											F												
19. lamp læmp	☐	_____	☐														I									F		
20. radio redio [redɪo]	☐	_____	☐																			I						
21. rain ren	☐	_____	☐													F						I						
22. carrot kɛrət	☐	_____	☐									F										I						
23. lion laɪən	☐	_____	☐													F	I											
24. leaf lif	☐	_____	☐					F									I											
25. bus bʌs	☐	_____	☐		I									F														
26. seal sil	☐	_____	☐											I			F											
27. fish fɪʃ	☐	_____	☐					I										F										
28. sun sʌn	☐	_____	☐											I		F												

Page 3 Subtotal Words Correct ☐

	p	b	m	w	f	v	θ	ð	t	d	s	z	n	l	ʃ	tʃ	dʒ	j	r	k	g	h	ɚ	cl.
Page 3 Subtotals Initial Errors																								
Page 3 Subtotals Final Errors																								

■ FIGURE 5.1 Two-position speech sound test that samples words in initial and final position.

Source: Sample items from phonetic inventory portion of the *Bankson-Bernthal Test of Phonology (BBTOP)* (Bankson and Bernthal, 1990b). Used with permission of PRO-ED.

Pollock (1991) delineated the following suggestions regarding vowel sampling:

1. Clients should be provided with multiple opportunities to produce each vowel.
2. Vowels should be assessed in a variety of different contexts, including (a) monosyllabic and multisyllabic words, (b) stressed and unstressed syllables, and (c) a variety of adjacent preceding and especially following consonants.
3. Limits for the range of responses considered correct or acceptable should be established since cultural influences may affect what is considered "correct."
4. Recommended vowels and diphthongs to be assessed include the following:

Nonrhotic

/i/	/ou/
/ɪ/	/ɔ/
/ei/	/ɑ/
/ɛ/	/ʌ/ə/
/ae/	/aɪ/
/u/	/aʊ/
/ʊ/	/ɔi/

Rhotic

/ɝ, ɚ/	/ɔɚ/
/ɪɚ/	/ɑɚ/
/ɛɚ/	

To compensate for the lack of formal vowel assessment procedures, it is suggested that clinicians transcribe whole-word responses to the stimuli from commonly used phonological tests. In order to conduct a comprehensive review of vowels and diphthongs, it may be necessary, however, to supplement existing stimuli with additional vowels, diphthongs, and contexts not included in standard tests. For a comprehensive review of vowel disorders, refer to Ball and Gibbon (2001).

A number of phonological/articulation tests are commercially available. Despite the similarities between such tests, certain stimulus and response features differentiate one test from another. For example, one test may present items in a developmental sequence, another may organize the analysis according to place and manner of articulation, and a third test may emphasize colored line drawings that are especially attractive to young children or include actual photographs.

Although speech sound tests usually use pictures or photographs to elicit spontaneous responses, in some instances, toys or imitation tasks are used to elicit responses. Studies comparing responses elicited via imitation with those elicited through spontaneous picture-naming have produced inconsistent results. Investigators studying children between the ages of 5 and 8 years have reported that responses elicited via imitation tasks yield a greater number of correct responses than those elicited via spontaneous picture-naming (Siegel, Winitz, and Conkey, 1963; Smith and Ainsworth, 1967; Carter and Buck, 1958; Snow and Milisen, 1954). Other investigators who studied children ranging in age from 2 to 6 years reported no significant differences in results from elicitation via picture-naming and imitation (Templin, 1947; Paynter and Bumpas, 1977). It is best to simply assume that children, especially of school age, will do better on imitation as compared to spontaneous picture-naming tasks.

Harrington, Lux, and Higgins (1984) studied responses to different types of picture-naming tasks and reported that children produced fewer errors when items were elicited via photographs as compared to line drawings. These data again suggest that different response elicitation procedures frequently produce different findings; however, the clinical significance of such differences tends to be minimal. The clinician should be mindful that for a given client, the nature of the test stimuli may have a bearing on responses obtained.

In spite of their widespread use, single-word tests have a number of limitations. Such measures do not allow children to use their "own" words but rather a set of predetermined and sometimes complex syllable and word shapes. The use of multisyllabic test words may make more demands on a child's productions and elicit more errors than would monosyllabic words or the words used in a child's own spontaneous speech. Ingram (1976) reported that when initial-occurring fricative and affricate word pairs were similar in stress pattern and syllable structure, phoneme productions tended to be similar, but when syllable structure and/or stress of the pairs differed, monosyllabic words were more likely to be produced correctly than were multisyllabic words. Clinicians should recognize that syllable shape and stress patterns of stimulus words may affect speech sound productions. The clinician should also keep in mind that citation tests primarily consist of nouns because they can be pictured; thus, citation tests do not reflect the parts of speech used in connected conversational speech.

Another difficulty with tests designed to elicit a sample via picture-naming is that they often elicit only a single production of a given sound in each of either two or three word positions. During phonological development, inconsistency in production is common, even in the same stimulus word. Since the production of a sound may fluctuate, the client's customary articulatory patterns may be difficult to determine with only one to three samples of a sound. The clinician can increase the number of sound samples obtained through a single-word test by transcribing all the sounds in each stimulus (lexical) item, instead of focusing only on one or two sounds in each stimulus item. They can also add words that include particular phonemes in order to provide the testee additional opportunities to produce a sound of interest.

As a supplement to standard phonological analyses that are segmentally oriented, Ingram and Ingram (2001) outlined two measures based on whole-word productions. They pointed out that during the acquisition process, children attempt to learn and say words, not phonemes/segments, and thus word-oriented measures can assist the clinician to better understand a child's phonological system and the child's learning. Ingram and Ingram suggest that selection of target words for instruction should include an assessment of the complexity of the words to ensure that new sounds are introduced in word forms within the child's word system—that is, words within his or her vocabulary or those he or she can approximate. The goal of therapy is to expand not only the sound system and syllable shapes but also to increase the child's overall word complexity. The researchers proposed a metric called "phonological mean length of utterance" (PMLU) that attempts to do what mean length of utterance does in language assessment. This metric examines the number of correct consonants produced at the word level, a number that increases with the length of the child's productions. A second metric—proportion of whole-word proximity (PWP)—was assumed to be highly correlated with word intelligibility. The PWP is calculated by dividing the PMLU of the child's production by the PMLU of the fully correct production of the same word. Ingram and Ingram (2001) give the example of zucchini [zukini], with a PMLU of 9 (i.e., one point for each segment and one extra point for each of the three consonants). The child produces [zim] with a PMLU score of 6 (i.e., three segments, two points for each consonant). The PWP is then .67 (6 divided by 9). These two alternative measures are used to determine whole-word correctness, complexity, intelligibility, and variations. It is of note that although Schmitt, Howard, and Schmitt (1983) reported a significant correlation between score on whole-word accuracy and articulation scores, Bankson and Bernthal (1990b) reported that many children's "whole-word correct" score varied from what would have been predicted from segmental and process scores, although no statistical analysis of the correlation was reported.

Summary. Single-word samples, including speech sound tests, provide an efficient and relatively easy method for obtaining a sample of speech sound productions. Although they can be a valuable part of the phonological assessment battery, they should not constitute the only sampling procedure. Among their limitations are the small number of phonetic contexts sampled, the failure to reflect the effects of conversational context, the questionable representativeness of single-word naming responses, and the variability factors such as syllable shape, prosody, word familiarity, and parts of speech (e.g., nouns, verbs). To increase the number of phonetic contexts sampled through such tests, the clinician is encouraged to transcribe entire stimulus words rather than just the target sound in the word.

Stimulability Testing

Rationale. Another sample of speech sound productions frequently included in a test battery is obtained through stimulability testing—that is, sampling the client's ability to repeat the correct form (adult standard) of error sounds when provided with "stimulation." Traditionally, this testing has examined how well an individual imitates, in one or more phonetic contexts (i.e., isolation, syllables, words, phrases), sounds that were produced in error during testing. Although descriptions of what constitutes stimulability testing have varied, a commonly used procedure is one in which the examiner asks the respondent to imitate an auditory and/or visual model of a sound in one or more phonetic environements. A typical way of cueing the client is for the examiner to tell the client to "watch and listen to what I am going to say, and then you say it." In more recent years, investigators have gone beyond imitation to include more additional cueing such as placement instruction and visual/tactile imagery. Glaspey and Stoel-Gammon (2005) have developed a detailed procedure for doing stimulability testing that includes systematically varying phonetic environments and cueing procedures. They have labeled their form of testing as a "scaffolding" procedure, including directions and scoring for this type assessment. It should be recognized, however, that there are few standardized procedures for conducting stimulability testing. Some tests, such as the *Goldman-Fristoe Test of Articulation*, include a stimulability subtest. See Figure 5.2 for an example of a stimulability test for sounds in isolation and syllable productions that was developed by Adele Miccio (personal communication).

   Stimulability testing has been used (1) to determine whether a sound is likely to be acquired without intervention, (2) to determine the level and/or type of production at which instruction might begin, and (3) to predict the occurrence and nature of generalization. In

Stimulability Probe												
Name:												
Transcriber:												
Date:												
Sound	Iso	#__i	i__i	i__#		#__ɑ	ɑ__ɑ	ɑ__#	#__u	u__u	u__#	% Correct
b												
w			▨			▨			▨			
tʃ												
k												
s												
h			▨			▨			▨			
r												
d												
f												
θ												
l												
ʃ												
v												
z												
ð												
m												
p												
n												
g												
j			▨			▨			▨			
dʒ												
t												
Probe: "Look at me, listen, and say what I say."												

■ **FIGURE 5.2** Example probe for stimulability of sounds absent from a child's phonetic inventory.

Source: Used with permission of Adele Miccio.

other words, these data are often used when making decisions regarding case selection and determining which speech sounds to target in treatment.

Investigators have reported that the ability of a child to imitate syllables or words is related to normal phonological acquisition as well as to the probability of a child spontaneously correcting his or her misarticulations (Miccio, Elbert, and Forrest, 1999). Pre-test and post-test comparisons with kindergarten and first-grade children have indicated that untreated children with high stimulability skills tended to perform better than children with low stimulability scores. For participants who were not stimulable, direct instruction on speech sounds was found to be necessary, as children would not self-correct their errors. It has also been reported that good stimulability suggests more rapid progress in treatment (Carter and Buck, 1958; Farquhar, 1961; Irwin, West, and Trombetta, 1966; Sommers et al., 1967). Carter and Buck (1958) reported, in a study of first-grade children, that stimulability testing can be used for such prognostic purposes. They inferred that first-grade children who correctly imitated error sounds in nonsense syllables were more likely to correct those sounds without instruction than children who were not able to imitate their error sounds. Kisatsky (1967) compared the pre- to post-test gains in articulation accuracy over a six-month period of two groups of kindergarten children, one identified as a high stimulability group and the other as a low stimulability group. Although neither group received articulation instruction, results indicated that significantly more speech sounds were self corrected by the high stimulability group in the six-month post-test when compared to the low stimulability group.

It can be inferred from these studies that individuals with poor stimulability skills should be seen for treatment, as it is unlikely that such children will self-correct their speech sound errors. Children with good stimulability skills tend to show more self-correction on their speech sound errors, but this finding is not true for all children. As a result, stimulability is but one factor used in determining treatment decisions and targets for treatment. In summary, the prognosis for individuals who are stimulable is more favorable than that for individuals who are not stimulable or who initiate their error sounds. Likewise, a child can be expected to make faster progress on sounds in which he or she is stimulable than on sounds that are not stimulable.

Stimulability has also been found to be an important factor in generalization. Elbert and McReynolds (1978) noted that generalization of correct /s/ production to a variety of contexts occurred as soon as the children learned to imitate the sound. In addition, Powell, Elbert, and Dinnsen (1991) reported that stimulability was the most decisive variable that they examined in explaining generalization patterns and could be used to explain and predict generalization patterns. They concluded that clinicians should target nonstimulable sounds first, as nonstimulable sounds are unlikely to change while many stimulable sounds may self-correct during treatment, even without direct instruction on those stimulable sounds.

Elicitation Procedures. As stated earlier, the examiner typically asks the client to look at the examiner's mouth or watch it in a mirror, listen to what is said, and then imitate the production. The examiner does not point out where teeth, tongue, or lips may be during production; the examinee is simply encouraged to listen and observe a production. If the client is unsuccessful at imitating the sound, some examiners engage in cueing or trial instruction, providing directions for how to make sounds. The latter information is also used in selecting targets and determining the direction of treatment.

Stimulability testing usually includes imitative testing of those sounds produced in error in word and/or conversational samples. Some articulation tests include a place on the scoring form to record stimulability results, particularly for sounds in isolation. Clinicians will usually want to assess imitation in isolation, nonsense syllables (usually prevocalic, intervocalic, and postvocalic positions), and monosyllabic words (again in across-word positions). The number of productions required at each level will vary from one client and/or examiner to the next. Cooperation of the child, number of sounds produced in error, and success with the imitative task are factors the clinician should consider when deciding how extensive the stimulability assessment will be.

For example, in the case of a client with a /θ/ for /s/ error or ([θʌn] for [sʌn]), the client could be asked to initiate /s/ as follows:

1. Isolation: /s/ 6 tries
2. Nonsense syllables:

si	iʃi	iʃ
sa	aʃa	aʃ
su	uʃu	uʃ

3. Words:

sail	bicycle	ice
sun	baseball	horse
seal	missile	bus

For a client with multiple errors, individual sounds may be assessed only in isolation (two productions), with two syllables, and with one or two words because of time constraints.

Summary.   Stimulability testing is useful in identifying those individuals most likely to need phonological intervention (those with poor stimulability scores), and for determining stimulus items for initiation of instruction. Stimulability scores have been found to have prognostic value for identifying those speech sound errors a child will likely self-correct, and/or that will generalize most quickly in therapy.

Contextual Testing

Rationale.   As indicated earlier, speech sound errors, especially in children, may be variable and inconsistent. Sounds are often easier to produce in some contexts as opposed to others, thus accounting for some of the inconsistency in production, especially during the phonological acquisition period. Knowledge of the consistency of phonological errors is often a factor taken into consideration when deciding on the need for therapy, but is more frequently used for making treatment decisions such as choosing sounds or sound patterns to work on in therapy or deciding on a particular phonetic context that may facilitate accurate sound production.

Assessing contextual influences is based on the concept that sound productions influence each other in the ongoing stream of speech. McDonald (1964a) and others have suggested that valuable clinical information can be gained by systematically examining a sound as it is produced in varying contexts. McDonald coined the term *deep test* to refer to the practice of testing a sound in a variety of phonetic contexts. Coarticulatory effects consist of mechanical constraints associated with adjacent sounds and simultaneous pre-programming adjustments for segments later in the speech stream. This overlapping of movements (preprogramming) may extend as far as six phonetic segments away from a given sound (Kent and Minifie, 1977). Although the primary influence would appear to be sounds immediately preceding or following a target sound (Zehel, Shelton, Arndt, Wright, and Elbert, 1972), the result is that segments may be produced correctly in one context but not in another. Such information is of value to the clinician who seeks to establish a particular segment in a client's repertoire.

Elicitation Procedures.   The first published instrument for sampling contextual influences on sounds was the *Deep Test of Articulation* (McDonald, 1964b), a series of phoneme-specific tasks designed to assess individual speech sounds in approximately 50 phonetic contexts. This test is predicated on the hypothesis that when the consonants preceding or following the sound of interest are systematically varied, the client may produce the target sound correctly in at least one phonetic context.

More recent materials that have been developed to assess consistency-contextual influences include the *Secord Contextual Articulation Tests (S-CAT)* (Secord and Shine, 1997a) and the *Contextual Test of Articulation* (Aase, Hovre, Krause, Shelfhout, Smith, and Carpenter, 2000). The S-CAT consists of three components: (1) Contextual Probes of Articulation Competence (CPAC), (2) Storytelling Probes of Articulation Competence (SPAC), and (3) Target Words for Contextual Training (TWAC). The CPAC and SPAC are designed to assess 23 consonants and vocalic /ɝ/ in various phonetic contexts through word and connected speech, samples, and can be used with clients from preschool through adult. The *Contextual Test of Articulation* tests 5 consonant sounds and 15 consonant clusters through sentence completion items in 7 vowel contexts.

In addition to published contextual tests, an informal contextual analysis may be done by reviewing a connected speech sample for contexts in which a target sound is produced correctly. Occasionally, facilitating contexts can be found in conversation that are not observed in single words or word-pairs. Phonemes may also be examined in various morphophonemic alterations to determine the effect of morpheme structure on phonological productions. Such alterations may be examined by having the client produce a sound in differing morphophonemic structures. For example, if word-final obstruent /g/ has been deleted in /dɔg/ (i.e., [dɔ]), the examiner might assess whether or not /g/ is produced in the diminutive /dɔgi/. Likewise, if the child misarticulates /z/ in the word /roz/, the examiner might observe /z/ production in the morphophonemic context of /rozəz/. In this example, such testing may allow the clinician also to determine whether the error is a sound production problem or a problem marking plurality (a language related difficulty).

Consonants may also be examined for correct phoneme productions in the context of consonant clusters. Although it is true that in most instances a consonant is more likely to be produced correctly as a singleton rather than in consonant clusters, it is not unusual for sounds to be produced correctly in the context of a cluster even when misarticulated in a singleton context. For example, one may find a correct /r/ or /s/ production in a cluster, even though it may consistently be in error in a singleton context.

Summary.   Contextual testing is conducted to determine phonetic contexts in which a sound error may be produced correctly. These contexts may then be used to identify a starting point for remediation. Contextual testing is also used as a measure of consistency of misarticulation.

Error Pattern Identification

For children with multiple errors, the assessment battery often includes a formal measure designed to identify sound error patterns and error sounds within sound classes.

Rationale. Many clinicians employ what has historically been referred to as a *phonological process analysis* to facilitate error pattern delineation in clients who evidence multiple speech sound errors. A phonological *pattern* (now the preferred term rather than *process*—which is also still used, however) is typically defined as a systematic sound change or simplification that affects a class of sounds, a particular sequence of sounds, or the syllable structure of words. Response elicitation procedures are often identical to that employed in citation testing (i.e., the client names pictures to produce single-word responses), but may also involve engaging a client in conversational speech. The type of scoring and analysis of either type of sample is designed to identify the presence of phonological process/phonological patterns across error sounds. This type of analysis is based on the assumption that children's speech sound errors are not random, but represent systematic variations from the adult standard. Phonologic patterns that describe several individual speech sound errors are identified through such procedures. When doing a pattern analysis, clinicians compare the child's productions with the adult standard and then categorize individual errors into phonologic patterns.

One of the reasons pattern analysis procedures have appeal is that they provide a description of the child's overall phonological system. For example, if a child leaves /p, b, k, g, t, s, and z/ off the ends of words, he or she may be described as evidenced a "final consonant deletion" process. Khan (1985) furnished another illustration of a phonological process/pattern. A child who substitutes /wawa/ for *water* might be described in a traditional substitution analysis as substituting [w] for /t/ and substituting [a] for final /ɚ/. On the basis of what we know about phonological acquisition, the [wawa] for *water* substitution is more accurately described as syllable reduplication, a common pattern seen in young children. The child in this instance is probably repeating the first syllable of the word *water* /wa/ rather than using sound substitutions for target sounds in the second syllable. In this example, the child is also demonstrating knowledge of syllable structure, since *water* contains two syllables, as does /wawa/.

A second reason for doing a pattern analysis is the potential for facilitating treatment efficacy. When a pattern reflecting several sound errors is targeted for treatment, there is the potential for enhancing rapid generalization across sounds related to that pattern by working on one or more sounds that reflect that pattern, and looking for generalization to other sounds also a part of the error pattern.

Systems of pattern analysis, whether based on a place-manner-voicing analysis, distinctive feature analysis, or the more commonly employed phonological process analysis procedures, are most appropriate for the client who has multiple errors. The intent of the analysis is to determine if there are patterns or relationships among speech sound error productions. If only a few speech sounds are in error, one need not do a pattern analysis of a child's speech. For example, if a client is misarticulating only two consonants, /s/ and /ʃ/, the clinician would not do a pattern analysis. In this instance, the clinician would develop a remediation plan where both consonants are targeted for direct instruction.

Phonological patterns identified during analysis are used for target selection in treatment. For example, if a child has eight speech sound substitutions reflecting three error patterns (e.g., stopping of fricatives, gliding of liquids, and fronting), remediation would likely focus on the reduction of one or more of these phonological patterns. The modification of one or more speech sounds (exemplars) reflecting a particular error pattern frequently results in generalization to other speech sounds reflecting the same error pattern. For example, establishment of final /p/ and /f/ may generalize to other stops and fricatives deleted in word-final position. Another example of a pattern-oriented remediation strategy would be to target for instruction all speech sounds that appear to be simplified in a similar manner, such as fricatives being replaced with stops (i.e., stopping). In this instance, the clinician might focus on the contrast between stops and fricatives. By focusing on sounds that reflect a similar error pattern, treatment should be more efficient than if it focuses on individual sounds without regard to phonological patterns.

Elicitation Procedures.   Several analysis procedures have been published that are based on identifying phonologic processes/patterns. Phonologic analysis procedures have been published by Hodson (2003), Dawson and Tattersall (2001), Khan and Lewis (1986, 2002), Bankson and Bernthal (1990b), and Smit and Hand (1997). Through each of these single-word measures, phonologic patterns can be identified. In addition to these published analysis procedures, phonologic productions recorded during connected speech sampling and/or single-word testing can be analyzed for the presence of error patterns. It should also be pointed out that several computer-based programs may assist the clinician in analyzing error patterns (e.g., Hodson, 2003; Masterson and Bernhardt, 2001).

Summary

Instruments, designed to identify phonological patterns/processes facilitate identification of commonalities among error productions. The unique nature of these tests is in the type of analysis they facilitate, as opposed to the type of samples obtained. A more detailed description of phonological patterns, instruments that have been developed to assess these patterns, and analysis procedures related to pattern identification, will be presented later in this chapter.

Criteria for Selecting Phonological Assessment Instruments

Formal test instruments selected by the clinician should be appropriate to the individual being tested and provide the information desired by the clinician. When selecting commercially available test instruments for phonological assessment, the clinician will want to consider the sample the instrument is designed to obtain, the nature of the stimulus materials (e.g., how easily recognized are the target pictures or objects?), the scoring system, and the type of analysis facilitated by the instrument. Practical considerations in test selection include the amount of time required to administer the instrument and analyze the sample obtained, as well as the cost for purchasing the test. The following variables need to be taken into consideration when selecting a test instrument to include in the battery.

Sample Obtained

A factor to consider in selecting a test instrument is the adequacy or representativeness of the speech sample obtained. Variables to consider include the specific consonants, consonant clusters, vowels, and diphthongs tested, as well as the units in which sounds are to be produced (i.e., syllables, words, sentences). In addition, stimulus presentation and type of sample elicited (e.g., picture-naming, sentence completion, imitation, delayed imitation, conversation) should also be considered in selecting instruments.

Material Presentation

Another practical factor in selecting commercially available tests is the attractiveness, compactness, and manipulability of materials. Size, familiarity, and color of stimulus pictures and appropriateness to the age of the client may influence the ease with which the clinician obtains responses to test stimuli. In addition, the organization and format of the scoring sheet are important for information retrieval. Tests with familiar and attractive stimulus items and score sheets that facilitate analysis are desirable.

Scoring and Analysis

Because the scoring and analysis procedures that accompany a test instrument determine the type of information obtained from the instrument, they are important considerations in test selection. Different assessment instruments currently available are designed to facilitate one or more of the following types of analysis: (1) phonetic and/or phoneme analysis of consonant and vowel sounds of the language; (2) sound productions in a variety of word positions and phonetic contexts; (3) place, manner, voice analysis; (4) phonological pattern/process analysis; (5) age appropriateness of phonological productions; and (6) speech sound stimulability. A practical consideration relates to how much time may be required to complete an analysis versus the value of information obtained.

Transcription and Scoring Procedures

Methods for Recording Responses

The recording systems used by clinicians vary according to the purposes of testing, the transcription skills of the examiner, and personal preferences. The type of response recording the examiner employs will, however, determine the type of analysis the clinician is able to do with the sample obtained. In turn, management decisions, which frequently include a recommended treatment approach, may be significantly influenced by the type of analysis conducted.

In the least sophisticated scoring procedure, phonological productions are simply scored as correct or incorrect, based on the examiner's perception of whether the sound produced is within the acceptable adult phoneme boundary. This type of scoring is sometimes used to assess day-to-day progress but is not recommended when doing a phonological assessment designed to determine the direction of treatment because more detailed description is required for this purpose.

The most common transcription system for recording sound errors is the *International Phonetic Alphabet (IPA)*, which includes a different symbol for each phoneme. As indicated in Chapter 2, more than 40 such symbols are utilized to identify the phonemes of the English language. This broad transcription system supplemented with a set of *diacritics* (narrow markers) usually provides sufficient detail for speech-language clinicians to adequately describe speech sound productions. For example, in a broad transcription of the word *key*, one would transcribe the initial segment with the symbol /k/. A more precise transcription of the initial /k/ would include the diacritic for aspiration [ʰ] following word initial [kʰ] because aspiration occurs in production of /k/ in word-initial contexts. The aspiration modifier [ʰ] in this transcription represents one example of a diacritic. Use of diacritics, sometimes called a *close* or *narrow transcription system*, allows for recording specific topographical dimensions of individual segments, and is recommended when broad transcription does not adequately describe an error. For example, if /s/ in the word /sʌn/ is lateralized (air emitted sideways rather than forward), the diacritic for lateralization is placed under the /s/, thus [ʂʌn]. A list of common symbols and diacritics for clinical use is presented in Table 5.1.

Diacritic markers are used to describe the speech of individuals whose speech sound productions cannot be adequately described by broad phonetic symbols. For example, in assessing the phonological status of an individual with a cleft condition who is unable to

▨ TABLE 5.1   Symbols and Diacritics

[x]	voiceless velar fricative, as in *Bach*
[Φ]	voiceless bilabial fricative
[β]	voiced bilabial fricative
[ʔ]	glottal stop, as in [mʌʔi]
ɾ[w]	r with [w] like quality

Stop Release Diacritics

[ʰ]	aspirated, as in [tʰap]
[⁼]	unaspirated, as in [p⁼un]

Diacritics for Nasality

[˜]	nasalized, as in [fæ̃n]
[⁓̸]	denasalized
[˷]	produced with nasal emission

Diacritics for Length

[ː]	lengthened

Diacritics for Voicing

[̥]	partially devoiced, as in [spuṇ]

Diacritics for Tongue Position or Shape

[̪]	dentalized, as in [tɛṋθ]
[̪]	lateralized, as in [ʂop]

achieve velopharyngeal closure for certain speech sounds, diacritics indicating nasal emission (šnail), or nasalization (bǽn), may be useful in the description of the client's production of such segments. Similarly, when assessing the articulation of an individual with impaired hearing, symbols to indicate appropriate vowel duration (e.g., [si:] for lengthened), devoicing (e.g., [b̥]), and denasalization (e.g., rǽn) are recommended if these characteristics are present in productions. Likewise, with developmental articulation errors characterized by lateralization (e.g., [ɬ]), dentalization (e.g., [s̪]), and devoicing (e.g., [n̥]), diacritics should be utilized.

Accuracy of Transcriptions

One of the major concerns regarding transcription of responses relates to accuracy. Clinicians must be concerned with whether their transcriptions are a valid representation of a client's productions. In making transcriptions, clinicians rely primarily on auditory perceptual judgments. These judgments are sometimes supplemented with physiological measures (such as air pressure and flow information) and acoustical measures (such as that obtained from spectrographic analysis). These three types of data may not always be consistent with each other. For example, a glottal substitution for a stop in word-final position may be identified via a spectrographic analysis, and yet the glottal production may not be heard by a listener and thus will be transcribed as a deletion (omission). It must be recognized, however, that even the more objective measures of speech segments (i.e., acoustical and physiological recordings) are not devoid of human interpretation and no one-to-one correspondence exists between a phoneme production, perception, and/or acoustical and physiological measurements. For most aspects of clinical phonology, auditory perceptual judgments by the examiner remain the primary basis for intervention decisions, although acoustical and physiological analysis can be useful. Because of the dependence on perceptual judgments, it is important for clinicians to establish the reliability of their perceptual judgments.

Interjudge Reliability. Traditionally, clinicians have used agreement between two independent transcribers as a means of establishing reliability of judgments. *Interjudge agreement* or *reliability* is determined by the comparison of one examiner's transcriptions with those of another and is essential for reporting the results of phonological research. In addition, for students beginning to make judgments about accuracy of phonological productions, establishing interjudge reliability with a more experienced person can assist in the development of accurate judgments. A commonly used method to determine interjudge reliability, called *point-to-point agreement*, compares the clinicians' judgments on each test item. The number of items judged the same is divided by the total number of items to determine a percentage of agreement between judges. As an example, if two judges were to agree on 17 of 20 items and disagree on 3, they would divide 17 by 20 and get 0.85, which would then be multiplied by 100 to obtain an interjudge reliability index of 85 percent agreement. Such point-to-point or item-by-item reliability is a typically employed method for establishing agreement between judges in phonological research.

Sometimes transcriptions are made by two or more examiners independently but simultaneously, with the final transcript arrived at by consensus (Shriberg, Kwiatkowski, and Hoffman, 1984). Discussion between examiners regarding what is heard occurs prior to a "final" judgment. This procedure, which typically involves a panel of examiners listening to tape-recorded responses, is used in situations that are difficult to judge. Obviously, some independence of judgment is lost in such a procedure.

Shriberg and Lof (1991), in a study of point-to-point reliability of judgments of broad and narrow phonetic transcription, reported that for interjudge and intrajudge reliability, average agreement for broad transcriptions exceeded 90 percent, and for narrow transcriptions, between 65 and 75 percent.

Intrajudge Reliability. Along with knowing that his or her judgments are in agreement with those of another examiner, the clinician will also want to know that his or her standards for judgments are consistent over time. Comparison of judgments made when scoring the same data on two separate occasions is referred to as *intrajudge reliability*. High reliability on such a measure is an indication that the examiner is consistent in his or her judgments. Recordings of responses are used to determine this type of reliability, because two judgments are made of the same responses.

Phonologic Assessment in Young Children

Phonologic evaluation of young children (infants and toddlers) must be done within the broader context of evaluating overall communicative behavior. Since phonologic development is integrally related to development of cognition, language, and motor skills, obviously phonological development reflects other aspects of a child's development. However, for purposes of this text, it is useful to isolate phonologic considerations from the overall communication process. The following paragraphs will present information related to this component of communication development that is not discussed elsewhere in our discussion of phonologic assessment.

There is much variability among young children in terms of the speech sounds and/or specific phonemes produced at a given age. Such variability makes it difficult to formulate strict developmental expectations and guidelines for phonology in infants and toddlers. One of the first assessments of phonologic development, especially with children at risk for developmental delay, involves determining whether the infant is progressing normally through the stages of infant vocalization. Speech sound productions emerge within the context of infant vocalizations at the prelinguistic level. Information presented in Chapter 3 regarding the characteristics of these stages is helpful in knowing about sound productions that typically occur during this developmental period, including the gradual shift from prelinguistic to linguistic behavior that usually occurs during the first year.

The point in time and/or development when clinicians frequently become involved in assessing phonology in young children occurs after they have acquired approximately 50 words (completion of the transition stage), or are putting two words together. This usually occurs between 18 and 24 months. For these children, clinicians are usually interested in determining how a child is doing in comparison to age, peers, and/or the adult standard. For younger children, or those with limited vocal repertoires, the interest is directed to describing whatever sounds they may employ for communication regardless of correct usage. In normal developing children, first words typically occur at about 12 months of age, the transition stage occurs between 12 and 18 months, and two or three words are put together in sequence (strings) around 24 months. In children with phonological delay, obviously these stages may occur at a later chronological age. Phonologic analysis in young children is inextricably bound to development of the child's lexicon. Procedures for eliciting vocalizations from young children depend on the level of the child's development, and can include a range of activities such as stimulating vocalizations during caregiving and feeding activities; informal play with a caregiver, sibling, or clinician; structured play; interactive storytelling; sentence repetition; delayed imitation of a story told by the clinician; narrative generation (about a favorite book); and spontaneous conversation.

Stoel-Gammon (1994) indicated that at age 24 months, children may be categorized into three groups: (1) those who are normal in terms of linguistic development (85 percent of children); (2) those who are slow developing (late talkers), but evidence no major deviations from patterns of normal acquisition; and (3) those whose developmental patterns deviate substantially from the broadest interpretation of norms in terms of order of acquisition or achievement of certain milestones. She indicated that the second and third groups together constitute 15 percent of the population. Children in the second group should be monitored to be certain that they "catch up" with the normal group. Stoel-Gammon indicated that children falling into this category would likely be those who, at 24 months, have a vocabulary smaller than 50 words, have a phonetic inventory with only 4 to 5 consonants and a limited variety of vowels, and who, otherwise, are following the normal order of phoneme acquisition and do not have unusual error types. Children in the third group are those who should be considered for an early intervention program.

The type of phonological analysis usually employed during the early stages of speech sound acquisition is termed an independent analysis of phonological behavior. An independent analysis identifies the speech sounds produced by a child without reference to appropriateness of usage relative to the adult standard. This type of analysis is appropriate for the assessment of both normal and delayed phoneme acquisition. For those children who have progressed to the point where they have enough language that intelligibility is a concern (beyond 50 words in their vocabulary), a relational analysis may also be employed. In relational analyses, the child's phonological productions are compared with the adult standard.

An independent analysis of phonology is typically based on a continuous speech sample and is designed to describe a child's productions without reference to adult usage. Analysis of a child's productions as a self-contained system include the following (Stoel-Gammon and Dunn, 1985):

1. An inventory of sounds (consonants and vowels) classified by word position and articulatory features (e.g., place, manner, voicing).
2. An inventory of syllables and word shapes produced (e.g., CVC, CV, VC, CCV).
3. Sequential constraints on particular sound sequences.

As stated earlier, a relational analysis of phonological productions is typically used with children in the 2-year age range evidencing normal language development, as well as with older children with phonological delay. Most of the assessment information presented elsewhere in this chapter pertains to relational analyses.

Summary.   Phonological evaluations with infants and toddlers are done within the context of an overall communication assessment since phonological development is integrally related to other aspects of development such as cognition, motor development, and other aspects of linguistic development. Informal assessment involving independent analyses is typically done with very young children and for those with limited verbal repertoires. Usually, these include an inventory of sounds, syllables and word shapes produced, phonological contrasts employed, and sequential contrasts. Once a child has a vocabulary of approximately 50 words, relational analysis may also be employed as part of the assessment battery.

RELATED ASSESSMENT PROCEDURES

The assessment of a child with a phonologic problem includes testing and data-gathering procedures supplemental to those focusing directly on phonologic behavior. Information is gathered in order to provide a more comprehensive picture of an individual client and thereby contribute to a better understanding of his or her phonological status. It may also influence treatment recommendations that are made regarding a given client.

These additional assessment procedures often include a case history; an oral cavity examination; and hearing, language, fluency, and voice screenings. These procedures can aid the clinician in the identification of factors that may contribute to or be related to the delay or impairment of phonology. Data gathered from these additional measures may lead to referral to other specialists and/or influence treatment decisions. If, for example, a child has a problem with closure of the velopharyngeal port, referral to a cleft palate team may result in pharyngeal flap surgery prior to speech intervention.

Presence of suspected sensory, structural, or neurological deficiencies must be corroborated by appropriate related personnel (e.g., audiological, medical) and recommendations from those sources must be taken into consideration as part of the assessment. Any of these factors may be important in decisions regarding the need for therapy, the point at which therapy should begin, and the treatment to be prescribed. Although they are routinely screened in phonologic evaluations, language, fluency, and voice screening will not be covered in this text.

Case History

To facilitate an efficient and effective assessment, a case history is obtained from the client or a parent prior to the phonological assessment. This allows the clinician to identify (1) possible etiological factors; (2) the family's or client's perception of the problem; (3) the academic, work, home, and social environment of the client; and (4) medical, developmental, and social information about the client. Case history information is usually obtained through a written form completed by the client or parents. It is frequently supplemented by an oral interview. Specific questions on the phonological status of a young child might include the following: (1) Did your child babble? Can you describe it? (2) When did your child say his or her first words? What were they? When did he or she start putting words together? (3) Describe your child's communication problem, and your concerns about it. (4) How easy is your child to understand? By the family? By strangers? (5) What sounds and words does your child say? (6) What do you think caused your child's speech difficulty? (7) Is there a family history of speech difficulties, and how would you describe them?

Although case histories obtained from the client or the client's family are products of memory and perception and thus may not reflect total accuracy, parents and clients in general are reliable informants. In spite of shortcomings, the case history provides the clinician with important background information that frequently influences assessment decisions and subsequent management recommendations.

Oral Cavity Examination

Oral cavity (oral peripheral) examinations are administered to describe the structure and function of the oral mechanism for speech purposes. In particular, dentition is observed for bite and missing teeth; hard and soft palates are examined for clefts, submucous clefts, fistulas, and fissures. Size, symmetry, and movement of the lips; size and movement of the tongue; and symmetry, movement, and functional length of the soft palate are assessed.

To examine the intraoral structures, it is recommended that the client be seated immediately in front of the clinician with his or her head in a natural upright position and at a level that allows easy viewing. The examiner should wear surgical gloves. If the client is a child, the examiner may have the child sit on a table or the examiner can kneel on the floor. Although it might seem that the oral cavity would be viewed best when the client extends his or her head backward, such a position can distort normal relationships of the head and neck. The client's mouth usually should be at the examiner's eye level. A flashlight or other light source, together with a tongue blade, will aid in the examination. Observations should start at the front of the oral cavity and progress to the back. Since the oral cavity examination is important in identifying possible structural abnormalities, a description of how an examination is conducted is presented below. For a more complete presentation of procedures for conducting an oral-mechanism examination, see St. Louis and Ruscello (2000).

Dentition

For the examiner to evaluate the occlusal relationship (i.e., alignment of upper and lower jaws), the client should have the first molars in contact with each other since the occlusal relationship of the upper and lower dental arch are made with reference to these molar contacts. The upper dental arch is normally longer and wider than the lower dental arch; therefore, the upper teeth normally extend horizontally around the lower dental arch; and the maxillary (upper) incisors protrude about one-quarter inch in front of the lower teeth and cover about one-third of the crown of the mandibular incisors. Such dental overjet or overbite is the normal relationship of the dental arches in occlusion.

The teeth are said to be in open bite when the upper teeth do not cover part of the lower teeth at any given point along the dental arch. Mason and Wickwire (1978) recommended that, when evaluating occlusal relationships, the clinician should instruct the client to bite on the back teeth and to separate the lips. They further stated that

> while in occlusion, the client should be asked to produce several speech sounds in isolation, especially /s/, /z/, /f/, and /v/. Although these sounds may not normally be produced by the client with teeth in occlusion, the standardization of airspace dimensions and increases in pressure in the oral cavity can unmask a variety of functional relationships. For example, the child who usually exhibits an interdental lisp may be able to articulate /s/ surprisingly well

with teeth together. This occluded position can also unmask and/or counteract habit patterns related to the protrusion of tongue and mandible on selected sounds. (p. 15)

Mason and Wickwire also suggested that when an individual with excessive overjet has difficulty with /s/, he or she should be instructed to rotate the mandible forward as a means of adaptation to the excessive overjet. As pointed out in Chapter 4, however, dental abnormality and speech problems are frequently unrelated, and thus a cause-and-effect relationship between occlusion deviation and articulation problems should not be assumed.

Hard Palate

The hard palate (i.e., the bony portion of the oral cavity roof) is best viewed when the client extends his or her head backward. Normal midline coloration is pink and white. When a blue tint on the midline is observed, further investigation of the integrity of the bony framework is indicated. Such discoloration may be caused by a blood supply close to the surface of the palate and is sometimes associated with a submucous cleft (an opening in the bony palatal shelf). But when a blue tint is seen lateral to the midline of the hard palate, it usually suggests only an extra bony growth, which occurs in approximately 20 percent of the population.

Where a submucous cleft of the hard palate is suspected, palpation (rubbing) of the mucous membrane at the midline of the most posterior portion of the hard palate (nasal spine) is recommended. Although many speech-language pathologists note the height of the hard palatal vault, it probably has little relationship to articulation deviations. The contour or height of the palatal vault may influence certain articulatory contacts, but most individuals with high palatal vaults use compensatory movements that allow for adequate speech sound production.

Soft Palate or Velum

The soft palate should be evaluated with the head in a natural upright position. When the head is not in that position, changes in the structural relationship in the oral cavity area may prevent the viewing of velar function as it occurs during speech.

Mason and Wickwire (1978) cautioned that the assessment of velar function, especially velar elevation, should not be done with the tongue protruded or with the mandible positioned for maximum mouth opening. They recommended a mouth opening of about three quarters of the maximum opening since velar elevation may be less than maximum when the mouth is open maximally.

The coloration of the soft palate, like that of the hard palate, should be pink and white. A midline bluish tint should alert the clinician to the possibility of a submucous cleft of the velum, in which case the surface of the velum is covered with mucous membrane, but the underlying layer of periosteum is absent.

The critical factor in velar function is the effective or functional length of the velum, not the velar length per se. Effective velar length is the portion of tissue that fills the space between the posterior border of the hard palate and the pharyngeal closure. Effective velar length is only one factor in adequate velopharyngeal sphincter function and provides little or no information concerning the function of the sphincter's pharyngeal component (described below), another critical factor for adequate velopharyngeal valving.

The final velar observation typically made is velar symmetry and evaluation. The elevation and posterior movement of the velum is also partially obstructed from view in an intraoral exam. But when the velum does not elevate to the plane of the hard palate during sustained vowel phonation, an inadequately functioning velopharyngeal sphincter should be suspected. It should also be remembered that if the observation is made with the tongue protruded, velar elevation can be restricted.

The posterior-most appendage or extension of the velum is the uvula, which has little or no role in speech production. However, a *bifid* uvula should alert the clinician to other possible anatomical deviations. A bifid uvula appears as two appendages rather than one and is occasionally seen in the presence of submucous clefts and other abnormal anatomical findings.

Fauces

The next area to observe in the oral cavity is the faucial pillars and the tonsillar masses. Only in rare instances are these structures a factor in speech production. The presence or absence of tonsillar masses is noted and, if present, their size and coloration are observed. Redness or inflammation may be evidence of tonsillitis, and large tonsillar masses may displace the faucial pillars and reduce the isthmus.

Pharynx

The oropharyngeal area is difficult to view in an intraoral examination. The pharyngeal contribution to velopharyngeal closure cannot be assessed through intraoral viewing because pharyngeal valving occurs at the level of the nasopharynx, a level superior to that which can be observed through the oral cavity. In some individuals, movement of tissue to form a prominence or ridge (Passavant's Pad) can be seen on the posterior wall of the pharynx; Passavant's Pad is not visible at rest but can usually be seen during sustained phonation. Passavant's Pad is present in approximately one-third of the individuals with cleft palates but is otherwise rare. Since its presence reflects a compensatory mechanism, the examiner should be alert to possible velopharyngeal valving problems. The presence of Passavant's Pad may suggest that adenoidal tissue is needed for velopharyngeal closure, and this factor should be considered in surgical decisions regarding adenoidectomies.

The pharyngeal gag response has been identified as a useful procedure to obtain an idea of the functional potential of the velum. Gagging usually results in maximum velar excursion and maximum movement of the pharyngeal walls. Gagging can be induced by pressing firmly on the base of the tongue or by touching the velum with a tongue blade. We recommend that elicitation of the gag response be used only in very rare instances since many clients have a strong aversion to the procedure, and velar function during gagging generally has little relationship to velopharyngeal valving during speech. Elicitation of a gag may provide some useful information in cases where lack of innervation and a paresis of the pharyngeal or palatal function is suspected.

Considerable research has been conducted in the development of instrumental measures that can help in the assessment of velopharyngeal adequacy and function. Such measures are used to supplement clinical perceptions related to the adequacy of velopharyngeal function. Inadequate velopharyngeal function frequently is associated with hypernasal resonance, weak production of pressured consonants (i.e., stops, fricatives, and affricates), and nasal emission of air. A number of direct and indirect instrumental procedures can help to assess velopharyngeal function—for example, nasometer, videofluoroscopy, nasopharyngoscopy, and airflow (aerodynamic) measures. For more information about such techniques, see chapters in Bzoch (2004).

Tongue

As pointed out in Chapter 4, the tongue is a primary articulator, and individuals are able to modify tongue movements to compensate for many structural variations in the oral cavity. In terms of tongue size, two problematic conditions are occasionally found. The first, termed *macroglossia*, is an abnormally large tongue. Although the incidence of this condition is relatively low, historically some have associated it with Down syndrome. Research data, however, indicate normal tongue size in this population, but low muscle tone in the tongue and an undersized oral cavity may be present. The condition where the tongue is abnormally small in relation to the oral cavity is termed *microglossia*, but this condition rarely, if ever, causes a speech problem.

It has been pointed out that tongue movements for speech activities show little relationship to tongue movements for nonspeech activities. Unless motor problems are suspected, little is gained by having the client perform a series of tongue movements used for nonspeech activities. Protrusion of the tongue or moving the tongue laterally from one corner of the mouth to the other may provide information about possible motor limitations or problems in control of the tongue.

The rapid speech movements observed in diadochokinetic tasks (syllabic repetition—e.g., pʌ pʌ pʌ, pʌ tʌ kʌ) provide some information with respect to speech function. The absolute number of syllables that an individual can produce in a given unit of time usually bears little relationship to articulatory proficiency except when gross-motor problems are present. For a discussion of the relationship between diadochokinetic testing and articulation, see Chapter 4. Mason and Wickwire (1978) suggested that the clinician focus on the pattern of tongue movement and the consistency of contacts during diadochokinetic tasks.

A short lingual frenum can restrict movement of the tongue tip. Most individuals, however, acquire normal speech in spite of a short lingual frenum. If the client can touch the alveolar ridge with the tongue tip, the length of the frenum is probably adequate for speech purposes. In the rare instance where this is not possible, surgical intervention may be necessary.

Summary

In an oral cavity examination, in which the clinician notes an inadequacy of structure or function that might contribute to speech sound errors, he or she has several options: (1) refer the client to other professionals (e.g., otolaryngologist, orthodontist, cleft palate team) for assessment and possible intervention; (2) engage in further observation and testing to verify the earlier observation and note its impact on speaking skills; and (3) provide instruction related to compensatory or remedial behaviors.

Audiological Screening

The primary purpose of audiological screening is to determine whether a client exhibits a loss or reduction of auditory function, which could be an etiological factor associated with a phonological disorder. Audiological screening is usually conducted with pure tones and/or impedance audiometry prior to phonological assessment.

Pure tone screening typically involves presentation of pure tone stimuli at 500, 1,000, 2,000, and 4,000 Hz at a predetermined intensity level. Usually, a 20 dB HL is used for screening, but this level may be altered to compensate for ambient noise in the room. The pure tone frequencies used in screening are those considered most important for perceiving speech stimuli. The loudness of the pure tone stimuli reflects threshold levels needed to function adequately in the classroom.

Impedance screening measures eardrum compliance (movement of the eardrum) and middle-ear pressure as air pressure is altered in the external auditory canal. This screening test yields basic information about the functioning of the tympanic membrane by eliciting the acoustic reflex. The acoustic reflex can be measured by presenting a relatively loud signal to the ear and observing the presence or absence of a change in the compliance of the eardrum. Screening of the acoustic reflex usually involves the presentation of a 1,000 Hz signal at 70 dB above a person's threshold. The acoustic reflex is a contraction of the stapedial muscle when the ear is stimulated by a loud sound and serves as a protective device for the inner ear. The client who fails a pure tone or impedance screening test should be referred to an audiologist for a complete audiological assessment.

Summary

As indicated in Chapter 4 in the discussion of hearing as it relates to speech sound productions, it is critical to know the status of a client's hearing. There is some indication that recurrent middle ear problems can contribute to phonological delay and speech sound disorders. In the case of more severe auditory impairments, there is frequently a correlation between extent of hearing loss and level of speech and language development. Given this relationship, audiological screening must be a routine part of phonological assessment procedures.

Speech Sound Perception/Discrimination Testing

A review of the literature concerning the relationship between speech sound discrimination and articulation is presented in Chapter 4. The information presented there provides background for the assessment of speech sound perception, which is discussed here.

In the earlier years of the speech-language pathology profession (1920 to 1950), clinicians assumed that children with articulation errors were unable to perceive the difference between the standard adult production and their own error production, and then inferred that many phonological problems were the result of faulty perception. As a result of this assumption, speech sound discrimination testing that covered a wide variety of sound contrasts became a standard procedure in the assessment battery. These general discrimination tests did not examine contrasts relevant to a particular child's error productions (e.g., target sound vs. error sound—*rabbit* vs. *wabbit*), but as indicated, sampled a wide variety of contrasts. An example of a general test of discrimination is the *Goldman-Fristoe-Woodcock Test of Auditory Discrimination* (Goldman, Fristoe, and Woodcock, 1970). Research findings have cast doubt on the relationship between general speech sound discrimination and phonological disorders. The result has been that today, general speech sound discrimination tests are rarely used in clinical assessment. This testing is, however, recommended for those few clients suspected of having a generalized perceptual problem (e.g., inability to differentiate a wide variety of minimal pair sound contrasts). The type of testing recommended for clinical use is a phoneme task based on error production(s).

Locke's Speech Perception/Discrimination Testing

The *Speech Production Perception Task* (Locke, 1980b) is a perceptual measure designed to assess a child's perception of his or her articulatory errors and involves no preselected stimuli, but rather stimuli based on the child's error productions. The format for this task, along with an example of the scoring sheet, appear in Table 5.2.

■ **TABLE 5.2** Speech Production Perception Task

Child's Name _____ Sex: M F Birthdate: _____ Age: _____ Yrs. _____ Mos. _____

Date _____		Date _____		Date _____	
Production Task		Production Task		Production Task	
Stimulus	Response[*]	Stimulus	Response	Stimulus	Response
/θ ʌ m/ →	/f ʌ m/	/r e i k/ →	/w e i k/	/ʃ u/ →	/s u/
SP /θ/ RP /f/	CP /s/	SP /r/ RP /w/ CP /l/		SP /ʃ/ RP /s/ CP /t/	
Stimulus-Class	*Response*	*Stimulus-Class*	*Response*	*Stimulus-Class*	*Response*
1 /s/ - CP	yes NO	1 /r/ - SP	YES no	1 /s/ - RP	yes NO
2 /f/ - RP	yes NO	2 /l/ - CP	yes NO	2 /t/ - CP	yes NO
3 /θ/ - SP	YES no	3 /r/ - SP	YES no	3 /t/ - CP	yes NO
4 /θ/ - SP	YES no	4 /l/ - CP	yes NO	4 /ʃ/ - SP	YES no
5 /f/ - RP	yes NO	5 /w/ - RP	yes NO	5 /ʃ/ - SP	YES no
6 /s/ - CP	yes NO	6 /w/ - RP	yes NO	6 /s/ - RP	yes NO
7 /s/ - CP	yes NO	7 /r/ - SP	YES no	7 /s/ - RP	yes NO
8 /θ/ - SP	YES no	8 /w/ - RP	yes NO	8 /ʃ/ - SP	YES no
9 /f/ - RP	yes NO	9 /r/ - SP	YES no	9 /t/ - CP	yes NO
10 /θ/ - SP	YES no	10 /l/ - CP	yes NO	10 /ʃ/ - SP	YES no
11 /f/ - RP	yes NO	11 /l/ - CP	yes NO	11 /t/ - CP	yes NO
12 /s/ - CP	yes NO	12 /w/ - RP	yes NO	12 /s/ - RP	yes NO
13 /f/ - RP	yes NO	13 /t/ - SP	YES no	13 /ʃ/ - SP	YES no
14 /θ/ - SP	YES no	14 /l/ - CP	yes NO	14 /s/ - RP	yes NO
15 /s/ - CP	yes NO	15 /w/ - SP	YES no	15 /ʃ/ - SP	YES no
16 /f/ - RP	yes NO	16 /r/ - SP	YES no	16 /t/ - CP	yes NO
17 /θ/ - SP	YES no	17 /w/ - RP	yes NO	17 /t/ - CP	yes NO
18 /s/ - CP	yes NO	18 /l/ - CP	yes NO	18 /s/ - RP	yes NO
RP _____ CP _____ SP _____		RP _____ CP _____ SP _____		RP _____ CP _____ SP _____	

[*]The correct response is in uppercase letters.

Source: Adapted by permission from J. Locke, "The Inference of Speech Perception in the Phonologically Disordered Child Part II: Some Clinically Novel Procedures, Their Use, Some Findings." *Journal of Speech and Hearing Disorders, 45* (1980b): 447.

Preliminary to the presentation of the *Speech Production Perception Task*, the child's speech sound errors must be identified. The child's error productions and the corresponding adult standard (correct) forms are then used to construct the perception task. In this procedure, the adult norm is identified as the stimulus phoneme (SP), the child's substitution or deletion as the response phoneme (RP), and a perceptually similar "control phoneme" is identified as (CP). For example, if the client substitutes [wek] for /rek/, the stimulus production (SP) would be *rake* /r/, the response production (RP) would be *wake* /w/, and an appropriate control production (CP) would be *lake* /l/, since /l/ is a liquid as is /r/.

To administer the task, the examiner presents a picture or an object to the child and names it, either the correct or stimulus phoneme (SP), the client's incorrect response phoneme (RP), or a control phoneme. The number of correct responses to the three types of stimulus items (SP, RP, CP) are tabulated. A similar 18-item test is constructed for each sound substitution in which perception is to be examined in-depth.

Phonological Contrast Testing

As can be ascertained from information presented in the preceding paragraphs, the type of perceptual testing recommended is the assessment of a client's perception of phonological contrasts related to his or her error productions. Perceptual testing usually involves the client's differentiating the adult standard production from his or her error production and/or assessment of the child's perception of minimal pair phonological contrasts related to his or her error sound (e.g., *lake-rake*, where /r/ is the sound produced in error). In-depth perceptual testing of an error sound requires numerous phonemic pairings, all focusing on contrasts with the target sound.

Contrast testing is also useful with individuals learning English as a second language. Frequently, it is difficult for such people to hear sound differences that involve sounds not used in their native language. For example, native Japanese have trouble differentiating /r/ and /l/, and Spanish speakers sometimes have trouble differentiating /ɪ/ and /i/.

Assessment of a child's awareness of phonological contrasts provides the clinician with data relative to the child's phonemic system at a perceptual level. Most clinicians improvise assessment tasks requiring the child to indicate awareness that certain contrasts are in his or her perceptual repertoire. For example, a child may be shown pictures of the following pairs of words which contrast s/t, s/ʃ, and s/θ, and be asked to pick up one picture from each pair as it is named.

sea	sea	some
tea	she	thumb

Summary

If it is suspected that a child's phonological errors may be related to faulty perception, perceptual testing is appropriate. The primary concern relates to the child's ability to differentiate between the adult standard and his or her error productions. Tests based on the child's specific errors and tests of phonemic contrasts are recommended for this purpose, and are usually developed for the client by the clinician. Although our understanding of the relationship between phonological productions and perception is incomplete, it appears that improving perceptual skills may be useful in helping some children to improve their phono-logical productions (Rvachew, 1994). For individuals who are second language learners, perception testing is a very useful component to the assessment battery.

DETERMINING THE NEED FOR INTERVENTION

After the clinician has collected various types of phonological samples, the data gathered during the assessment are analyzed and interpreted to determine (1) whether there is a phonological problem; (2) the nature of the problem, if there is one; (3) whether the client should be seen for treatment; and (4) if treatment is indicated, a recommended plan of action. The primary goals of analyses are to score, sort, or otherwise organize data collected in order to describe phonological performance. The purpose of interpretation is to examine the results of the phonological analyses and determine what course of action should be taken. Based on the interpretation of the phonological analyses, the clinician must deter-mine whether the client needs instruction, and, if so, select target behaviors for treatment and appropriate intervention strategies. In summary, the clinician reviews responses to the phonological assessment tasks and interprets the analysis of these data in order to make appropriate and efficacious decisions.

In the case of children who will likely be receiving phonological therapy in the school under the provision of the Individual with Disabilities Education Act (IDEA), services are mandated only for those children whose speech and language interferes with their academic performance. As a result, in some school districts, services for a child with speech-language disorders may be directly tied to whether the speech-language impairment interferes with academic performance, whereas in other school districts, social acceptability may be used as a factor in selecting children to receive services. Qualifying children for phonological intervention requires the school-based speech-language pathologist to collaborate with a school-based diagnostic team to establish the need for services consistent with state and local eligibility criteria.

Intelligibility

An important consideration for determining the phonological status of an individual is the intelligibility or understandability of the client's spontaneous speech. The intelligibility of spontaneous speech is a reflection of the client's verbal communication competence and is a most important factor when determining the need for intervention and for evaluating the effectiveness of intervention strategies. Intelligibility of the speaker is the factor most fre-quently cited by both speech-language pathologists and naive listeners when judging the severity of a phonological problem (Shriberg and Kwiatkowski, 1982a). It should be pointed out that severity, which will be discussed later, and intelligibility, are different though related concepts.

Degree of speech intelligibility is a perceptual judgment made by a listener and is based, to a large extent, on the percentage of words in a speech sample that are understood. Intelligibility of speech reflects a continuum of judgments ranging from unintelligible (where the message is not understood) to totally intelligible (where the message is completely understood by the listener). Intermediate points along such a continuum might include the following: speech is usually unintelligible, speech is partially intelligible, speech is intelligible although noticeably in error, and speech sound errors are occasionally noticed in continuous speech. Furthermore, intelligibility may vary according to a number of variables, including level of communication (single words, conversation), topic under discussion, rate of speech, and familiarity of the listener with the speaker.

There is no standard procedure for quantifying the intelligibility of young children. Gordon-Brannan (1994) identified three general approaches for measuring intelligibility: (1) *open-set word identification* procedure, which calculates the percentage of words understood in a sample where the examiner transcribes a speech sample and determines the percentage of words identifiable; (2) *closed-set word identification*, wherein a listener identifies words repeated or read from prescribed word lists; and (3) *rating scale* procedures, which may take the form of either an interval scaling procedure, where a listener assigns a rating (number along a continuum of 5 to 9 points) or a direct magnitude scale, where a judgment of a speech sample is made relative to a standard stimulus. Although scaling procedures are often used because of their simplicity and efficiency, Schiavetti (1992) has pointed out that listeners have difficulty dividing interval scales evenly, and often it is difficult to establish reliability of listeners particularly in the middle part of a scale.

Factors influencing speech sound intelligibility include the number and types of speech sound errors, consistency of sound errors, frequency of occurrence of error sounds, and phonological patterns used. In general, the larger the number of a speaker's productions which differ from the adult standard, the more intelligibility is reduced. However, a simple tally of the number of sounds in error is not an adequate index of intelligibility. As Shriberg and Kwiatkowski (1982a) reported, there is a low correlation ($r = .42$) between the percentage of consonants correct and the intelligibility of a speech sample.

As stated, other factors in addition to the numbers of errors impact intelligibility. The nature of the clients' errors relative to the target is one such factor. For example, deleting a sound will affect intelligibility more than a distortion of the same sound will. Intelligibility is also affected by the consistency of misarticulated sounds and by the frequency with which an error sound occurs in the language. The more consistently a target sound is produced in error, and, likewise, the more frequently error sounds occur in the language, the more likely the listener will perceive the speaker's speech as defective.

Extraneous factors may influence intelligibility judgments. These factors include the listeners' familiarity with the speaker's speech pattern; prosodic factors such as speaker's rate, inflection, stress patterns, pauses, voice quality, loudness, and fluency; the linguistic experience of the listener; the social environment of the communication act; the message content; the communication cues available to the listener; and the characteristics of the transmission media. The complexity of these factors accounts for the finding that intelligibility ratings are not highly correlated with the percentage of consonants correct.

In case selection, a general principle of operation is that the poorer the ratings of intelligibility, the more likely the need for intervention. According to parent reports, normal developing 2-year-old children should be understood by a stranger 50 percent of the time (Coplan and Gleason, 1988). Vihman (2004) reported a study of normal development wherein her 3-year-old participants from well-educated families averaged over 70 percent intelligibility in conversation (range of 50 to 80 percent). Gordon-Brannan (1994) reported a mean intelligibility of 93 percent (range of 73 to 100 percent) with normal developing 4-year-old children. Commonly accepted standards for intelligibility expectations are as follows: 3 years, 75 percent intelligible; 4 years, 85 percent intelligible; and 5 years, 95 percent intelligible. Bowen (2002) suggested the following intelligibility (percentage of words understood in conversation with an unfamiliar adult) expectations: 1 year, 25 percent intelligible; 2 years, 50 percent intelligible; 3 years, 75 percent intelligible; and 4 years, 100 percent intelligible. She arrived at this percentage by dividing a child's age in years by 4. It should be pointed out that these percentages are in keeping with commonly accepted standards of intelligibility, particularly for 3- and 4-year-old children. These percentages do not reflect correct consonants, but simply the ability of a listener to understand what a speaker intended to say. It is generally recognized that a client 3 years of age or older who is unintelligible is a candidate for treatment.

Gordon-Brannan (1994), following a review of the literature concerning the assessment of intelligibility of children, suggested that calculating the actual percentage of words understood in a speech sample may be the most valid way to determine intelligibility. She suggested that the procedure could be enhanced by including orthographic transcription by a caregiver as a reliability check, and she also pointed out that although rating scales for judging speech intelligibility are less time consuming than determining percentage of words understood, such rating scales have not been validated or standardized for children with phonological deficits.

Another way of estimating intelligibility based on a conversational speech sample was suggested by Shriberg and Kwiatkowski (1980). The method is ultimately based on counting intelligible words, but these researchers suggested that even when word boundaries of the speaker are difficult to determine, transcribers can reliably count and record the number of syllables that were produced, and then group these syllables into words. They labeled their procedure an *Intelligibility Index (II)*. Based on the (1980) syllable identification and grouping procedures of Shriberg and Kwiatkowski, Flipsen (2006b) described expanded ways of doing such a count, and compared transcriber estimations based on these procedures. He reported that although the original II has practical efficiency, alternative procedures, though more complex, may be appropriate with certain types of clients. Flipsen concluded that intelligibility of conversational speech of children can be reliably quantified, and that clinicians and researchers need not limit themselves to less reliable and less valid scaling methods.

An example of one of the few published procedures for estimating speech sound intelligibility is the *Children's Speech Intelligibility Measure (CSIM)* developed by Wilcox and Morris (1999). This test involves a client imitating a list of words presented with responses tape recorded by the examiner. Words are drawn from a pool of 600 words that are categorized into 50 sets of 12 phonetically similar words. One word from each of the 50 sets is used as a target item for each CSIM administration. Because of this large pool of items, intelligibility estimates may be repeated with a new set of similar words for each measure. Following the tape recording, an independent judge listens to the tape and scores 50 words, selecting a response for each word from a list of 12 words that contain 11 phonetically similar foils. While this test produces a quantitative index of intelligibility, it is based on single-word productions, and because the listener must identify one word or another from a list, he or she has the possibility of selecting the correct response even though he or she did not understand the word produced. It does provide, however, a quantitative index of single-word production intelligibility that does not rely on clinician transcription of productions.

It is anticipated that further research in the area of measuring speech intelligibility in children will be conducted in the years ahead. For a more comprehensive review of procedures for evaluating the intelligibility of children's speech, see Kent, Miolo, and Bloedel (1994).

Severity

Severity of a phonological disorder refers to how significant the speech sound disorder is, with labels such as *mild, moderate*, and *severe* applied. Severity may also be looked at as representing the degree of impairment or "disability" in a particular client (Shriberg and Kwiatkowski, 1982a). Thus, severity of the phonological disorder is a second variable considered by speech-language clinicians in case selection decisions. Often, school systems take severity ratings into consideration when determining caseload size for individual clinicians, since clients with more severe problems require more clinician time.

Historically, a frequently employed way of arriving at severity has been for the clinician to make an impressionistic judgment as to degree of impairment by using a scale (numerical, continuum of disability) that is designed to represent degree of severity (mild to severe). Such scales have been used because of their time efficiency and the lack of more definitive ways of arriving at severity determination. Despite the importance of this estimation in terms of treatment decisions, there does not seem to be a clear consensus regarding the most valid way to arrive at level of severity of a phonological disorder. In a study of clinicians' judgments of severity, Flipsen, Hammer, and Yost (2005) reported that clinicians tend to use judgments of both individual segments as well as whole-word accuracy in making such determinations. They further reported, however, that there was such variability even among experienced clinicians in their perceptual ratings, that significant questions regarding the usefulness of measures arrived at in this manner should be raised. These investigators further suggested that when clinicians are making perceptual judgments, they attended to individual sounds (segmental data), including number, type, and consistency of errors, as well as whole-word accuracy,

A more objective way of arriving at a determination of the degree of severity was developed by Shriberg and Kwiatkowski (1982a). These researchers developed a widely used metric for quantifying the severity of involvement of children with a developmental phonological disorder. They recommended the calculation of percentage of consonants correct (PCC) as an index to quantify severity of involvement. Their research indicated that among several variables studied in relation to listeners' perceptions of severity, the PCC correlated most closely. The percentage of consonants correct requires the examiner to make correct–incorrect judgments of individual sounds produced in a continuous speech sample. Such judgments were found to be a fairly reliable measure for the classification of most children's phonological disorders as mild, mild-moderate, moderate-severe, or severe.

Procedures outlined by Shriberg and Kwiatkowski (1982a, p. 267) for determining PCC are as follows:

> Tape record a continuous speech sample of a child following sampling procedures. Any means that yield continuous speech from the child are acceptable, provided that the clinician

can tell the child that his exact words will be repeated onto the "tape machine" so that the clinician is sure to "get things right."

Sampling Rules

1. Consider only intended (target) consonants in words. Intended vowels are not considered.
   a. Addition of a consonant before a vowel, for example, *on* [hon], is not scored because the target sound /ɔ/ is a vowel.
   b. Postvocalic /r/ in fair [feir] is a consonant, but stressed and unstressed vocalics [ɝ] and [ɚ], as in *furrier* [fɝˑiɚ], are considered vowels.
2. Do not score target consonants in the second or successive repetitions of a syllable, for example, *ba-balloon*—score only the first /b/.
3. Do not score target consonants in words that are completely or partially unintelligible or whose gloss is highly questionable.
4. Do not score target consonants in the third or successive repetitions of adjacent words unless articulation changes. For example, the consonants in only the first two words of the series [kæt], [kæt], [kæt] are counted. However, the consonants in all three words are counted as if the series were [kæt], [kæk], [kæt].

Scoring Rules

1. The following six types of consonant sound changes are scored as incorrect:
   a. Deletions of a target consonant
   b. Substitutions of another sound for a target consonant, including replacement by a glottal stop or a cognate
   c. Partial voicing of initial target consonants
   d. Distortions of a target sound, no matter how subtle
   e. Addition of a sound to a correct or incorrect target consonant, for example, *cars* said as [karks]
   f. Initial /h/ deletion (*he* [i]) and final n/ŋ substitutions (*ring* [rin]) are counted as errors only when they occur in stressed syllables; in unstressed syllables they are counted as correct, for example *feed her* [fidɚ]; *running* [rʌnin].
2. Observe the following:
   a. The response definition for children who obviously have speech errors is "score as incorrect unless heard as correct." This response definition assigns questionable speech behaviors to an "incorrect" category.
   b. Dialectal variants should be glossed as intended in the child's dialect, for example, *picture* "piture," *ask* "aks," and so on.
   c. Fast or casual speech sound changes should be glossed as the child intended, for example, *don't know* "dono," and "*n*," and the like.
   d. Allophones should be scored as correct, for example, *water* [warɚ], *tail* [teɪɬ].
   Calculation of Percentage of Consonants Correct (PCC)

$$PCC = \frac{\text{Number of Correct Consonants}}{\text{Number of Correct Plus Incorrect Consonants}} \times 100$$

Based on research that related PCC values to listeners' perception of degree of handicap, Shriberg and Kwiatkowski recommended the following scale of severity:

85–100%	Mild
65–85%	Mild/moderate
50–65%	Moderate/severe
<50%	Severe

Shriberg, Austin, Lewis, McSweeney, and Wilson (1997a, 1997b) have described extensions of this widely employed PCC metric. These additional segmentally based extensions were developed to address concerns related to what some clinical phonologists perceived as limitations in the original procedure. Thus, the authors have presented additional formulas (e.g., Percentage of Vowels Correct (PVC); Percentage of Phonemes Correct (PPC); Percentage of Consonants Correct Adjusted (PPC-A) that address such variables as frequency of occurrence of sounds; types of errors, including omissions and substitutions; the nature of distortions; and vowel and diphthong errors.

Johnson, Weston, and Bain (2004) researched whether differences in PCC values would be obtained if the speech sample was based on sentence imitation, rather than the conversational task recommended by Shriberg and colleagues. They compared scores of 21 4- to 6-year-old children with speech delay that were derived from both an imitative sentence task and a conversational task. Johnson and associates reported that scores did not differ significantly, with results indicating clinical equivalency. They suggested that sentence imitation offered a valid and efficient alternative to conversational sampling, but cautioned that clinicians should consider individual child characteristics when choosing an imitative approach.

Quantitative estimates of severity, such as the PCC, provide the clinician with an objective means for determining the relative priority of those who may need intervention and a way to monitor progress/change.

Stimulability

Earlier in this chapter, procedures for conducting and interpreting stimulability testing were presented. As indicated, stimulability data are often used in making decisions regarding case selection. Investigators have reported that the ability of a child to imitate syllables and/or words containing a target sound is related to the probability that a child will spontaneously correct his or her misarticulations of that sound. The fact that a young child acquiring phonology can imitate error sounds correctly suggests that the child may be in the process of acquiring those sounds.

The use of stimulability testing for predicting spontaneous improvement or the rate of improvement in remediation has not been documented to the extent that definitive prognostic statements can be made, particularly with reference to an individual client.

Stimulability testing is only a general guide for the identification of clients who may correct their phonological errors without intervention. False positives (i.e., clients identified as needing instruction but who ultimately will outgrow their problems) and false negatives (i.e., clients identified as not needing instruction but who ultimately will require intervention) have been identified in all investigations focusing on stimulability as a prognostic indicator. These findings must be considered when results from stimulability testing are used to make predictive statements in clinical practice.

Error Patterns

After the examiner has reviewed a speaker's phonological productions in terms of intelligibility, severity, and stimulability, for those clients with multiple errors the next step is to further review the phonological samples for the presence of error patterns. Not only are individual sound productions reviewed for age appropriateness, but error patterns are also reviewed to determine if a child is using patterns/processes at a level appropriate to the child's age. In such procedures, the clinician reviews and categorizes errors according to commonalities among the errors, otherwise identified as phonological patterns/processes. As already discussed earlier in this chapter, determination of a child's phonological patterns may be based on a process assessment instrument designed to identify patterns, a connected speech sample, or a single-word articulation test.

Types of Pattern Analysis

Place-Manner-Voicing.   Perhaps the most simple type of pattern analysis involves classifying substitution errors according to place, manner, and voicing characteristics. A *place-manner-voicing analysis* facilitates the identification of patterns such as voiced for voiceless sound substitutions (e.g., voicing errors—/f/→[v] /t/→[d]), replacement of fricatives by stops (e.g., manner errors—/ð/→[d] /s/→/t/), or substitution of linguavelar sounds for linguaveolar sounds (e.g., place errors—/t/→[k] /d/→[g]). Another example would be a child whose speech patterns reflect correct manner and voicing but produce errors in place of articulation, such as fronting of consonants, for example, /k/→[t] /g/→[d]. In this instance, the child is "fronting" consonants that are produced more posteriorly.

Distinctive feature and phonological process analysis procedures are extensions of analyses based on place, manner, and voicing. These procedures are discussed next.

Distinctive Feature Analysis.   In this type of pattern analysis, speech sound substitutions are reviewed for presence or absence of particular distinctive features. As presented in Chapter 2, the idea underlying *distinctive features* is that a combination of elements or features characterize a given sound segment and that such features can distinguish one sound from other sounds. Distinctive features are based on acoustic, perceptual, and/or articulatory characteristics. From a clinical perspective, distinctive features most easily adapted to assessment and treatment of phonological problems are those based primarily on articulatory characteristics. Distinctive feature systems typically include between 13 and 16 binary (plus or minus feature value) characteristics that are used to distinguish speech sound segments.

Some of the applications that speech-language pathologists have made of distinctive feature analysis have been the subject of criticism. It has been suggested that distinctive features, although helpful in classifying sounds of languages, may not be suited to the analysis of speech sound errors. Since distinctive feature systems were developed to classify the speech sounds of languages, they do not accurately describe many nonstandard (error) productions (e.g., certain sound distortions). The binary nature of the distinctive features may not reflect the varied productions seen in the speech of children with phonological disorders. A further problem is that the features of a deleted target sound are scored as errors although the sound and, as a result, the features were never attempted. Furthermore, those features that rely on acoustical characteristics are often impractical clinically. For a critical discussion of the issues regarding the application of distinctive features to clinical analysis and intervention, refer to the papers by Walsh (1974), Parker (1976), and Foster, Riley, and Parker (1985).

Phonological Pattern/Process Analysis.   A third type of pattern analysis, sometimes called *phonological process analysis,* was described earlier in terms of case selection and is the most frequently employed type of pattern analysis. As already indicated, phonological pattern/process analysis is a method for identifying commonalities among errors. Since speech sound productions are affected by such factors as position in words, phonetic context, and syllable structure of words, these factors are reviewed for any patterns that occur across error sound productions. Before discussing interpretation of such analyses, we would like to review again some of the more common patterns (they were presented in Chapter 3 in terms of language development) observed in the speech of young children. Although process listings of different authors may vary, most resemble this listing.

Whole Word (and Syllable) Processes.   Whole word and syllable structure processes are changes that affect the syllabic structures of the target word.

1. *Final consonant deletion.*   Deletion of the final consonant in a word.

   e.g., *book*   [bu]
   cap   [ka]
   fish   [fɪ]

2. *Unstressed syllable deletion (weak syllable deletion).*   An unstressed syllable is deleted, often at the beginning of a word, sometimes in the middle.

   e.g., *potato*   [teto]
   telephone   [tɛfon]
   pajamas   [dʒæmiz]

3. *Reduplication.*   A syllable or a portion of a syllable is repeated or duplicated usually becoming CVCV.

   e.g., *dad*   [dada]
   water   [wawa]
   cat   [kaka]

4. *Consonant cluster simplification deletion.*   A consonant cluster is simplified in some manner. The cluster can be reduced to one member of the consonant cluster (i.e., cluster reduction), or a substitution may occur for one or more members of the cluster.

   e.g., *stop*   [tap]   *brown*   [bwon]   *milk*   [mɪ]
   park   [pak]   *snow*   [n̥ou]

5. *Epenthesis.*   A segment, usually the unstressed vowel [ə], is inserted.

    e.g., *black*   [bəlak]

         sweet   [səwit]

         sun   [sθʌn]

         long   [lɔŋg]

6. *Metathesis.*   There is a transposition or reversal of two segments (sounds) in a word.

    e.g., *basket*   [bæksɪt]

         spaghetti [pʌsgɛti]

         elephant [ɛfəlʌnt]

7. *Coalescence.*   Characteristics of features from two adjacent sounds are combined so that one sound replaces two other sounds.

    e.g., *swim*   [fɪm]   *tree*   [fɪ]

8. *Assimilatory (harmony) processes.*   One sound is influenced by another sound such that a sound assumes features of a second sound. Thus, the two segments become more alike or similar (hence the term harmony) or, frequently identical. These sound changes are sometimes termed *progressive assimilation* if the sound that causes the sound change precedes the affected sound (*gate* [geɪk]) and *regressive assimilation* if the sound that causes the sound change follows the affected sound (*soup* [pup]).

    a. *Velar assimilation.*   A nonvelar sound is assimilated (changed) to a velar sound because of the influence, or dominance, of the velar.

      e.g., *duck*   [gʌk]   (regressive assimilation)

         take   [kek]   (regressive assimilation)

         coat   [kok]   (progressive assimilation)

    b. *Nasal assimilation.*   A nonnasal sound is assimilated because of the influence, or dominance, of a nasal consonant.

      e.g., *candy*   [næni]   (regressive assimilation)

         lamb   [næm]   (regressive assimilation)

         fun   [nʌn]   (regressive assimilation)

    c. *Labial assimilation.*   A nonlabial sound is assimilated to a labial consonant because of the influence of a labial consonant.

      e.g., *bed*   [bɛb]   (progressive assimilation)

         table   [bebu]   (regressive assimilation)

         pit   [pip]   (progressive assimilation)

Segment Change (Substitution) Processes.   One sound is substituted for another, with the replacement sound reflecting changes in place of articulation, manner of articulation, or some other change in the way a sound is produced in a standard production.

    1. *Velar fronting.*   Substitutions are produced anterior, or forward of, the standard production.

      e.g., *key*   [ti]   (velar replaced by alveolar)

         monkey [mʌnti]   (velar replaced by alveolar)

         go   [do]   (velar replaced by alveolar)

2. *Backing.*   Sounds are substituted or replaced by segments produced posterior to, or further back in, the oral cavity than the standard production.

e.g., *tan*   [kæn]
  do   [gu]
  sip   [ʃɪp]

3. *Stopping.*   Fricatives or affricates are replaced by stops.

e.g., *sun*   [tʌn]
  peach   [pit]
  that   [dæt]

4. *Gliding of liquids.*   Prevocalic liquids are replaced by glides.

e.g., *run*   [wʌn]
  yellow   [jɛwo]
  leaf   [wif]

5. *Affrication.*   Fricatives are replaced by affricates.

e.g., *saw*   [tʃau]
  shoe   [tʃu]
  sun   [tʃʌn]

6. *Vocalization.*   Liquids or nasals are replaced by vowels.

e.g., *bird*   [bʌd]
  table   [tebo]
  mother   [mʌðo]

7. *Denasalization.*   Nasals are replaced by homorganic stops (place of articulation is similar to target sound).

e.g., *moon*   [bud]
  nice   [deis]
  man   [bæn]

8. *Deaffrication.*   Affricates are replaced by fricatives.

e.g., *chop*   [sap]
  chip   [ʃɪp]
  page   [pez]

9. *Glottal replacement.*   Glottal stops replace sounds usually in either intervocalic or final position.

e.g., *cat*   [kæʔ]
  tooth   [tuʔ]
  bottle   [baʔl]

10. *Prevocalic voicing.*   Voiceless consonants (obstruents) in the prevocalic position are voiced.

e.g., *paper*   [bepɚ]
  Tom   [dam]
  table   [debi]

11. *Devoicing of final consonants.* Voiced obstruents are devoiced in final position.

e.g., *dog* [dɔk]
nose [nos]
bed [bɛt]

Multiple Pattern Occurrence. The examples of phonological patterns given above typically included lexical items in which only a single pattern was used. In reality, the child may produce forms that reflect more than one process, including some that are not reflected in the definitions and descriptions above. A single lexical item may have two or even more processes interacting. When such productions occur, they are more complex and difficult to unravel than words which reflect a single process. For example, in the production of [du] for *shoe*, Edwards (1983) pointed out that the [d] for /ʃ/ replacement reflects the phonological pattern of (1) depalatalization, which changes the place of articulation; (2) stopping, which changes the manner of articulation; and (3) prevocalic voicing, which changes a voiceless consonant target to a voiced consonant. In the substitution of [dar] for *car*, the [d] for /k/ substitution is accounted for by the patterns of velar fronting and prevocalic voicing. The identification of the sequence of steps describing how interacting processes account for substitutions is called a *derivation* or *process ordering*.

Unusual Pattern Occurrence. As indicated throughout this book, a great deal of individual variation exists in the phonological acquisition of children. Although there are common developmental phonological patterns used by most children, the patterns observed across individuals vary. This is especially true in the speech of children with speech sound disorders. Unusual phonological patterns (e.g., use of a nasal sound for /s/ and /z/), called *idiosyncratic processes* or *patterns*, differ from the more common phonological patterns we have identified and are seen in both children with normal and delayed phonological development. The greatest variation in phonology occurs during the early stages of development and is probably influenced, in part, by the lexical items the child uses when acquiring his or her first words. When idiosyncratic patterns persist after age 3;0 to 3;5, they likely reflect a phonological disorder.

The preceding list of phonological patterns is not exhaustive but represents most of the common patterns seen in normally developing children. These phonological patterns have also been used in analyzing the sound errors of phonologically delayed children. Several procedures designed to assist the clinician in the identification of phonological patterns/processes in children's speech have been published in monograph or kit form. Included in these procedures are various groupings, as well as additions and deletions to the patterns/processes listed earlier. Table 5.3 reflects a modified version of Edwards's (1983) listing of the characteristics of published phonological assessment procedures.

Sound Preferences. Another type of sound pattern that some clinicians have reported is called *systematic sound preference*. In these situations, children seem to have a segment or two that they use for a large number of sounds or sound classes. Sometimes a particular sound is substituted for several or even all phonemes in a particular sound class (e.g., fricatives). Other children will substitute a single consonant for a variety of segments, such as [h] for /b, d, s, ʒ, z, dʒ, tʃ, ʃ, l, k, g, r/ (Weiner, 1981a). It has been postulated that some

■ TABLE 5.3 Characteristics of the Published Phonological Assessment Procedures

Basis of Comparison by Authors	Hodson (2003)	Khan-Lewis (2002)	Bankson and Bernthal (1990b)	Smit and Hand (1997)	Lowe (1986)
Stimuli	3-dimensional objects	Pictures from the *Goldman-Fristoe Test of Articulation*	Pictures from the *Bankson-Bernthal Test of Phonology*	Photographs from the *Smit-Hand Articulation and Phonology Evaluation*	Embedded target words-picture stimuli
Elicitation procedures	Object-naming; no set order	Picture-naming in citation form	Picture-naming in citation form	Photograph-naming in citation form	Delayed sentence imitation-picture stimuli supplemental
Sample size	50 single words	44 single words	80 single words	80 single words	50 words
Transcription	Broad transcriptions modified; audiotaped for reference	Narrow "on-line" and from recordings	Live and from recordings	Live and from recordings check sheet with options delineated	Live
Number of processes	30 deviations	12 developmental processes 3 nondevelopmental processes	10 most frequently occurring processes in standardization samples	11 most frequently occurring processes in standardization samples	15
Target population	Children with multiple articulation errors; unintelligible speech	Normally developing and phonologically disordered children	Normally developing and phonologically disordered children ages 3–6	Normally developing and phonologically disordered children ages 3–9	Normally developing and phonologically disordered children ages 3–9
Time (total)	±50 minutes	±35 minutes	±30 minutes	Not specified	10–15 minutes
Number of processes per word	Allows for multiple processes	Allows for multiple processes	Allows for multiple processes	Allows for multiple processes	Allows for multiple processes
Process descriptions	Number of occurrences tabulated across sounds and positions	Organized by sounds and word position	Organized by sounds and word position	Number of occurrences in test words	Number occurrences in test words
Frequency of occurrence	Calculation for 10 basic deviations	Frequency of each of the 15 processes calculated	Frequency of each of the 10 processes calculated	Percentage of occurrence in test words calculated	Frequency of each of the 15 processes calculated

children avoid the use of certain sounds in their productions and, instead simplify their sound productions.

Young children during the phonological acquisition stage simplify their productions as they learn the adult phonological system. The reasons that children simplify their productions likely include such factors as physiological and perceptual limitations/immaturities and a lack of linguistic knowledge. When such phonological simplifications (processes) persist in a child's productions, we identify these patterns as a way to describe the child's phonological system. It is difficult to determine the precise reason for the persistence of phonological patterns during normal sound acquisition.

Theoretical Considerations Regarding Phonological Patterns. An example demonstrating the inherent difficulty in arriving at an explanatory statement for a given phonological pattern was provided by Hoffman and Schuckers (1984). One explanation for the occurrence of a particular pattern might be that the child misperceives the adult word, for example, perceives [dɔg] as [dɔ]. A second explanation might be that the child's underlying word storage for dog is [dɔ]. A third possible explanation is that the child's perceptual system functions appropriately and the lexical match between what the child perceives and what he or she has stored is consistent with the adult standard, but he or she has a phonological production rule that calls for the deletion of word-final stops. A fourth possibility is that the child has a motor production problem; in this case, the child may have the appropriate perception but does not possess the necessary motor skill to make the articulation gesture to produce the sound.

Shelton (1986) has identified three different theoretical interpretations of phonological patterns in the speech-language pathology literature. One view is that phonological patterns constitute a taxonomy or listing of speech sound error patterns, a catalog of descriptors that can be used to identify the simplifications or modifications used by children. This view makes no speculations or assumptions regarding the child's underlying representations (mental images or internal knowledge of the lexical items) in relation to the adult standard; it simply describes behavior at the observable or surface level. This atheoretical perspective posits nothing about the operation of processes, the nature of phonological structure, the relationship of surface forms and underlying representations, or even the relationship of production and perception. This interpretation is the most widely accepted today.

A second view of phonological patterns assumes that the child has underlying representations of lexical forms that are similar to those of the adult surface forms. This view, which comes from work in normal phonological development, assumes that the child is attempting to produce the adult form of the word and has an adult-like mental image of the lexical item. The surface forms produced by the child, however, reflect immature development. The child changes or simplifies the target production in some manner during the production of the word. It is these simplifications that are identified as errors in the individual's speech. The mismatches between the child's productions and his or her underlying representations (which are the same as the adult standard) are expressed as phonological patterns.

The third theoretical position acknowledges the existence of underlying representations but makes no assumptions concerning their form. The clinician examines the child's surface forms (the child's articulatory productions) to determine the status or nature of the child's underlying representations. If a child uses a phoneme contrastively, it is assumed that he or she has the adult underlying form. If the child misarticulates a sound, and there is no evidence from phonological assessment or acoustical analysis that the sound is in the child's repertoire, it is not assumed the child has the adult-like underlying representation of the sound. For example, if a child says [dɔ] for [dɔg] but uses [g] in the diminutive doggy [dɔgi], one can assume that the child has the underlying form for [g] since /g/ is produced in the form [dɔgi]. On the other hand, if /g/ is not observed in any of the child's utterances, no assumption is made regarding the underlying form for /g/. Thus, this view of underlying structures differs from the second view, described above, in that it makes no assumptions concerning the underlying representations; the second assumes the child has the adult form.

Developmental Appropriateness

A fifth factor to consider in deciding if a client is a candidate for intervention is the age appropriateness of his or her phonological productions. If a child misarticulates sounds that are produced by 75 percent or 90 percent of children at that age (depending on which criterion is selected), or if a child's performance on a normed speech sound test is one or more standard deviations below the mean, or if a child evidences phonological processes that typically are eliminated by other children of his or her age, the child is often identified as having a developmental delay or disorder.

Two methods traditionally have been employed to compare articulation performance and chronological age: (1) the number of correct responses on a speech sound articulation test are tabulated and then compared with normative data for a given age level on the same test (e.g., *Bankson-Bernthal Test of Phonology*; Bankson and Bernthal, 1990a) and (2) a comparison is made of the child's individual segmental productions with developmental norms for individual sounds (e.g., Prather, Hedrick, and Kern, 1975; Iowa-Nebraska norms, Smit, Hand, Freilinger, Bernthal, and Bird, 1990).

The comparison of a child's segmental productions with developmental norms for individual sounds is one way norms are frequently used. Although this appears to be a simple task, one must be cautious when assigning an age norm to a particular sound. Normative data are statistical averages that reflect overall patterns of mastery. One must remember that children learn sounds at different rates and in different sequences. Thus caution is required in the application of normative data for individual sounds produced by an individual child.

As discussed earlier, investigators have attached an age expectation to specific speech sounds by listing the age levels at which 75 percent and/or 90 percent of the children in a normative group have mastered each sound tested. Sander (1972) pointed out that such normative data are group standards that reflect upper age limits (i.e., 75 percent or 90 percent of children at a particular age produce the sound) rather than average performance or customary production (50 percent of children at a particular age produce the sound). Sander also argued that "variability among children in the ages at which they successfully produce specific sounds is so great as to discourage pinpoint statistics" (p. 58).

Prather and colleagues (1975) reported speech sound acquisition norms for children from age 2 through 4 years on a test designed to elicit consonants in the prevocalic and postvocalic positions. With respect to the age levels at which 75 percent of the children had mastered specific sounds, these investigators reported earlier age levels than Templin (1957), although the sequence of acquisition was similar in both studies. They pointed out that the differences in findings could be due to their use of two-position versus Templin's three-position testing. A useful set of normative data for individual sound acquisition, which reflects an age range for sound development, is shown in Figure 5.3.

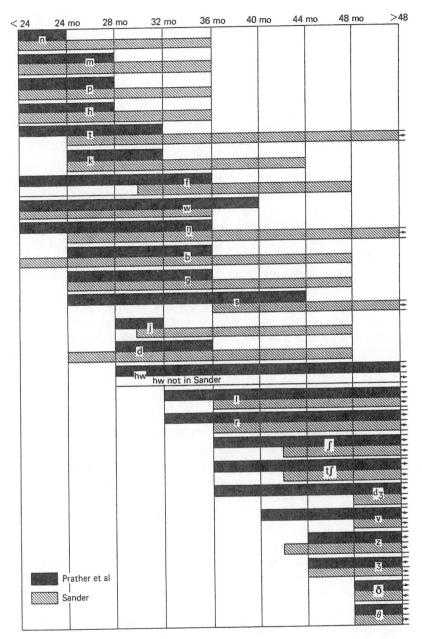

■ **FIGURE 5.3** Normative articulation data. The left-hand margin of each bar represents the age at which 50 percent of the children in normative studies used the specified sound correctly. The right-hand margin shows the age at which 90 percent of the children used the sound correctly. Data reported in the lower bars are from Sander (1972). Data in the black bars are from the work of Hedrick, Prather, and Tobin (1975).

Source: Adapted by permission from E. M. Prather, D. L. Hedrick, and C. A. Kern, "Articulation Development in Children Aged Two to Four Years," *Journal of Speech and Hearing Disorders, 40* (1975): 186.

Smit and colleagues (1990) gathered three-position data from children in two midwestern states. Using a 75 percent criterion level, they reported that children acquire sounds at ages equal to or younger than ages reported by Templin except for /ŋ/ and /r/, for which the 75 percent criterion was later than that reported by Templin. They also found that clusters tended to reach the 75 percent criterion at the same age or later than singletons contained in the clusters. It is interesting to note, however, the overall similarity between the data of Smit and colleagues and those of Templin gathered 33 years earlier.

The clinician should keep in mind that in using the data from any large group study, individual subject data are obscured. Although the precise sequence and nature of phonological development varies from one person to another, in general, certain segments are mastered earlier than others, and this information is used in determining presence of phonological delay and the direction of treatment. For example, if 6-year-old Kirsten says all the sounds usually produced by 75 percent of 3-year-old children, but is not yet using sounds commonly associated with 4-, 5-, and 6-year-olds, her phonological productions would be considered delayed. This developmental aspect of phonological acquisition makes age a useful factor in determining whether a child has a phonological delay.

A second commonly employed way of comparing phonology and chronological age is to compare a child's phonological performance with norms for a specific phonological measure (as opposed to individual segmental norms). In this procedure, the number of speech sound productions produced correctly on a specific test are compared with normative data for that instrument. In other words, the number of sounds that the child produces correctly are compared with normative data to determine whether a child's articulatory performance is typical for the child's age. This analysis is appropriate for children 8 years old and younger, since correct production of speech sound segments is usually expected by age 8 in typically developing children. This procedure is the basis by which many states and school districts determine if children with phonological delay and disorders qualify for services. Tests such as the *Goldman-Fristoe Test of Articulation* (2000), the *Arizona Articulation Proficiency Scale* (Fudala and Reynolds, 1986), and the *Bankson-Bernthal Test of Phonology* (1990b) are examples of tests that report normative data.

An additional way of looking at a child's individual speech sound productions from a developmental perspective is to review sound errors in terms of whether they tend to fall into one or another of the three developmental sounds classes (Shriberg, 1993) that were discussed in Chapter 3 (i.e., 8 early developing sounds, 8 middle developing sounds, 8 late developing sounds). By reviewing a child's age and the nature of his or her errors, an additional perspective relative to developmental appropriateness can be obtained.

The age appropriateness of certain phonological processes/patterns that may be present in a young child's speech is an additional normative factor taken into consideration in case selection. Several investigators have provided data that are relevant to young children's use of phonological processes. Preisser, Hodson, and Paden (1988), in a cross-sectional study, examined phonological processes used by young children. Between 24 and 29 months, the most commonly observed processes were cluster reduction, liquid deviation (which included deletions of a liquid in a consonant cluster, e.g., *black* → [bæk]), vowelization (e.g., *zipper* → [zɪpo]), and gliding of liquids (e.g., red → [wɛd]). Next most common were patterns involving the strident feature.

Roberts, Burchinal, and Footo (1990) observed a group of children between 2;5 and 8 years in a quasi-longitudinal study—that is, children were tested a varying number of times over the course of the study. They reported a marked decrease in the use of processes between the ages of 2;5 and 4 years. They also reported that at age 2;5, percentage of occurrence for the following processes was less than 20 percent: reduplication, assimilation, deletion of initial consonants, addition of a consonant, labialization shifts, methathesis, and backing. By age 4, only cluster reduction, liquid gliding, and deaffrication had a percentage of occurrence of 20 percent or more. Refer to Chapter 3 for a more complete summary of speech sound development.

Stoel-Gammon and Dunn (1985) reviewed studies of process occurrence and identified those processes that typically are deleted by age 3 and those that persist after 3 years. Their summary is:

Processes Disappearing by 3 Years	*Processes Persisting after 3 Years*
Unstressed syllable deletion	Cluster reduction
Final consonant deletion	Epenthesis
Consonant assimilation	Gliding
Reduplication	Vocalization
Velar fronting	Stopping
Prevocalic voicing	Depalatalization
	Final devoicing

Table 5.4 from Grunwell (1981) reflects "simplifying processes" used by young children in normal phonological development. The table is derived largely from data reported by Ingram (1976) and Anthony, Bogle, Ingram, and McIssac (1971) and is based on a relatively small number of subjects. The solid lines reflect typical ages at which particular processes are evidenced, and the broken lines reflect the approximate age at which the processes are modified or begin to disappear.

Bankson and Bernthal (1990b) reported data on the processes most frequently observed in a sample of over 1,000 children, 3 to 9 years of age, tested during the standardization of the *Bankson-Bernthal Test of Phonology (BBTOP)*. The BBTOP ultimately included the 10 processes that appeared most frequently in children's productions during standardization testing. The processes which persisted the longest in children's speech were gliding of liquids, stopping, cluster simplification, vocalization, and final consonant deletion. These data are almost identical to those reported by Khan and Lewis (1986) except they later (2000) found velar fronting persisted longer in young children's speech.

Comparison of age and phonological development is widely practiced, and such data must be taken into consideration in intervention decisions. Justifiable criticism has been made of using such data as the single criterion for case selection (Turton, 1980). Criticism is based on the following factors: (1) Speech sound developmental norms typically reflect upper age limits of customary consonant production (between 75 and 100 percent of children produce the sounds correctly) rather than average age estimates; (2) the norms are based on production in the initial, medial, and final positions of single words rather than spontaneous speech; (3) there is a great deal of variability across children; (4) norms frequently are based on a single production of a particular sound in one or two contexts; (5) norms represent a statement of average performance by age, but the resulting sequence of acquisition may not be applicable to a given individual; (6) although sounds generally appear to be acquired in a sequence, prior acquisition of certain sounds is not necessarily required for

■ **TABLE 5.4** Chronology of Phonological Processes

	2;0–2;6	2;6–3;0	3;0–3;6	3;6–4;0	4;0–4;6	4;6–5;0	5;0→
Unstressed Syllable Deletion							
Final Consonant Deletion							
Reduplication							
Consonant Harmony							
Cluster Reduction (Initial)							
Obstruent—Approximant							
/s/ + Consonant							
Stopping							
/f/							
/v/							
/θ/		θ → [f]					
/ð/				/ð/ → [d] or [v]			
/s/							
/z/							
/ʃ/		Fronting '[s] type'					
/tʃ, dʒ/		Fronting [ts, dz]					
Fronting/k, g, ŋ/							
Gliding r → [w]							
Context-Sensitive Voicing							

Source: Adapted by permission from P. Grunwell, "The Development of Phonology: A Descriptive Profile." *First Language*, *3* (1981): 161-191. Used with permission.

the learning of other sounds; and (7) the nature of the error may be a critical factor. For example, Stephens, Hoffman, and Daniloff (1986) reported that unlike most errors, lateralization of /s/ did not spontaneously improve with age. Our clinical experience is that lateralization of /s/ is a production that will not likely self-correct with maturation. We would concur with the suggestion of Smit and colleagues (1990) that lateralized /s/ errors be treated earlier than other /s/ errors because unlike most speech sound errors they do not generally spontaneously or self correct with age.

Process norms can also be helpful in determining need for intervention. In this case, one is looking for processes/patterns or simplifications that are not typically used at a particular age. If processes/patterns persist beyond the expected age level, or if a child uses unusual processes, their presence is one of the factors that should be taken into consideration in case selection.

Case Selection Guidelines and Summary

The first question that must be answered through analysis of phonological sampling procedures is whether there is a phonological problem that warrants intervention. By reviewing the intelligibility of the speaker, the severity of the phonological problems that may be present, the developmental appropriateness of the child's phonological productions, and the error patterns, such a question can be answered.

As a general guideline for initiating intervention, a child, in order to be identifiable for services, should be one standard deviation or more (some state guidelines call for 1.5 to 2 standard deviations) below his or her age norm on a standardized measure of phonology. The clinician should recognize, however, that this is only a general guideline and that other considerations, such as intelligibility, nature of the errors and error patterns, consistency of errors, speaker's perception of his or her problem, and other speech-language characteristics, may also be important in intervention decisions.

Children between ages 2.5 and 3 who are unintelligible are usually recommended for early intervention programs, which typically include parental education and assistance. Children age 3 years or older who evidence pronounced intelligibility and/or severity problems, or who evidence idiosyncratic phonological problems, are candidates for intervention. Children age 8 and below whose phonological performance is at least one standard deviation below the mean for their age are also candidates for intervention. Most children 9 years or older are also recommended for intervention if they have consistently produced speech sound errors—often residual distortion errors. Teenagers and adults who perceive that their phonological errors constitute a handicap should be considered for instruction. Likewise, children of any age should be considered for evaluation when they or their parents are concerned about their speech sound productions.

TARGET BEHAVIOR SELECTION

Once the need for intervention is established, sampling data are further reviewed to determine goals for intervention. The following paragraphs will delineate how the various components of the assessment battery are utilized to establish target behaviors for remediation.

Stimulability

As you will recall, stimulability testing consists of assessing client performance when the client is asked to imitate the adult form of speech sound errors in isolation, syllables, and words. Many clinicians have postulated that error sounds that can be produced through imitation are more rapidly corrected through intervention than sounds that cannot be imitated. McReynolds and Elbert (1978) reported that once a child could imitate a sound, generalization occurred to other contexts. Thus, imitation served as a predictor of generalization. Powell and colleagues (1991) also reported that stimulability explained many of the generalization patterns observed during treatment. They found that sounds that were stimulable were most likely to be added to the phonetic repertoire regardless of the sounds selected for treatment. Miccio and Elbert (1996) suggested that "teaching stimulability" may be a way to facilitate phonological acquisition and generalization by increasing the client's phonetic repertoire.

Intervention is usually initiated at the level of the most complex linguistic unit the client can imitate (i.e., isolation, syllable, word, phrase). Sounds from different sound classes are often chosen as exemplars, with stimulability data aiding in their selection. For example, if word-final stops, fricatives, and nasals are all deleted, the clinician might target one stimulable stop, fricative, and nasal as exemplars. Hodson (2007a), in her cycles approach to remediation, suggested selecting patterns on which the child is most stimulable in order to enhance the client's phonological repertoire.

Although there seems to be general agreement that more rapid generalization occurs for sounds on which the child is stimulable, some clinicians assign such sounds a lower priority for remediation. It has been reported that teaching sounds on which the child is not stimulable has the greatest potential to positively affect the child's overall phonological system although such sounds may be more difficult to teach (Powell et al., 1991). Thus, for children with multiple errors, greater gains in the overall phonological system may be made when intervention initially focuses on sounds not in the child's repertoire. This recommendation is in contrast to the notion that target selections should focus on sounds on which the client is stimulable, since therapy will move rapidly and the child will enjoy faster success (Secord, 1989; Diedrich, 1983).

It has been postulated (Dinnsen and Elbert, 1984) that imitation of words by the child may reflect correct underlying representations (storage of the adult form). One might speculate, then, that if a child is able to imitate a word, this performance may indicate that the child has acquired at a cognitive level the linguistic contrasts of the language necessary to produce a sound in at least some appropriate contrastive contexts. From this perspective, correct imitation is a reflection not only of phonetic or motor skill but also of the child's possession of the adult's (correct) underlying form of the error word. In a study of this issue, Lof (1994) concluded that stimulability testing reflects phonetic behavior only.

Frequency of Occurrence

Another factor used in target behavior selection is the frequency with which the sounds produced in error occur in the spoken language. Obviously, the greater the frequency of a sound in a language, the greater its potential effect on intelligibility. Thus, treatment will have the greatest impact on a client's overall intelligibility if frequently occurring segments produced in error are selected for treatment.

Table 5.5 lists the rank order and frequency of occurrence of the 24 most frequently used consonants in conversational American English (Shriberg and Kwiatkowski, 1983). These statistics are based on a collection of natural speech data from a variety of sources. Mines, Hanson, and Shoup (1978) noted a relatively high correlation among all frequency counts, based on both spoken and written expression. The consonants /n, t, s, r, l, d, ð, k, m, w, z/ occur very frequently in connected speech and errors on these sounds will adversely affect intelligibility. Other data reported in the table show that almost two-thirds of the consonants used are voiced, 29 percent are stops, 19 percent are sonorants, and 18 percent are nasals. Moreover, three of the six stops /t, d, k/, three of four sonorants /r, l, w/, and two of three nasals /n, m/ are among the 11 most frequently occurring consonants. Dental and alveolar consonants accounted for 61 percent of the productions and labial and labiodental sounds, 21 percent. In other words, over four-fifths of consonant occurrences are produced at the anterior area of the mouth.

■ **TABLE 5.5** Percentage of Occurrence of (Intended) English Consonants in Continuoius Speech

Sound	Rank	Mean %	Hoffmann (1982)	Irwin and Wong (1983)[a]	Carterette and Jones (1974)	Mader (1954)	Shriberg and Kwiatkowski (1982)	Shriberg and Kwiatkowski (1983)	Mines et al. (1978)
n	1	12.01	11.22	9.84	13.63	13.14	11.7	13.04	11.49
t	2	11.83	12.43	14.05	7.91	11.74	13.7	13.08	9.88
s	3	6.90	6.78	6.66	6.94	6.50	7.1	6.43	7.88
r	4	6.68	7.06	5.99	8.20	7.83	5.2	5.84	6.61
d	5	6.41	4.26	6.89	6.31	10.25	5.8	5.33	5.70
m	6	5.93	5.20	5.52	7.49	4.63	5.6	7.97	5.11
z	7	5.36	8.69	4.88	4.58	3.70	3.0	3.97	4.70
ð	8	5.32	6.90	6.04	4.42	6.40	4.1	4.04	5.37
l	9	5.25	3.42	5.41	4.96	5.55	5.6	5.59	6.21
k	10	5.13	4.60	5.20	4.96	4.25	6.0	5.57	5.30
w	11	4.88	4.19	4.70	5.57	5.33	4.8	4.79	4.81
h	12	4.38	7.47	5.17	3.37	3.33	4.2	4.97	2.23
b	13	3.28	2.84	3.40	3.18	2.97	3.5	3.92	3.24
p	14	3.12	2.98	3.12	2.12	2.73	3.9	3.90	3.07
g	15	3.08	3.93	3.29	2.90	2.38	4.1	2.93	2.02
f	16	2.07	2.38	1.64	2.21	1.83	2.4	1.37	2.65
ŋ	17	1.58	0.94	1.86	1.05	1.61	2.5	1.24	1.85
j	18	1.56	1.22	1.49	1.41	0.77	2.2	1.94	1.87
v	19	1.52	1.03	1.46	1.64	1.91	1.2	0.42	2.97
ʃ	20	0.93	0.87	1.14	0.84	0.84	1.5	0.38	0.95
θ	21	0.89	0.59	0.84	1.03	0.93	0.9	0.76	1.19
dʒ	22	0.58	0.62	0.50	0.53	0.69	0.6	0.19	0.95
tʃ	23	0.55	0.34	0.31	0.51	0.55	0.7	0.56	0.85
ʒ	24	0.03	0.01	0.01	0	0.01	0	0	0.15

[a]Data calculated from page 156, Table 8.4 to reflect only children ages 3, 4, and 6 years.

Source: L. Shriberg and J. Kwiatkowski, "Computer-Assisted Natural Process Analysis (NPA): Recent Issues and Data." In *Assessing and Treating Phonological Disorders: Current Approaches.* J. Locke (Ed.), *Seminars in Speech and Language, 4* (1983): 397. Used by permission.

Developmental Appropriateness

Earlier in this chapter, we discussed the role of normative data in case selection. That discussion is also relevant to target selection. Traditionally, clinicians have tended to select sounds for intervention that are earlier acquired and thus should already be in a client's repertoire. Research by Gierut, Morrisette, Hughes, and Rowland (1996) has suggested, however, that for children with multiple errors, treatment of later as opposed to earlier developing sounds results in greater overall improvement in a client's phonological system than does targeting early developing sounds. This finding is in keeping with other research (Dinnsen, Chin, Elbert, and Powell, 1990; Tyler and Figurski, 1994), which suggests that targeting sounds evidencing greater as opposed to lesser complexity is a more efficient way to proceed with phonological intervention. Data that do not support this assertion was reported by Rvachew and Nowak (2001). In a study of children with moderate or severe phonological delays, these investigators found that children who received treatment for phonemes that are early developing and associated with greater productive phonological knowledge showed greater progress toward acquisition of the target sounds than did children who received treatment for late-developing phonemes associated with little or no productive phonological knowledge. Further research appears warranted before a recommendation can be made regarding the efficacy of targeting early versus later developing sounds.

Some speech-language pathologists have suggested that target selection might be based on the concept of relating age and sound errors to the eight early, middle, and late developing sounds (Shriberg, 1993) that were discussed in Chapter 3. Bleile (2006) authored a book titled *The Late Eight*, which is a resource for teaching the late eight developing sounds (/θ, ð, s, z, ɝ, r, l, ʃ/). He indicated that these sounds are most likely to challenge school-age children and nonnative speakers, both children and adults.

In terms of processes/patterns, most clinicians would agree that targeting patterns that tend to be used early in acquisition (e.g., final consonant deletion) is better advised than targeting processes that tend to persist longer (e.g., gliding) during phonological acquisition because the early disappearing processes are more closely related to overall intelligibility. Age appropriateness is one factor to take into consideration in target selection; however, it should be pointed out that other variables discussed in this section should also be reviewed when selecting targets for phonological remediation. For older children in particular, other factors usually weigh more heavily in terms of target selection.

Contextual Analysis

As stated earlier, contextual testing examines the influence of surrounding sounds on error sounds. Contextual testing may identify facilitating *phonetic contexts*, which are defined as surrounding sounds that have a positive influence on production of error sounds. Thus, contextual testing provides data on phonetic contexts in which an error sound may be produced correctly, which information may be a helpful beginning point for treatment. Through the identification of such contexts, the clinician may find that a specific sound doesn't have to be taught, but rather should be isolated and stabilized in a specific context, since it is already in the client's repertoire. Both the client and clinician may save time and frustration that often accompany initial attempts to establish a speech sound by focusing first on a certain context in which a sound is produced correctly and then gradually shifting to other contexts.

For example, if a child lisps on /s/ but a correct /s/ is observed in the /sk/ cluster in [bɪskɪt] (biscuit), one could have the client say *biscuit* slowly, emphasizing the medial cluster (i.e., sk), and hopefully hear a good /s/. The client could then prolong the /s/ before saying the /k/ (i.e., [bɪs ss kɪt]), and ultimately say the /s/ independent of the word context (i.e., /sss/). This production could then be used to progress to other contexts using the stabilized /s/ production. In general, when contexts can be found where target sounds are produced correctly, using such sound contexts can be used efficiently in remediation. The number of contexts in which a child can produce a sound correctly on a contextual test may provide some indication of the stability of the error. It seems logical that the less stable the error, the easier it may be to correct. However, some clinicians find that a stable error pattern is easier to focus on than is a more "elusive error." The clinician can utilize contexts in which a segment is produced correctly to reinforce correct production and facilitate generalization to other contexts. If a client's error tends to be inconsistent across different phonetic contexts, one might assume that the chances for improvement are better than if the error tends to persist across different phonetic contexts or situations.

Phonological Process/Pattern Analysis

The comparison of a client's use of phonological processes/patterns with normative data regarding the use of phonological patterns or simplifications can also be used in target selection. The processes or patterns used by a phonologically delayed child can be compared with those that might be expected in the speech of normally developing children. Patterns that are not normally present in children of a particular age are those usually targeted for intervention. One caution, however, is that few data suggest that reduction in the use of phonological processes occurs in a prescribed order, although some processes tend to persist in older children and others tend to occur only in younger children. Moreover, no data are reported that suggest that the elimination or reduction of one process in a child's speech should occur before another process is targeted for treatment. There are, however, general trends that may be helpful in targeting processes for treatment, but a universally prescribed developmental order for process selection has not been established.

Hodson (2007a) suggested that clinicians focus on facilitating appropriate phonological patterns (rather than eliminating inappropriate patterns). For highly unintelligibile children, she suggested focusing on the most stimulable pattern in order that the child can experience immediate success. As a general guide, Hodson delineates the following potential primary targets for facilitation:

1. Syllableness (for omitted vowels, diphthongs, vocalic/syllabic consonants resulting in productions limited to monosyllables; using two-syllable compound words, such as *cowboy;* and then three-syllable word combinations, such as *cowboy hat*)
2. Singleton consonants in words (prevocalic /p, b, m, w/; postvocalic voiceless stops; pre- and postvocalic consonants, such as *pup, pop;* intervocalic consonants, such as *apple*)
3. /s/ clusters (word initial, word final)
4. Anterior/posterior contrasts (word-final /k/, word-initial /k/, /g/ for "fronters"; occasional /h/; alvolars/labials if "backers")
5. Liquids (word-initial /l/, word-initial /r/, word initial /kr/, /gr/—after the child readily produces singleton velars; word initial /l/ clusters—after child readily produces prevocalic /l/)

Target Behavior Selection Guidelines

Few Errors

For children evidencing a small number of sound errors that are likely to be phonetic in nature, the clinician may wish to work simultaneously on all error productions. For example, if a child misarticulates /s/, /z/, /r/, and /l/, the clinician may target /s/ and /r/ (assuming that the client will generalize from /s/ to /z/). If, however, a client is not able to handle multiple targets, one might wish to focus on a target that occurs most frequently in the language and/or that affects intelligibility the most. Age of the client, attention span, and length and/or frequency of treatment sessions are variables to take into consideration in determining how many and which targets to focus on at any point in time.

Multiple Errors

For children with multiple phonological errors, target selection has some similarity to selection for clients with a small number of errors. However, some additional components and considerations exist. The first step for determining targets in clients with multiple errors is to determine the patterns or processes that are evident. In the preceding paragraphs we presented the listing of Hodson's (2007a) suggested priorities for identifying target patterns for remediation.

When patterns have been identified for intervention, one is then faced with selecting specific sounds that need to be focused on in order to facilitate production of a particular pattern. The expectation is that a selected target(s) or exemplar(s) will generalize to other sounds and patterns related to that target. For example, if final consonant deletion is identified as the first target process, one must then choose a sound, or perhaps two or more sounds, to work on in the word-final position. Sound selection in this instance would be similar to the method identified earlier for choosing among sounds when there is a small number of errors (i.e., stimulability, frequency of occurrence of a target, developmental order).

In more recent years, these time-honored ways of selecting individual sound targets have been challenged because data have been provided (Gierut, 2001, and other work by Gierut and colleagues) that would suggest that other criteria for target sound selection may be more appropriate in terms of efficiency of treatment. More specifically, there are data to suggest that by targeting the following, a greater impact may be made on a child's overall sound system:

1. Later developing as contrasted with early developing sounds
2. Nonstimulable as contrasted with stimulable sounds
3. Clusters as contrasted with singletons
4. Difficult to produce as contrasted with easy to produce

Although many clinicians would suggest that these criteria for target selection should come into play after target processes have first been identified, some suggest that one could employ these criteria without reference to overall patterns present in a child's errors. However, the nature of sound collapses may also influence target sound selection. For example, if /w/ is used for /r/, /l/, /s/, /z/, /θ/, /ð/, /h/, one might attempt to initially target /s/ or /h/ to establish a contrast between /w/ and another sound in another sound class.

OTHER FACTORS TO CONSIDER IN CASE SELECTION: INTERVENTION DECISIONS

Dialectal Considerations

As will be discussed in detail in Chapter 8, the linguistic culture of the speaker is a factor that must be considered when deciding on the need for speech-language intervention, particularly for those clients from ethnic or minority populations, where standard English may not be the norm. *Dialect*, as discussed in Chapter 8, refers to a consistent variation of a language, reflected in pronunciation, grammar, or vocabulary, that is used by a particular subgroup of the general population. Although many dialects are identified with a geographical area, those of greatest interest to clinicians are often dialects related to sociocultural or ethnic identification.

The phonological patterns of a particular dialect will differ from the general cultural norm, but these variations reflect only differences and not delays or deficiencies in comparison to the so-called standard version of the language. To view the phonological or syntactic patterns used by members of such subcultures as delayed, deviant, or substandard is totally inappropriate. As Williams (1972) put it years ago, "The relatively simple yet important point here is that language variation is a logical and expected phenomenon, hence, we should not look upon nonstandard dialects as deficient versions of a language" (p. 111). This perspective has obvious clinical implications: Persons whose speech and language patterns reflect a cultural dialect should not be considered for remediation unless their phonological patterns are outside the cultural norm for the region or ethnic group, or the individual wishes to learn a standard dialect.

Phonological differences may also occur in the speech of individuals within subcultures. The language patterns of inner-city African Americans in New York City, for example, may be quite different from those in New Orleans. One cannot use normative data based on General American English (GAE) to judge the phonological status of individuals of some subcultures, and one should not assume that members of certain subcultures have homogeneous linguistic patterns, especially when geographic or ethnic factors are considered. Again, you are referred to Chapter 8 for further information on this topic.

Clinicians need to know about a child's linguistic and cultural background in order to make appropriate assessment-related decisions, including the need for intervention and instructional goals. Peña-Brooks and Hegde (2000) suggest that clinicians need to know:

1. The language and phonologic characteristics, properties, and rules of the linguistically diverse child's primary language
2. How the primary language affects the learning of the second language
3. How to determine whether there are language or phonologic disorders in the child's first language, second language, or both

In the event that a speaker or the speaker's family wishes to modify their dialect or accent, the clinician may wish not only to use traditional sampling methods to describe the child's phonology but also to employ measures specifically designed to assess the dialect and nonnative speaker's use of English phonology. Instructional decisions are then based on samples obtained and the variations that exist between Standard English and the person's dialect or accent.

Social-Vocational Expectations

Another factor to consider in the analysis and interpretation of a phonological sample is the attitude of the client or the client's parents toward the individual's phonological status. In cases where a treatment recommendation is questionable, the attitude of a client or family may be a factor in decisions for or against intervention. This is particularly the case in older children and beyond. Extreme concern over an articulatory difference by the client or the client's parents may convince the clinician to enroll an individual for instruction. For example, the child who has a frontal lisp and also has a name that begins with /s/ may feel very strongly that the error is a source of embarrassment. Crowe-Hall (1991) and Kleffner (1952) found that fourth- and sixth-grade children reacted unfavorably to children who had even mild articulation disorders. There are many reports in the literature wherein elementary children have recounted negative experiences in speaking or reading situations when they produced only a few speech sounds in error. Even "minor distortions" can influence how one is perceived. Silverman (1976) reported that when a female speaker simulated a lateral lisp, listeners judged her more negatively on a personality characteristics inventory than when she spoke without a lisp.

The standard for acceptance of communication depends, to a large extent, on the speaking situation. People in public speaking situations may find that even minor distortions detract from their message. Some vocations—for example, radio and television broadcasters—may call for very precise articulation and pronunciations, and thus, some individuals may feel the need for intervention for what may be relatively minor phonetic distortions. We suggest that if an individual, regardless of age, feels handicapped by speech errors, treatment should usually be provided.

Computer-Assisted Phonological Analysis

Any discussion of phonological analysis and interpretation would be incomplete without calling attention to the fact that there are computer-based programs designed to assist with the analysis of phonological samples in clients who exhibit multiple errors. Masterson, Long, and Buder (1998) indicated that there are two primary reasons for using a computer-based analysis of a phonological sample: (1) it saves time and (2) it provides greater detail of analysis than one typically produces with traditional paper and pencil (manual) analysis procedures. Computer phonological analysis (CPA) software involves inputting phonetic transcriptions from a computer keyboard and/or selecting from predetermined stimuli, displaying the data on the screen, and ultimately printing results of an analysis. Analyses often include both relational and independent analyses of consonants and vowels, word position analysis, syllable shapes used, patterns among errors, and calculation of percentage of consonants correct. Each of the current programs has its own strengths and limitations, and undoubtedly future procedures will add new and helpful procedures for clinicians.

The Computerized Articulation and Phonology Evaluation System (CAPES) (Masterson and Bernhardt, 2001) is a good example of a computer system that was developed to elicit and analyze phonological productions. It elicits 47 single-word responses through digitized photographs presented on the computer. The clinician can tape record responses or record responses on-line. Following the initial 47 word productions, additional items of increasing word complexity are included based on the nature of the client's responses in the first items. These additional items are referred to as the Individual Phonological Evaluation (IPE). The end result of this assessment program is that the clinician has data that reflect the client's omission, substitution, and distortion errors for each consonant and consonant sequence in the intial, medial, and final positions of words, as well as vowel productions. Analyses that describe the client's productions in terms of word length, syllable stress, word shape, place-manner-voice features, and phonological processes/patterns can also be generated. On the basis of these data, the program suggests treatment goals, though of course the clinician has a detailed enough speech sample to develop his or her own goals as well as intervention program.

In a study of time efficiency of procedures for phonological and grammatical analysis, comparing manual and computerized methods, Long (2001) reported that without exception, for both phonology and language, computerized analyses were completed faster and with equal or better accuracy than were manual analyses. Phonological analyses included the evaluation of variability, homonymy, word shapes, phonetic inventory, accuracy of production, and correspondence between target and production forms. Long further indicated that time needed for analyses, both computer and manual, was affected by the type of analysis, the type of sample, and the efficiency of individual participants.

A listing of some of the current CPA software programs is as follows:

Hodson Computer Analysis of Phonological Patterns (HCAPP). Hodson, B. (2003). Wichita, KS: Phonocomp Software.

Computerized Profiling (Version CP941.exe). Long, S. H., Fey, M. E., and Channell, R. W. (2002). Cleveland, OH: Case Western Reserve University.

Interactive System for Phonological Analysis (ISPA). Masterson, J., and Pagan, F. (1993). San Antonio, TX: The Psychological Corporation.

Programs to Examine Phonetic and Phonological Evaluation Records (PEPPER). Shriberg, L. (1986). Hillsdale, NJ: Erlbaum.

Computerized Articulation and Phonology Evaluation System (CAPES). Masterson, J., and Bernhardt, B. (2001). San Antonio, TX: The Psychological Corporation.

▒ CASE STUDY

Assessment: Phonological Samples Obtained

Client

Kirk

Age

3.0 years

Reason for Referral

Parental referral due to Kirk's poor intelligibility when speaking

Case History/Speech and Hearing Mechanisms Status

The case history submitted by the parents and supplemented with the examination interview revealed normal motor and language development; however, speech sound development was delayed. Hearing screening indicated that hearing was within normal limits. A speech mechanism examination indicated normal structure and function.

Language.   Vocabulary, syntax, and pragmatics appeared normal based on case history, language sample obtained, and social interaction between Kirk and the examiner. Language skills, as measured by the *Peabody Picture Vocabulary Test* and the *Preschool Language Scale*, indicated language within normal limits. Poor intelligibility made it difficult to assess expressive morphosyntactic structures; however, a spontaneous speech sample obtained through storytelling evidenced four 6-word utterances, a seemingly rich vocabulary, and appropriate concepts for a 3-year-old child. Based on these data, Kirk's language skills were determined to be within normal limits.

Fluency and Voice.   Fluency was regarded as normal. However, a hoarse voice was noted. It was determined that vocal quality should be monitored over time by the parents and clinician to determine whether a problem was developing.

Phonological Samples Gathered

- *Conversation/Connected speech sample* of 180 words was obtained, with Kirk telling the story of "The Three Little Pigs." This story was used becaue Kirk was familiar with the story and words in the story were known to the examiner, thus facilitating phonological analysis.
- *Single-word productions* were obtained through the *Bankson-Bernthal Test of Phonology (BBTOP)*. All consonants and vowels produced by Kirk in the stimulus words were transcribed.
- *Stimulability testing* was done in isolation, syllables, and words for all target sounds produced in error.

Phonological Results and Analysis.   The transcription of the connected speech sample and the single words from BBTOP were analyzed with the Proph phonological analysis component of the Computerized Profiling (Long, Fey, and Channell, 2002) program. Individual sound transcriptions were entered into the program and served as the basis for the analysis.

Phonological Analysis Outcomes.   The percentage of consonants correct (PCC) was determined based on the connected speech sample. The PCC value was 34 percent, which translates to a rating of "severe" (i.e., level of disability) for connected speech.

Segmental Analysis.   Segmental analysis revealed numerous sound substitutions, particularly the use of /d/ in place of fricatives, affricates, and some clusters. In addition, there were inconsistent initial and final consonant deletions, including deletion of the initial /h/, /r/, and /l/. Other substitutions included /f/ for /s/ and some prevocalic voicing. These errors were evidenced in both single-word productions and in running speech, though greater accuracy was reflected in single-word productions. Table 5.6 reflects consonant

■ TABLE 5.6 Consonant Singleton Productions in Single-Word Productions Including Percent Accuracy of Production

Target	Error Productions			
	Error	Initial	Error	Final
p		100%		100%
b		100%		100%
m		100%		100%
w	ø	0%		
f	/d/	0%	/s/	0%
v	/d/	0%		100%
θ	/d/	0%	/t/	0%
ð	/d/	0%		
t		100%		100%
d		100%		100%
s	/d/	0%	/f/	50%
z	/d/	0%	/v/	0%
n		100%		100%
l	ø	0%	/o/	0%
ʃ	/d/	0%	/f/	0%
tʃ	/d/	0%		100%
ʤ	/d/	0%		
j	ø	0%		
r	ø	0%		
k		100%		100%
g		100%		100%
h	ø	0%		

singleton transcriptions from single-word productions. Figures in the table indicate percent accuracy of production.

Stimulability Analysis.   Kirk was instructed to "look at me, listen to what I say, and then you say it," followed by a model of the correct sound. Imitative testing (stimulability) was conducted for all sounds produced in error. Responses were solicited for sounds in isolation, syllables, and the initial position of words.

Kirk was stimulable for most error sounds in isolation, syllables, and initial word position. He did not imitate clusters that were in error. The following sounds were not stimulable: /ʃ/, /tʃ/, /z/, /ʤ/, /r/, and /ɝ/. The /s/ was stimulable only in isolation even though it was observed in the word-final position of some words during testing.

Pattern Analysis.   A phonological process analysis was completed through the Proph program to determine error patterns that were evidenced in the single-word as well as connected speech sample of Kirk. This analysis revealed that the most prevalent process was stopping, with all fricatives and affricates impacted by this pattern (occurred in 85 percent of possible occasions in connected speech and with 44 percent occurrence in stimulus words from the BBTOP, particularly initial position). The most prevalent example of stopping was the use of /d/, which was substituted for initial /f/, /v/, /θ/, /ð/, /s/, /z/, /ʃ/, /tʃ/, /dʒ/, and the clusters /sl/, /sn/, and /fl/. Kirk used frication (e.g., /s/, /f/, although inappropriately) when producing some single words. A diagram of his sound collapses for /d/ is as follows:

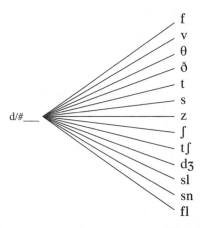

Clusters were simplified approximately 75 percent of the time in both isolated words and connected speech samples. Less frequently occurring patterns included *context sensitive voicing* (prevocalic voicing), and *initial consonant deletions*. Prevocalic voicing occurred in less than 25 percent of possible instances and initial consonants deletions less than 12 percent. Process analysis scoring on the BBTOP revealed similar error patterns.

Vowel Analysis.   The Proph program assesses vowel accuracy, and as might be expected for his age, Kirk's vowel productions were almost entirely accurate in both running speech and single-word productions. Inconsistent misarticulations were observed on the vowels /ɛ/ and /ʊ/ in running speech.

Summary

These data reflect a 3-year-old boy with a speech sound disorder that, according to his PCC, BBTOP norms, and examiner subjective evaluation, is severe in nature. Although intelligibility was not formally measured, understanding his verbal productions was difficult even for family members. Most of Kirk's errors were sound substitutions, with some deletions in both initial and final word positions. Substitution errors were predominately the /d/ being substituted for fricatives and affricates. The presence of initial consonant deletions is developmentally an unusual process, but it is present only for the aspirate /h/ and liquids. Final consonant deletion is a process usually eliminated by age 3 and was observed only occasionally in Kirk's speech. Inconsistencies in all types of error productions were noted.

Speech sound errors for which Kirk was not stimulable included the fricative /ʃ/, the affricates /tʃ/, and /dʒ/, the prevocalic /r/, and the vowelized /ɝ/. These error consonants will likely need to be stabilized in isolation and/or syllables, and will require motor practice in single words before they are incorporated into word-pairs that reflect relevant sound contrasts. For /h/ and /k/, which were easily stimulated at the word level, it is likely that Kirk needs instruction in how these sounds are used contrastively in the language, or it may be necessary only to monitor these sounds to make sure they are acquired.

Assessment: Interpretation

Case Selection

Phonological intervention is warranted for Kirk. Factors that influenced this recommendation are as follows:

1. Normative data indicate that most normal developing 3-year-old children are approximately 75 percent intelligible. Although Kirk has just turned 3, we would nonetheless expect him to be more intelligible than he is. Intelligibility was not formally determined in our assessment battery, but observational data, as well as reports from his family, indicate that much of Kirk's speech is unintelligible. This factor weighed heavily in our decision regarding Kirk's need for intervention.

2. With a PCC value in running speech of less than 40 percent, Kirk's phonological impairment is regarded as severe in nature. This rating relates to level of handicap reflected in his speech.

3. Phonological analysis evidences numerous substitution errors, some deletions, and several inappropriate phonological patterns. Positive indicators regarding Kirk's phonological status include the fact that he uses almost all vowels and some consonants correctly in his speech and is stimulable (with effort) for many of his error segments. His good vocabulary and the length of his utterances suggest that his linguistic deficits are confined to articulation and phonology, another positive indicator.

4. Intervention appears favorable because Kirk is stimulable for many of his error sounds, is highly verbal, and is not reluctant to speak for fear of negative consequences.

Target Sound Selection

Because Kirk has numerous misarticulations, and because these errors fall into patterns, target selection should begin with a review of these patterns. The error pattern that occurred most frequently was that of stopping, with several initial sounds, predominately fricatives and glides, collapsed into /d/. He also evidenced voicing of voiceless consonants in the initial position, gliding of liquids, and cluster reductions.

Although stopping is a process that persists in children sometimes past the age of 3, it is unusual for a child of this age not to be using more fricatives in speech. Most children are expected to use /f/ correctly by this age, and many are using the /s/ as well. Because the frication feature, including its correct usage, is diminished in Kirk's speech, reduction of stopping is the phonologic target of choice for initial therapy. The other two patterns evidenced in Kirk's speech (i.e., voicing, gliding) will be focused on later, largely because voicing does not have a great impact on intelligibility, and gliding occurred relatively infrequently and does not affect Kirk's intelligibility as much as stopping.

Intervention suggestions for Kirk are discussed in detail in Chapter 7. In terms of target selection, we would suggest focusing on several error sounds in each lesson. Kirk's good attention span and good language skills will hopefully facilitate his ease handling multiple treatment goals. We would suggest address the sound collapses reflected in the /d/

replacement for numerous fricatives, other stops, and clusters. Perhaps the multiple oppositions approach developed by Williams (1993, 2006) could be used as a treatment strategy.

Because Kirk is very young, one might choose to focus on only one or two sounds in the early sessions to avoid confusion among targets. As progress is made, additional targets can be identified. If one chooses to focus on one or two target sounds at a time, our suggestion for a priority focus is /f/. This is a highly visible sound and one that develops early, would address Kirk's stopping pattern, and frequently develops in final position prior to initial position. Kirk already uses the sound as a substitution for other fricatives in the final position; for example, he says /tif/ for /ti/ but /lis/ for /lif/. A second treatment target, likely one to work on simultaneously, is the correct use of /s/. The /s/ is in Kirk's repertoire; however, it is used inappropriately. As stated already, length of attention span, including ability to focus on multiple sounds and/or sound contrasts simultaneously will influence the choice of treatment approach. This issue is addressed further in Chapter 7.

Summary

Kirk is a child who needs phonological intervention. Intelligibility, severity, and developmental level of his phonology support this decision. On the basis of his phonological samples, teaching frication to reduce stopping, producing sounds correctly in word-initial position, and further increasing Kirk's phonological repertoire are priority goals for initiating therapy.

■ QUESTIONS FOR CHAPTER 5

1. What are the purposes of phonological assessment?
2. Identify criteria for selecting a phonological assessment instrument.
3. Discuss the strengths and limitations of single-word testing and conversational sampling.
4. What is the nature and purpose of stimulability testing?
5. When might a clinician employ phonological perception testing as part of testing?
6. Discuss how the following factors may be utilized in case selection:
   a. Intelligibility
   b. Severity
   c. Stimulability
   d. Error patterns
   e. Developmental appropriateness
7. Discuss how the following factors might influence target behavior selection:
   a. Stimulability
   b. Frequency of occurrence
   c. Developmental appropriateness
   d. Contextual analysis
   e. Phonological process analysis
8. Differentiate between intelligibility and severity.
9. How do dialectal considerations influence intervention decisions?

Remediation Procedures

NICHOLAS W. BANKSON

James Madison University

JOHN E. BERNTHAL

University of Nebraska–Lincoln

PETER FLIPSEN JR.

Idaho State University

BASIC CONSIDERATIONS

The typical long-range objective of remediation for phonological disorders with a client not exhibiting significant cognitive/physical limitations is spontaneous use of speech sounds that reflect the adult standard of his or her linguistic community. Once a speech-language clinician has determined that an individual's phonology is disordered or otherwise warrants intervention, assessment data are used in the planning of management strategies to accomplish this instructional objective. As described in Chapter 5, phonological analyses are designed to assist the clinician in identifying appropriate target behaviors for instruction. After specific goals and objectives for intervention have been determined, the clinician is then faced with the task of determining the type of treatment approach that is best suited for an individual client. Before discussing specifics of particular treatment approaches in the next chapter, we focus in this chapter on some basic underlying concepts that must be taken into consideration when developing a treatment plan. Although the focus of the chapter is on disordered phonology, concepts and principles described may also be useful in terms of instruction related to other speech/language disorders as well as accent/dialect modification (speech sound differences).

Framework for Conducting Therapy

Before clinical speech instruction is initiated, regardless of the disorder being treated, certain administrative or organizational factors should be considered as part of developing the framework from which specific treatment methodologies will emerge. In this section, we review several overarching variables to be considered as a first step in treatment planning.

Temporal Sequencing of Instructional Components

Once intervention objectives have been determined, the clinician formulates a treatment plan that spells out activities that will be used in accord with the moment-to-moment temporal sequence of instructional components. The typical sequence of clinical speech instruction components is:

Antecedent events (AE)	Delineation of stimulus events designed to elicit particular responses (e.g., auditory/visual modeling or pictures presented by the clinician, followed by a request for the client to imitate the model or name a picture)
Responses (R)	Production of a target behavior (often a particular sound in isolation or in a given linguistic and/or social context)
Consequent events (CE)	Reinforcement or feedback that follows the response (the clinician says "good" if a response is accurate, or may say "try again" if inaccurate: tokens to reinforce correct responses)

Antecedent events are the stimulus events presented during or just prior to a response. Such events typically consist of a verbal model, a picture, printed material, or verbal instructions designed to elicit particular verbal responses. For example, if a client is working on the /s/ phoneme at the word level, the clinician may show the child a picture of soap, and ask the child, "What do we wash with?" The child may be further asked to "say the word three times," or to "put it in a sentence." The type of antecedent events will vary depending on whether the clinician is seeking to establish a motor behavior or is trying to help the client use a motor behavior in accord with the phonological rules of the language.

Responses are the behaviors the clinician has targeted for the client. These may range from approximations of the desired behavior (e.g., movement of the tongue backward for production of /k/), to production of the correct behavior (e.g., /k/ in connected speech). The clinician is concerned with the functional relationship between an antecedent event and a response or, in other words, the likelihood that a given stimulus will elicit the desired response. Movement to the next level of instruction is often contingent on a certain number of correct responses. It is important in phonologic training that clients have the opportunity to produce many utterances in the course of a therapy session. A high rate of utterances provides the opportunity for both the clinician's external monitoring and the client's automatization of the response. It is usual that responses are stabilized on one level of complexity before proceeding the next level (e.g., sounds are often easier to produce in syllables than in words; word production is easier than it is in phrases).

The third aspect of the temporal sequence for instruction is *consequent events* (CE). Consequent events are events that occur following a particular response, and usually are labeled reinforcement or punishment. Whether or not a response is learned (and how quickly it is learned) is closely related to what happens following the occurrence of a behavior or response. The most frequently used consequent event in clinical speech instruction is positive *reinforcement*. Tangible consequents such as tokens, points, chips, and informal reinforcers such as a smile or verbal feedback are used. Consequent events intended to reinforce should immediately follow the correct or desired behavior and should only be used when the desired or correct response is produced. Reinforcement is defined by an increase in a behavior following the presentation of consequent events. Providing a reinforcement after an incorrect behavior sends the "wrong message" to the speaker, reinforces an incorrect response, and does not facilitate learning of correct responses. Formal use of "punishment" as a consequence seldom is used in phonological treatment.

Instructional steps are organized so that a sequential series of antecedent events, responses, and consequent events are followed as one moves through therapy. See Table 6.1 for an example.

Goal Attack Strategies

An early treatment decision relates to the number of treatment goals targeted in a given session. Fey (1986) described three "goal attack strategies" applicable to children with phonological disorders. The first strategy is called a *vertically structured treatment program*, in which one or two goals or targets are trained to some performance criterion before proceeding to another target. Treatment sessions of this type involve a high response rate for a single target, involving lots of repetition of that target. The traditional approach to treatment of phonological disorders, to be described in detail later in this book, is an example of a vertically structured program. In this approach, one or two phonemes are targeted for treatment and are worked on until they are produced in conversation before training is initiated on other target sounds. For a client who exhibits five different phonologic processes, the clinician may target one process and focus treatment on one or two sounds related to that process/pattern until some criterion level is reached before proceeding to the next target process. Elbert and Gierut (1986) termed this vertical type of strategy *training deep*. The assumptions behind the vertical strategy are that (1) mass practice on a restricted number of target sounds with a limited number of training items will facilitate generalization to other nontrained items and (2) some clients are best served by focusing on one goal or target rather than many.

A second instructional strategy is a *horizontally structured treatment program* (Fey, 1986; Williams, 2000b), or what Elbert and Gierut (1986) have called *training broad*. Using this strategy, the clinician addresses multiple goals in each session. Thus, more than

■ **TABLE 6.1** Sequential Series of Antecedent Events, Responses, and Consequent Events

Step	Anecedent Event	Response	Consequent Event
1	Clinician: Put your tongue behind your teeth, have the tip of your tongue lightly touch the roof of your mouth as if you were saying /t/, and blow air. Say /s/.	/t/	Clinician: No, I heard /t/.
2	Clinician: Keep your tongue tip a little bit down from the roof of your mouth and blow air. Say /s/.	/s/	Clinician: Good! Perfect!
3	Now say /s/ 3 times.	/s/, /s/, /s/	Clinician: Great!
4	Now say /sa/.	/sa/	Clinician: Super!

one goal may be incorporated into each session, and goals may change across sessions. By working on several sounds in the same session, the client will presumably learn commonalities or relationships among sound productions and treatment will be more efficient. In other words, the client receives less training about more aspects of the sound system than in the vertical approach. The concept behind training broad is that limited practice, with a range of exemplars and sound contrasts, is an efficient way to modify a child's phonological system. The goal is to expose the child to a wide range of target sound productions so that this broad-based training will facilitate simultaneous acquisition of several treatment targets.

A third strategy (Fey, 1986), which combines aspects of the vertical and horizontal approaches, is a *cyclically structured treatment program* (Hodson and Paden, 1991; Hodson, 2007a). In this approach, a single phonemic target (related to a particular phonological pattern) is addressed for a single session or week. The following session or week another goal is addressed. The movement from goal to goal is essentially a horizontal approach to treatment, whereas the focus on a single sound for a session or week may be viewed as vertical. Historically, the most common strategy employed in remediation was the vertical approach, but many clinicians now favor the horizontal or cyclical approach, especially once clients have a sound in their repertoire (i.e., they can produce a sound at the motor level with some consistency). Our preference with children who produce multiple errors is the cyclical approach, although all three approaches have been shown to improve phonological productions. For clients who evidence a small number of errors, such as misarticulate /r/, /s/, /l/, or /θ/ (residual errors), a vertical approach is preferable.

Scheduling of Instruction

Another basic consideration in planning for phonological intervention relates to the scheduling of treatment sessions. Relatively little is known about the influence that scheduling of instruction has on remediation efficacy, and sufficient research has not been reported to determine which scheduling arrangements are most desirable. In addition, it is often not practical to schedule treatment sessions on an "ideal" basis. Scheduling of treatment may be related to age of the client, attention span of the client, severity of the disorder, and practical realities such as availability of instructional services, size of a clinician's caseload, and treatment models employed by a school system (e.g., pull-out versus classroom-based instruction). Investigators who have studied scheduling have generally focused on the efficacy of intermittent scheduling versus block scheduling of treatment sessions. *Intermittent scheduling* usually refers to two or three sessions each week over an extended period of time (such as eight months), whereas *block scheduling* refers to daily sessions for a shorter temporal span (such as an eight-week block). Several investigators have compared dismissal rates associated with intermittent and block scheduling, primarily for public school students with articulation disorders (Van Hattum, 1969). Based on these studies, Van Hattum reported that block scheduling was a more efficient way to achieve articulatory/phonological progress than was intermittent scheduling. Unfortunately, however, variables such as articulation disorder severity, stimulability, and treatment methodology employed were not well enough controlled to make definitive clinical recommendations from these investigations.

Bowen and Cupples (1999) described a scheduling protocol where children were seen once weekly for approximately 10-week blocks, followed by approximately 10 weeks without treatment. They reported positive results with this treatment schedule. It should be pointed out, however, that their treatment included multifaceted components including parent education. The specific influence of the break in treatment schedule on treatment outcome is unknown; however, this study reflects a contemporary approach that utilizes a form of block scheduling.

Although control experiments on scheduling are lacking, suggestions for scheduling of phonological intervention seem appropriate:

1. Scheduling of intervention four to five times per week for 8 to 10 weeks may result in slightly higher dismissal rates than intermittent scheduling for a longer period of time, the greater gains being made early in the treatment process.
2. Intensive scheduling on only a short-term basis does not appear to be as appropriate with clients who have severe articulation/phonological disorders and need ongoing services.
3. Scheduling a child for three 20-minute sessions appears to yield better results than one 60-minute session.

Pull-Out versus Classroom-Based Instruction

Basic considerations related to phonological intervention relate to the place and format whereby services will be delivered. One issue is the matter of whether treatment will be provided through a *pull-out model* (the client is instructed in a treatment room) or *inclusion model* (the client is instructed in a classroom setting), or a combination of the two. Historically, the pull-out model was the choice for articulation/phonological treatment. In recent years, an increased emphasis has been placed on integrating speech and language services within the classroom. The opportunity to incorporate a child's phonological instruction with the academic curriculum and communication events associated with a child's daily school routine is the optimal way to enhance the efficiency and effectiveness of therapy. Furthermore, classroom inclusion capitalizes on the opportunity for collaboration among regular educators, special education educators, speech-language pathologists, and other professionals within a child's educational environment.

Masterson (1993) suggested that classroom-based approaches for school-age children allow the clinician to draw on textbooks, homework, and classroom discourse to establish instructional goals, target words, and instructional procedures. For preschoolers, classroom activities such as crafts, snacks, and toileting are similarly helpful activities for language and phonological instruction. In addition, for preschool and early primary-grade children, classroom-based phonological awareness activities may provide the clinicians with the opportunity to extend services to all children in a classroom as they collaborate with teachers. Masterson (1993) further indicated that classroom-based approaches may be most useful for treating conceptual- or linguistic-based errors, as opposed to errors that require motor-based habilitation. Instruction in the context of the classroom setting is typically less direct than that involved in a pull-out model and requires collaborative efforts between the clinician and the classroom teacher. The vocabulary used in the curriculum can be used by the speech clinician as the basis for target practice words. Classroom instruction is particularly appropriate when a client is in the generalization, or "carryover," phase of instruction, in which academic material and other classroom activities allow for an emphasis on communication skills and intent. It is likely that both of these models (i.e., pull-out; classroom inclusion) may be appropriate for a given client during the course of intervention, depending on where they are on the treatment continuum.

Clinicians must determine whether clients are treated individually or in a small group. Although group instruction is sometimes conducted because of large caseloads, reports have indicated that group instruction may well be as effective as individual instruction in remediating articulation disorders (Sommers et al., 1964; Sommers et al., 1966).

Sommers and colleagues (1964) reported that 50-minute group instruction based on the pull-out model resulted in as much articulatory change as 30-minute individual instruction when both group and individual sessions were conducted four times per week for 4 weeks. In a subsequent study (Sommers et al., 1966), similar results were obtained from group sessions held 45 minutes each week and individual instruction sessions held 30 minutes each week over a period of 8.5 months. These investigators concluded that group and individual sessions were equally effective and that the results were not influenced by the grade level (fourth to sixth grade versus second grade) or the severity of the phonologic disorder. When children with speech sound disorders are grouped, such groups usually consist of three or four clients of about the same age who work on similar target behaviors. Unfortunately, such group sessions frequently have a tendency to become regimented so that all individuals work on the same activity, the same target behavior, and the same level of behavior; they are sometimes even given the same homework assignments.

It should be pointed out that *group instruction* should be different from *individual instruction in a group*. When assigned a group of clients, the clinician may simply work with each client individually while remaining group members observe. Group instruction can and should be structured so that individuals in the group can benefit from interaction with other members and from activities that involve the entire group. For example, individuals can monitor and reinforce each other's productions and can serve both as correct models for each other and as listeners to see whether the communication intent of the message is met.

It is our suggestion that a combination of group and individual sessions may be advantageous for most individuals with phonologic problems. Furthermore, instructional groups should usually be limited to three or four individuals whose ages do not exceed a three-year range. Some would suggest that when children are learning the motor skills involved in production of a given sound, individual instruction is perhaps the best environment, if only for relatively short sessions or a part of a session. Once a sound is in the child's production repertoire, group and classroom activities can easily be incorporated into the instructional plans.

Intervention Style

A final consideration before we begin our discussion of specific therapy approaches is intervention style. In addition to selecting target behaviors to be used in treatment, the clinician must also consider the management mode or style most appropriate for a given client. A key issue here is the amount of structure that may be prescribed for or tolerated by a given client.

Shriberg and Kwiatkowski (1982b) described the structure of treatment as a continuum ranging from drill (highly structured therapy) to play (little structure to therapy), with combinations of these two end-points as in-between stages on the continuum. These authors described the following four modes of management:

1. *Drill.* This type of therapy relies heavily on clinician presentation or some form of antecedent instructional events, followed by client responses. The client has little control over the rate and presentation of training stimuli.
2. *Drill play.* This type of therapy is distinguished from drill by the inclusion of an antecedent motivational event (e.g., activity involving a spinner; card games).
3. *Structured play.* This type of instruction is structurally similar to drill play. However, training stimuli are presented as play activities. In this mode, the clinician moves from formal instruction to playlike activities, especially when the child becomes unresponsive to more formal instruction.
4. *Play.* The child perceives what he or she is doing as play. However, the clinician arranges activities so that target responses will occur as a natural component of the activity. Clinicians may also use modeling, self-talk, and other techniques to elicit responses from a child.

Shriberg and Kwiatkowski (1982b) conducted several studies with young children with phonological disorders to compare the relative effects of these four treatment modes. They reported that drill and drill play modes were more effective and efficient than structured play and play modes. In addition, drill play was as effective and efficient as drill.

Clinicians' evaluation of the four modes indicated that they felt drill play was most effective and efficient for their clients, and they personally preferred it. They also urged that three factors be considered when making a choice of management mode: (1) a general knowledge of the child's personality, (2) the intended target response, and (3) the stage of therapy (Shriberg and Kwiatkowski, 1982b).

It should be kept in mind that details regarding the organization of intervention sessions are impacted by the presence of additional communication impairments, particularly language disorders. Because language and phonological disorders often both occur in young children, decisions discussed above related to planning therapy are influenced by the severity of disorders in each of these areas, and their priority for treatment. Instruction for children with phonological and other language impairments is discussed in Chapter 7.

Summary

Before deciding on a specific treatment methodology, the clinician must make several administrative decisions that interact significantly with treatment approaches and, potentially, clients' progress. These include the following:

1. What is the severity of the problem, and how many targets will you select to be incorporated into treatment planning?
2. Which targets need to be focused on at a motor level and which may be approached from a rule or phonological basis?

3. How many targets will I work on in a given session, and how long will I stay with a target before I move on to another?
4. How frequently will therapy sessions be held, and how long will each session last?
5. Will instruction be individual or in a small group? If it is conducted in a school environment, will it be pull-out, classroom based, or a combination of the two? Is drill and practice the best approach, or play, or a combination of the two?
6. For children with both phonological and language impairments, how should intervention be structured (e.g., an integrated approach; target each area separately)?

MAKING PROGRESS IN THERAPY: MEASURING CLINICAL CHANGE

As discussed in Chapter 5, there are a variety of ways of measuring speech sound skills that allow clinicians to determine whether intervention is necessary. Measurement doesn't end at that point, however. Speech-language pathologists also need to be able to measure progress (or lack of progress) so they can decide when therapy is no longer necessary or if what they are doing in therapy needs to change.

Tools for Measuring Change

Norm-referenced tests such as the *Goldman-Fristoe Test of Articulation*, the *Photo Articulation Test*, and the *Bernthal-Bankson Test of Phonology* are very widely used to determine eligibility for therapy. And they work very well for that purpose. It is very tempting to simply readminister these tests on a regular basis and look for changes in scores. This is not, however, a wise practice, for a couple of reasons. First, there is a statistical problem with such a practice known as *regression to the mean*, which will be discussed later. Second, and from a more practical standpoint, such tests typically give only a limited sample of the child's speech. They often include only a single word that tests performance on each sound in each word position (e.g., word-initial /s/). It is possible that when such a test is readministered, the child might remember having problems with that particular word during testing and may have overpracticed it. The child may then appear to have mastered the sound, but will not necessarily be able to produce that same sound in other words. On the other hand, the child may have become hypersensitive to that particular word because of his or her failure and may continue having difficulty with it even when he or she is perfectly capable of producing that sound in many other words.

To get around this limitation of norm-referenced tests, clinicians can create what is known as a *probe* (sometimes called a *generalization probe*) for each target sound being worked on in therapy (see Elbert, Shelton, and Arndt, 1967). Such probes include several words (typically 8 to 15) that contain the target sound. The S-CAT probes (Secord and Shine, 1997a) discussed in Chapter 5 could easily be used or adapted for this purpose. The selected probe words are ones not used in therapy, but rather are brought out on a regular basis to see how the child is doing. Using words that are not practiced in therapy helps determine whether the child is really learning the sound and incorporating that sound into his or her sound system. Having that sound in the system allows the child to produce any word containing that sound, even if that word has seldom been encountered before. Without such probes, clinicians can never be certain that the child isn't simply memorizing the set of speech movements for the particular words being practiced in therapy. Probes generally are not administered during each treatment session because clinicians don't want the child to become overly familiar with the probe items. A more typical practice is to administer the probes every 4 or 5 sessions, once a month, or at the point where the child reaches some predetermined production criterion.

Determining What Caused the Change

Change either happens or it doesn't. Clinicians administer probes and determine whether the child is adding the sounds being worked on to his or her sound system. If there is no change, the speech-language pathologist has to decide whether to continue with the intervention plan or change it. On the other hand, if the SLP sees change, he or she is pleased because the goal is for the clients to develop normal speech sound skills and to be able to produce fully intelligible speech. But in an age of accountability and *evidence-based practice*, seeing change happen is not enough. Clinicians are increasingly being asked to demonstrate that the change occurred as a result of what they did and not as a result of something else.

The obvious question at this point is: What else might have caused the change? If the clinician provided intervention and the child improved, didn't the clinician cause it? Perhaps, but there is a very real possibility that the change had nothing whatsoever to do with what the professional did. There are many other influences that could have resulted in the change. Before we discuss what those influences might be, however, we should answer the more obvious question: So what? If the child improves, doesn't everyone win? Certainly, the clients and their families and friends will be happy with the result. But if something else besides the SLP's intervention caused the change, then the therapy may not have been necessary, and the SLP may have just wasted a lot of his or her valuable time—time that could have been devoted to other clients on his or her ever-expanding caseload. And unless the clinician is independently wealthy and providing services for free, that's also time that someone, somewhere, had to pay for, whether it's the taxpayers who fund the school district or clinic, an insurance company, or the client's family. The bottom line is that SLPs are more and more being asked to demonstrate that they were the ones who caused the change.

Other Sources of Clinical Change

If you enter a room and flip on a light switch and a light goes on, you generally assume that it was your action of flipping the switch that caused the light to go on. But what if there was a motion sensor in the room that turns on the light? Your act of flipping the switch on may just have been coincidental. It was the movement of you coming into the room that actually turned on the light. Or what if the light was really turned on by sound activation? Your footsteps or the noise of turning the door handle as you entered the room was what turned on the light. Again, your flipping the switch on would have been just coincidental. Or what if the light were controlled by a wireless device held by a friend who was with you, and your friend actually turned on the light using that device just as you flipped the switch? Once again, your act of flipping on the switch may have been just a coincidence. The light just happened to come on right after you flipped the switch. Finally, what if there was a timer on the light and you just happened to flip on the switch exactly as the timer was turning the lights on? Again, it may just have been a coincidence.

Clearly, this is a pretty silly example. We all know that most of the time when we flip on a light switch and the light goes on, we caused the light to go on. But in clinical situations, things are not always so clear. There really are a number of different things (sometimes called *extraneous effects*) that might have caused the change instead of or in addition to the clinician's intervention. Gruber, Lowery, Seung, and Deal (2003) identified several such effects that all practicing clinicians need to be aware of. One of the first ones we think of when we work with children is normal development or maturation. With children, it is always possible that something about the child (e.g., his fine-motor skills, her auditory discrimination skills, his grasp of a particular phonemic contrast) may have improved on its own so that the child is now capable of producing the sound that the clinician and child happen to have been working on. It may have had nothing to do with the intervention. This is part of what Gruber and colleagues call the *natural history effect* or the normal course of a condition over time. For children, the natural history effect includes things like normal development and the typical pattern of change seen in genetic syndromes. For adults, the natural history effect includes things like normal recovery from neurological insult or the expected changes seen over time from a degenerative disease such as Parkinson's.

A second extraneous effect is the well-known *placebo effect* in which improvement results from the mere fact that any intervention is being applied. Gruber and associates (2003) document a wide range of studies (in speech-language pathology and other disciplines) demonstrating this effect. Any attention being paid to the speech of young children has the potential to lead to the child also focusing on his or her speech and making changes that have nothing to do with the specific intervention that is being applied. Such changes may be temporary or even permanent. A variation on the placebo effect is the *Hawthorne effect* in which the client improves because the client becomes convinced that the treatment he or she is receiving will work. A fourth extraneous effect discussed by Gruber and associates is the experimenter or *Pygmalion effect* in which the client interprets subtle or not so subtle signals from the clinician that the clinician believes change will occur. For all three of these latter effects (placebo, Hawthorne, Pygmalion), the client may put forth extra effort or extra focus on what the client and the SLP are working on. Or perhaps the client or his or her family reports improvement to the clinician when in fact there is none. Clinicians can't monitor clients' speech all the time, so they often rely on reports from the client or client's family to help determine therapy success.

Finally, there is the extraneous effect known as *regression to the mean*. This is a statistical (but very real) phenomenon in which anyone who achieves an extremely low or extremely high score on some measurement will produce a subsequent score on that same measurement that is closer to the average (or the mean). People vary in their behavior from moment to moment, and that is certainly true of children with speech sound disorders. When the SLP measures a child's performance on a norm-referenced test, the SLP obtains a sample of the child's behavior. If at one point the child produces a very low score, part of the reason for that low score may be because he or she was not necessarily performing at his or her best on that particular day. Indeed, the child may have been performing at his or her worst. Statistically speaking, when the clinician measures the performance at a later time, the probability is very high that the child will have a better day and his or her score will go up (i.e., be closer to the mean). The higher score may have nothing to do with a change in the child's skill resulting from therapy.

In addition to the extraneous effects discussed by Gruber and colleagues (2003), there are also potential influences from outside "therapy" sources. Some children, for example, may be attending private therapy in addition to receiving services from clinicians in the public schools. Alternatively, parents or teachers, who are often aware of the intervention goals, may be emphasizing correct articulation in their interactions with the child, such as during book-reading activities. Such additional input is certainly a potentially positive influence, but it only serves to complicate the question of what caused the change.

As can be seen from this discussion, clinicians simply cannot assume that any observed change is due to their therapy. It is the clinician's job to try to control for these effects so that the clinician can demonstrate that he or she is not just wasting everyone's valuable time.

Controlling for Extraneous Effects

There are a variety of things that might be done to control for these extraneous effects. For researchers who are studying the effects of various treatments, a matched control group is typically used. This is a group of very similar children who either receive no treatment (usually hard to justify) or who receive an alternative treatment. The two groups are compared on how well they do. As a clinician, however, you usually won't have access to groups of children with similar problems that you can compare. And ultimately, you will be interested only in whether a particular child is making progress anyway. The typical solution is to have the child act as his or her own control. That means you measure change on several targets at the same time, but you provide treatment only for some of those targets (perhaps only one depending on your choice of goal attack strategy). You then compare progress on treated targets against progress on untreated targets. Ideally, the untreated target(s) would share few if any features with the target. Once the child achieves mastery on the target(s) being treated, additional (formerly untreated) targets are then introduced into the treatment sessions. This approach is sometimes called a *multiple baseline* approach and is illustrated in Figure 6.1 with a hypothetical example of a child who needed to improve his production of both /s/ and /r/. On the horizontal axis of each half of the figure is the session number where the probes were presented and performance measured. On the vertical axis of the top half is the percentage correct for /s/ and on the vertical axis of the bottom half is the percentage correct for /r/. Sessions 1 through 3 are "baseline" sessions in which no treatment was provided and, as shown, no improvement was noted for either target. Such baseline measurements are important to establish that the behavior you are measuring is not beginning to change on its own. During sessions 4 through 7, treatment was provided for /s/ (Treatment I), but not for /r/. Notice an increase in the percentage correct for /s/ but no change in percentage correct for /r/. At that point, treatment changed to a focus on /r/, and an improvement is seen in the percentage correct for /r/ during sessions 8 through 11.

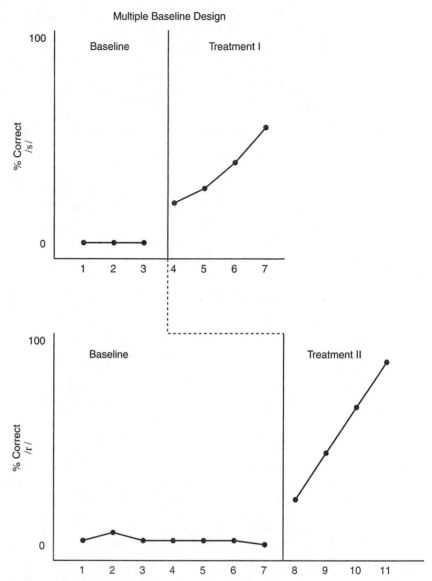

■ FIGURE 6.1 A multiple baseline design for investigating the effects of a phonological intervention procedure.

So, how does this approach account for extraneous effects? Well, we saw change when treatment was applied, but no change when treatment was not applied. And when the focus of treatment changed to a new target, we saw change on the new target. It appears that only the treatment was responsible for the change. If any extraneous effects were operating, we would expect improvement on at least some (if not all) of targets that were not receiving treatment.

Is Significant and Important Change Occurring?

It's one thing to demonstrate that change is occurring as a result of treatment; it's quite another to say that the degree or quality of the change is significant or important. Olswang and Bain (1994) suggest that the clinician can answer yes to this question only if generalization is occurring. The nature of generalization and how to measure it will be discussed in the next section.

MAKING PROGRESS IN THERAPY: GENERALIZATION

Once target behaviors are in a client's repertoire and can be produced on demand, the next task is to facilitate generalization to other linguistic contexts and nonclinical settings. Generalization is a process that is facilitated rather than taught, and it is relevant to correction of all phonologic errors whether they be viewed as motor and/or linguistic in nature. Generalization is a critical and all-important step in the learning process for all children who receive treatment for phonologic disorders. Our discussion of generalization includes an introduction to the concept, followed by a review of (1) across-position generalization, (2) across-context generalization, (3) across-linguistic unit generalization, (4) across-sound and feature generalization, and (5) across-situation generalization.

Generalization has been defined by Stokes and Baer (1977) as

> The occurrence of relevant behavior under different non-training conditions (i.e., across subjects, settings, people, behavior, and/or time) without the scheduling of the same events in those conditions as had been scheduled in the training conditions. Thus, generalization may be claimed when no extra training manipulations are needed for extra training changes (p. 350).

In other words, generalization (sometimes called *transfer*) is the principle that learning one behavior in a particular environment often carries over to other similar behaviors, environments, or untrained contexts. For example, if one learns to drive in a Ford Taurus, there is a high probability that one can also drive a Honda Accord. Generalization of training occurs from the driving apparatus in the Taurus to the driving apparatus in the Honda. In terms of articulation remediation, if a client learns to produce /f/ in the word *fish*, [f] production will probably generalize to other words that contain /f/, such as *fun*. If generalization did not occur, it would be necessary to teach a sound in every word and context—an impossible task. The clinician must rely on a client's ability to generalize in order to effect a change in the use of speech sounds. Generalization, however, does not occur automatically, nor do all persons have the same aptitude for it. People vary in their ability to achieve generalization, but certain activities can increase the likelihood of generalization.

One type of generalization is *stimulus generalization*, which occurs when a learned response to a particular stimulus is evoked by similar stimuli. The importance of reinforcement in such generalization cannot be overemphasized. Behaviors that have been reinforced in the presence of a particular stimulus may be said to have generalized when they occur in the presence of novel but similar stimuli, even though the response was not reinforced. Consider this example: A client who utilizes the process of "velar fronting"

(/t/ for /k/ substitution) has been taught to produce /k/ correctly at the word level in response to the auditory stimulus, "Say kangaroo." The client is later shown a picture of a kangaroo and asked to name it, but no model is provided. If the client says "kangaroo" with [k^h] produced correctly in response to the picture (i.e., the model is no longer necessary for a correct production), stimulus generalization has occurred.

Response generalization is another type of generalization that is especially relevant to speech sound remediation. This is the process in which responses that have been taught carry over to other behaviors that are not taught. An example of response generalization is as follows: A client with /s/ and /z/ errors is taught to say [s] in response to an auditory model of [s]. He or she is then presented with an auditory model [z] and asked to imitate it. If the client emits a correct [z], response generalization has occurred. Such generalization is well documented in the literature, including an early study by Elbert, Shelton, and Arndt (1967) in which children with /s/, /z/, and /r/ errors were taught to say [s] correctly. Generalization was evident by correction of the untrained /z/, which has many features in common with /s/. However, no generalization to the untrained [r] was noted. Obviously, sounds in the same sound class and having similar features with the target sound are those where response generalization is most likely to occur.

Several other types of generalization may also occur during speech sound remediation, including generalization from one position to another, from one context to another, to increasingly complex linguistic levels, to nontrained words, to other sounds and features, and to various speaking environments and situations. Clinicians often attempt to facilitate generalization by sequencing instructional steps from simple to more complex behaviors. By proceeding in small, progressive steps, the clinician seeks to gradually extend the behavior developed during the establishment period to other contexts and situations.

The amount of training required for the different types of generalization has not been established and seems to vary considerably across subjects. Elbert and McReynolds (1978) have reported data from five children indicating that from 5 to 26 sessions were required before across-word generalization occurred. They speculated that the error patterns exhibited by children affected both the time required and the extent of transfer that occurs.

For those clients who begin remediation with an established target behavior in their repertoire, generalization may be the primary task of instruction. Following is a discussion of the various types of generalization that are expected in the articulation remediation process.

Across-Word Position/Contextual Generalization

Generalization of correct sound productions across-word positions is well documented (Elbert and McReynolds, 1975, 1978; Powell and McReynolds, 1969). This term refers to generalization from a word position that is taught (initial, medial, or final) to a word position that is not taught. By teaching a sound in a particular position (e.g., initial position), generalization may occur to a second position (e.g., final position). Speech-language pathologists have traditionally taught target sounds first in the initial position of words, followed by either the final or medial position. One rationale for beginning with the initial position is that, for most children, many sounds are first acquired in the prevocalic position (the most notable exception is certain fricatives that appear first in word-final position).

In the process of investigating a particular approach to articulation remediation (paired-stimuli), Weston and Irwin (1971) examined position generalization. They observed in children with pre- and postvocalic substitutions that when a sound was taught in the pre-vocalic position, generalization usually occurred to the postvocalic position. Similarly, they observed that sounds taught in the postvocalic position usually generalized to the prevocalic position.

Ruscello (1975) studied the influence of training on generalization across-word positions. Two groups, each containing three participants, were presented training programs that differed with respect to the number of word positions practiced in each session. Ruscello reported significantly more generalization across-training sessions for those subjects who practiced a target sound in the initial, medial, and final word-positions than the group who practiced a target sound only in the word-initial position. Weaver-Spurlock and Brasseur (1988) also reported that simultaneous training of /s/ in the initial, medial, and final positions of familiar words was an effective training strategy for across-position generalization to nontrained words.

Olswang and Bain (1985) reported different amounts of position generalization for /s/ and /l/ in two participants. For both speakers, improvement in initial /l/ had little influence on final /l/. In other words, improvement on initial /l/ did not seem to facilitate improvement of final /l/. By contrast, when /s/ was trained in one word position in one subject, it seemed to facilitate production of the sound to other positions. They attributed the differences in position generalization between /l/ and /s/ to the greater allophonic variation between initial and final /l/ (i.e., initial and final /l/ are produced differently) compared to that of initial and final /s/. Wolfe, Blocker, and Prater (1988) reported that generalization of sounds in the medial word position may be related to whether the word reflects a sound in the traditional medial position (e.g., /k/ in *bacon*), or is related to inflection (e.g., /k/ in *picking*). In their study, greater generalization occurred with medial inflection, which they attributed to factors of coarticulation, perceptual salience, and representational integrity of the word.

It can be inferred from the available data that generalization from initial to final position is just as likely to occur as generalization from final to initial. A preferred word position that would maximally facilitate position generalization has not been established. Thus, the word position in which a target sound is trained does not seem to be a factor in position generalization. In terms of clinical management, unless the pattern of errors suggests a particular word position for initial training (such as final consonant deletion), it is recommended that the clinician train the word position that the client finds easiest to produce, check for generalization to other positions, and then proceed to train the other word positions if generalization has not already occurred. Except for selected fricative sounds (those that develop earliest in the final position), the easiest position to teach is the initial position. However, contextual testing may result in the identification of singleton or cluster contexts that are facilitating for an individual child.

Technically, position generalization may be viewed as a type of contextual generalization. The term *contextual generalization*, however, also refers to phonetic context transfer—for example, generalization from /s/ in *ask* to /s/ in *biscuit* or to /s/ in *fist*. This type of generalization where a production transfers to other words without direct treatment is an example of response generalization as previously described. When preliminary testing has indicated specific contexts in which an error sound may be produced correctly, clinicians will frequently attempt to stabilize such productions—that is, see that a target sound can be consistently produced correctly in that context—and then provide instruction designed to facilitate generalization of the correct sound to other contexts. As with all types of generalization, the client must exhibit transfer to untrained contexts at some point for the remediation process to be complete. In a study of phoneme generalization, Elbert and McReynolds (1978) reported that although facilitative phonetic contexts have been posited as a factor in generalization, their data did not support the idea that certain contexts facilitate generalization across subjects. Instead, they found a great deal of variability in facilitative contexts across subjects. The authors also reported that once a child imitated the sound, generalization occurred to other contexts. They concluded that the client's position of the sound in his or her productive repertoire had more to do with generalization than did contextual factors.

Elbert, Powell, and Swartzlander (1991) examined the number of minimal word-pair exemplars necessary for phonologically impaired children to meet a generalization criterion. They reported that for their subjects (primarily preschool children), generalization occurred using a small number of word-pair exemplars (five or less for 80 percent of the children) but there was substantial variability across subjects. The occurrence of response generalization subsequent to teaching a small number of exemplars is consistent with findings from previous treatment reports (Elbert and McReynolds, 1978; Weiner, 1981b).

Across-Linguistic Unit Generalization

A second type of generalization involves shifting correct sound productions from one level of linguistic complexity to another (e.g., from syllables to words). For some clients, the first goal in this process is to transfer production of isolated sounds to syllables and words; others begin at the syllable or word level and generalize target sound productions to phrases and sentences.

Van Riper and Erickson (1996) recommended that the transfer sequence be initiated with sounds in isolation, followed by syllables, words, and finally sentences. This hierarchy of production complexity is the usual treatment sequence in traditional therapy. Instruction at the transfer phase of the instructional continuum begins at the highest level of linguistic complexity at which a client can produce a target behavior on demand. Instruction progresses from that point to the next level of complexity. When sounds are taught in isolation, the effects of coarticulation are absent, and therefore the potential for generalization to syllables and words may be diminished. This notion received some support from a study reported by McReynolds (1972), in which the transfer of /s/ productions to words was probed after each of four sequential teaching steps: (1) /s/ in isolation, (2) /sa/, (3) /as/, and (4) /asa/. Although no transfer to words was observed following training on /s/ in isolation, over 50 percent transfer to words was observed following training on /sa/. It should be recognized, however, that the training of /s/ in isolation prior to syllables may have had a learning effect and influenced the generalization observed following syllable instruction. Some clinicians prefer initially to teach sounds in isolation or in syllables rather than in words in order to decrease interference from previous learning.

Van Riper and Erickson (1996) and Winitz (1975) recommended that sounds be taught in nonsense syllables or nonsense (nonce) words before they are practiced in meaningful words, thereby reducing the interference of previously learned error productions of the target sound. This view is in contrast with the language-based perspective that phonologic contrasts should be established at the word level because *meaningful* contrasts are a key to acquisition. Powell and McReynolds (1969) studied generalization in four participants who misarticulated /s/. They reported that when two of the individuals were taught consonant productions in nonsense syllables, transfer of the target sound to words occurred without additional training. The other two individuals had to be provided instruction for generalization from nonsense syllables to words to occur.

Elbert, Dinnsen, Swartzlander, and Chin (1990) reported that when preschool children were taught target sounds within a minimal pair contrast training paradigm, generalization occurred to other single-word productions as well as to conversational speech. Based on a three-month post-treatment probe, they reported that participants continued to generalize to other nontrained productions.

In summary, it appears that some clients generalize from one linguistic unit to another without specific training; others require specific instructional activities for transfer from one linguistic unit to another. The process of generalization across linguistic units varies across individuals as do all types of generalization.

Across-Sound and Across-Feature Generalization

A third type of generalization is observed when correct production of a target sound generalizes from one sound to another. Generalization most often occurs within sound classes and/or between sounds that are phonetically similar (e.g., /k/ to /g/; /s/ to /z/ and /ʃ/). Clinicians have long observed that training on one sound in a cognate pair frequently results in generalization to the second sound (e.g., Elbert et al., 1967). McNutt (1994), in a study of bilingual children, reported that correction of /s/ in English generalized to correction of a defective /s/ in French.

Generalization of correct production from one sound to another is expected when remediation targets are selected on the basis of place, manner, and voicing analysis, distinctive feature analysis, or phonologic process/pattern analysis. Often in these approaches, target behaviors are selected that reflect features or processes/patterns common to several error productions. It is assumed that generalization will occur from exemplars to other error sounds within the same sound class or, in some instances, across sound classes. For example, an underlying assumption of distinctive feature analysis and remediation is that features generalize from one sound production to another production containing the same features. This type of generalization can be seen in the client who initially did not correctly produce any sounds containing [+ stridency], yet after learning to produce /s/, was able to correctly articulate /ʃ/ and /z/, which also contain the feature [+ stridency].

A client can learn a feature and transfer the feature without necessarily correcting a sound. For example, a client who substitutes stops for fricatives may learn to produce /f/ and overgeneralize its use to several fricative sounds. Although the client no longer substitutes stops for fricatives, he or she now substitutes /f/ for other fricatives (e.g., [sʌn] → [fʌn]; [ʃou] → [fou].

Although the same number of phonemes is in error, the fact that the client has incorporated a new sound class into his or her repertoire represents enhancement of the child's phonological system (Williams, 1993).

McReynolds and Bennett (1972) studied three speakers who received training to facilitate feature generalization. Instruction for each subject focused on a specified sound that was selected to reflect a particular feature. Specifically, one person was taught an exemplar containing the [+ stridency] feature, another the [+ voicing] feature, and the third the [+ continuancy] feature. Feature generalization to other error sounds was assessed through deep testing of nontrained phonemes. Results for the three individuals indicated that the feature generalized to several sounds even though training was limited to a single sound exemplar.

Frequently, the establishment of feature contrasts is part of the effort to reduce and eliminate process usage and homonomy (in which one sound is substituted for several sounds in the language). The notion of feature and sound generalization, like other types of generalization, is critical to the remediation process. During the 1990s, several studies of children with multiple speech sound errors were conducted wherein data were collected regarding the impact on generalization of various types of treatment targets. Results of these studies are relevant to our discussion of across-sound and across-feature generalization.

In a study related to teaching stimulable versus nonstimulable sounds, Powell, Elbert, and Dinnsen (1991) reported that teaching a nonstimulable sound prompted change in the target sound and other errored stimulable sounds. However, teaching a stimulable sound did not necessarily lead to changes in untreated stimulable or nonstimulable sounds. The implication of this study is that treatment of nonstimulable sounds may lead to increased generalization and thus have a more widespread impact on the child's overall sound system.

Gierut, Morrisette, Hughes, and Rowland (1996) examined generalization associated with teaching early developing sounds versus later developing sounds. They reported that children taught later developing sounds evidenced change in the treated sound, with generalization occurring both within and across sound classes. For those taught early developing sounds, improvements were noted on the target sound within class sounds, but not across class sounds.

Studies of generalization associated with teaching sounds evidencing "least" versus "most" knowledge of sounds in the sound system (Dinnsen and Elbert, 1984; Gierut, Elbert, and Dinnsen, 1987) have indicated that treatment focused on least knowledge resulted in extensive systemwide generalization, wherein treatment of most knowledge contributed to focused but limited change in a child's overall sound system. Studies comparing generalization associated with teaching phonetically more complex sounds to those less phonetically complex sounds (Dinnsen, Chin, Elbert, and Powell, 1990; Tyler and Figurski, 1994) have evidenced that more extensive changes were obtained when treatment was focused on more complex phonetic distinctions between error sounds as compared to simpler distinctions between sounds.

As a follow-up to the studies reported in the preceding paragraphs, Rvachew and Nowak (2001) studied the amount of phonological generalization associated with treatment targets that reflected early developing and greater phonological knowledge, as contrasted with later developing and little or no productive phonological knowledge. In contrast to previous findings, these investigators reported that greater treatment efficiency was associated with phoneme targets that reflected early developing and greater productive phonological knowledge. Further investigation is necessary before definitive statements may be made with regard to the issue of targeting early versus later acquired sounds, and more versus less phonological knowledge.

Powell and Elbert (1984) investigated the generalization patterns of two groups of children with misarticulations. Specifically, they wanted to see if the group receiving instruction on earlier developing consonant clusters (stop + liquid) would exhibit generalization patterns different from those of the group receiving instruction on later-developing consonant clusters (fricative + liquid). The authors reported that no clear overall pattern was observed; instead, the six participants exhibited individual generalization patterns. All participants evidenced some generalization to both the trained and untrained consonant clusters. The most interesting finding was that generalization to both cluster categories occurred on the final probe measure in five of six participants regardless of the treatment received. Powell and Elbert (1984) attributed generalization across sound and classes in part to good pre-treatment stimulability skills.

Weiner (1981b) also reported across-sound generalization in teaching final consonants in children who deleted final consonants. He trained speakers to produce word-final stops and reported generalization to word-final fricatives.

Across-Situations Generalization

The fourth and final type of generalization to be discussed in this chapter, called *situational generalization*, involves transfer of behaviors taught in the clinical setting to other situations and locations, such as school, work, or home. This type of generalization is critical to the remediation process because it represents the terminal objective of instruction (i.e., correct phonologic productions in conversational speech in nonclinical settings). Such generalization has also been called *carryover* in the speech-language pathology literature.

Most clinicians focus on activities to facilitate situational transfer during the final stages of remediation. Some, including the authors, have argued that clinicians should incorporate these activities into early stages of instruction. For example, once a client can produce single words correctly, efforts should be made to incorporate these words into nonclinical settings. A major advantage of providing phonological instruction in the classroom setting (inclusion model) is the opportunity to incorporate treatment targets into a child's natural communicative environment. For example, if a child's science lesson incorporates a word containing a target sound (such as /s/), the teacher or clinician can provide the opportunity for the child to utilize his or her new speech sound in words like *sun, solar, ice, estimate, season, summer*, and so on. Although much emphasis is placed on facilitating situational generalization, little experimental data are available to provide specific guidance to the clinician.

Studies by Costello and Bosler (1976), Olswang and Bain (1985), and Bankson and Byrne (1972) have shown that situational generalization is facilitated through treatment, but the extent of such transfer varies greatly from one individual to another. Costello and

Bosler (1976) investigated whether certain clinical situations were more likely to evidence generalization than others. They recorded the transfer that occurred from training in the home environment to probes obtained in the following four settings:

1. A mother administered the probe while sitting across from her child at a table in a treatment room of the speech clinic.
2. An experimenter (who was only vaguely familiar to the child) administered the probe while sitting across from the child at the same table in the same room as setting 1.
3. The same experimenter administered the probe while she and the child were seated at separate desks facing each other in a large classroom outside the speech clinic.
4. A second experimenter (unknown to the child prior to the study) administered a probe while she and the child were alone and seated in comfortable chairs in the informal atmosphere of the clinic waiting room.

Although all three participants generalized from therapy to one or more of the above testing settings, there was no evidence that one setting was more likely to evidence generalization than another. It may be that generalization variables differ so much from person to person that it is impossible to predict which environments are most likely to facilitate situational transfer.

Olswang and Bain (1985) monitored situational generalization for three 4-year-old children in two different settings during speech sound remediation. They examined connected speech samples recorded in conversational activities in a clinic treatment room and connected speech samples audio recorded by parents during conversational activities at home. They reported similar rates and amounts of generalization of target sounds for both settings.

Bankson and Byrne (1972) reported that four out of five clients generalized correct sound production in words from a motor-based remediation procedure to conversational samples gathered both in the training setting (school) and the home environment. Although the amount of generalization seen in the home and school training probes varied from day to day for each subject, the daily fluctuations were consistent between settings for each subject. The overall extent to which generalization occurred varied greatly across individuals and from day to day.

One strategy that has been suggested to facilitate situational generalization is the use of self-monitoring (self-evaluation). Self-monitoring techniques have included hand raising (Engel and Groth, 1976), charting (Diedrich, 1971; Koegel, Koegel, and Ingham, 1986), and counting of correct productions, both within and outside the clinic (Koegel, Koegel, Van Voy, and Ingham, 1988). Bennett, Bennett, and James (1996) suggested the following steps to facilitate self-monitoring:

1. External monitoring and verbal feedback
2. External monitoring with cues provided for revision (e.g., raise hand)
3. Self-revision by client when errors occur
4. Anticipating when errors may occur
5. Automatic usage of correct production

Koegel and colleagues (1988) examined generalization of /s/ and /z/ in seven children. They reported that when children self-monitored their conversational productions in the clinic, no generalization of the correct target production outside the clinic occurred. However, when children were required to monitor their conversational speech outside the clinic, "rapid and widespread generalization" occurred across subjects, although at slightly different rates. They reported high levels of generalization for all children. In contrast, when Gray and Shelton (1992) field tested the self-monitoring strategy of Koegel and colleagues (1988), the results did not replicate the positive generalization treatment effect reported by the latter.

Shriberg and Kwiatkowski (1987), in a retrospective study of efficacy of intervention strategies, identified self-monitoring procedures as a potentially effective component to facilitate generalization to continuous speech. In a subsequent experimental study, Shriberg and Kwiatkowski (1990) reported that seven of the eight preschool children generalized from such self-monitoring instruction to spontaneous speech. They concluded, however, that although self-monitoring facilitated generalization, it varied in terms of type, extent, and point of onset.

Despite a paucity of data on situational generalization, available evidence indicates that, as with other forms of generalization, the extent to which it occurs in different settings varies greatly among individuals. There is also the suggestion that situational generalization may be influenced by age and how well developed the child's phonologic system is (Elbert et al., 1990).

Several investigators have suggested that productive phonologic knowledge (accuracy and consistency of sound production) influences children's generalization learning (Dinnsen and Elbert, 1984; Elbert and Gierut, 1986; Gierut et al., 1987; Gierut, 1989). They have inferred that phonologic knowledge accounts for some of the individual differences that occur in generalization. Gierut and colleagues (1987) reported that greater generalization occurred in sounds where children exhibited more knowledge (correct productions in a wide array of contexts) as opposed to less knowledge (correct productions in fewer contexts; more positional constraints), but the greatest generalization occurred on those sounds for which training was provided. They also reported that when intervention was directed toward sounds where the child evidenced the least phonologic knowledge, generalization learning occurred across the child's phonologic system. These investigators recommended that clinicians choose sounds for treatment that reflect the least phonologic knowledge (inventory constraints). Even though training on sounds in which children showed most knowledge facilitated greater generalization within a sound class, training on sounds for which children exhibited least knowledge resulted in more broad-based generalization. Gierut and colleagues (1987) inferred from these findings that training on sounds in which children displayed least knowledge (e.g., no correct production of a sound) resulted in more systemwide changes and reorganization of the child's phonologic system than did training on sounds in which children showed most knowledge (e.g., inconsistent productions).

Williams (1991) examined generalization of nine children on /s/ and /r/ sounds for which they exhibited least phonologic knowledge as reflected by inventory constraints (i.e., the children did not produce /s/ and /r/ on a conversational sample or on a 306-item probe test). The misarticulated [s] and [r] were trained in consonant clusters. Williams reported three different generalization and learning patterns across the subjects and hypothesized that differences in generalization reflected different levels of phonological knowledge, even though all error targets were classified in the least phonologic knowledge category (sound is not in child's repertoire). Williams questioned if Gierut and colleagues' (1987) category of least knowledge was too broad to capture subtle differences in children's knowledge and recommended acoustical measurements to supplement transcription to further differentiate the amount of phonologic knowledge demonstrated for sounds in the least knowledge category of this system. This observation is consistent with recommendations from Weismer, Dinnsen, and Elbert (1981), Smit and Bernthal (1983), and Tyler, Edwards, and Saxman (1990).

Parental Assistance with Generalization

Clinicians have long recognized that the generalization process in phonologic remediation might be facilitated if individuals from the client's environment could be drawn into the generalization phase of the treatment process. The assumption has been that persons significant to the client, including parents, spouse, teachers, or peers, could engage in activities designed to extend what the clinician was doing in the clinical setting. Several programs include instructional activities designed for parents to use with their children at home (Bowen and Cupples, 1999; Mowrer, Baker, and Schutz, 1968; Gray, 1974). Sommers (1962) and Sommers and colleagues (1964) studied several variables related to articulation instruction. Greater improvement between pre- and post-test scores was reported for children whose mothers were trained to assist with instruction than for a control group of children whose mothers had not received training. Carrier (1970) reported a study comparing a group of 10 children 4 to 7 years old who participated in an articulation training program administered by their mothers and a similar control group who received minimal assistance from their mothers. The experimental group obtained significantly higher scores on four phonologic measures than the control group. Other investigations in which parents provided directed articulation instruction for their children (Shelton, Johnson, and Arndt, 1972; Shelton, Johnson, Willis, and Arndt, 1975) reported that parents can be utilized to enhance phonological intervention.

The clinician must be sensitive to the role parents and other nonprofessionals can assume in the treatment process and must keep several things in mind. For example, parents can (1) provide good auditory models of target words, (2) have their child(ren) practice target words that the child(ren) can easily produce correctly, and (3) reinforce correct productions. First, if parents are to judge the accuracy of sound productions, they must be able to discriminate the sounds correctly. Second, the clinician must demonstrate to the parents the procedures to be used in the program; then the parents must demonstrate to the clinician the same procedures to ensure that they can carry them out. Third, the clinician must recognize that parents have only a limited amount of time; consequently, programs should be designed for short periods. Fourth, written instructions of the specific tasks should be provided to the caregivers/parents. Finally, clinicians should keep in mind that parents probably function better as monitors of productions than as teachers. Often parents lack the patience and objectivity necessary to teach their own children. However, if parents or other individuals in the child's environment have the desire, skill, time, and patience to work with their children, the clinician may have a helpful facilitator of the generalization process.

Generalization Guidelines

1. For most rapid context and situational generalization, begin instruction with target behaviors (sounds) that are stimulable or in the client's repertoire.

2. For children with multiple errors, there are data to support each of the following as ways to facilitate generalization:
   a. Nonstimulable sounds are treated before stimulable sounds.
   b. More phonetically complex sounds are treated before those less complex.
   c. Late developing sounds are treated before early developing sounds.
   d. Sounds evidencing least knowledge are treated before those evidencing most knowledge.
   e. Early developing sounds that also reflect greater productive knowledge are treated before later developing sounds with less productive knowledge.

3. Because word productions form the basis of position generalization, productions at this level should be incorporated into the instructional sequence as soon as possible. When teaching a sound, utilize words and syllable shapes within the child's lexicon.

4. The more features that sounds have in common, the more likely that generalization will occur from one to another. For example, teaching [ɝ] usually results in generalization to the unstressed [ɚ] and the consonantal [r]; teaching one member of a cognate sound-pair, such as [s], usually results in the client's correction of the cognate [z].

5. Teaching a distinctive feature in the context of one sound, such as frication in [f], may result in generalization of that feature to other untreated sounds, such as [z].

6. Data are lacking to support a particular order for teaching sounds in various word positions to facilitate generalization. Beginning with the word position that is easiest for the client is an often used starting point.

7. When selecting sounds to target phonologic patterns, select target sounds from across sound classes in which the pattern occurs to increase the likelihood of generalization across the phonological system.

8. Nonsense syllables may facilitate production of sounds in syllable contexts during establishment of sound production because nonsense syllables pose less interference with previously learned behaviors than do words.

9. Meaningful words may generalize more rapidly than nonsense syllables because they reflect phonemic contrasts and may be reinforced in the environment.

10. Activities to facilitate situational generalization are advised as soon as the client can say a sound in words, rather than waiting until sounds are produced at the sentence level. In the case of preschool children, generalization frequently takes place without a plan to facilitate situational generalization in treatment.

11. Parents and others in the child's environment can be used effectively to facilitate phonologic change in children.

Dismissal from Instruction

The final phase of phonologic instruction occurs when the client habituates new target behaviors and otherwise assumes responsibility for self-monitoring of target phonologic productions. This phase of therapy is an extension of the generalization phase.

During the final phase of therapy, sometimes referred to as the *maintenance phase*, clients decrease their contact with the clinician. Shelton (1978) labeled the terminal objective of articulation remediation as *automatization* and described it as automatic usage of standard articulation patterns in spontaneous speech. The term *automatization* implies that phonologic productions can be viewed as motor behavior that develops into an automatic response. When phonologic errors are linguistic in nature, maintenance may be viewed as the mastery of phonologic rules or phonemic contrasts. In reality, both the motor production and phonologic rules become part of a person's everyday productive behavioral responses by this point in treatment. The maintenance phase may be considered complete once the client can consistently use target behaviors in spontaneous speech.

To determine the extent to which a client has maintained target behaviors, the clinician must assess a client's behavior during conversational speech. Diedrich (1971) suggested that three-minute "talk" samples are a good way to monitor correct and incorrect speech productions during conversation.

During maintenance, the client usually receives intermittent reinforcement for the new speech patterns because this type of schedule results in behavior that is most resistant to extinction. Clients are also required to monitor their own articulation productions during maintenance. Having the client keep track of target productions during specified periods of the day is a procedure that can be used to self-monitor target production.

Information from the learning literature offers insights into the maintenance or retention of newly acquired phonologic patterns. *Retention*, in the context of phonologic remediation, refers to the continued and persistent use of responses learned during instruction. Once an individual learns a new phonologic pattern or response, he or she must continue to use (retain) the response. In clinical literature, retention is sometimes discussed in terms of intersession retention and sometimes in terms of habitual retention. *Intersession retention* refers to the ability to produce recently taught responses correctly. Speech clinicians frequently observe "between-session forgetting" in many clients. This is an instance where the decision concerning parental assistance with therapy is useful. Short practice sessions between therapy sessions may improve intersession retention. *Habitual retention* is the persistent and continued use of the response after instruction has been terminated. The term *maintenance* is frequently used to refer to this phenomenon. Speech clinicians occasionally dismiss clients from instruction only to have them return for additional therapy some months later. Such individuals obviously did not habituate or retain their newly learned responses. Mowrer (1977) pointed out that lack of intersession retention is a particular problem with mentally retarded children.

Sommers (1969) reported that articulation errors are susceptible to regression. In a follow-up study of 177 elementary school children who had been dismissed from articulation instruction during a six-month period, he found that approximately one-third had regressed. Based on conversational samples of target sound productions, 59 percent of those who had worked on /s/ and /z/ had regressed, but only 6 percent of those who had worked on /r/ had regressed. He did not report dismissal criteria or the level of performance prior to dismissal.

In contrast, Elbert and colleagues (1990) reported that for preschool children, learning continued to improve on both single-word and conversational speech samples obtained three months post-treatment. These data support the idea that young children are actively involved and continue to learn the phonologic system even after treatment was terminated. It appears that phonologic errors in preschool children are less habituated than in older school-age children and easier to correct.

Winitz (1969) proposed that interference, which results in competition between the error sound and the newly acquired sound, may explain why individuals forget articulatory responses. Winitz pointed out that the years of motor production practice using an incorrect articulatory gesture, such as /t/ for /tʃ/, will interfere with the individual's ability to produce a newly learned /tʃ/. Similarly, speech clinicians frequently observe individuals who, during the early stages of /s/ instruction, insert a /θ/ following a newly learned /s/ in a word context (e.g., [sθup]).

Mowrer (1982) pointed out several factors that have been shown to influence the degree to which information will be retained, whether in the child who is dismissed from therapy but returns for lack of long-term maintenance or in the child who seems to have forgotten previous learning between sessions. First, the meaningfulness of the material used to teach the new responses may affect retention, although there is little empirical evidence in the articulation learning literature on this point. In general, as the meaningfulness of the material increases, the rate of forgetting tends to decrease, and thus the use of meaningful material is recommended during remediation. Thus, names of friends, family members, pets, familiar objects, and classroom vocabulary are appropriate choices. Although meaningfulness of material may be an important aid to long-term retention, the clinician may find, as stated earlier, that nonmeaningful material (e.g., nonsense syllables) may be useful during earlier phases of instruction (i.e., establishment). Leonard (1973) reported that when /s/ had been established in meaningful words, fewer training trials were required to transfer to other words than when nonsense items were utilized. But this finding on generalization must be distinguished from the finding presented earlier in our discussion of interference—that acquisition or establishment of new responses can be accomplished in fewer trials with nonsense items than with meaningful items.

A second factor believed to affect retention is the degree or extent to which something has been learned. In general, the greater the number of trials during the learning process, the greater the retention. Retention improves when some overlearning of verbal material takes place. To avoid unnecessary practice, it is important to determine the minimum amount of learning needed to provide a satisfactory level of retention. The optimum point for stopping instruction occurs when additional training does not produce sufficient change in performance to merit additional practice; however, there are little data to guide the clinician about where this point may be.

A third factor affecting retention is the frequency of instruction or the distribution of practice. Retention is superior when tasks are practiced during several short sessions (distributed practice) than during fewer, longer sessions (massed practice). On the basis of this fact, frequent, short practice sessions are recommended. In his review of this topic, Mowrer

(1982) concluded: "On the basis of controlled learning experiments in psychology alone, it could be recommended that clinicians could increase retention by providing frequent instruction; but bear in mind that no data are available from speech research that confirms this recommendation ... the important factor in terms of frequency of instruction is not how much instruction ... but the total number of instruction periods" (p. 259).

A fourth factor shown to affect retention is the individual's motivational state. The more motivated a person, the greater the retention of the material that has been learned. Little, if any, experimental work reported in the phonologic literature has attempted to examine motivational state during speech instruction.

Dismissal Criteria

The maintenance phase provides a period for monitoring retention, and it is during this period that dismissal decisions are made. Limited data on dismissal criteria have been reported, and thus evidence is lacking to support a single dismissal criterion. Elbert (1967) suggested dismissal might be based on two questions: (1) Has the maximum change in this individual's speech behavior been attained? (2) Can this individual maintain this level of speech behavior and continue to improve without additional speech instruction? Whatever criteria are used for dismissal, they should be based on periodic samples of phonologic behavior over time. The maintenance phase provides the final opportunity for the clinician to monitor, reinforce, and encourage the client to assume responsibility for habituation of the new speech patterns.

Diedrich and Bangert (1976) reported data on articulatory retention and dismissal from treatment. Some of the children studied were dismissed after reaching a 75 percent criterion level for correct /s/ and /r/ productions, as measured on a 30-item probe word test plus a three-minute sample of conversational speech. Four months later, 19 percent of the children had regressed below the 75 percent criterion level. No greater retention was found, however, among those children who remained in treatment until achieving higher than 75 percent criterion level on the probe measure. Diedrich and Bangert concluded that most speech clinicians tend to retain children with /s/ and /r/ errors in articulation instruction longer than necessary.

Maintenance and Dismissal Guidelines

1. Dismissal criteria may vary depending on the nature of the client's problem and the client's age. Preschool children with multiple errors generally require less stringent dismissal criteria than older children because they have been reported to continue to improve phonological productions without instruction once they begin to incorporate a new sound(s) into their repertoire. School-age and older clients who evidence residual errors /r/, /s/, and /l/ may require more stringent dismissal criteria in order to retain the new behavior.
2. During the maintenance phase, clients assume increased responsibility for self-monitoring their production and maintaining accurate production.
3. The reinforcement schedule should continue to be intermittent during maintenance, as is the situation during the latter stages of generalization.

4. It has been suggested that clinicians may tend to keep many clients enrolled for phonologic remediation longer than is necessary. In other words, the cost-benefit ratio for intervention may significantly decline after a certain point is reached in treatment.

▮ QUESTIONS FOR CHAPTER 6

1. When in the treatment process would it be appropriate to use continuous versus intermittent reinforcement?

2. What are critical considerations in selecting consequent events?

3. Describe vertical, horizontal, and cyclical structured treatment programs.

4. Describe and give examples of three types of phonological generalization.

5. Present five expectations relative to phonological generalization.

Treatment Approaches

JOHN E. BERNTHAL

University of Nebraska–Lincoln

NICHOLAS W. BANKSON

James Madison University

PETER FLIPSEN JR.

Idaho State University

In Chapter 6, we discussed concepts and principles that underlie phonological remediation. These principles and considerations are applicable to all the treatment approaches that will be discussed in this chapter.

As discussed in Chapter 4, historically, speech-language pathologists approached the correction of speech sound errors from the standpoint of teaching a motor behavior. Most clinicians viewed speech sound errors as an individual's inability to produce the complex motor skills required for the articulation of speech sounds. Since the 1970s, clinicians have also viewed speech sound disorders from a more linguistic (phonological) perspective. The linguistic perspective is based on the recognition that some individuals produce speech sound errors because they have not learned to use certain phonologic rules, especially sound contrasts, in accord with the adult norm. In other words, many error productions reflect a client's lack of rules for appropriate sound usage rather than an inability to produce the sounds.

Although it is convenient to dichotomize *motor/articulation* and *linguistic/phonologic* aspects of phonology for organization purposes, normal sound usage involves both the production of sounds at a motor level and their use in accordance with the rules of the language. Thus, the two skills are intertwined and may be described as two sides of the same coin. At a clinical level, it is often difficult or impossible to determine whether a client's errors reflect a lack of motor skills to produce a sound, a lack of linguistic knowledge, or deficiencies in both. It may be that, in a given client, some errors relate to one factor, some to another, and some to both.

Even though a disorder may be perceived as relating primarily to either the motor or linguistic aspects of phonology, instructional programs typically involve elements of both. It should be recognized that although it is often difficult to determine whether a given instructional procedure is primarily a motor-based or a linguistic-based technique, some activities undoubtedly assist the client in both the development of linguistic knowledge and the development of appropriate motor skills. Both motor and linguistic aspects of phonology are a part of most therapy programs. One notable exception may be the case of residual errors (e.g., /r/, /l/, /s/) where a motor approach is the treatment of choice since the child's knowledge of the linguistic aspects of the sound can usually be assumed (e.g., the child uses distorted or lateralized [s] in situations where /s/ is the target). By careful observation of a client and the nature of his or her problem, the clinician may be able to determine when one type of intervention should be emphasized.

Although we sometimes categorize the treatment approaches presented in this chapter as primarily motor or linguistic, that does not mean that the approaches were necessarily developed from a particular theoretical perspective. Many phonologic treatment approaches have emerged from pragmatic origins and continue to be used simply because "they work." In the pages that follow, several approaches to remediation are described. Some of these can be related to theory, some are atheoretical, and others lie somewhere in between. In the summary of each approach, we provide a "Background Statement" that reflects our perception of the theoretical perspective from which the approach has emerged. A challenge for the future is to develop, refine, and revise theories that provide rationale, support, explanations, and direction for intervention procedures.

Regardless of the treatment approach used, it is important to examine the evidence that supports a particular treatment. The American Speech-Language-Hearing Association has stated that members who hold a Certificate of Clinical Competence should engage in evidence-based practice. This statement goes on to say that individuals "must demonstrate knowledge used in research and the integration of research principles into evidence-based practice . . . [and] must demonstrate comprehension of the basic and applied research design" (ASHA, 2005, p. 6).

One generally accepted method that investigators have used to examine the evidence and the efficacy of treatment research and outcomes is to do a meta-analysis in which a complete body of literature is analyzed to determine outcomes across studies and determine an overall effect of treatment. Law, Garrett, and Nye (2004) conducted a meta-analysis of data from studies that spanned a number of years, in which participants were randomly assigned to either an experimental group or a control group. They reported that when comparing the groups receiving phonological intervention to those receiving no treatment, the intervention group performed better on outcome assessment measures. This positive treatment effect was seen when measuring the percentage of consonants correct in conversation as well as on speech sound articulation (criterion) measures.

Although these studies spanned a time frame of over two decades and reflected different interventions, there was adequate support for the authors to conclude that intervention by speech-language pathologists with children with speech sound disorders results in positive outcomes when compared to individuals who do not receive therapy. In addition, such outcomes can be obtained using a variety of treatment approaches and procedures.

The question of which particular treatment approaches are more efficacious (i.e., results in better outcomes) is one where we have very limited data and few answers. Likewise, we need additional data to determine if one subgroup of children with speech sound disorders responds better to one treatment approach or procedure than another.

TREATMENT CONTINUUM

Treatment can be viewed as a continuum of activities comprising three stages: establishment, facilitation of generalization, and maintenance. This continuum, which comes from the motor learning literature, is applicable to most types of speech and language disorders and constitutes a framework for a wide variety of specific teaching techniques and procedures. The goal of the first phase of instruction, called *establishment*, is to elicit target behaviors from a client and then stabilize such behaviors at a voluntary level, and/or establish phonologic contrasts. Establishment procedures are often based on production tasks, as in the example of a clinician teaching a child who does not produce /l/ where to place his or her tongue to say /l/. In addition, for a child who can say /l/ but deletes it in the final position (e.g., *bow* for *bowl*), the contrast between word-pairs, such as *bow* and *bowl* or *so* and *soul*, may need to be taught during the establishment phase. Once the client is able to readily produce the correct form of sound and is aware of how it is used contrastively, he or she is ready to move into the generalization phase of instruction.

The second phase of instruction is called *generalization*. As discussed in Chapter 6, it is designed to facilitate transfer or carryover of behavior at several levels—positional generalization, contextual generalization, linguistic unit generalization, sound and feature generalization, and situational generalization. The treatment process includes instructional activities or strategies designed to facilitate generalization or carryover of correct sound productions to sound contrasts, words, and speaking situations that have not been specifically trained. An example of a context generalization activity would be practicing /s/ in a few key words (e.g., *see, sit, seek*) and then determining whether /s/ is produced correctly in other words. An example of a situational generalization activity would be practicing /l/ in sentences in the treatment setting and then observing whether the child uses /l/ in words, phrases, and sentences produced in his or her classroom or home.

The third and final phase of remediation, *maintenance*, is designed to stabilize and facilitate retention of those behaviors acquired during the establishment and generalization phases. Instructional activities related to the generalization and maintenance phases of treatment generally overlap. Frequency and duration of instruction are often reduced during maintenance, and the client assumes increased responsibility for "maintaining" and self-monitoring correct speech patterns. The client may also engage in specific activities designed to habituate or automatize particular speech patterns. A maintenance activity may consist of a client's keeping track of his or her /s/ productions at mealtime or use of r-clusters during five-minute phone conversations every evening for a week. It should be pointed out that although establishment, generalization/carryover, and maintenance have been identified as discrete phases of treatment, in practice there may be considerable overlap among these phases.

A commonly used or traditional approach to remediation has been to focus on correcting one or two sounds, moving them through the treatment continuum to the maintenance phase, and then initiating the correction of other sound(s). As indicated earlier, most clinicians prefer to focus on several error sounds or phonologic patterns simultaneously, proceeding along the treatment continuum with several segments or patterns.

Clients may enter the treatment continuum at different points, the exact point being determined by the individual's articulatory/phonological skills. Consider these two examples: Mark is able to produce a sound correctly in words and is able to perceive the target contrastively. Mark therefore begins instruction at the generalization stage, and would likely focus on incorporating target words into phrases. Kristy is able to produce a sound imitatively in syllables, perceives the sound contrast in word-pairs, but fails to incorporate the target production of the sound into words. She also enters the treatment continuum at the generalization stage, but at an earlier point than Mark. In her case, the clinician will seek to establish the target sound in a set of target words, selected on the basis perhaps of facilitating context, or even vocabulary items used in her classroom. For Mark, the clinician will facilitate generalization to phrases and sometimes other contexts. For Kristy, the clinician will facilitate generalization from syllables to words, including words not specifically focused on in a therapy session. The clinician must identify not only the appropriate phase of the treatment continuum but also the appropriate level within a phase at which to begin instruction.

MOTOR LEARNING PRINCIPLES

The treatment approaches described in the next two major sections of this chapter were designed to focus primarily on the motor skills involved in producing target sounds and frequently include perceptual tasks as part of the treatment procedures. Most of them represent variations of what is often referred to as a *traditional approach* or *motor-based approach* to remediation. Treatment based on an articulation/phonetic or motor perspective focuses on the placement and movement of the articulators in combination with auditory stimulation (e.g., ear training and auditory bombardment). This remediation approach involves the selection of a target speech sound or sounds, with instruction proceeding through a sequence of increasingly complex linguistic units (e.g., isolation, syllables, words, phrases) until target sounds are used appropriately in spontaneous conversation. Thus, speech production is viewed as a learned motor skill, with remediation requiring repetitive practice at increasingly complex motor and linguistic levels until the targeted articulatory gesture becomes automatic.

Ruscello (1984) has indicated that phonological errors may be modified in two ways when viewed from a motor perspective: (1) movements may be taught to replace incorrect movements or (2) movements may be taught where they were formerly absent. On the basis of the literature related to motor skill learning, Ruscello has outlined the following critical features in motor skill development:

1. *Cognitive analysis.* A mental or cognitive analysis is important in the early phase of movement formation. In this process, the learner evaluates his or her anticipated performance mentally and then incorporates those adjustments necessary for appropriate

execution of the movement. Once stabilization of the movement occurs, cognitive planning is minimized. This internalization of a skilled movement is thought to contribute to the generalization of skilled movement across a variety of contexts. Based on experimental data, Ruscello and Shelton (1979) reported that such mental planning was helpful in the acquisition of articulatory skills in a treatment paradigm.

2. *Practice.* Practice is the key variable thought necessary for mastery of any skilled motor behavior. As the learner practices a particular motor skill, modifications based on internal and/or external feedback are made so that accuracy of performance is increased. A motor skill is best practiced in limited contexts until correct execution of the movement is achieved. Early treatment sessions involve discrete productions, such as isolated sound or word practice, while later sessions introduce more advanced tasks in the context of continuous discourse.

3. *Stages of motor skill development.* Initially there is a "sluggishness" in the execution of motor skills because the learner is acquiring the movement. With practice, the motor skill is perfected and stabilized. Ultimately, the skill becomes a part of the learner's repertoire of skilled movements and becomes automatic for the speaker.

4. *Feedback.* Sensory feedback processes (internal and external) are described in the motor learning literature as being of great importance in the early development of a skill. When the individual perfects a skill pattern through practice, the error response is diminished and feedback becomes less important.

The focus of such motor learning in this context is on the development of gestures for the production (articulation) of speech sounds and not on nonspeech oral-motor exercises designed to strengthen the speech mechanism. The use of oral-motor exercises that are not relevant to speech movements have not been proven to be effective in the treatment of speech sounds. We have been unable to find any reports in peer-reviewed outlets that nonspeech oral-motor exercises are helpful in the remediation of speech sound disorders with the possible exception of some cases of dysarthria (Smit, 2004; Forrest, 2002; Lof, 2006).

TEACHING SOUNDS: ESTABLISHMENT OF TARGET BEHAVIORS

The first phase of remediation for clients who do not produce target behaviors on demand, or who have perceptual and/or production difficulty with particular adult phonologic contrasts, is called *establishment.* While the teaching of sounds may be viewed as motor-oriented therapy, perceptual training (i.e., discrimination training, minimal pairs contrasts, and auditory bombardment) may be incorporated in both motor and linguistic oriented treatments. During the establishment phase of instruction, the clinician seeks to teach target behaviors and establish the awareness of phonological contrasts. Thus, the focus in this treatment phase is usually the production of a sound in isolation, syllables, words, and/or discrimination of a sound and the perception of sound contrasts in words. Clients who enter the treatment continuum at the establishment phase often include those who (1) do not have a specific sound in their repertoire and are not stimulable; (2) produce a sound in their repertoire, but only in a limited number of phonetic contexts, and are unable to readily produce the segment on demand; (3) do not perceive the sound in minimal pairs; and (4) produce a sound on demand but do not easily incorporate the sound into syllabic units, particularly combining the consonant with a following or preceding vowel.

Two basic teaching strategies are used to establish sound productions. The first involves discrimination/perceptual training prior to direct production training. The second involves initiating treatment with a production focus and makes the assumption that the client learns to discriminate and perceive the sound as an indirect benefit of production training. Perceptual training may be described as including minimal contrast training (e.g., sorting word-pairs such as *two* and *tooth* into two categories that reflect the presence of the final consonant and the deletion of the final consonant) as well as traditional discrimination tasks (e.g., discrimination of [s] from [θ]) and auditory stimulation—that is, the child listens only (does not produce) to 5-10 words with the target sound produced correctly.

Discrimination/Ear Training and Perceptual Training of Sound Contrasts

The type of perceptual training that historically was used most commonly is called *ear training* or *speech sound discrimination training*. Instructional tasks designed to teach discrimination stem from the traditional motor approach to articulation treatment and typically involve making same-different judgments about what is heard (e.g., "Tell me if these are the same or different: *rake-wake*").

Van Riper and Emerick (1984), Winitz (1975, 1984), Powers (1971), and Weber (1970) recommended that discrimination training occur prior to production training during the establishment phase of the treatment continuum. Sounds produced in error should be the focus of speech sound discrimination training since, as discussed in Chapter 4, little, if any, relationship has been reported between an individual's misarticulation of speech sounds and performance on general speech sound discrimination tasks (Locke, 1980). However, Overby (2007) reported that a group of second-grade children with speech sound disorders had lower overall scores on a speech perception task than typically developing children. She did not find, though, a consistent pattern or relationship of the specific speech sound errors children made and performance on the speech perception task for the specific speech sound error.

Traditionally, speech sound discrimination training has focused on judgments of external (clinician-produced) speech sound stimuli. Speech sound discrimination training procedures are often sequenced so that the client goes from judgments of another speaker's productions to judgments of one's own sound productions.

Winitz (1984) suggested that auditory discrimination training precede articulation production training and also be concurrent with production training at each stage of production (e.g., isolation, syllable, word, sentence, conversation) until the client can make the appropriate speech sound discrimination easily at that level. The idea that perceptual training should precede production training is based on the assumption that certain perceptual distinctions are prerequisites for establishing the production of a speech sound in the child's phonologic system, although this assumption is not universally accepted.

Perceptual instruction is frequently an inherent aspect of production training. For example, when a client is asked to say *house* and he or she says *hout*, the clinician may say, "No, not *hout* but *house*." In this instance, although instruction is production oriented, perceptual training is an inherent part of the task.

A critical question to be answered is whether speech sound discrimination/perceptual training has a positive impact on the establishment or production of a target sound. Williams and McReynolds (1975) reported that when children were taught to produce a sound, they also learned to discriminate the sound. They also found that sound discrimination training alone did not result in improvement in production. Rvachew (1994) reported that a speech perception training program involving a computer based word-pair training program facilitated sound production learning. This study varied from earlier studies, however, in that subjects received both production and perceptual training simultaneously, rather than one preceding or following the other. Although there is a lack of evidence about the precise nature of the relationship between sound discrimination and the establishment of correct productions, it has frequently been assumed that perceptual training is an inherent part of production treatment. Later in this chapter we will talk about a therapy approach that emphasizes contrasts between word-pairs, such as *so* versus *soul*; *tea* versus *teeth*.

Methodology for Traditional Discrimination/Ear Perceptual Training (Van Riper and Erickson, 1996)

1. *Identification.* Call the client's attention to the target sound—what it sounds like, what it looks like as you observe the lips and mouth—and, as best you can, help them be aware of kinesthetic sensations, or what it feels like inside the mouth. For some children, it may help to label the sound and have an appropriate picture or object to go with the sound (e.g., /f/ is the angry cat sound; /t/ is the ticking sound; /k/ is the throaty sound).

   After auditorily stimulating the child with repeated productions of the target sound, then ask the child to raise his or her hand, ring a bell, or otherwise indicate when he or she hears the target sound in isolation. Intermingle the target with other sounds. Initially, the other sounds should have several feature differences from the target in terms of voicing, manner, and place of production (e.g., /s/ and /m/). However, as instruction progresses, the number of feature contrasts between the target and the other sounds should be fewer (e.g., /s/ and /θ/).

2. *Isolation.* Have the client again listen for the target sound, by identifying it in increasingly complex environments. Begin by having the child raise his or her hand, show a happy face, or otherwise indicate when he or she hears the sound in a word (begin with the initial position). Progress to hearing it in phrases and sentences. This step might also include practice identifying the presence of a sound at the middle or end of the word. Note that this step is very difficult for young children before they have learned to read, and is not usually included unless the child has a good grasp of the concept's beginning and end.

3. *Stimulation.* Provide the client an appropriate auditory model of the target sound in both isolation and words. This activity might include limited amplification and varying stress and duration of the target sound. This type of activity is advocated by Hodson and Paden (1991) as part of the cycles approach to remediation and in the treatment program is referred to as "auditory bombardment" or auditory stimulation.

4. *Discrimination.* Ask the client to make judgments of correct and incorrect productions you produce, in increasingly complex contexts (i.e., words, phrases, sentences). In this activity, the client is comparing someone else's production with his or her own internal image of the correct form of a sound. For example, if a child substitutes /θ/ for /s/, the clinician might say: "Here is a picture of a thun. Did I say that word right? Did you see my tongue peeking out at the beginning of the word? Did you hear /θ/ instead of /s/? See if I am right when I name this picture (picture of school): *thcool, thcool*. Did I say that correctly?"

Making judgments of another speaker is an easier task than making judgments about one's own productions. Winitz (1975) suggested that for clients who are not stimulable for a particular sound, speech sound discrimination such as that presented above is an important prerequisite to motor production. As indicated earlier, however, this concept has not been strongly supported by empirical research.

Methodology for Perceptual Training of Sound Contrasts

One aspect of the influence of linguistics on clinical phonology has been its impact on the nature of perceptual training that should either precede or be a part of phonological treatment. Rather than focus on discrimination between sounds, the phonological perspective suggests that perceptual training should focus on minimal pair contrast training. This training was proposed by LaRiviere, Winitz, Reeds, and Herriman (1974), and focuses on the client's differentiation of minimally contrasting word pairs. They recommended that when consonant clusters are reduced, the child be taught to sort contrasting word pairs (e.g., *led-sled*) into categories that reflect simplification of a consonant cluster and those that reflect appropriate production of the target consonant cluster (e.g., *sick* versus *stick*). Another example of such training is a task for final consonant deletion in which the client picks up pictures of "tea" and "teeth" as they are randomly named by the clinician. The intent of this training is to develop a perceptual awareness of differences between minimal pairs (in this case, the presence or absence of a final consonant in the word) and serve to establish the appropriate phonologic contrasts. Perceptual training is widely employed, and a method for using it is presented here. The topic is further described later in this chapter when minimal pair intervention strategies are discussed.

1. *Introduction of a minimal pair.* Present to the client a word that contains the target sound. For example, if the child is substituting /t/ for the fricative /ʃ/, the word *shoe* might be used in a perceptual training activity. The child listens as the clinician points to five identical pictures of a shoe, and names each one.

   Next, present to the client a second word, along with associated pictures of the word, which contains a contrasting sound that is very different from the target sound (i.e., has several different features from the target sound.) For example, *shoe* might be contrasted with *boo* (ghost picture). The phonemes /ʃ/ and /b/ differ in voicing, manner, and place of articulation. For this step, the clinician will identify the original five pictures of a shoe plus the five pictures of "boo."

2. *Contrast training.* Practice differentiating the two contrasting words at a perceptual level. Line up the 10 pictures, 5 of which are of a shoe, and 5 of boo. Ask the client

to hand you the picture you name. Make random requests for either *boo* or *shoe*. If the child can readily do this, he or she has established at a perceptual level the contrast between /ʃ/ and /b/. If the child has difficulty with this task, this activity should be repeated, possibly with different words. Once the child can do this task, contrast training should be repeated with a minimal pair involving the target and error sound (e.g., *shoe-toe; shop-top*).

When the clinician is satisfied that the client can discriminate the target sound from other sounds and that he or she can perceive the target in minimal pairs involving the target sound and error sound, the client is ready for production training. It should be pointed out that in our experience, many children readily discriminate accurately through external monitoring tasks—that is, discriminate the clinician's productions although they may not produce the contrast.

In summary, many speech clinicians teach their clients to perceive the distinction between the target and error sounds or to identify phonemic contrasts as part of the establishment process. Such activities may precede and/or accompany production training. As stated earlier, routine discrimination/perceptual training in treatment has been questioned because many individuals with phonologic disorders do not reflect discrimination problems. In addition, production training, unaccompanied by direct perceptual training, has been shown to modify phonologic errors. The type of perceptual training that appears most useful during the establishment phase is that of phonemic contrast training, as described above.

Production Training

For many clients, clinicians begin phonologic intervention at the establishment phase and focus on helping a client learn to produce a target sound. Whether perceptual training precedes or is interwoven with production training, the goal during this phase of training is to elicit a target sound from a client and stabilize it at a voluntary level.

When a sound is not in a person's repertoire, it is sometimes taught in isolation or syllables rather than words. It should be remembered that some speech sounds, such as stops, are difficult to teach in isolation since stops by their physical nature are produced in combination with vowels or vowel approximations. Glides, likewise, involve production of more than the glide when they are produced. Fricatives can be taught in isolation because they are sounds that can be sustained (e.g., s-s-s-s-s-s). Stops and glides are usually taught in CV contexts (e.g., stop + schwa = /gə/).

Whether sounds should be taught initially in isolation, syllables, or words is a matter of some controversy. McDonald (1964a) urged that syllables be used in production training since the syllable is the basic unit of motor speech production. Some clinicians (e.g., Van Riper and Emerick, 1984) argued that because isolated sounds are the least complex units of production and afford the least interference between the client's habitual speech sound error and the learning of a correct (adult) production, they should be taught first. Words sometimes elicit interference from old error patterns and in such cases may not be a good place to initiate instruction. Others advocate words (lexical items) as the best place to begin instruction because the client can benefit from contextual influences in meaningful productions, and because of the communicative benefits that accrue from the use of "real words." The clinician can determine the level of production that is most facilitative for correct production and then determine whether interference from previous learning is a problem.

Four methods are commonly employed by speech-language clinicians to establish the production of a target sound: imitation, phonetic placement, successive approximation, and contextual utilization. Each of these approaches is discussed below:

1. *Imitation.* We recommend that the clinician attempt to elicit responses through imitation as an initial instructional method for production training. Usually, the clinician presents several auditory models of the desired behavior (typically a sound in isolation, syllables, or words), instructs the client to watch his or her mouth and listen to the sound that is being said, and then asks the client to repeat the target behavior. Sometimes, the clinician may wish to amplify the model through an auditory trainer.

   Procedures for Eliciting a Sound through Imitation

   CLINICIAN: Watch my mouth and listen while I say this sound—/θ/ (repeat it several times). Now you say it.
   CLINICIAN: That's right, I heard the /θ/ sound. Now say this—/θa/ (repeat it several times).
   CLINICIAN: Good, now say /θi/. (Proceed to have the client combine /θ/ and a couple of other vowels.)
   CLINICIAN: Now say *thumb* (repeat it several times).

   Productions are sometimes tape recorded by the clinician so that the client's productions may be played back for self-evaluation. Clients may also be asked to focus on how a sound feels during correct production and to modify their productions to maintain this kinesthetic awareness.

   When an individual can imitate a target sound, the goal during establishment is simply to stabilize target productions. Subsequent instruction will begin at the most complex linguistic level at which the client is able to imitate, whether it be isolation, syllables, or words. The level at which a client can imitate may already have been determined during stimulability testing, but it should be rechecked at the initiation of instruction. Even if the client was not stimulable on a sound during assessment, it is recommended that the clinician begin remediation by asking the client to imitate target productions using auditory, visual, and tactile cues.

2. *Phonetic placement.* When the client is unable to imitate a target sound, the clinician typically begins to cue or instruct the client regarding where to place his or her articulators to produce a particular sound. This type of instruction is called phonetic placement.

   Procedures for Using the Phonetic Placement Technique to Teach Sounds

   a. Instruct the client where to place the articulators to produce a specific speech sound (e.g., for /f/, tell the client to place his or her upper teeth on his or her lower lip and blow air over the lip; for /sh/, tell the client to pull the tongue back from the upper teeth past the rough part of the palate, make a groove in the tongue, round the lips, and blow air).

b. Provide visual and tactile cues to supplement verbal description (e.g., model the correct sound, and provide verbal cueing as the client attempts the sounds: "Remember to lightly touch the lower lip as you blow air for /f/; remember the groove as you blow air for the /ʃ/.").

c. It may be helpful, depending on the maturity level of the client, to analyze and describe differences between the error production and the target production. Sometimes clinicians like to use pictures or drawings reflecting placement of the articulators as part of the instruction.

The phonetic placement method has probably been used as long as anyone has attempted to modify speech patterns. Over three-fourths of a century ago, Scripture and Jackson (1927) published *A Manual of Exercises for the Correction of Speech Disorders,* which included phonetic placement techniques for speech instruction. These authors suggested:

a. Mirror work

b. Drawings designed to show the position of the articulators for the production of specific sounds

c. "Mouth gymnastics"; that is, movements of the articulators (lips and tongue) in response to models and verbal cues and instructions

d. The use of tongue blades to teach placement of sounds, and straws to help direct the airstream

The phonetic placement approach involves explanations and descriptions of idealized phoneme productions. The verbal explanations provided to the client include descriptions of motor gestures or movements and the appropriate points of articulatory contact (tongue, jaw, lip, and velum) involved in producing the target segments. This approach to teaching sounds frequently is used alone or in combination with imitation, plus successive approximation and context utilization (described below). Appendix B describes techniques for teaching various consonants, some of which utilize phonetic placement cues.

Application of the Phonetic Placement Procedure for Teaching /s/

a. Raise the tongue so that its sides are firmly in contact with the inner surface of the upper back teeth.

b. Slightly groove the tongue along the midline. Insert a straw along the midline of the tongue to provide the client a tactile cue as to the place to form the groove.

c. Place the tip of the tongue immediately behind the upper or lower teeth. Show the client in a mirror where to place the tongue tip.

d. Bring the front teeth (central incisors) into alignment (as much as possible) so that a narrow small space between the rows of teeth is formed.

e. Direct the airstream along the groove of the tongue toward the cutting edges of the teeth.

3. *Successive approximation.* Another procedure for teaching sounds that is in some respects an extension of using phonetic placement cues involves shaping a new sound from one that is already in a client's repertoire, or even a behavior the client can perform, such as elevating the tongue. Complex behavioral responses such as speech sound productions often need to be broken down into a series of successive steps or approximations that lead to the production of the target behavior(s). A teaching method that utilizes successive approximation is termed *shaping*. The first step in shaping is to identify an initial response that the client can produce and one that is related to the terminal goal. One common way that this method can be initiated is by the modification of other speech sounds already in the repertoire. Instructional steps move successfully through a series of graded steps or approximations, each progressively closer to the target behavior. Shaping has been found to be an efficient method for teaching complex behavioral tasks but requires careful planning in the sequencing of events to be used for treatment.

Shaping Procedure for Teaching /s/

a. Make [t] (the alveolar place of constriction is similar for both /t/ and /s/).
b. Make [t] with a strong aspiration on the release, prior to the onset of the vowel.
c. Prolong the strongly aspirated release.
d. Remove the tip of the tongue slowly during the release from the alveolar ridge to make a [ts] cluster.
e. Prolong the [s] portion of the [ts] cluster in a word like oats.
f. Practice prolonging the last portion of the [ts] production.
g. Practice "sneaking up quietly" on the /s/ (delete /t/).
h. Produce /s/.

Shaping Procedure for Teaching /ɝ/ (Shriberg, 1975)

a. Stick your tongue out (model provided).
b. Stick your tongue out and touch the tip of your finger (model provided).
c. Put your finger on the bumpy place right behind your top teeth (model provided).
d. Now put the tip of your tongue "lightly" on that bumpy place (model provided).
e. Now put your tongue tip there again, and say [l] (model provided).
f. Say [l] each time I hold up my finger (clinician holds up finger).
g. Now say [l] for as long as I hold my finger up, like this: (model provided for five seconds). Ready. Go.
h. Say a long [l] but this time as you are saying it, drag the tip of your tongue slowly back along the roof of your mouth—so far back that you have to drop it. (Accompany instructions with hand gestures of moving fingertips back slowly, palm up.) (p. 104)

These examples for /s/ and /ɝ/ reflect ways that clinicians capitalize on successive approximations: by shaping behavior from a sound in the client's repertoire (e.g., /t/), and by shaping from a nonphonetic behavior in the client's repertoire (e.g., protruded tongue). Once the client produces a sound that is close to the target, the clinician can use other techniques, such as auditory stimulation, imitation, and phonetic placement cues, to reach the target production. Descriptions of other ways to elicit various sounds are provided in Appendix B and are frequently discussed on the Internet phonology listserv (www.phonologicaltherapy@yahoogroups.com) or refer to Secord, Boyce, Donahue, Fox, and Shine (2007).

4. *Contextual utilization.* Another procedure used to establish a sound involves isolating a target sound from a particular phonetic context in which a client may happen to produce a sound correctly, even though he or she typically produces the sound in error. As indicated in Chapter 5, correct sound productions can sometimes be elicited through contextual testing since sounds are affected by phonetic and positional context, and some contexts may facilitate the correct production of a particular sound. In Chapter 5, contextual testing was recommended for some clients selected for remediation. The intent of such testing is to identify environments where correct production of target behaviors occurs.

Correct consonant productions may occasionally be observed in clusters even when absent in singletons. Therefore, clusters should be included in contextual testing. Curtis and Hardy (1959) reported that more correct responses of /r/ were elicited in consonant clusters than in consonant singletons. Williams (1991) reported when teaching /s/ in clusters, the sound generalized to /s/ in singletons, which is consistent with the notion that teaching sounds in more complex contexts will generalize to less complex contexts. Hodson (2007b) supports this idea by suggesting the targeting of /s/ in clusters during treatment has the potential to facilitate widespread change within a child's phonological system. If a context can be found in which the target behavior is produced correctly, it can be used to facilitate correct production in other contexts.

Procedures for Teaching Sounds through Context Utilization

If /s/ is produced correctly in the context of the word-pair "bright sun," the /t/ preceding the /s/ may be viewed as a facilitating context.

a. Ask the client to say *bright sun* slowly and prolong the /s/. Demonstrate what you mean by saying the two words and extending the duration of /s/ (e.g., *bright— ssssssssun*).
b. Next ask the client to repeat *bright—ssssssink*, then *hot—ssssssea*. Other facilitating pairs may be used to extend and stabilize the /s/ production.
c. Ask the client to just say /s/ without the "lead-in."

Using phonetic/linguistic context as a method to establish a sound allows the clinician to capitalize on a behavior that may already be in the client's repertoire. This procedure also represents a form of shaping, because one is using context to help the client isolate and stabilize production of an individual phoneme.

Establishment Guidelines

Individual variations among clients preclude a detailed set of specific instructions applicable to all clients; however, the following are general guidelines for establishment:

1. Perceptual training, particularly contrast training employing minimal pairs, is suggested as part of establishment when there is evidence that the client is unable to perceive appropriate phonologic contrasts or that the error pattern is based on a phonologic rule.

2. When teaching production of a target sound, look for the target sound in the client's response repertoire through stimulability (imitation) testing, contextual testing (including consonant clusters, other word positions, and phonetic contexts), and observation of a connected speech sample. Our recommended hierarchy for eliciting sounds that cannot be produced on demand is (a) imitation (verbal stimulation), (b) phonetic placement, (c) successive approximation (shaping), and (d) contextual utilization. Stabilize correct productions and use them as a starting point for more complex linguistic units and contexts.

BEYOND TEACHING SOUNDS: TREATMENT APPROACHES WITH A MOTOR EMPHASIS

Traditional Approach

Teaching a sound may be the first step in intervention, but correction of phonologic errors involves stages of the treatment continuum that go beyond establishment. Several treatment approaches are designed to move a client through a multistep process toward correct production of target sounds. The *traditional approach* to articulation therapy was formulated during the early decades of the 1900s by pioneering clinicians of the field. By the late 1930s, Charles Van Riper had assimilated these treatment techniques into an overall plan for treating articulation disorders and published them in his text titled *Speech Correction: Principles and Methods* (originally published in 1939 and modified in subsequent editions). As an outgrowth of his writings, the traditional approach is sometimes referred to as the "Van Riper method."

The traditional approach is motor oriented and was developed at a time when those receiving treatment were typically school-age clients, often with residual errors. At that time, clinicians were seeing few children with language disorders and caseloads included more children with mild disorders than at present. However, the traditional approach was successfully used with clients representing a range of severity. The traditional approach to articulation therapy is still widely used and is appropriate for individuals with residual errors that typically are articulatory in nature.

The traditional approach progresses from the speaker's identification of error productions to the establishment of correct productions, and then moves on to generalization and finally to maintenance. As Van Riper and Emerick (1984) stated:

> The hallmark of traditional articulation therapy lies in its sequencing of activities for (1) sensory-perceptual training, which concentrates on identifying the standard sound and discriminating it from its error through scanning and comparing; (2) varying and correcting the various productions of the sound until it is produced correctly; (3) strengthening and stabilizing the correct production; and finally (4) transferring the new speech skill to everyday communication situations. This process is usually carried out first for the standard sound in isolation, then in the syllable, then in a word, and finally in sentences. (p. 206)

A characteristic of this approach is its emphasis on perceptual training. During this part of therapy, the client is not required to produce the sound, but rather, instruction is designed to provide a perceptual standard by which the client can contrast his or her own productions. Thus, perceptual training becomes a precursor to production training. Procedures for doing perceptual training were presented earlier in this chapter in our discussion of methods for teaching sounds and will not be repeated here.

The primary ingredient of traditional instruction is production training, with the focus on helping a client learn to produce a sound on demand. Production training usually includes four sequential instructional phases wherein a target sound is (1) produced in isolation (the target sound is elicited in isolation or, in the case of stops and certain glides, in a CV context such as /pa/; (2) produced in syllables (the sound is produced in CV, VC, and VCV syllables); (3) produced in words (the target sound is produced in a word or lexical context in initial, final, and medial positions); and (4) produced in increasingly complex syntactic utterances (i.e., phrases, sentences, conversational speech).

Instructional Steps for Traditional Production Training (Secord, 1989; Van Riper and Erickson, 1996)

1. *Isolation.* The first step in the traditional method is to teach a client to produce a sound in isolation. An explanation for beginning with production of the target sound in isolation is the assumption that the articulatory gestures of a sound are most easily learned when the sound is highly identifiable and in the least complex context. The goal at this level is to develop a consistently correct response. Specific techniques for teaching sounds were discussed earlier and are included in Appendix B. It should be pointed out that training should begin at whatever level of sound complexity a child can produce—isolation, sound clusters, syllables, or words.

2. *Nonsense syllables.* The second step involves teaching the client to produce a sound in a syllable. The goal at this step is consistently correct productions in a variety of nonsense syllable contexts. A suggested sequence for syllable practice is CV, VC, VCV, and CVC. It is also suggested that the transition from the consonant to the vowel should be accomplished with sounds that are similar in place of articulation. For example, an alveolar consonant such as /s/ should be facilitated in a high front vowel context, as in [si]. The clinician might also wish to use the target sound in nonsense clusters.

3. *Words.* The third step involves having a client produce a sound in meaningful units—that is, words. This step begins once the client can consistently produce the target sound in nonsense syllables. Instructions at this level should begin with monosyllabic words, with the target consonant (assuming instruction is focusing on consonants as opposed to vowels) in the prevocalic position (CV). Instruction then moves to VC, CVC, CVCV, monosyllabic words with clusters, followed by more complex word forms. Table 7.1 reflects a hierarchy of phoneme production complexity at the word level as presented by Secord (1989).

   Once a core group of words is established in which the client is readily able to produce the target sound, the clinician seeks to expand the small set of core words to a somewhat larger set of training words. Usually target words are selected on the basis of meaningfulness to the client (e.g., family names, places, social expressions, words from the academic curriculum), but other factors such as phonetic context and syllable complexity should also be taken into consideration, just as they were for the initial set of core words.

■ **TABLE 7.1**   Substages of Word Level Stabilization Training

Substage	Syllables	Examples for /s/
1. Initial prevocalic words	1	*sun, sign, say*
2. Final postvocalic words	1	*glass, miss, pass*
3. Medial intervocalic words	2	*kissing, lassie, racer*
4. Initial blends/clusters	1	*star, spoon, skate*
5. Final blends/clusters	1	*lost, lips, rocks*
6. Medial blends/clusters	2	*whisper, outside, ice-skate*
7. All word positions	1–2	(any of the above)
8. All word positions	any	*signaling, eraser, therapist*
9. All word positions; multiple targets	any	*necessary, successful*

Source: Secord (1989).

4. *Phrases.* Once the client can easily produce a target sound in words, instruction shifts from single-word productions to practicing a target sound in two- to four-word phrases. This level of production represents a complexity level between single words and sentence-level productions. This is especially true if carrier phrases are employed. *Carrier phrases* are phrases where only a single word is changed with each repetition (e.g., I see the *car*; I see the *cup*; I see the *cane*.). In phrase-level productions, one should begin with phrases where only one word contains the target sound. As the client produces a target sound in a single word, the clinician may wish to add a second word in the phrase that contains the target sound.

5. *Sentences.* An extension of phrase-level productions is sentence-level practice. Just as practice at other levels has involved careful sequencing of task complexity, this principle also holds at this level. Consideration should be given to factors such as phonetic context, syllable structure of words, and number of words in the sentence. The following sequence of sentence levels is suggested:

    a. Simple short sentence with one instance of the target sound.
    b. Sentences of various lengths with one instance of the target sound.
    c. Simple short sentences with two or more instances of the target sound.
    d. Sentences of various lengths with two or more instances of the target sound.

6. *Conversation.* The final step in production training involves using a target sound in everyday speech. At this point, the clinician is seeking to facilitate generalization of productions that have already proceeded through more structured production tasks. Initially, generalization situations are structured so that the client produces his or her sound correctly in situations where the speech is monitored. Activities such as role playing, talking about future plans, attempting to get information, interviewing, and oral reading can be used at this level. Following structured conversations, subsequent activities are more spontaneous and free and sometimes characterized as "off-guard" type conversations. The intent is to provide activities to facilitate transfer that approximates real-life situations. Activities should include speaking situations where the client focuses not on self-monitoring but on what he or she says. Telling personal experiences, talking about

topics that evoke strong feelings, and taking part in group discussions are used at this stage of instruction. Some clinicians include "negative practice" to help to stabilize a new response. In negative practice, a client deliberately produces a target sound incorrectly and then contrasts it to a correct production; Van Riper and Erickson (1996) stated that such deliberate productions of error sounds increased the rate of learning.

At this point, the clinician also seeks to facilitate the carryover of conversation to situations beyond the therapy environment. It is suggested that such situational generalization be encouraged once the client can produce a target sound at the word level. By encouraging transfer in earlier stages of instruction, it is assumed that generalization beyond the word level will be significantly enhanced and will perhaps decrease the amount of time needed at the phrase, sentence, and conversational levels.

Summary of the Traditional Approach

Background Statement. The underlying assumptions of the traditional approach to remediation include the following: (1) Faulty perception of speech sounds may be related to speech sound errors and (2) speech sound errors may be viewed as an inadequate motor production of speech sounds. Thus, the traditional approach relies heavily on motor production practice combined with activities related to discrimination/perceptual training.

Unique Features. The traditional approach to articulation remediation, until the 1980s, constituted the basic methodology employed by most clinicians for instruction and treatment of speech sound errors and is still widely used today. The traditional method focuses on motor learning of individual speech sounds. The approach provides a complete instructional sequence for correcting articulatory errors. It can be modified to fit the needs of clients of all ages. Perceptual training is recommended as a precursor to or an accompaniment of direct work on sounds.

Strengths and Limitations. This approach has been widely used over time and forms the basis of several current treatment approaches. Its widespread usage is likely related to the logical sequence of training tasks, the success that accrues through motor practice, and the adaptability and applicability of the approach. It may not, however, be the most efficacious approach for clients with multiple errors.

Research Support. This approach has stood the test of time because it has "worked" for many clinicians, with many clients. Many investigators have reported phonological change in association with intervention that has been based on this approach; however, comparative studies between the "traditional approach" and others are limited. The emphasis on external discrimination training as part of the treatment process for all children has been questioned because of the difficulty involved in separating discrimination training and production training, as well as the lack of data to support its effectiveness. The traditional approach is appropriate for the treatment of clients who have a limited number of errors that are articulatory based. Elements of this approach (e.g., increasing the linguistic complexity of the training tasks by moving from words to phrases and sentences; perceptual training; auditory bombardment/auditory stimulation) are also utilized in many linguistic approaches to remediation.

Context Utilization Approaches

Contextual or sensory-motor based approaches to intervention have been advocated by some clinical phonologists (McDonald, 1964a; Hoffman, Schuckers, and Daniloff, 1989). Treatment suggestions related to these approaches are based on the recognition that speech sounds are not produced in isolation, but rather in syllable-based contexts, and that certain phonetic contexts may be facilitative of correct sound usage. McDonald suggested that instruction for articulatory errors be initiated in a context(s) where the error sound can be produced correctly. He provided an example of a child with a /s/ distortion who produced [s] correctly in the context of *watchsun*. He suggested the following sequence of instructions after *watchsun* was identified as a context where /s/ was correctly produced: (1) Say *watchsun* with "slow-motion" speed; (2) say *watchsun* with equal stress on both syllables, then with primary stress on the first syllable, and then with primary stress on the second syllable; (3) say *watchs* and prolong [s] until a signal is given to complete the bisyllable with [ʌn]; (4) say short sentences with the same facilitating context such as "Watch, sun will burn you." The sequence is repeated with other sentences and stress patterns. The meaningfulness of the sentence is not important since the primary focus of the activity is the movement sequences.

Following the above steps, the client is instructed to alter the movement patterns associated with the correct /s/ by changing the vowel following the segment in a suggested sequence such as:

watch-sun	*watch-sat*
watch-sea	*watch-soon*
watch-sit	*watch-sew*
watch-send	*watch-saw*

The next step is to practice words that include a second context using words like *teach, reach, pitch, catch,* and *beach* that would be used in combination with one-syllable words beginning with /s/ and followed by a variety of vowels (such as *sand, sun, said,* and *soon*). Various sound combinations are practiced with different rates and stress patterns and should eventually be practiced in sentence contexts.

Hoffman and associates (1989) described another variation of a contextual approach that involves a sequenced set of production-based training tasks designed to facilitate the automatization of articulator performance. The basic assumption behind their suggestions is that "revision of over learned, highly automatic behavior is possible through carefully planned and executed performance rehearsal" (p. 248). Intervention is seen as involving instruction and practice of motor articulatory adjustments to replace previously learned (incorrect) productions. The paragraphs that follow present the sequence of tasks and instructional activities these authors suggest.

Prior to working directly on error targets, the clinician elicits, via imitation, sound segments that the client can produce correctly. Such "stimulability tasks" provide the client with an opportunity to experience success in a speech task as well as the opportunity to observe and imitate the clinician's productions. It is suggested that the clinician not only model the correct form of sounds in the child's repertoire but also distort such productions through excessive movements (e.g., lip rounding for /m, p, f/) for the purpose of giving the client the opportunity to practice manipulation of the articulators in response to the clinician's model. Such activity will hopefully facilitate the client's skill at identifying, comparing, and discriminating the clinician's and his or her own sound productions.

Following stimulability tasks, the client needs to learn the articulatory adjustments necessary for correct target sound production. It is suggested that the clinician be able to repeat sentences using error productions similar to those of the client in order to be aware of the motoric acts involved in the client's misarticulations. The emphasis at this point is on doing interesting things with the speech mechanism (e.g., view their productions in the mirror or listen to recordings of themselves).

Rehearsal involves four levels of complexity: nonsymbolic units, words and word pairs, rehearsal sentences, and narratives. Once the narrative level is reached, rehearsal can include a mixture of the four levels.

Practice with *nonsense syllables* provides practice with articulatory gestures that were begun during pretraining. Nonsymbolic instruction focuses on target productions in VC, CV, VCV, and VCCV syllables. It is asserted that production of nonsymbolic units imposes minimal constraints on the speaker by allowing him or her to focus on the speech task rather than morphology, syntax, and semantics. Table 7.2 reflects nonsymbolic sound unit rehearsal matrices. The authors suggest that motoric success at this rudimentary level facilitates success at more linguistically and socially complex levels.

TABLE 7.2 Nonsymbolic Sound Unit Rehearsal Matrices

V	C		V	C	V		C	V		V	C	C	V
i	s		i	s	i		s	i		i	t	s	i
a	s		i	s	a		s	a		i	t	s	a
u	s		i	s	u		s	u		i	t	s	u
æ	s		i	s	æ		s	æ		i	t	s	æ
			a	s	i					a	t	s	i
			a	s	a					a	t	s	a
			a	s	u					a	t	s	u
			a	s	æ					a	t	s	æ
			u	s	i					u	t	s	i
			u	s	a					u	t	s	a
			u	s	u					u	t	s	u
			u	s	æ					u	t	s	æ
			æ	s	i					æ	t	s	i
			æ	s	a					æ	t	s	a
			æ	s	u					æ	t	s	u
			æ	s	æ					æ	t	s	æ

Word and word-pair practice is the next step in the program. Initial targets should reflect a transition from nonsymbolic units to meaningful units that encompass the nonsymbolic syllables already practiced. Practice activities at this level are designed to encourage the client to assume responsibility for recognizing and judging the adequacy of his or her performance. Table 7.3 reflects a list of words and word-pairs by word-position that might be used at this level.

The next step in the program involves *rehearsal sentences*. At this stage, the client repeats the clinician's model of sentences that includes words practiced at the word level followed by practice on a word containing the target segment and then embedding it in a spontaneously generated sentence.

The final step in this program involves using a target sound in *narratives* that can be illustrated, acted out, or read. A series of clinician-generated narratives are employed—for example, for a preschool client, "This is Poky the turtle. Today is his birthday. He is 6 years old. He says, 'It's my birthday.' What does he say?" This is followed by the client saying "It's my birthday." Through such narratives, practice of the target sound is embedded in communicative tasks. The clinician may have a client practice individual sentences from these narratives for additional practice at the sentence level.

Although this program has been presented as a series of steps or levels, the authors point out that these steps should overlap. Throughout the program the client is the primary judge of adequacy of productions, describing the movement patterns and articulatory contacts.

Summary of Contextually Based Approaches

Background Statement.   The theoretical concept underlying contextual approaches is that articulatory errors can be corrected by extensive motor practice of articulatory behaviors, with syllabic units as a basic building block for later motor practice at more complex levels. To employ this approach, a sound must be in the client's repertoire.

Unique Features.   The emphasis on imitated, repetitive productions is a unique aspect of this approach. The systematic variation of phonetic contexts in productions of both sounds produced correctly and error sounds targeted for remediation sets this approach apart from others. A major value of context testing is to identify contexts that may be useful in therapy.

TABLE 7.3   Word and Word-Pair List for [s]

Prevocalic		Intervocalic	Postvocalic	
Initial	**Cluster**	**Medial**	**Final**	**Word-Pair**
Sam	scat	passing	pass	Jack sat
seed	ski	receive	niece	jeep seat
soup	scooter	loosen	loose	room soon
saw	scar	bossy	toss	cop saw
sit	skit	kissing	miss	lip sip
sign	sky	nicer	mice	right side

Strengths and Limitations.   A major strength of this approach is that it builds on behaviors (segmental productions in particular phonetic contexts) that are in a client's repertoire and capitalizes on syllables plus auditory, tactile, and kinesthetic awareness of motor movements. It may be particularly useful for clients who use a sound inconsistently and need methodology to facilitate consistent production in other contexts. The concept of syllable practice and systematic variation of phonetic contexts and stress may be useful to any training method that includes syllable productions.

Research Support.   Contextual testing, designed to locate facilitating contexts, can be used with clients who have difficulty with stimulability. Published clinical investigations that provide support for the efficacy of using a context facilitation approach to intervention are lacking.

Summary of Motor Approaches to Remediation

The treatment approaches described on the previous pages focus on the development and habituation of the motor skills necessary for target sound productions, with the traditional approach to remediation forming the basis of these approaches. An underlying assumption is that motor practice leads to generalization of correct productions to untrained contexts and to automatization of behaviors. Motor approaches to remediation are especially appropriate for phonetically based errors but are frequently employed in combination with procedures that will later be described under linguistic-based approaches.

Remediation Guidelines for Motor Approaches

1. A motor approach to remediation is recommended as a teaching procedure for clients who evidence motor production problems with individual segments such as /s/, /l/, /r/, and other residual errors. It can also be incorporated into treatment programs for clients reflecting linguistic or pattern-based errors, especially if the patterns reflect motor constraints (e.g., prevocalic voicing or certain cluster simplifications). Instruction should be initiated at the linguistic unit level (isolation, syllable, word) at which a client can produce target sounds.
2. Perceptual training, especially contrast training, is recommended as part of a motor remediation program, especially for those clients who evidence perceptual problems related to their error sounds.
3. Addressing multiple errors in a given treatment session (i.e., horizontal and cyclical approaches) is recommended for clients with multiple errors.

Core Vocabulary Approach

The core vocabulary approach targets children with severe but inconsistent speech sound production (i.e., different sound substitutions across productions and ≥ 40 percent variable productions) (Dodd, Crosbie, and Holm, 2004). The researchers classify children with "inconsistent speech disorders" as one of four subgroups of children with speech sound disorders. These children have speech characterized by variable productions of words or variable phonological features across contexts and also within the same context. The researchers hypothesize that the reason for such children's unstable phonological system reflects a deficit in phonological planning (i.e., phoneme selection and sequencing). They differentiate this subgroup of children with inconsistent speech sound disorders from childhood apraxia of speech (CAS), although inconsistency is present in both types of disorders. Dodd and colleagues state that the core vocabulary approach is "the treatment of choice" for children with inconsistent speech sound productions who may be resistant to contrast treatment or traditional therapy. They suggest that core vocabulary treatment results in a systemwide change by improving the consistency of whole-word production and addressing speech processing deficits.

The core vocabulary procedure includes the following steps:

1. The child, parents, and teacher select a list of approximately 50 words that are "functionally powerful" for the child and that includes names (family, friends, teachers, pets), places (*school, library, shops, toilet*), function words (*please, sorry, thank you*), foods (*drinks, soda, hamburger, cereal*), and the child's favorite things (*games, Batman, sports*). Words are chosen because they are used frequently in the child's functional communication.

2. Each week 10 of the functional 50 words are selected for treatment. The clinician teaches the child his or her best production using cues or teaching the word sound-by-sound. If the child is unable to produce a correct production of the word, developmental errors are permissible. The child is required to practice the 10 words during the week and at the therapy sessions with a high number of responses per session. Teachers and parents are to reinforce and praise the child for "best" word production in communication situations. The intent is to make sure the 10 words are said the same way each time rather than to target correct productions. If a child produces a word different from his or her best production, the clinician would imitate the word and explain that the word was said differently and how it differed from the best production. However, the clinician does not ask the child to imitate the target word but rather provides information about the best production, because when a child imitates "it doesn't require the child to use [his or her] own phonological plan."

3. At the end of the weekly sessions (twice weekly), the child is asked to produce the words three times. Words produced consistently are then removed from the list of 50 words. Inconsistently produced words remain on the list and the next week's words are randomly chosen from the 50-word list. Once every two weeks, untreated words from the 50-word list are selected as probe words. The probe words are elicited three times each to monitor generalization.

Crosbie, Holm, and Dodd (2005) reported on a study comparing treatment using a phonological contrast approach to treatment with a core vocabulary treatment approach. Eighteen children ages 4;8 to 6;5 with severe speech disorders received two 8-week blocks of both of the intervention treatments. All of the children increased their accuracy of production of consonants (PCC) as well as their consistency of the production. They reported that core vocabulary intervention resulted in more change in children with "inconsistent" speech sound disorders and that the "contrast therapy" resulted in greater changes in children with "consistent" speech disorders.

■ LINGUISTIC-BASED APPROACHES TO INTERVENTION

A second category of treatment approaches to disordered speech is linguistic or phonologically based instruction. Whereas motor approaches may be described as phonetically based and focus on teaching sounds one at a time, linguistic approaches are focused more on teaching sound contrasts and appropriate phonological patterns in children with multiple errors. As such, linguistic-based intervention focuses on strategies for reorganizing the child's phonological system. Although a linguistic-based approach is most suitable for children with multiple speech sound errors, elements of the approach can be and continue to be used in combination with more traditional or motor-based approaches.

The primary focus of linguistic approaches to remediation is the establishment of adult phonological rules in a client's repertoire (e.g., distinctive features, contrast rules, and phonotactic rules). Treatment programs designed to facilitate acquisition of linguistic rules are not associated with a single unified method; however, two primary characteristics are associated with linguistically oriented phonological approaches. The first characteristic relates to the behaviors targeted for treatment, the second to the instructional procedures themselves.

As discussed in Chapter 5, selection of target behaviors is based on phonological errors as they relate to patterns that may describe the errors. Following pattern or phonological process identification, individual sound(s), called *exemplars*, are chosen that are likely to facilitate generalization from the exemplar to other sounds related to a particular error pattern. Treatment is then designed to facilitate the acquisition of appropriate sound contrasts and/or sequences, with the expectation that generalization will occur to other sounds that are part of the same pattern (e.g., in targeting final consonant deletion, teaching a couple of final consonants is assumed to generalize to other final consonants that are also deleted).

Most treatment protocols that are based on a linguistic model employ minimal contrast word-pairs, which involve minimal or maximal feature contrasts (Weiner, 1981b; Gierut, 1989; Fey, 1992). For example, minimal pairs such as bu*s*-buc*k* and bu*s*-bu*t* represent minimal pairs with greater and lesser contrasts, respectively, because of the differences in place and manner of articulation between /s/ and /k/ (greater differences because of place and manner contrasts), and /s/ and /t/ (because /s/ and /t/ differ only in manner).

The primary focus of linguistic approaches has been to (1) establish sound and feature contrasts and (2) replace error patterns with appropriate phonological patterns. Linguistic approaches have targeted elimination of homonyms (one word used for two referents—for example, *shoe* used for both *chew* and *shoe*), establishment of new syllable and word shapes, and establishment of new sound classes and feature contrasts.

Distinctive Feature Approaches

Distinctive features may be considered subphonemic elements of phonemes that determine the linguistic contrasts between sounds and sound classes. In other words, unique bundles of distinctive features underlie the distinctions among phonemes in a language. For a review of information concerning distinctive features, refer to Chapters 1 and 5.

The intent of instructional programs based on distinctive features is to establish a feature that is lacking in a client's repertoire. For example, lack of frication may describe several sound production errors; for example, the client may use stops for fricatives (e.g., /t/ for /s/). Distinctive feature instructional programs usually focus on the establishment of a particular feature through teaching a sound containing that feature, since features are subphonemic units of sounds and cannot be taught independently. It is then assumed that the newly established feature will generalize from the exemplar sound to other members of the sound class in which the feature may be absent (e.g., + continuant generalizes from target /f/ to /θ/, /s/, and /ʃ/).

McReynolds and Bennett (1972) reported data indicating that features established in one sound (exemplar) will generalize to other sound segments in which the target feature is absent. They inferred from this finding that remediation based on distinctive features should be an efficient treatment approach, since by teaching a feature in one sound you may correct several error sounds. Generalization seems to be significantly influenced by the similarity between the sound selected for training and other error sounds (e.g., sound classes). In general, the more features two sounds share, the more potential there is for generalization to occur from one sound to a second sound. For example, in teaching /s/, one can assume generalization to /z/ and perhaps to other fricatives but not to /r/.

McReynolds and Bennett (1972) described instructional procedures designed to teach a feature contrast that was absent in a child's productive repertoire. In Phase 1, production focused on nonsense syllables that contained the target feature (e.g., + continuant) in the initial position (e.g., *fɑ*). In Phase 2, the child was taught to produce a sound containing the target feature in the final position of a nonsense syllable (e.g., *ɑf*). For example, in phase 1 if [+ continuant] was the feature contained in the first sound taught, [− continuant] might be the feature selected for the second or contrast sound (e.g., [fi] vs. [pi], [fa] vs. [pa], [fʌ] vs. [pʌ], and [fo] vs. [po]). Phase 2 was identical except for the position of the target sound. In the example above, the child used stops instead of fricatives/continuants (e.g., *fun* was said *tun; show* was said *toe*, etc.). In Phase 1, the client was taught the continuant /f/ and then was taught to produce it in the initial position of a nonsense syllable (e.g., fi, fæ, fa, fo). Step 2 focused on having the child produce pairs of nonsense syllables that reflected the + continuant/− continuant contrast (e.g., *fɑ-pɑ; fi-pi*). In Phase 2, the two steps were repeated except /f/ was taught in the final position (e.g., *af; af-if*).

Blache (1989) published a distinctive feature approach to remediation of phonological delay. The approach is organized into four basic steps:

Step 1. Discussion of words. Determine whether the child knows the meaning of lexical items (words) to be used in therapy. Once a minimal pair contrast has been selected to teach a distinctive feature, it is important to determine if the child understands both lexical items in the word-pair. For example, if the word-pair selected is the letter *T* and the word *key*, the child might be asked: "Which one opens the door? Which one is a letter of the alphabet? Which one goes into a lock? Which one do you write?" (See Figure 7.1.)

Step 2. Discrimination testing and training. The child is tested to determine if he or she can perceive the feature contrast. The clinician presents one word of a minimal pair, for example, *fan-pan* or *bear-pear*. The child is instructed to point to the picture that the clinician has named. A criterion of seven consecutive correct responses is used to determine that the child perceived the contrasting word-pairs.

■ **FIGURE 7.1** Exemplars illustrating six different distinctive features contrasts.

Step 3. Production training. After the client has demonstrated that he or she perceives the minimal contrast, the next step is to establish the feature in a production task. In this step, the child is instructed to say the word and the clinician points to the picture of the word the client pronounced. The client should always be able to correctly pronounce one word of the pair but may not be able to pronounce the other member of the word-pair; thus, a correct production of an error sound may not be required at this stage. Production training continues until the client can use the target feature in a correct production of a target sound.

Step 4. Carryover training. Once the child is able to pronounce the target word, the word is placed in longer and more complex linguistic environments. The word is used with the indefinite article *a* in varied phonetic contexts, two-word expressions, three-word carrier phrases, and so on, until the word is used in meaningful social situations in the school and home.

Blache (1989) recommended a sequence of feature comparisons that were hypothesized as successive steps from larger to finer contrasts. An example of a suggested sequence for the stop-nasal sound class is presented in Table 7.4.

An example of a distinctive feature program designed to teach + frication was presented by Weiner and Bankson (1978) and is presented here:

1. Introduction of the concept of "dripping" sounds (stops) and "flowing" sounds (fricatives).
2. Identification of words that begin with dripping as compared to flowing sounds.
3. Imitation of words containing fricatives in the initial position, with such fricatives emphasized through prolongation of initial sound (e.g., *f-f-f-f*ish). Following his or her production, the client was required to judge whether the word began with a dripping (e.g., /k/) or flowing (e.g., /f/) sound. Feedback was provided for both production and identification.
4. Repetition of Step 3 without exaggeration of the word-initial fricative.
5. Presentation of a 20-item picture-naming task in which each item began with a fricative.

These investigators reported that as a result of this instructional program, a subject who used stops for fricatives learned to use fricatives in single-word responses.

Summary of Distinctive Feature Approaches

Background Statement. Distinctive feature approaches to phonological remediation are based on the theory that speech sounds are comprised of bundles of features, each phoneme having a unique and individual set of features that characterize segmental productions. Further, if a client has several sounds in error, an efficient instructional strategy may be to identify or teach an exemplar that contains the absent feature(s), and monitor generalization from that exemplar to other sounds containing the same feature(s) that is in error.

■ **TABLE 7.4** Contrast Ordering for Stop-Nasal Sound Class

No.	Pair	Feature	Sample Words
1.	[t-k]	front-back lingual	*tea-key, tape-cape, ten-Ken*
2.	[n-]	front-back lingual	*win-wing, fan-fang, ton-tongue*
3.	[p-b]	voiced-voiceless	*pea-bee, pig-big, pat-bat*
4.	[t-d]	voiced-voiceless	*toe-doe, time-dime, tot-dot*
5.	[k-g]	voiced-voiceless	*curl-girl, coat-goat, cap-gap*
6.	[b-m]	nasal-nonnasal	*beet-meat, bat-mat, bike-Mike*
7.	[d-n]	nasal-nonnasal	*D-knee, deck-neck, dot-knot*
8.	[g-]	nasal-nonnasal	*wig-wing, bag-bang, log-long*
9.	[b-d]	labial-lingual	*big-dig, bark-dark, bow-dough*
10.	[d-g]	front-back lingual	*deer-gear, date-gate, doe-go*

Source: "A Distinctive Feature Approach" by S. E. Blache, in *Assessment and Remediation of Articulatory and Phonological Disorders* (p. 377). N. Creaghead, P. Newman, and W. Secord, eds., Columbus, OH: Charles E. Merrill, 1989.

Unique Features. This approach is designed to capitalize on patterns (features) of commonalities among error productions. Although features are taught in sounds, feature analysis and remediation represent an endeavor to correct several sounds simultaneously by teaching a feature in one target sound with the assumption that it will generalize to other sounds containing the target feature.

Strengths and Limitations. An attraction of therapy based on distinctive features is the targeting of phonological patterns that may underlie several individual errors. A major limitation, as pointed out in earlier discussion, is that distinctive features were not designed for clinical intervention. Rather, features were derived as a classification system in order to describe the sound segments across language systems. As a result, some sounds produced in error by individuals with phonological disorders cannot be described within this framework. The feature classification systems that have been applied clinically tend to be useful for sound substitutions, but difficult to use with sound omissions and distortions. In spite of the fact that distinctive feature approaches are not frequently employed, they encompass the concepts of pattern analyses and treatment focused on linguistic contrasts.

Research Support. Data to support a distinctive feature approach to therapy may be gleaned from studies that have included the treatment approaches described here. McReynolds and Bennett (1972) reported that all three of their subjects reflected distinctive feature generalization from the exemplar sounds to other sounds, although the amount of feature generalization varied across subjects. Similarly, Weiner and Bankson (1978) reported that their subject generalized [+ frication] to nontrained items. Costello and Onstein (1976) reported that their distinctive feature instructional approach was successful in teaching a subject to generalize the [+ continuant] feature. These data support the finding that feature generalization is seen with distinctive feature approaches to remediation. The number of subjects involved in these studies was small, and additional data regarding the efficiency of this approach are needed.

Minimal Pair Contrast Therapy

A signature approach of linguistic-based remediation is *minimal pair contrast therapy.* Contrast therapy employs pairs of words that differ only by a single phoneme (e.g., *bat-pat, move-mood, sun-ton*). As stated earlier, the underlying concept of this type of therapy is that by focusing on word-pairs that typically differ by a single phonemic contrast, the client will be taught that different sounds signal different meanings in words. The phonemic contrasts are related either to feature differences between sounds (e.g., *pat-bat* differ by the voicing feature; *pat-fat* differ by the continuant feature), or syllable shape (e.g., *bow-boat* differ by presence or absence of the final sound; *key-ski* differ by the presence or absence of the initial sound(s) in the syllable initiation—cluster vs. non-cluster). Investigators have reported changes in children's phonological systems (Weiner, 1981; Elbert and Gierut, 1986; Gierut, 1989, 1990; Williams, 1991) following training with word-pair contrasts. Contrast therapy focuses on the establishment of sound contrasts necessary to differentiate one word from another. While this communication-oriented therapy emerged from a linguistic orientation, it is also used in traditional treatment approaches.

An example of a contrast approach to treatment can be observed through remediation strategies employed with a client who deletes final consonants. In this instance, stops may be produced correctly in word-initial position, but deleted in word-final position (lack of syllable closure). In such a circumstance, the clinician can assume that the final consonant deletions are probably not a production (phonetic) problem. Rather, final consonant deletion in this case likely reflects a conceptual rule related to syllable structure (use of the open syllable). Treatment for this rule would focus on getting the client to recognize that the presence of a consonant in word-final position is a necessary contrast to distinguish certain word-pairs in the language (e.g., *two-tooth*; *bee-beet*). In this instance, the motoric production of a target consonant is already within a child's productive repertoire, and thus motor production of the sound is not the focus of instruction. Rather, the focus of instruction is the development of cognitive awareness of final consonant contrasts/syllable closure.

The most commonly employed type of contrast training typically contrasts a substituted or deleted sound with a target sound. For example, if a client substitutes /t/ for /k/ in word-initial position, contrast training words might include *tea-key* and *top-cop*. Similarly, if a child deletes the final /t/, contrast pairs might include *bow-boat* and *see-seat*. Minimal contrast instruction is appropriate when two or more contrasting sounds in the adult language are collapsed into a single sound unit with the result that feature contrasts are not produced (e.g., /t/ replaced /k/), or segments are deleted, such as in final consonant deletions. Training is designed to establish sound contrasts that mark a difference in meaning.

Minimal contrast instruction, as discussed earlier in this chapter, typically focuses first on perception of contrasts and then production of contrasts. A training task that focuses on perceptual training utilizing contrast pairs was first proposed by La Riviere and colleagues (1974). In this procedure, subjects are taught to identify words where the target sounds and errors are presented in word-pairs. For example, if a child deletes /s/ in /s/ clusters (cluster simplification), the clinician names several pictures representing minimal pair words like *spool-pool* or *spill-pill* to the client. The client is then required to pick up items named by the clinician, or perhaps sort each lexical item into one or two categories (/s/ singletons or /s/ clusters).

A production-based task would require the client to produce minimal pairs. For example, a client who deletes final consonants might ask the clinician to give him or her the picture of either a *bee* or a *beet*, then be reinforced by the clinician's response for the appropriate production. In this task, the client must be able to produce the distinction between *bee* and *beet*. As stated earlier, the reverse of this procedure (i.e., the clinician asks the client to give him or her certain pictures) can be used to establish perceptual contrasts (i.e., the distinction between *bee* and *beat*).

Weiner (1981b) reported a study where minimal contrast training was used to reduce the frequency of selected phonological patterns. He used minimal pairs in activities where accurate word productions were required for the child to communicate successfully. For example, Weiner used a game to teach final [t] in a minimal contrast format. He placed into minimal pairs such words as *bow* and *boat*. Sample stimuli consisted of several pictures of *bow* and several pictures of boat. The instructions for the game were as follows:

"We are going to play a game. The object of the game is to get me to pick up all the pictures of the *boat*. Every time you say boat, I will pick one up. When I have all five, you may paste a star on your paper." If the child said *bow*, the clinician picked up the *bow* picture. At times he would provide an instruction, e.g., "You keep saying *bow*. If you want me to pick up the *boat* picture, you must say the [t] sound at the end. Listen, *boat, boat, boat*. You try it. Okay. Let's begin again" (p. 98)

Weiner (1981b) reported that such training established additional phonological contrasts in the child's repertoire and then generalization to nontrained words. A variety of word lists (e.g., Bleile, 1995) and treatment materials (e.g., Bird and Higgins, 1990; Palin, 1992; Price and Scarry-Larkin, 1999), are available commercially to assist clinicians in finding contrasting word pairs and pictures for treatment.

Protocol for Employing a Minimal Pair Training Procedure

1. Select a sound contrast to be trained based on the client's phonological errors. For example, if the child substitutes /t/ for /ʃ/ (stopping), one might select *tea-she, toe-show*, and *tape-shape* as target contrast words reflecting the stopping pattern. Select five pictures for each of the contrast words.
2. Engage the client in minimal contrast training at a perceptual level (e.g., "I want you to pick up the pictures that I name. Pick up _____.").
3. Pretest the client's motor production of each of the target words containing the error sound, and if necessary instruct him or her in production of the target phoneme.
4. Have the client imitatively produce each target word.
5. Engage the client in minimal contrast training at a production level (e.g., "I want you to tell me which picture to pick up. Every time you say *show*, I will pick up this picture").
6. Engage the client in a task that requires him or her to incorporate each of the contrast words in a carrier phrase (e.g., "I want you to point to a picture and name it by saying 'I found a _____' ").
7. Continue the carrier phrase task, incorporating each of the contrasting words into the phrase (e.g., "I found a *tea* and a *she*").

Clinicians can use their creativity and clinical knowledge to modify a protocol such as that just presented. As stated earlier, there are descriptions in the literature of minimal pair treatment approaches as well as several commercially available sets of materials designed to facilitate this treatment approach. It should be mentioned that for those instances where meaningful minimal pairs cannot be found to reflect a particular contrast, "near minimal pairs" are sometimes used (e.g., *van-shan*), wherein one word may not have meaning. In this instance, the clinician may point to an abstract drawing and, as in the example above, say, "This is a *shan*." Thus, the child is taught a nonsense but contrasting word to use in the minimal pair activity.

Thus far we have focused on using minimal pairs that involve error and target sound contrasts. Sometimes minimal pairs involve the target sound and another sound, not necessarily the error production. Often it may be helpful to work on contrasts between the target sound and one or more other sounds which contain several feature differences from the target. When choosing such word pairs, the sound contrasts may represent a minimal or maximal sound opposition. When sound contrasts in minimal pairs contrast by a single feature, this is referred to as *minimal opposition contrasts*. On the other hand, a *maximal opposition contrast* reflects several feature contrasts between a target sound and the second sound. For example, if a child replaces /ʃ/ with /t/, the target words might be *shoe* and *moo* rather than *shoe* and *two*. In this case, /ʃ/ and /m/ are more dissimilar than are /ʃ/ and /t/, and thus the phoneme contrasts reflect a greater number of feature differences (maximal opposition) rather than fewer feature differences (minimal opposition). An underlying assumption of the maximal contrast approach is that phonological oppositions of greater disparity will facilitate more change in the client's acquisition of feature contrasts and the contrast between the word pairs will be more salient and thus easier for the client to perceive. Examples of minimal and maximal oppositions are as follows:

Minimal Oppositions	*Feature Differences*
*s*un—*t*on	manner of production
*th*umb—*s*um	place of production
*ch*ew—*sh*oe	manner of production

Maximal Oppositions	*Feature Differences*
*ch*ain—*m*ain	manner of production, nasality, place of production
*c*an—*m*an	manner of production, nasality, place of production
*g*ear—*f*ear	manner of production, voicing, place of production

The treatment methodologies outlined earlier for minimal contrast therapy are applicable to maximal contrast training.

The use of maximal oppositions is supported by data from Gierut (1989, 1990). Her research indicated that for children with multiple errors, maximal contrast training facilitated a greater overall change in the phonological system than did minimal contrast training. In her research, the sound contrasted to the target sound was a phoneme that was already in the subject's phonological repertoire, not one that had to be taught before being used in the minimal pair. Nonetheless, by focusing on maximal oppositions, greater generalization to other sounds occurred than with minimal opposition minimal pairs. In other studies, where two new target sounds were paired and introduced at the same time (Gierut, 1991, 1992; Gierut and Neumann, 1992), this strategy resulted in more generalization to other sounds than did pairs where the target sound was paired with substitute sound or the target sound with a known sound.

Multiple Oppositions Therapy

A treatment methodology that represents a variation of the minimal contrast approach is the multiple oppositions approach (Williams, 1993, 2000a, 2000b, 2003). *Multiple oppositions* is a treatment approach that simultaneously contrasts several target sounds with a comparison sound. This approach is in contrast to the singular contrastive approach (i.e., including either minimal or maximal oppositions), which addresses sound errors or collapses one at a time. The multiple oppositions approach is designed for children with multiple sound errors characterized by severe to profound phonological impairments.

The underlying premise behind this approach is that multiple errors produced by children evidencing numerous phoneme collapses (i.e., one sound is used in place of two or more other sounds), are best treated with a "systematic" view as opposed to individual sound focus. The goal is to help a child reorganize his or her sound system by focusing on numerous minimal contrast pairs designed to help the child recognize the nature of his or her phoneme collapses. For example, if a child substitutes /t/ in the final word position for each of the following sounds—/k/, /tʃ/, /s/—treatment might focus on contrasting the word *bat* with *back, batch* with *bass, ate* with *ache*, and *H* with *ace*. In these examples, instead of focusing on a single contrast (e.g., *bat-back*), the procedure would use three minimal pair contrasts in the same activity (i.e., *bat-back; bat-batch; bat-bass*). A treatment session might also include instructional activities related to additional phoneme collapses. Lessons are centered on words evidencing "multiple oppositions" related to error targets. Eventually instruction moves from focusing only on contrastive word pairs to using sounds in increasingly complex linguistic structures.

A list of a child's phoneme collapses followed by sets of contrasting training items focusing on multiple oppositions (Williams, 2000a, 2000b) can be found in Figure 7.2.

Data reported by Williams (1993, 2000a, 2000b) indicated that by using the enlarged treatment sets included in the multiple oppositions approach with severely impaired children, clinicians were able to expand the number of phonemic contrasts. She hypothesized that through such an approach, the greatest amount of change will occur in the smallest amount of time with the least effort. Williams (2006) has developed a software program, *Sound Contrasts in Phonology (SCIP)*, that includes contrasting vocabulary items available for multiple oppositions therapy.

Metaphon Therapy

Howell and Dean (1991) indicated that children with phonological disorders who fail to respond well to minimal pair therapy need to be taught the characteristics of sounds as a way to facilitate development of sound contrasts in their phonological repertoire. Instruction is designed to teach the awareness and skills necessary to succeed with minimal pair therapy. It structures treatment to facilitate children's development of metaphonological skills, that is, the ability to pay attention to the phonological structure of language. Investigators have reported that children with phonological disorders do not perform as well as their normal developing peers on metaphonological tasks (Kamhi, Friemoth-Lee, and Nelson, 1985). Metaphon therapy focuses on feature differences between sounds in order to develop an awareness that sounds can be classified by characteristics such as duration *(long-short)*, manner *(noisy-whisper, stopping-flowing)*, and place *(front-back)*.

Therapy begins by teaching these basic concepts, followed by teaching how these concepts apply to sounds in general. Treatment then moves to identifying features across target speech sounds and then focuses on word pairs, which incorporate targeted sound contrasts. The second phase of therapy is designed to transfer the metaphonological knowledge gained in the first phase to communication situations wherein the client must convey his or her intended message through appropriate use of sound contrasts.

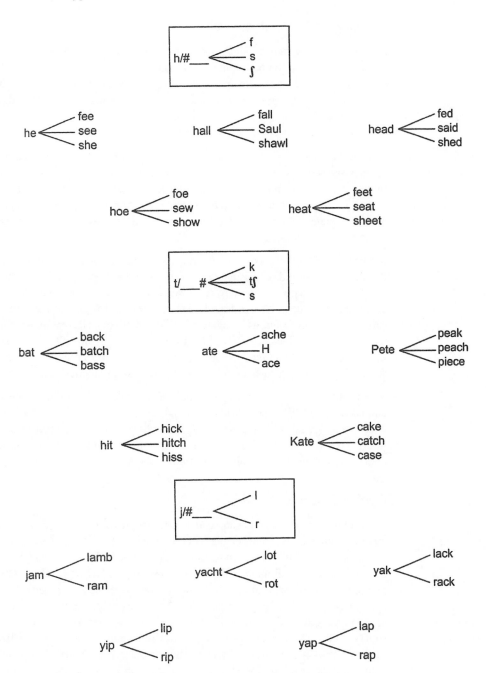

■ **FIGURE 7.2** Phoneme collapses with related minimal pair treatment sets focusing on multiple oppositions.

Summary of Minimal Pair Contrast Training

Background Statement.   The establishment of sound contrasts (contrast training) is a linguistic approach to phonological remediation. Instruction typically involves perceptual and production tasks of word-pairs that reflect phonemic contrasts described as minimal, maximal, or multiple oppositions. Contrast training procedures facilitate the reorganization of the phonological system to reduce the use of phonemic collapses and to establish additional phonemic contrasts and syllable shapes.

Unique Features.   Contrast training can be communication oriented by requiring the listener-speaker to select the appropriate word of the word-pair in order for communication intent to occur. That is, the listener-speaker must perceive and produce a particular phonemic contrast in order to communicate (act or get someone else to act appropriately) with the listener. It is focused on the ways sounds are used in the language (i.e., to signal contrasts in meaning).

Strengths and Limitations.   The approach is designed for clients who collapse sounds and do not contrast sounds consistent with the rules of the language. It is particularly useful with children who evidence numerous misarticulations or phonological rules that are not consistent with the adult standard. It is recommended for use with any client who needs to establish phonemic contrasts, regardless of whether errors have a motor component or not. Clinicians need to have a plan for fitting contrast training in with other treatment activities, including practice with increasingly complex linguistic utterances. Contrasting word-pairs can be focused on a single sound contrast pair or simultaneously on multiple contrasts.

Research Support.   Data to support the efficacy of contrast training are available (Ferrier and Davis, 1973; Weiner, 1981; Elbert and Gierut, 1986; Gierut, 1989, 1990, 1991, 1992; Gierut and Neumann, 1992; Williams, 1993, 2000a, 2000b). It is anticipated that research in this area will be ongoing and will assist in developing a stronger theoretical base for understanding and treating phonological disorders.

Cycles Approach

The cycles approach (Hodson and Paden, 1991) represents a linguistic approach designed for children with multiple sound errors. This approach targets deficient phonological patterns for instruction, uses sounds to teach appropriate phonological patterns, and moves through these targets in a sequential manner that is not based on a criterion level of performance before moving onto another sound and/or pattern. The cycles approach helps children to acquire appropriate phonological patterns, rather than focusing on helping children eliminate inappropriate patterns or deviations. The procedures followed in a cycles approach treatment session typically include (1) auditory stimulation of a target sound with amplification (the client focuses attention on auditory characteristics on the target sound); (2) production practice (to help the child develop new kinesthetic images); and (3) participation in experiential play activities involving picture and object naming tasks that incorporate the target pattern into word productions. A cycle is completed after a set of targeted patterns (usually three or four patterns per cycle) focusing on targets sounds in words related to each pattern. Subsequent cycles incorporate patterns that are inconsistent with the adult standard.

The remediation plan is organized around treatment cycles that range from 5 to 16 weeks, depending on the client's number of deficient patterns and the number of stimulable phonemes within each pattern. Hodson's (1989, 2007) suggestions for treating behaviors through a cycles approach include the following:

> Each phoneme (or consonant cluster) within a pattern is targeted for approximately 60 minutes per cycle (i.e., one 60-minute, two 30-minute, or three 20-minute sessions) before progressing to the next phoneme in that pattern and then on to other deficient phonological patterns. Within each cycle, a pattern is the focus of instruction for two to four weeks, with a different phoneme targeted each week. Furthermore, it is desirable to provide stimulation for two or more target *phonemes* (in successive weeks) within a pattern before changing to the next target *pattern* (i.e., each deficient phonological pattern is stimulated for two hours or more within each cycle). Only *one* phonological pattern is targeted during a beginning cycles session allowing the child to focus on a specific pattern. Patterns are not intermingled until a child has made progress in therapy and can attend to more than one pattern in a session (e.g., final /k/ in the same session as initial /st/) until the third or fourth cycle.

A cycle is complete when all phonological patterns selected for remediation at a given point in time have been treated. Following completion of one cycle, a second cycle begins that will again cover those patterns not yet emerging and in need of further instruction. Phonological patterns are recycled until the targeted patterns emerge in spontaneous utterances. Hodson (1989) indicated that three to six cycles of phonological remediation, involving 30 to 40 hours of instruction (40 to 60 minutes per week) are usually required for a client with a disordered phonological system to become intelligible.

Hodson recommended that deviations (processes) targeted for remediation should occur in at least 40 percent of the instances in which the opportunity for their occurrence is present in the *Hodson Assessment of Phonological Patterns* (Hodson, 2003). Phonological patterns are targeted for remediation based on the child's "phonological deficiencies" and the patterns on which he or she is stimulable.

An example of target selection and implementation of the cycles approach is the following. If fronting of velars occurs at least 40 percent of the time and if velars are stimulable, the appropriate use of velars could be selected as a target pattern for remediation. Initially, a target velar (e.g., final /k/) would be selected as an instructional target and, following the instructional sequence delineated below, activities related to this sound would be focused on for approximately one hour. Following work on this sound, a second velar (e.g., initial /g/) could be targeted. Following work on this pattern, a second pattern would be selected as part of this cycle (e.g., /s/ clusters).

Hodson (2007b) has identified "optimal primary target patterns for beginning cycles" and "potential secondary target patterns." The potential primary targets are (1) syllableness (omission of the syllabi nuclei: vowels, diphthongs, vocalic/syllabic consonants); (2) singleton consonants when consistently omitted in a word position (i.e., in CV, VC, CVC, or VCV; (3) /s/ clusters either in word-initial or word-final position; (4) anterior/posterior contrasts where the child either lacks velars or alveolars/labials and either fronts or backs sounds; and (5) liquids /l/, /r/, /kr/, /gr/, and /i/ clusters all in word-initial positions.

Potential secondary target patterns are not targeted until the child has acquired the following patterns in spontaneous speech: (1) syllableness, (2) basic word structure, (3) anterior/posterior contrasts, and (4) some evidence of stridency, suppression of gliding, and substitution for liquids in spontaneous utterances.

Secondary target patterns are (1) palatals (i.e., /j/, /t/, /ʒ /, /tʃ/, /dʒ/), /ɚ/, /ɝ/, and word-medial /r/; (2) other consonant sequences (some which may be primary targets, such as /s/ cluster in word final position, /s/ plus stop in word-medial position (basket), glide clusters (tw, kj), liquid clusters /tr/, and CCC /skw, skr/; and (3) singleton stridents, such as /f, s/, voicing contrasts (prevocalic, vowel contrasts, assimilations, and any other deviations).

Hodson also recommends against targeting the following in preschool children: voiced-final obstruents /b, d, g, v, z, ð, ʒ, dʒ/, post vocalic /l/, word-final /ɴ/, unstressed syllables, and /θ, ð/.

The instructional sequence for each session is as follows:

1. *Review.* At the beginning of each session, the prior week's production practice word cards are reviewed.

2. *Listening activity.* This step requires listening for about 30 seconds while the clinician reads approximately 20 words containing the target pattern. This auditory stimulation is done at the beginning and end of each session using two different word lists and includes the use of amplification (mild gain assistive listening device). The clinician may also demonstrate the error and contrast it with the target.

3. *Target word cards.* The client draws, colors, or pastes pictures of three to five carefully selected based on phonetic environment target words for the lesson on 5" × 8" index cards. The name of the picture is written on each card and the child says each word prior to it being selected as a target word to evaluate it for difficulty.

4. *Production practice.* The client participates in experiential play production practice activities. The client is expected to have a very high success rate in terms of correct productions. Shifting activities every 5 to 7 minutes helps to maintain a child's interest in production practice. The client is also given the opportunity to use target words in conversation. Production practice incorporates auditory, tactual, and visual stimulation and cues as needed for correct production at the word level. Usually, five words per target sound are used in a single session. The client must produce the target pattern in words in order to get his or her turn in the activity.

5. *Stimulability probing.* The target phoneme in the next session for a given pattern is selected based on stimulability probing (checking to see what words a child can imitate), which occurs at this point in the treatment session.

6. *Listening activity.* Auditory bombardment with amplification is repeated, using the word list from the beginning of the session.

7. *Phonological awareness activities.* Activities such as rhyming and syllable segmentation are incorporated for a few minutes each session as many of these children with speech sound disorders are "at risk" for later developing literacy skills. See Chapter 9 for a review of the relationship among children with speech sound disorders, phonological awareness skills, and literacy skills.

8. *Home program.* Parents are instructed to read a word list to the child and then the child names the words on the picture cards used in the auditory bombardment/simulation task to the child at least once a day. The five cards used during the session for production practice are also sent home for the child to practice daily. This activity should only take about 2 minutes each day.

The client is not required to meet a criterion level prior to moving on to treatment of other patterns within a cycle. When patterns persist, they are recycled for treatment at a later time.

Summary of Cycles Approach

Background Statement. The cycles approach is based on the phenomenon of gradualness (moving ahead, recycling, moving ahead) as observed in normal phonological acquisition. The emphasis on acquisition of phonological patterns stems from a linguistic perspective of phonological behavior. Production practice of target sounds along with auditory stimulation (listening tasks) reflect aspects of a more traditional approach to intervention.

Unique Features. The most distinctive feature of this approach is its focus on shifting and cycling of remediation targets and the fact that a phoneme related to a particular pattern is focused on for a given length of time rather than a set criterion level of performance, with a new target being worked on after an hour of instructional time. Focusing on pattern acquisition rather than on elimination of inappropriate patterns is a developmentally sound way to conceptualize intervention.

Strengths and Limitations. The attributes identified above are all strengths of this approach. Although it was designed for unintelligible children, aspects of this approach can be used with less severely impaired clients. The cycles approach has been adapted for use with children with cleft palate (Hodson, Chin, Redmond, and Simpson, 1983), developmental dyspraxia (Hodson and Paden, 1991), and recurrent otitis media and hearing impairments (Gordon-Brannan, Hodson, and Wynne, 1992), as well as developmental delay.

Research Support. The authors have a wealth of clinical experience to support this approach to intervention and report good success with unintelligible children. This approach, like many others, represents a composite or "package" of various instructional components. However, it has seen widespread adoption among clinicians for unintelligible and phonologically delayed children.

Teaching Phonology through Broader-Based Language Approaches

Children with severe phonologic disorders frequently have difficulty with other aspects of language (Camarata and Schwartz, 1985; Panagos and Prelock, 1982; Hoffman et al., 1989; Paul and Shriberg, 1982; Fey, Cleave, Ravida, Long, Dejmal, and Easton, 1994; Tyler, Lewis, Haskill, and Tolbert, 2002; Tyler and Watterson, 1991). The relationship between phonology and morphosyntax has been shown to be strong, and this relationship impacts clinical practice. Impairments of phonology that coexist with other language impairments suggest that many children have a generalized difficulty in the language learning process. Although the precise nature of the relationship between phonology and other aspects of language is unknown, it has been suggested that phonologic delay, especially when it coincides with other language impairments, can be at least partially remediated by employing a language-based intervention approach (Gray and Ryan, 1973; Matheny and Panagos, 1978; Hoffman, Norris, and Monjure, 1990; Tyler et al., 2002). Hoffman and colleagues (1990) stated that research continues to show that higher level language organization has an effect upon sound production. As a result of this finding, they suggest that remediation of speech disorders outside of a more generalized context of language development may not be the most efficacious way to treat children with speech sound disorders

Others have indicated that the efficacy of a language-based approach to treating phonological disorders may be related to the degree of severity of the phonological impairment (Fey et al., 1994; Tyler and Watterson, 1991), although results reported by Tyler and colleagues (2002) did not support this view. However, many clinicians use a language-based approach to remediation for children with mild phonological problems and language delay/disorders, while for those with more severe phonological disorders, instruction may need to be focused specifically on phonology as well as the language problem. It may be that as children with severe phonological disorders progress in treatment, instruction may be more language based. The following paragraphs delineate possible ways to use language-based therapy to ameliorate a phonological disorder.

Norris and Hoffman (1990) described a storytelling language-based approach to phonologic intervention based on client generation of narratives. Preschool children constructed verbal stories in response to pictures from action-oriented children's stories and shared these with a listener(s). The clinician's primary role was to engage the child in constructing and talking about the pictures. The goal for each child was to produce meaningful linguistic units, syllable shapes, phonemes, and gestures that are shared with a listener. The clinician seeks to expand each child's language-processing ability by asking children to produce utterances that exceed their current level of functioning.

Norris and Hoffman (1990, 2005) believe that language-oriented intervention should be naturalistic and interactive as the clinician seeks to simultaneously improve semantics, syntax, morphology, pragmatics, and phonology since they all are components of language. In such an approach, perceptual and motor cues are embedded within communication-based intervention with sound and production cues integrated within the constellation of language processes. In terms of treatment priorities, phonology is the last component emphasized since intelligibility is a concern only after children have expressive language. Such child-clinician interactions should be based on spontaneous events or utterances and communicative situations that arise in the context of daily play routines and instructional activities. They outline three steps for intervention:

1. Provide appropriate organization of the environment/stimulus materials for the child to attend to, which enables the clinician to alter language complexity systematically throughout the course of therapy.
2. Provide a communicative opportunity, including scaffolding strategies that consist of various types of prompts, questions, information, and restatements that provide support to the child who is actively engaging in the process of communicating a message.

3. Provide consequences or feedback directly related to the effectiveness of the child's communication.

Norris and Hoffman (1990) described an "interactive storytelling" technique in which the clinician points to a picture and models language for the client, then gives the child an opportunity to talk about the event. If the child miscommunicates the idea, the adult provides feedback designed to assist the child in reformulating the message. The clinician can use three primary responses with the child:

1. *Clarification.* When the child's explanation is unclear, inaccurate, or poorly stated, the clinician asks for a clarification. The clinician then supplies relevant information to be incorporated in the child's response, restates the event using a variety of language forms, and asks the child to recommunicate the event. Hoffman and colleagues (1990) presented the following example of this type of response: If a child described a picture of a man cooking at a grill by saying, "Him eating," the clinician might say:

   No, that's not what I see happening. The man isn't eating yet, he's cooking the food. See his fork, he is using it to turn the food. I see him—he is cooking the food. He will eat when he's done cooking, but right now the food is cooking on the grill. He is cooking the food so that they can eat. (p. 105)

   Then the clinician provides an opportunity for the child to restate the information (e.g., ". . . so tell that part of the story again"). Thus, feedback is based on meaning rather than structure.

2. *Adding events.* If the child adequately reports an event, the clinician points out another event to incorporate in the story using a variety of language models. The child is then given the opportunity to retell the story. In an example from Hoffman and colleagues (1990), the clinician points to specific features in the picture and says something like:

   That's right, the man is cooking. He is the dad and he is cooking the hamburgers for lunch. Mom is putting plates on the table. Dad will put the hamburgers on the plates. So you explain the story to the puppet. (p. 105)

3. *Increasing complexity.* If the child adequately describes a series of events, the clinician seeks to increase the complexity of the child's story by pointing out relationships among events such as motives of the characters, cause-effect relationships among the individual events, time and space relationships, and predictions. The child is given the opportunity again to reformulate his or her own version of the story. Another example from these authors is: If the child said, "The daddy is cooking hamburgers and the mommy is setting the table," the clinician might prompt the child to link these two events in time and space by saying:

   That's right, mommy and daddy are making lunch for the family. When daddy finishes cooking the hamburgers he will put them on the plates, so tell that part of the story to the puppet. (p. 105)

Although such interactive storytelling focuses on syntax, semantics, and narrative language skills, correct phonological models and feedback are also being provided the child.

As discussed in Chapter 5, investigators who have studied the effect that language-based intervention has on disordered phonology have reported conflicting results. In a study conducted by Fey and colleagues (1994), 30 preschool children displaying mild to severe speech and language impairments received either clinician or parental language intervention. Treatment in both settings focused on language-based stimulation in highly naturalistic tasks that were designed to facilitate grammar (i.e., making sandwiches, planting beans, play, etc.).

Baseline and treatment measures of phonology and expressive grammar were obtained at regular intervals. The results indicated that although gains in the children's grammatical output were observed, phonologic gains remained insignificant. Fey and colleagues (1994) stated, "We found no support for our prediction that effective facilitation of grammar would lead to spontaneous improvements in phonological output in children with speech and language impairments" (p. 605).

Fey and colleagues (1994) indicated that the lack of an indirect effect of language-based intervention on phonology could have resulted from the intervention style employed and the severity level of the speech and language impairments. Their subjects appeared to be more severely involved than those of Hoffman and associates (1990). Fey and colleagues (1994) concurred with the findings of Tyler and Sandoval (1994), who also reported that language-based instruction had little effect on children with moderate to severe problems in both domains. Both of these studies concluded that clinical attention needed to be focused on both speech and language when impairments in these areas coexisted. This could be accomplished by simultaneously treating phonology and grammar (integration) or by shifting intervention focus from one area to another (alternating language and phonology instruction).

An investigation by Tyler and colleagues (2002) suggests that the matter of cross-domain generalization between language and phonology is not yet resolved. These investigators, using children with moderate to severe language and phonological disorders, studied the extent to which intervention focused on morphosyntax facilitates gains in phonology, and conversely, the extent to which intervention focused on phonology facilitates gains in morphosyntax. In contrast to reviews reported by Fey and associates (1994), their data indicated that intervention focusing on morphosyntax resulted in phonological improvement; however, the reverse did not occur. These investigators employed a 12-week block of morphosyntactic instruction and a 12-week block of phonological instruction with two groups, counterbalancing the order in which the blocks were presented. These authors suggested that clinicians should consider targeting morphosyntax first when using a block intervention sequence for children with concomitant morphosyntactic and phonological impairments.

Tyler, Lewis, Haskill, and Tolbert (2003) reported a subsequent study to assess phonological and morphosyntactic change in children with co-occurring speech and language impairments comparing four different strategies for treatment across the two treatment domains: (1) children in first condition received a 12-week block of phonological intervention followed by a 12-week block on morphosyntax; (2) the second condition was the same as the first but the interventions were reversed; (3) an alternating condition was employed in which phonology and morphosyntax intervention was alternated weekly; and (4) a simultaneous condition was used where phonology and morphosyntax was treated at each session. Tyler and colleagues reported that although none of the four strategies was superior to another in showing gains in phonological performance, the alternating strategy was greatest in showing gains in morphonsyntax, but it was not clear if one strategy was superior to another. The authors pointed out that the relatedness of the goals across the two domains may be a factor in selection of a strategy. Whether the morphological problem is due to phonological factors or is independent of the morphological problem might determine the strategy of choice for a given child.

Issues of sample size, degree of severity, and type of instruction appear to have influenced the nature of research findings in the area of cross-domain generalization and may account for the conflicting findings. At this time, our recommendation, based on current data, would be to target both domains and to use an alternating strategy for children with both language and phonological delay.

Summary of Teaching Phonology through Broader-Based Language Approaches

Background Statement. Language-based approaches are generally founded on two basic premises: (1) phonology is a part of the overall language system and should be treated in a language/communication context and (2) improvement in phonologic behaviors occurs when instruction is focused on higher levels of language (morphosyntax, semantics).

Unique Features. This approach emphasizes a communication-oriented therapy that focuses on narratives, semantics, and syntax on the assumption that such emphasis will facilitate phonological development/remediation.

Strengths and Limitations. From a theoretical perspective, the rationale behind this approach is attractive (i.e., teaching higher-level language communication context will result in phonological improvement). Research results are conflicting concerning the validity of this approach with clients evidencing moderate to severe phonological impairment. Nonetheless, for some phonology clients, this concept is useful. In addition, when any client is at the point in treatment where carryover of connected speech is the goal, these approaches can be very useful.

Research Support. Preliminary data from Hoffman and colleagues (1990) suggested that a whole language approach was a more efficacious approach to language-phonology intervention than was phonologic intervention alone, but their subjects appeared to have mild phonologic delay and were small in number (one set of twins). Research of Fey and colleagues (1994) and Tyler and Sandoval (1994) indicated that for children with more severe phonological impairments, direct instruction in phonology may be necessary to see improvement in phonologic behavior. However, Tyler and colleagues (2002) reported that a morphosyntactic intervention approach, delivered in a 12-week block, resulted in cross-domain (i.e., morphosyntax to phonology) improvement.

Remediation Guidelines for Linguistic Approaches

1. A linguistic approach, particularly the use of minimal pairs, is recommended when there are multiple sound errors that reflect phonologic error patterns. This approach is particularly useful with young children who are unintelligible.

2. Once error patterns have been identified, a review of the child's phonetic inventory will assist in the identification of target sounds (exemplars) to facilitate correct pattern usage. This review usually includes stimulability and may also include phonetic contexts, which facilitate correct production of a target, frequency of occurrence, and developmental appropriateness.

3. Selection of training words should reflect the syllabic word shapes the child uses. For example, if the child uses only CV and CVCV syllable shapes, multisyllabic target words would not be targeted. This guideline is obviously inappropriate if the focus on remediation is on syllable structure simplifications and/or word structure complexity.

4. Treatment efficiency may be increased by selecting target words that facilitate the reduction of two or more patterns simultaneously. For example, if a child uses stopping and deletes final fricatives, the selection of a final fricative for training may aid in the simultaneous reduction of the processes of stopping and final consonant deletion.

5. When errors cross several sound classes (e.g., final consonant deletion may affect stops, fricatives, and nasals), select exemplars that reflect different sound classes.

6. Instruction related to phonologic patterns may focus on appropriate use of a phonologic rule and less on the phonetic accuracy of sounds used in treatment. For example, if a child deletes final consonants but learns to say [dɔd] for [dɔg], the /d/ for /g/ replacement might be overlooked during the *initial* stage of instruction because the child has begun to change his or her phonologic system to incorporate final consonant productions.

7. The cycles approach has been shown to be an effective way to treat children with multiple errors.

8. Minimal contrast therapy usually focuses on both perception and production. When using contrast therapy, minimal pairs with maximal feature differences between contrasting sounds (maximal oppositions) and contrasting two target sounds may be the most efficient way to establish contrasts and impact the child's entire sound system than are word-pairs that reflect few feature differences (minimal oppositions).

9. For children with many sound collapses, a multiple oppositions approach may be an efficient way to impact the child's overall sound system.

10. Teaching behaviors from a linguistic perspective often incorporates selected methods used in more traditional approaches.

11. Treatment focused on morphosyntax and other aspects of language may result in positive changes in phonology. For example, working on plurals and other morphological endings may reduce the deletion of final consonants, thereby indicating that in such cases the perceived phonological error could be related to difficulty with morphological rules.

12. Correction of phonologic errors based on treatment of language behavior may or may not be an effective strategy for facilitating changes in the phonology of a child with moderate or severe phonologic impairment. More encouraging results have been reported in children with mild phonological delay.

ORAL-MOTOR ACTIVITIES AS PART OF ARTICULATION INSTRUCTION

Background

Some clinicians advocate the use of oral-motor training as a precursor to teaching sounds or to supplement articulation instruction. The rationale behind this concept has been that immature or deficient oral-motor control and/or strength may underlie poor articulation, and that differential control of the articulators is necessary or helpful before the rapid, precise, and sequential movements involved in correct articulatory productions are performed. Thus, remediation for articulation disorders should consider including oral-motor instruction as part of a therapy program. It is questionable whether most children identified as having a functional articulatory disorder (disorder of unknown etiology) lack the basic oral-motor skills necessary for articulation. Based on the fact that most clients learn correct speech sound productions without oral-motor training, such exercises have been called into question. Data are lacking to support the use of oral-motor activities as a part of articulation therapy if such activities involve no speech activities. See Forrest (2002) and Lof (2006) for a critical critique of such techniques.

It is highly questionable if nonspeech oral-motor training activities should be a part of therapy. It should be pointed out that oral-motor instruction is advocated not only for articulation disorders but also for disorders of developmental apraxia, feeding, swallowing, and other oral-myofunctional disorders (Marshalla, 1996). There are those who see oral-motor exercises as a useful precursor to phonological instruction for children with severe phonological impairments.

Rationale

Motor pattern development in children progresses from gross generalized reflexive patterns toward movements requiring finer motor control. In terms of speech sound productions, jaw movements become differentiated from head movements, lip and tongue movements become differentiated from the jaw, the tongue tip from the tongue body, the tongue back from the tongue body, and the tongue's lateral margins from the tongue body. Thus, it is hypothesized that differentiated use of each articulator is necessary for normal speech. As the child gets older, he or she develops independent movement of the tongue tip/blade and tongue body, which is necessary for the coarticulation of speech sound productions. It is hypothesized that differentiated movements of the oral structures are necessary for normal articulatory functioning, and when they are lacking, oral-motor instruction may be appropriate.

Assessment

Advocates of the use of nonspeech motor activities recommend that before a client with a phonological disorder is a candidate to receive oral-motor instruction as a component of therapy, the clinician must determine that there is a deficiency in terms of oral-motor awareness and skills. We would not recommend the assessment of any nonspeech motor skills in children with speech sound disorders since there are no data, which suggests there is a generalization from nonspeech motor activities to speech.

Treatment

Guidelines for oral-motor instructional activities are reported by Marshalla (1996) and Meyer (2000). Their programs are designed to address not only articulation but also oral-myofunctional disorders related to swallowing, drinking, and feeding. These authors suggested brushing the tip and sides of the tongue to increase tactile awareness of the oral areas; activities to help stabilize the jaw, such as having the child hold a tongue depressor between his or her teeth while speaking, having the client open his or her mouth and move the tongue up and down without moving the jaw, and having the child say "guh" like a frog without allowing the jaw/chin to move. These suggestions represent a sampling of what is included in oral-motor instruction, but data are lacking to support such nonspeech-based oral-motor instruction.

Summary

A central concern for speech-language pathologists is twofold: (1) Are there data to support the need to engage in oral-motor activities as part of articulation/phonological instruction? (2) If so, what procedures are recommended? With regard to the first concern, it is our view that there are few, if any, data to support oral-motor instruction as a part of articulation therapy. Clinicians who deal with oral-motor deficiencies and related articulation impairments report only anecdotal support for oral-motor therapy. We caution against jumping on the "bandwagon" of those who see oral-motor activities as a creditable treatment strategy for children with severe phonological disorders. Careful evaluation including, among other things, determining whether a problem relates to phonological rules, faulty phonological perception, developmental verbal dyspraxia, and/or deficiencies in speech mechanism as part of the evaluation of any child with a severe speech sound disorder.

INTERVENTION FOR CHILDREN WITH CHILDHOOD APRAXIA OF SPEECH

The topic of childhood apraxia of speech (CAS) was introduced in Chapter 4 in our discussion of classification and factors related to the presence of speech sound disorders. In this section, we address issues relevant to clinical assessment and intervention with this subpopulation of individuals with phonological impairment.

As noted in Chapter 4, we unfortunately still don't have a clear sense of how CAS differs from other speech sound disorders. The 2007 ASHA position statement provides a starting point, however. From that perspective, CAS is viewed as primarily a problem of planning and programming of speech sound production that manifests itself in errors of both precision and consistency of production. Children with CAS have difficulty reaching precise speech sound targets and may produce the same word in different ways on multiple attempts. Children with CAS may also have associated (comorbid) neuromuscular problems (i.e., dysarthria) and/or other types of apraxia such as oral or limb apraxia (i.e., problems with nonspeech movements). The position statement also indicates that CAS is likely a problem that is neurological in nature and may result from known neurological impairments such as cerebral palsy, or it may be associated with complex neurobehavioiral disorders such as autism, Fragile X syndrome, or Rhett syndrome. However, the origin is in many cases unknown (idiopathic).

Consistent with the idea of problems with planning and programming of speech output, Velleman and Strand (1994) have stated that children with CAS may be capable of producing the individual aspects of speech production (i.e., articulatory postures, phonemes, words), but have great difficulty "bridging among the various elements that constitute language performance" (p. 120). Put another way, CAS likely includes not only difficulty with phonology but also with other aspects of language.

In regard to higher levels of language, Velleman (2003) noted that many of these children often demonstrate receptive language skills that are superior to their expressive abilities. Lacking such a gap, another diagnosis such as specific language impairment may be more appropriate (although CAS may coexist in some cases). The possibility of higher-level language problems in children with CAS is also supported by Gillon and Moriarty (2007), who reported an increased risk for reading and spelling difficulty. It should also be noted that many children with CAS also manifest social and behavioral problems (Ball, 1999). This may be a consequence of the significant difficulty that many of these children appear to have in making themselves understood (i.e., having greatly reduced intelligibility).

Assessment

Assessment of this population is not unlike that used with any child with a phonologic disability and, in addition to a standard articulation/phonological battery, typically includes a case history, a hearing screening, and a screening for other areas of communication (language, voice, fluency). There are, however, specific aspects of evaluation of the CAS population that warrant elaboration.

The oral mechanism examination should be particularly thorough in order to determine whether comorbid dysarthria or oral apraxia are present. It should include an assessment of strength, tone, and stability of the oral structures (e.g., can the child move the tongue independently of the mandible?). Does the child do anything special to stabilize the mandible, such as thrust it forward?). A review of the child's feeding history may be of interest in this regard. Young children, in particular, may exhibit uncoordinated feeding patterns without dysphagia. Overall motor skills, both automatic and volitional, including the ability to perform imitative and rapidly alternating tongue movements, plus diadochokinetic rates should be a part of the assessment. As noted previously, one feature that is emerging as potentially unique to CAS is difficulty with transitions between sounds. While static articulatory positions (sounds in isolation) may be produced correctly, rapid combinations of movements frequently are difficult for this population. The rapid successive movements (e.g., syllable to syllable) of connected speech entail constant approximations of specific articulatory targets because there are no absolute or static positions associated with speech sounds. For children with CAS, the inherent dynamic overlapping movement involved in producing sequential motor speech elements is a problem. Velleman and Strand (1994) indicated that sequencing difficulties may not manifest themselves in phonemic sequencing errors per se, but rather are more evident at the articulatory level, affecting the relative timing of glottal and articulatory gestures. These latter factors result in perceived errors of voicing and vowels, especially diphthongs.

Strand and McCauley (1999) proposed using an utterance hierarchy for assessment. In their procedure, evaluation proceeds among levels of utterance types—for example, connected speech from conversation, picture description, and narrative; diadochokinetic tasks; imitative utterances including vowels (V), consonant-vowel (CV), and vowel-consonant (VC) combinations; CVC when the first and last phoneme are the same and when they are different; and repetition of words of increasing length, multisyllabic words, phrases, and sentences of increasing length.

In analyzing speech performance, the clinician must keep in mind the nature of CAS as a disorder involving the hierarchical levels of speech and language, including motor planning for syllable sequencing. Movements, transitions, and timing should be observed as speech is produced at a variety of linguistic levels from simple to complex. For children with a limited verbal repertoire, an independent phonological analysis of a speech/language sample is recommended. For those with more normal verbal skills, a traditional phonologic assessment battery (relational analysis) is recommended, with particular attention to the analysis of speech sounds within syllabic units. In this instance, a connected speech sample is critical because it will allow the examiner to review syllable and word shapes produced by the child. In order to evaluate consistency of productions, particular attention should be paid to words that occur multiple times in the sample.

Phonologic assessment should also include imitation of words that increase in number of syllables (e.g., *please, pleasing, pleasingly*). Because children with CAS evidence problems with the dynamic organization of communication efforts, it is not unusual for problems to be present with the suprasegmental (e.g., phrasal stress) aspects of speech. Coordinating the laryngeal and respiratory systems with the oral mechanism is often very difficult. This problem may result in difficulty with varying intonation contours, modulation of loudness, and maintaining proper resonance. Vowels may be prolonged because the child needs time to organize coordination for the next series of speech sound movements. Recall also that the 2007 ASHA position statement cited excessive and equal stress as another emerging feature of CAS.

In an assessment of children with suspected CAS, the clinician should be sensitive not only to apraxia but also to possible dysarthria. It may be prudent to refer more seriously impaired children with suspected dysarthria and/or CAS to a pediatric neurologist to determine the status of current neurological functioning. Seizure history, associated limb apraxia, presence of oral apraxia, and general knowledge of neurological functioning, may influence the overall management program for a given child and thus warrant such a neurological referral.

Recommended Assessment Battery for CAS

1. Case history (including review of feeding history)
2. Hearing screening/testing
3. Screening of voice and fluency characteristics
4. Speech mechanism examination
   a. Structure and function
   b. Strength, tone, stability
   c. Diadokokinetic rate and function
5. Connected speech sample
   a. Segmental productions
   b. Syllable and word shape productions
   c. Phonologic patterns present
   d. Intonation, vocal loudness, resonance
   e. Analysis of consistency (words occurring more than once)
6. Segmental productions (citation form testing; independent analysis for those with a limited phonological repertoire)
   a. Consonants, vowels, and diphthongs
   b. Syllable shapes used
7. Intelligibility—how well the acoustic signal is understood with and without context
8. Stimulability testing (include multiple opportunities)
   a. Segments
   b. Syllables
   c. Words with increasing number of syllables
9. Phonological awareness assessment
10. Interpersonal skills
    a. Social interaction
    b. Behavioral interactions
    c. Academic/community interactions
11. Language evaluation
    a. Comprehension and production
    b. Sound productions at various semantic and syntactic levels

Tests specifically designed for use in the assessment of children with suspected CAS are the *Screening Test for Developmental Apraxia of Speech* (Blakely, 2001), the *Apraxia Profile* (Hickman, 1997), and the *Kaufman Speech Praxis Test for Children* (Kaufman, 1995). Data reported by Ball, Beukelman, and Bernthal (2002) indicated that examination of the child's social and behavioral interactions, academic performance, and written language were useful components when assessing a child with CAS. The *Diagnostic Evaluation of Articulation and Phonology* (Dodd, Hua, Crosbie, Holm, and Ozanne, 2006) includes a consistency subtest which may also be useful with this population.

Treatment

Velleman (2003) noted that there is relatively little empirical research to support the use of any particular treatment program with children who have CAS. However, it appears that neither traditional motor approaches nor linguistic approaches work well for these children. Indeed, a slow response to intervention has been suggested by some clinicians as a diagnostic marker for CAS; that is, perhaps very slow progress in therapy is a characteristic of children with CAS. Velleman noted a diagnosis of CAS on the basis of slow progress in therapy would be unwise because slow progress may simply reflect poorly applied therapy and may not necessarily mean that there was a mistake in the original diagnosis.

Given what we know about CAS, two aspects of therapy would appear to require particular attention: short-term goals and production units. Rather than focusing on individual speech sounds, a major short-term therapy goal is to build a functional vocabulary for the child with CAS. Often these children have significant intelligibility problems, and efforts need to be directed toward building a core of intelligible words to facilitate the communication process. To the extent possible, production activities suggested here should include attention to syllabic structures and combinations of these syllables so that the child gains verbal building blocks for words. Some elements of the previously discussed core vocabulary approach may be appropriate for children with CAS. Recall that in Chapter 4 we noted that some children with speech sound disorders of unknown origin share the pattern of inconsistency seen in children who might be classified as having CAS.

Relative to production units, a focus of instructional activities should be is on the motor-planning component of the disorder. Rather than using drill motor activities that focus on repetition of the same sounds or syllables, a variety of speech and language motor planning activities should be provided to practice transitions and timing movements required in the dynamic process of ongoing speech. Emphasis is placed on shifting the stimulus materials to incorporate a wider variety of syllable sequences. For example, one could start by having a child name a succession of animals with one-syllable names (e.g., *bat, bear, bird, bug*), then shift to animals with two-syllable names (e.g., *baboon, beaver, camel*), then increase to three-syllable names (e.g., *buffalo, butterfly, bandanna*). Names could then be combined, with an emphasis on being able to do the motor planning necessary to accommodate shifts and variations in syllable sequencing that represent increasing linguistic complexity. Rosenbeck, Kent, and LaPointe (1984) also recommended continually shifting the segmental targets in a succession of syllables beginning with CV or VC, repeating the patterns, and then systematically varying the CV pattern and moving into word combinations.

Strand and Skindner (1999) recommended integral stimulation methods that included tactile and proprioceptive monitoring of articulatory configurations, movement paths, practice with movements, and to provide knowledge of results to the child. They suggested that more frequent distribution of sessions may result in better motor learning (e.g., 2 hours of therapy per week is better distributed in 4 half-hour sessions than in 2 1-hour sessions). They also suggested choosing stimuli for treatment that are useful and meaningful to the child, to allow the child to experience successful communication. They emphasized the importance of stimulus selection, including length and phonetic context of the target words.

Square (1999) outlined three additional types of interventions, including tactile-kinesthetic, rhythmic and melodic facilitation, and gestural cueing. In "touch-cueing" (Bashir, Grahamjones, and Bostwick, 1984), the clinician touches a particular area of the face or neck as each sound in a sequence is produced. Children learn the sound associated with each touching cue. Thus, children can be presented with simultaneous touch, auditory, and sometimes visual cues as they produce sounds in various movement patterns. The "touch-cue" method is an example of a tactile-kinesthetic approach. Another tactile-kinesthetic approach is *Prompts for Restructuring Oral Muscular Phonetic Targets (PROMPT)* developed by Chumpelik (1984). This approach specifies jaw height, facial-labial contraction, tongue height and advancement, muscular tension, duration of contractions, and airstream management for phoneme production. An example of a rhythmic and melodic facilitation approach is known as *Melodic Intonation Therapy* (Helfrich-Miller, 1984). This program uses stimuli that progress over a hierarchy of difficulty while being intoned with Signed English use as a pacer.

A set of guidelines for working with clients with CAS is presented in Table 7.5 (Velleman and Strand, 1994). Because of the possible difficulties with written language in this population, it might also be worth considering the addition of some form of

---

■ **TABLE 7.5**   Basic Principles of a Speech Production Treatment Program for Children with DVD

1. Main focus of treatment should be syllable structure control and organization within a variety of dynamic linguistic contexts.
2. A successful program is one that will facilitate correct production of varying syllable shapes and the organization of these shapes into longer and increasingly complex phonotatic patterns.
3. A sound-by-sound treatment plan that emphasizes phoneme production in isolation prior to moving to words and phrases does *not* address the hierarchical dynamic movement problem in DVD.
4. Auditory discrimination training does *not* address the problem.
5. Frequent, short sessions with breaks are most successful. Because DVD is a dynamic disorder, system fatigue is a problem.
6. Sessions should be divided into short parts:
   a. Warm-ups: Imitation of body and/or oral motor sequences.
   b. Practicing the scales: Syllable sequence drill activities. Establish consistent connected syllable productions from within the child's repertoir. Include sequences that vary articulatory positions, for example, from front to back ([b ʌ d ʌ g ʌ] or "buttercup") or vice versa ([gʌ dʌ bʌ] or "go to bed").
   c. Learning the song: Meaningful single-word activities to include a core group of words that would increase overall intelligibility of speech.
   d. Changing the song: Short sentence activities starting with a key carrier phrase and changing one word, gradually increasing in length and complexity.

Source: Adapted from Velleman, S., and K. Strand, "Developmental verbal dyspraxia." In J. Bernthal, and N. Bankson (Eds.), *Child Phonology: Characteristics, Assessment, and Intervention with Special Populations* (pp. 110–139). New York: Thieme Publishers, 1994. Used by permission.

phonological awareness training (McNeill, 2007). For children who are very young or severely impaired, gestures and pantomime may be encouraged. An augmentative communication system assessment may be desired, particularly for school-age children who are unintelligible. Such assessment should target the various systems that may be appropriate for facilitating language development, reading, spelling, and written language. Facilitating communication through these techniques is often viewed as a means to develop verbal communication as well as other aspects of language. Perhaps the most comprehensive set of instructional materials for treating clients with motor planning difficulties is the *Nuffield Centre Dyspraxia Programme* (1994), which was developed at the Royal National Throat Nose and Ear Hospital in London, England. Other programs commercially available may provide assistance in organizing treatment strategies; however, it is important to remember that individualized programs designed specifically for a child based on his or her assessment performance will likely result in the most effective interventions and progress. Another useful source for treatment suggestions for children with CAS is Velleman (2003).

CASE STUDY

Intervention Recommendations

In Chapter 5, we discussed the speech samples obtained from Kirk, with an analysis and interpretation of his test data. We now discuss how one might proceed in developing an intervention plan based on that interpretation. As you recall, Kirk is a 3-year-old child with multiple errors who is in need of phonological intervention because of poor speech intelligibility. You might wish to review the case study report at the end of Chapter 5 at this time. As you move through the discussion that follows, bear in mind that the steps involved and the variables taken into consideration are applicable with many clients with phonological impairments.

First Consideration: Do I Use a Motor or Phonological Approach to Intervention, or Both?

For most error sounds, with the exception of /ʃ/, /tʃ/, /dʒ/, /r/, and /ɝ/, Kirk is stimulable. Some of the stimulable sounds were more easily imitated than others. Because he could imitate most of his error sounds, a major goal of instruction will be to help Kirk learn to use sounds contrastively, or in other words, diminish his sound collapses, by using sounds appropriately in word contrasts. This goal is phonologically oriented, but instruction must also include teaching or stabilization of the motor production of sounds that he cannot consistently imitate on demand. Thus, therapy will include both sound contrast training and motor production activities.

Second Consideration: How Many Targets Should I Address in a Session?

Because Kirk has multiple error sounds, a focus on several targets is suggested, either within a single lesson, or across lessons within a three- or four-week time frame (cycles or horizontal approach). We have already stated that Kirk's difficulties seem to be primarily phonological: He can produce many sounds but just isn't using them appropriately. He also has a production problem with /ɝ/ and may also need motor practice with some of the other consonants. This means that in lesson planning, we will probably want to allow time for motor practice activities to teach the production of sounds as well as activities that focus on using sounds contrastively. Even though instructional activities may be considered phonological as opposed to motor oriented, they involve production practice. It is suggested that treatment sessions for Kirk should address: (1) error patterns, beginning with stopping and the sound collapses reflected in that pattern (i.e., /d/ replacing several other sounds and clusters such as /s, z, tʃ, θ/ and clusters sl, sn, fl); and (2) instruction and production practice for sounds that are not stimulable or readily produced on demand (e.g., /ɝ/, /ʃ/, /s/, /tʃ/).

Third Consideration: How Should I Conceptualize the Overall Treatment Program?

Because Kirk has so many sounds in error, and because some of those sounds are not stabilized at an imitative level, it is suggested that the clinician begin a session by spending about 5 minutes engaged in what has been identified as "sound stimulation/practice," an activity designed to enhance Kirk's stimulability for all error sounds. Kirk is young and still acquiring phonemes, so it seems advisable to provide him the opportunity to produce a variety of sounds that are not produced correctly in his conversational speech. Sound stimulation can include not only practice on error sounds (e.g., /ɝ/, /s/, /f/) but also sounds that he does say correctly (/p/, /h/, /f/). Successful production of such sounds may facilitate his willingness to try other sounds he has made in error.

Kirk should make five attempts to produce each sound target during sound stimulation, using a cueing hierarchy for those in error, based on the level of support necessary to produce a sound (e.g., modeling, phonetic placement, or selected context). After five attempts, another sound is practiced. With only five attempts, the client is not overwhelmed with repeated failures if he or she cannot produce a sound. It is hoped that by briefly focusing in each session on production of a variety of sounds and levels of complexity (i.e., isolation, syllables, words), a child will acquire the skill to imitate the sound when given an auditory and/or visual model. Production in this type of activity is a building block for focusing on phonological contrasts and for facilitating generalization when a child is stimulable. Following sound stimulation/production practice, the treatment program will focus on Kirk's need to establish sound contrasts.

One treatment option for addressing Kirk's errors is to use a cycling approach, wherein one or more sounds are targeted in a given lesson to help him learn to use a particular phonological pattern (e.g., frication because he currently substitutes stops for most fricatives). In a subsequent lesson, other fricatives related to that process would be focused on, continuing until most of the fricatives have been practiced. At this point, another pattern would be targeted, including one or more sounds in a given lesson (e.g., use of final consonants). This cycling approach may employ auditory bombardment, perceptual training of minimal pairs, and sound production of minimal pairs, including drill and play activities. The linguistic complexity of activities is increased as progress is made (e.g., going from words to phrases to sentences to conversation).

An alternative treatment approach that specifically addresses sound contrasts is to teach multiple oppositions that simultaneously address the collapse of numerous sounds to /d/. Instruction might initially focus on sound collapses that include sounds in Kirk's repertoire and then, as other sounds are established, expand to other sound collapses. In the following example, solid lines indicate initial collapses to focus on because the sounds are in Kirk's repertoire; broken lines reflect targets that can be addressed as additional sounds are added to Kirk's repertoire.

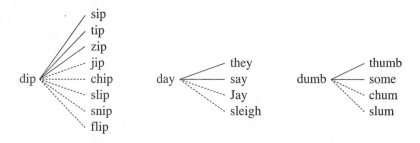

Another way to approach Kirk's stopping pattern is the use of focused minimal pairs rather than the multiple-oppositions approach. This method is a more traditional approach to using minimal pairs to establish sound contrasts; that is, focusing on a single pair and then progressing to other minimal pairs to establish other contrasts in his system. Instruction would begin with a minimal pair evidencing maximal opposition between a target sound and a contrasting sound. For example, instruction might first focus on the word-pair *seal-meal*, and once Kirk can produce that pair, go to *seal-veal*, and finally *deal-seal*. The hope is that by initially contrasting /s/ with /m/ (sounds that evidence several feature differences from /d/), such practice will facilitate more rapid acquisition of other sound contrasts.

Fourth Consideration: How Do Instructional Goals Relate to the Treatment Continuum and Specific Instructional Steps?

The treatment continuum was discussed earlier, including establishment, generalization, and maintenance, with generalization being the focus of much of what we do in therapy. In the case of Kirk, the /ɝ/ or other nonstimulable sounds will require an establishment activity such as sound stimulation mentioned above. His other error patterns (i.e., initial consonant deletion; stopping; final consonant deletion) will fit into the generalization phase of the continuum because he is stimulable on many of the sounds required to eliminate these patterns. Earlier we discussed how in each stage of the treatment, continuum therapy comprises a sequence of steps and activities that include antecedent events from the clinician, responses from the client, and consequating events from the clinician based on client responses. One of the initial planning tasks is to determine how one is going to sequence antecedent events (e.g., verbal instruction, pictures, printed symbols, game activity) and consequating events (e.g., verbal reinforcement, tokens, back-up reinforcers).

Table 7.6 outlines components of therapy sessions based on the preceding considerations. Included is a possible way to construct therapy. Remember that good clinical practice involves creativity, flexibility, and letting client performance guide day-to-day therapy.

■ TABLE 7.6 *Summary of Intervention Sequencing for Kirk*

Component	Procedure	Rationale
Sound Stimulation/ Practice	Ask the client to produce a variety of sounds five times each (both incorrect and correct sounds). Provide auditory models and cueing as necessary.	Generalization has been shown to be highly influenced by a child's stimulability. Therefore, we must help children acquire all the sounds at a motor level. Brief practice periods serve to encourage continued attempts at sounds that may be particularly difficult.
Production Activities	Focus on teaching frication and final consonant usage. Focus on one or two sounds per session, moving from /f/ to /m/ to /s/, and other stimulable sounds. Use minimal pairs at a perceptual level before practice on pairs at a production level. Drill/Play games and activities are recommended. Use a listening task to introduce each sound. Consider using multiple opposition contrasts for the /d/ collapses.	Cycling across patterns and sounds is helpful for children with multiple errors. Kirk is young and still developing his sound system, and he has a good attention span. Therefore, he could benefit from shifting focus from week to week. Multiple oppositions can be helpful for phoneme collapses and are recommended because Kirk is stimulable on many of the collapses.
Increasing Linguistic Complexity	When Kirk can produce word targets accurately, including minimal pairs, shift production to phrases and then sentences. In addition, progress from targets occurring only once in a word or phrase to more complex productions involving more than one occurrence, and competing sounds.	To reach the terminal objective of spontaneous use of appropriate speech sounds and patterns, Kirk must be able to use his new speech sounds and patterns in increasingly complex linguistic units.
Situational Generalization	Bring persons in the child's environment into activities to reinforce Kirk's new speech skills. Using target names, preschool vocabulary, and frequently used words as a focus may be helpful. Arrange for Kirk to "use" his new speech in the classroom and home.	Focusing on situational generalization as early as possible will help this young client generalize the new language skills to his environment. Increased intelligibility will be powerfullyreinforced by the environment.

■ QUESTIONS FOR CHAPTER 7

1. How would one assess auditory perception in a child suspected of having difficulty with sound contrasts?

2. Outline a traditional approach to articulation therapy and specify for whom it is appropriate.

3. Outline a linguistic approach to phonological intervention and specify for whom it is appropriate.

4. What characteristics distinguish children with CAS from other phonological delayed children and what distinguishes their treatment?

5. Discuss how one can use minimal pairs in phonological treatment.

6. Outline the procedures for a cycles approach to therapy.

Language and Dialectal Variations

BRIAN A. GOLDSTEIN
Temple University

AQUILES IGLESIAS
Temple University

Speech patterns used by individuals in our society vary as a function of language, age, socioeconomic status, and geography. Speech patterns also vary as a function of an individual's ability to acquire and produce the speech patterns of his or her community. As speech-language pathologists (SLPs), it is our responsibility to sort out the array of patterns that are typical of a child's speech community from those that are indicative of a speech sound disorder (defined as including both segment- and pattern-based errors). Information on variations in speech patterns seen within and across particular speech communities is necessary to conduct least-biased phonological assessments that reflect the characteristics of the child's speech community. For example, if members of a child's speech community consist of individuals who are bilingual (Spanish and English) and the variety of English spoken in the child's community is African American English (AAE), then the child will most likely speak a variety of English that has been influenced by both AAE and Spanish. Assessment of such a child must take into account the influence that AAE and Spanish might have on the child's phonological patterns. Sensitivity to and knowledge of variation are also required to adequately serve those individuals who elect to modify the language variety that they speak. In the following sections, we will examine phonological variation within and across languages and show how this information can be used to conduct least-biased assessment and plan for intervention.

DIALECT

Dialects are mutually intelligible forms of a language associated with a particular region, social class, or ethnic group. General American English, Southern White Standard, Appalachian English, Caribbean English, African American English, Eastern American

English, and Spanish-influenced English are just some of the dialects spoken in the United States. No dialect of any language is superior to any other because all thoughts can be expressed using any dialect of any language. This is not to say that all varieties of a language carry the same prestige. Some varieties of a language, specifically those used by the dominant groups in any socially stratified society, will be considered to have higher prestige (Wolfram, 1986), promulgated within the educational system (Adler, 1984), and valued by the private sector of the society (Shuy, 1972; Terrell and Terrell, 1983).

The promulgation of General American English (GAE; the prestige dialect in the United States) within the educational system and by contact through broadcast media between members of different regional dialects has decreased differences between dialects *(dialect leveling)*. At the same time, lack of linguistic contact among groups due to geographical or socioeconomic reasons has resulted in a linguistic isolation that has increased the distance between dialects (Labov, 1991). In addition, the increased immigration and ethnic isolation that have occurred among some subgroups have further increased the number and pervasiveness of dialects. The courts' acknowledgment of the rights of linguistic minority populations has resulted in greater acceptance of varieties other than General American English. For example, *Martin Luther King Junior Elementary School Children et al.* v. *Ann Arbor School District* (1978) provided for the use of children's home language, including African American English, in the educational process. At least in terms of dialects, the "melting pot" hypothesis appears to be a myth for certain segments of our society.

Regardless of whether dialects are becoming more or less like each other, people hold many different myths about dialects. Wolfram and Schilling-Estes (1998) have indicated a number of myths held about dialects and have countered those myths with corresponding facts (see Table 8.1).

Speakers of a particular dialect do not always use all of the features present in their dialect. A speaker's use of particular features depends on the context and interlocutors *(register)*. *Registral varieties* are dependent on the participants, setting, and topic. For example, one would typically use one register when talking to friends about an enjoyable weekend and use another variety when speaking to a police officer about a speeding violation. The extent to which particular individuals use the available features of their dialect *(dialect density)* may depend on factors such as socioeconomic status and geography. Sometimes the differences in dialect density are associated with socioeconomic status; a sociolinguistic phenomenon referred to by Wolfram (1986) as *social diagnosticity*. Wolfram (1986) observed the frequency of occurrence of selected AAE features among the speech of individuals representing four socioeconomic groups: upper middle class, lower middle class, upper working class, and lower working class. His research revealed that certain AAE linguistic features showed *gradient stratification* across the four groups. That is, individuals in lower socioeconomic groups used more of the available features of that dialect than individuals in higher socioeconomic groups. Washington and Craig (1998) found this same effect for 5- and 6-year-old, AAE-speaking boys. For example, the lack of realization of postvocalic *r* (e.g., /sɪstɚ/ → [sɪstə]) is an example of gradient stratification because all socioeconomic groups use this phonological feature, albeit with different levels of frequency. On the other hand, certain AAE features show a pattern of usage referred to as *sharp stratification*, which refers to linguistic features that more clearly differentiate socioeconomic groups, based on significant differences in frequency of usage. One example

▥ **TABLE 8.1**   Dialect Myths and Facts

Myth	Fact	Example
A dialect is a variety spoken by someone else.	Everyone speaks some dialect of a language.	Although there is a dialect form often referred to as the "standard" (e.g., Standard or General American English), it is usually a form not actually spoken by anyone in an invariable form. There is variation to one extent or another used by all speakers.
Dialectal features are always distinct and noticeable.	Some dialectal features are shared by many different dialects.	The weakening of postvocalic *r* (e.g., /moɚ/ → [moə]) is exhibited by speakers of African American English, Eastern American English, and Southern American English.
Dialects arise from ineffective tries at speaking the correct form of the language.	Speakers of dialects acquire those features by interacting with members of the speech community in which they live.	Some native speakers of Spanish often use characteristics of African American English because speakers of both varieties live in the same community (Poplack, 1978).
Dialects are random changes from the "standard."	Dialects are precise and show regular patterns.	In many dialects of the American South, /ɪ/ and /ɛ/ are pronounced as [ɪ] before nasals; /pɪn/; /pɛn/ → [pɪn].
Dialects are always viewed negatively.	Dialects are not inherently viewed negatively (or positively, for that matter); prestige of any dialect is derived from the social prestige of its speakers.	Ramirez and Milk (1986) found that bilingual teachers rated the local Mexican dialect of Spanish as less prestigious than the general dialect of Spanish. The dialect of English spoken by the British monarchy, however, is often perceived as prestigious.

of this type of stratification is the substitution of [f] for /θ/. The use of this feature contrasts middle-class with working-class groups, as working-class groups use the feature much more frequently than middle-class speakers. Wolfram has indicated that features revealing sharp stratification are of greater social diagnosticity than those showing gradient stratification.

Geography may also play a role in the likelihood of a specific dialect feature being expressed. For example, Hinton and Pollock (1999) examined the occurrence of vocalic and postvocalic American English /ɹ/* in African American English speakers from two geographic regions (Davenport, Iowa and Memphis, Tennessee). Overall, they found that speakers in Davenport were more likely than speakers in Memphis to maintain the rhotic quality of vocalic and postvocalic /ɹ/.

---

*For purposes of this chapter, the symbol /ɹ/ is used to represent the rhotic sound found in General American English and its dialects. The symbol /r/, as specified by the International Phonetic Alphabet Association, is used to designate the alveolar trill.

▓ CHARACTERISTICS OF AMERICAN ENGLISH DIALECTS

In addition to GAE, there are a number of dialects of English spoken in the United States. This chapter focuses on five common dialects: African American English, Eastern American English, Southern American English, Appalachian English, and Ozark English. Most of the available literature on these dialects focuses on their characteristics rather than on their development.

African American English

African American English (AAE) is a variety of American English that is spoken by many, but not all, African Americans. Other groups who have contact with AAE speakers also speak it. For example, English-speaking Puerto Rican teenagers in East Harlem, New York, have been found to use features of AAE (Wolfram, 1974). Wolfram found that the degree of contact that the teenagers had with AAE speakers greatly influenced the number of AAE features in their speech. Those individuals with the most contact showed the greatest number of features in their speech. Poplack (1978) examined the use of AAE, Puerto Rican Spanish, and Philadelphia English variants in the speech of sixth-grade Puerto Rican boys and girls. She found that the Puerto Rican boys tended to use more features of AAE, and the girls used more features of Philadelphia English. Poplack concluded that the specific variants used by the children were more related to "covert prestige" than to their linguistic environment, with the boys assigning more prestige to AAE speakers and the girls assigning more prestige to Philadelphia English. The results of both of these studies support the notion that use of dialect features is influenced by patterns in the speech community and that speech patterns are greatly affected by peer interaction.

Like all dialects, AAE is systematic with rule-governed phonological, semantic, syntactic, pragmatic, and proxemic systems. There are two major hypotheses accounting for the origin of African American English (Poplack, 2000; Wolfram and Schilling-Estes, 1998). The Creole Hypothesis assumes that AAE descended from Plantation Creole (Wolfram, 1994; Wolfram and Schilling-Estes, 1998), a language that developed from a mixture of languages brought into contact during the slave trade period. Plantation Creole was commonly used by African Americans on plantations in the South but was not spoken by European Americans at the time. Over time, AAE has further spread and changed. The exodus of African Americans from the southeast to the northeast and other parts of the United States in the early 1900s brought AAE to the urban areas of the North (Stewart, 1971). In many cases, individuals from a particular state tended to migrate to particular cities (e.g., South Carolinians moving to Philadelphia). The restricted social environments in which many African Americans lived, in addition to the continued contact with their southern families and communities, reinforced the use of AAE. In its evolution, AAE has undergone a decreolization process showing fewer links to its creole past and acquiring features that are not traceable to the original Creole (e.g., stopping of interdental fricatives) (Wolfram and Schilling-Estes, 1998).

An alternative hypothesis, the Anglicist Hypothesis, states that African American English is considered a dialect of English. That is, AAE can be traced to the varieties of English spoken in Britain (Wolfram and Schilling-Estes, 1998). Thus, slaves who were brought to the United States eventually "learned the regional and social varieties of surrounding white speakers" (Wolfram and Schilling-Estes, 1998, p. 176). These authors argue that the Creolist Hypothesis was favored until the 1980s, when written and recorded narratives of ex-slaves were discovered. At present, current evidence favors the Anglicist Hypothesis.

A number of linguistic features distinguish AAE from General American English. The major phonological features that distinguish these two varieties are listed in Table 8.2 (compiled from Bailey and Thomas, 1998; Hyter, 1996; Pollock, Bailey, Berni, Fletcher, Hinton, Johnson, and Weaver, 1998; Rickford, 1999; Stockman, 1996a; Wolfram and Schilling-Estes, 1998). These features are always optional, are not used in each possible phonetic context, and are not produced by all AAE speakers. For example, the simplification of word-final clusters tends to occur when one of the consonants is an alveolar and the other (i.e., the deleted consonant) is a morphological marker (Stockman, 1996a). Hence, some AAE speakers may not differentiate between the present and past tense of the same verb (e.g., *miss* and *missed* are pronounced as [mɪs]), but would retain the cluster in a word such as *mist*.

Features of AAE extend to suprasegmental phenomena as well (Hyter, 1996; Stockman, 1996a). For example, AAE speakers may place stress on the first rather than second syllable (Detróit → Détroit), use a wide range of intonation contours and vowel elongations, and produce more level and falling final contours than rising contours.

■ TABLE 8.2 Major Phonological Features Distinguishing African American English and General American English

Pattern	Example(s)
Word-final consonant cluster reduction (particularly when one of the two consonants is an alveolar)	/tɛst/ → [tɛs]
Deletion of /ɹ/	/sɪstɚ/ → [sɪstə]
	/kærəl/ → [kæəl]
	/pɹʌfɛsɚ/ → [pvfɛsə]
Deletion of /l/ in word-final abutting consonants	/hɛlp/ → [hɛp]
Deletion of nasal consonant in word-final position with nasalization of preceding vowel	/mun/ → [mũ]
Substitution of [ɪ] for /ɛ/ before nasals	"pin" /pɪn/ and "pen" /pɛn/ pronounced as [pɪn]
Substitution of [k] for /t/ in initial /str/ clusters	/stɹit/ → [skɹit]
Realization of /θɹ/ as [θ]	/θɹo/ → [θo]
Substitution of f/θ and v/ð in intervocalic position	/nʌθiŋ/ → [nʌfiŋ]
	/beðiŋ/ → [beviŋ]
Substitution of f/θ in word-final position	/saʊθ/ → [saʊf]
Realization of /v/ as [b] and /z/ as [d], in word-internal position before syllabic nasals	/sɛvən/ → [sɛbən]
Stopping of word-initial interdentals	/ðe/ → [de]
	/θɑt/ → [tɑt]
Metathesis	/æsk/ → [æks]

Phonological Development in AAE

In comparison to the investigation of phonological skills in speakers of General American English, less information exists on the development of AAE phonology. Existing studies have examined phonological development in typically developing AAE-speaking children and AAE-speaking children with speech sound disorders. Major findings indicate that AAE-speaking children tend to produce the same phonetic inventory as speakers of GAE (Stockman, 1996a); show great intersubject variability; exhibit systematic error patterns; and demonstrate differences in both the type and quantity of speech errors exhibited by typically developing speakers and those with speech sound disorders.

Preschoolers speaking AAE and GAE often exhibit similar phonological patterns although with different frequencies. Seymour and Seymour (1981) compared the performance of 4- and 5-year-old African American and White children. They reported that both groups evidenced phonological variations typically associated with AAE (e.g., f/θ in medial and final positions; d/ð in initial and medial positions; b/v in initial and medial positions). The AAE features, however, occurred more frequently in the productions of the African American children. Thus, both groups produced the same type of substitutions, but the frequency of their use differed between the two groups. These results suggested that for the children they studied, the contrast between AAE and General American English was *qualitatively* undifferentiated at this age. The same result has also been demonstrated for phonological processes (Haynes and Moran, 1989).

Stockman (2006a) examined the production of syllable-initial consonants in seven typically developing AAE-speaking children ages 2;8 to 3;0. All seven children produced 15 syllable-initial, singleton consonants (/m, n, p, b, t, d, k, g, w, j, l, ɹ, f, s, h/) at least four times in at least two different words. These 15 segments represent the minimal competence core of phonemes that are invariant in AAE and GAE (Stockman, 1996a). Accuracy for the group of segments in the minimal competence core exceeded 80 percent (range = 81 to 99 percent) compared to less than 80 percent (range = 14 to 76 percent) for sounds not in the core (i.e., the segments that vary between AAE and GAE). Error patterns included voicing errors, liquid gliding, stopping, and fronting. All seven children produced syllable-initial consonant clusters, totaling 19 types. Of the 19 types, 15 were of the oral stop + sonorant or fricative + sonorant variety. The children also produced /s/ + stop clusters and one three-member cluster, /skr-/. Results show that the phonetic skills of young AAE-speaking children are similar to those of same-aged children speaking GAE.

Pearson, Velleman, Bryant, and Charko (in submission) examined the phonological skills of 537 children ages 4 to 12 acquiring AAE and 317 children of the same age acquiring Mainstream (i.e., General) American English (MAE). They found that children acquiring AAE and MAE showed commensurate mastery (accuracy greater than or equal to 90 percent) of most singleton consonants in initial position—(/b/, /t/, /k/, /g/, /m/, /n/, /h/, /j/, /w/, /dʒ/, /ʃ/, /tʃ/, /l/). However, children acquiring AAE mastered some initial segments (e.g., /ɹ/ and /s/), initial clusters (kl-, pl-, kr-, gr-, pr-, sp-, st-, and skr-), and some final singletons (/s/ and /z/) earlier than did children acquiring MAE. Finally, acquisition of /d/ and /ð/ by AAE speakers occurred after that of MAE speakers. In final position, results were similar in that speakers of AAE and MAE generally showed comparable skills. By 6 years of age, AAE speakers mastered all consonants except /t/, /d/, /θ/, and /ð/; MAE speakers had mastered all consonants except /θ/ and /ð/. It should be noted that MAE speakers mastered /ð/

at age 8 compared with age 12 for AAE speakers. However, AAE speakers mastered /s/ and /z/ by age 4, compared to age 6 for MAE speakers. Finally, speakers of AAE tended to master a number of initial clusters (e.g., /kl/, pɹ/) earlier than MAE speakers, but MAE speakers mastered final clusters (e.g., /ks/, /nt/) before AAE speakers.

In a follow-up study with this same group of participants, Velleman, Pearson, Bryant, and Charko (in submission) examined the relationship between phonetic and phonotactic (e.g., syllable structure) development in AAE and MAE speakers. Results indicated that AAE speakers showed more advanced phonological skills related to segments than to phonotactics. The authors predicted this finding, given that AAE speakers have less over-all exposure to structures such as final singleton consonants, final clusters, and iambic words (i.e., words like *gi-RAFFE* that have a weak-strong stress pattern). Taken together, the results from these two studies indicate that AAE speakers may be placing greater emphasis on segmental rather than phonotactic learning, which in turn leads to mastery of some later developing consonants by AAE speakers before MAE speakers.

Variability across children has been found to be a hallmark of AAE phonological development. Seymour and Seymour (1981) reported considerable interchild variability among AAE speakers. Neither were all of the target features present in each AAE speaker nor were they equally distributed among the speakers. Although there is variability in phonological development between AAE-speaking children, the context for error patterns exhibited by these children has been found to be systematic. For example, although AAE-speaking children delete final consonants, they do not do so arbitrarily. Stockman (1996a, 2006b) noted that alveolar consonants were more likely than either labials or velars to be deleted; oral stops and nasals were more likely than fricatives to be deleted; and final consonants preceding a consonant were more likely to be deleted. In addition, the absence of final consonants may be marked by lengthening or nasalizing the vowel that preceded the absent consonant (Moran, 1993). Bryant, Velleman, Abdualkarim, and Seymour (2001) found that AAE-speaking children were more likely to delete one element of a word-final cluster if a more sonorous element preceded a less sonorous element. For example, words ending in /sk/ clusters (more sonorous element preceding less sonorous element) were more likely to undergo deletion than /ks/ clusters (less sonorous element preceding more sonorous element). In addition, their results indicated that in the clusters in which a more sonorous element preceded a less sonorous one, the most sonorous element was preserved. For example, AAE-speaking children would produce *desk* /dɛsk/ as [dɛs] and not [dɛk].

Developmental differences between typically developing AAE speakers and those with speech sound disorders have been found to be quantitatively and qualitatively different. Bleile and Wallach (1992) compared the articulation of nonspeech-delayed and speech-delayed AAE-speaking children ranging in age from 3;6 to 5;5. Head Start teachers who shared the same racial and linguistic background as the children differentiated the two groups of children. Data analysis was based on non-AAE phonological patterns exhibited by the children in a picture-identification, single-word test. The delayed and nondelayed groups demonstrated differences in the type and quantity of their speech errors. Speech-delayed children had a larger number of (1) stop errors (especially velars), (2) fricative errors in all positions (especially fricatives other than /θ/), and (3) affricate errors in all positions. Nonspeech-delayed participants evidenced greater devoicing of final /d/, sonorant errors, and errors related to /ɹ/. Both groups of children produced a large number of consonant cluster errors, with the speech-delayed children exhibiting a larger number of cluster errors. Bleile and Wallach (1992) concluded that a combination of characteristics, rather than a single indicator, appears to be the most reliable index of speech delay in African American English speakers, just as it is with children who do not speak AAE.

Eastern American English and Southern American English

Eastern American English and Southern American English, described by Labov (1991) as northern and southern dialects, are two geographical variations of GAE. The Eastern American dialect runs generally from Vermont to the north, parts of Iowa and Minnesota to the west, and New Jersey to the south (Wolfram and Schilling-Estes, 1998). The Southern American dialect runs generally from Maryland to the north, Texas to the west, and Florida to the south (Wolfram and Schilling-Estes, 1998). Although these two dialects share many of the same features, they can also be differentiated from each other through differences in the production of both vowels and consonants (see Table 8.3) (compiled from Parker and Riley, 2000; Small, 2004; Wolfram and Schilling-Estes, 1998).

TABLE 8.3   Common Dialectal Variations in English

Pattern	Example		Dialect
Vowels			
Tense → Lax	/i/ → [ɪ]	/rili/ → [rɪlɪ]	SAE
	/u/ → [ʊ]	/rut/ → [rʊt]	EAE
Lax → Tense	/ɪ/ → [i]	/fɪʃ/ → [fiʃ]	SAE
	/ɛ/ → [e]	/ɛg/ → [eg]	SAE
	/æ/ → [ɑ]	/hæf/ → [hɑf]	EAE
Vowel Neutralization	/ɪ/; /ɛ/ → [ɪ]	/pɪn/; /pɛn/ → [pɪn]	SAE
Diphthong Reduction	/aɪ/ → [ɑ]	/paɪ/ → [pɑ]	SAE
a/ɔ		[fɔt] → [fɑt]	SAE, EAE
Lowering	/ɔ/ → [ɑ]	/fɔɚ/ → [fɑɚ]	SAE, EAE
Derhoticization	/ɚ/ → [ə]	/fɔɚ/ → [fɔə]	SAE, EAE
"r" Deletion		/kɑɚ/ → [kɑ]	SAE, EAE
"r" Addition	/ə/ → [ɚ]	/lɪndə/ → [lɪndɚ]	EAE
Consonants			
Velar Fronting	/ŋ/ → [n]	/ɹʌnɪŋ/ → [ɹʌnɪn]	SAE
/j/ Addition		/nu/ → [nju]	SAE, EAE
Voicing Assimilation	/s/ → [z]	/gɹisi/ → [gɹizi]	SAE
Glottalization	/t/; /d/ → [ʔ]	/batəl/ → [baʔəl]	EAE
[t]; [d] for /θ/; /ð/	/θ/ → [t]	/θɪŋk/ → [tɪŋk]	EAE
	/ð/ → [d]	/ðɪs/ → [dɪs]	EAE

Key: SAE = Southern American English; EAE = Eastern American English.

Appalachian English and Ozark English

Two other common geographical dialects of English are Appalachian English (AE) and Ozark English (OE). Christian, Wolfram, and Nube (1988) indicate that AE and OE are related linguistically, with OE showing many similar features as AE. Given the phonological similarities of these two dialects, they will be discussed together. Appalachian English is spoken generally in the area of parts of Kentucky, Tennessee, Virginia, North Carolina, and West Virginia (parts of the Carolinas, Georgia, and Alabama may also be included). Ozark English is spoken in an area encompassing northern Arkansas, southern Missouri, and northwestern Oklahoma.

Christian and colleagues (1988, pp. 153–159) have outlined the characteristics of Appalachian English (AE) and Ozark English (OE) in Table 8.4. Only the most common features are outlined (see Christian et al., 1988, and Flipsen, 2007, for more details).

As was the case for AAE in African American speakers, not all features of AE and OE will be utilized by every speaker, used in every situation, or produced in every context. For example, the rule noted as *intrusive t*, in which [t] may be added to words ending in /s/ or /f/, is usually limited to a small set of words. Most commonly, the rule takes effect on the words *once* and *twice*. In addition, the number of words exhibiting this rule seems to be more extensive in AE than OE.

■ **TABLE 8.4** Characteristics of Appalachian English and Ozark English

Rule	Example
Epenthesis Following Clusters	
CCC# → CCəC#	/gosts/ → [gostəs]
Intrusive *t* (more common in AE)	
/s/# → [st]	/wʌns/ → [wʌnst]
/f/# → [ft]	/klɪf/ → [klɪft]
Stopping of Fricatives	
/θ/ → [t]	/θɑt/ → [tɑt]
/ð/ → [d]	/ðe/ → [de]
Initial *w* Reduction	
/w/ → ø	/wɪl/ → [ɪl]
Initial Unstressed Syllables	
IUS → ø	/əlaʊd/ → [laʊd]
h Retention	
ø → [h]	/ɪt/ → [hɪt]
Retroflex *r*	
/ɹ/ → ø (post-consonantal)	/θɹo/ → [θo]
/ɹ/ → ø (intervocalic)	/kæɹi/ → [kæi]
Lateral *l*	
/l/ → ø before labials	/wʊlf/ → [wʊf]

PHONOLOGY IN SPEAKERS OF LANGUAGE VARIETIES OTHER THAN ENGLISH

Prior to the arrival of Europeans, what is now the continental United States was a polyglot area with over 200 languages or dialects spoken (Leap, 1981). Over the past 600 years, immigrants to this area have brought their culture and language. Historically, the general trend for most immigrants to the United States was to use their home language as their primary language of communication. By the third generation, though, immigrants tended to lose their language of origin (Veltman, 1988). Some immigrant groups, however, have maintained the use of their home language (also termed *first* or *primary language*) from generation to generation with reinforcement from new immigrants and travel to their country of origin. In total, there are almost 47 million individuals older than 5 years in the United States who speak a language other than or in addition to English, almost 55 percent of whom speak English less than "very well" (U.S. Bureau of the Census, 2000). The number of individuals speaking a language variety other than English in the United States is likely to increase in the coming years. It is estimated that by the year 2050, if birth rates and current immigration trends continue, the percentage of individuals of Asian descent will almost triple, the percentage of individuals of Hispanic/Latino descent will almost double, and the percentage of Native Americans will increase to about 1 percent (for information on Native American languages, see Goldstein, 2000) (U.S. Bureau of the Census, 2000). The percentage of Whites will decrease to slightly over one-half the population.

There has been a realization that, although English is the most common and dominant language spoken in the United States, other languages have a right to coexist in our linguistically plural society. For example, *Lau* v. *Nichols* (1974) and the *Lau* Remedies (1975) mandated that federally funded schools must eliminate language barriers in school programs that excluded nonnative English speakers. The *Individuals with Disabilities Education Act* (IDEA, 2004) required that the native language commonly used in the home or learning environment be utilized in all contact for a child with a disability.

The current number and future increase of individuals from culturally and linguistically diverse populations mean that SLPs will likely encounter speakers of languages and language varieties other than English. To complete appropriate phonological assessments that guide the intervention process for children whose home language is not English, SLPs need to gather segmental, prosodic, syllabic, and developmental information. In this section, the characteristics of pidgins, creoles, and Spanish and Asian languages along with information about phonological acquisition and development in speakers of Spanish and Asian languages will be described. Although languages other than Spanish and those of Asia are spoken in the United States (e.g., Arabic) (Amayreh and Dyson, 1998, 2000; Dyson and Amayreh, 2000), we focus on those languages given that the majority of children in the schools use those languages (Kindler, 2001).

Pidgins and Creoles

Language is always changing. This change is represented in all areas of language—phonology, syntax, semantics, lexicon, and pragmatics. This change may take place because of a number of factors such as geography, social prestige, and the introduction of new vocabulary (Crystal, 1997). Pidgins and creoles are two examples of language change.

A *pidgin* is a communication system used by groups of people who wish and need to communicate with each other but have no means to do so. They use a limited vocabulary and "simplified" syntactic structure compared with their two native languages (Crystal, 1997). Pidgins are not simply degraded natural languages but come to have rules all their own. In fact, some pidgins—for example, Tok Pisin in Papua New Guinea—have become the most widely used linguistic variety in the country. Crystal notes, however, that a pidgin often has a short life (perhaps a few years) and disappears when the need for a common communication system ceases to exist. He also suggests that a pidgin may develop into a creole.

A *creole* is a pidgin that becomes the mother tongue of a community. Thus, pidgins and creoles are two points on the same language development continuum Crystal (1997). In essence, a creole is a pidgin that serves as primary input to the next generation of speakers. That is, a pidgin becomes a creole when it is passed on to child speakers. Compared with pidgins, creoles show increased complexity in syntax, phonology, lexicon, semantics, and pragmatics (Muyksen and Smith, 1995). Creoles tend to show rules that were not exhibited in their pidgin ancestor (Holm, 1988).

Common Creoles in the United States

There are four main creoles that SLPs may encounter: Gullah, Hawaiian Creole, Louisiana French Creole, and Haitian Creole. In this section, we will briefly outline their phonological characteristics.

Gullah (or *Geechee* or *Sea Island Creole* as it is sometimes called) is spoken by approximately 250,000 to 300,000 speakers mostly on the barrier islands off the coasts of South Carolina and Georgia (Holm, 1989). This English creole is closely related to other creoles such as Sierra Leone Krio, Cameroons Creole, Jamaican Creole, the Creole of British Guiana, and the Creoles of Surinam (Cunningham, 1992). The origin of this creole is debated. Some believe that Gullah arrived in the American colonies from the west coast of Africa as a fully developed creole (Nichols, 1981). Others link its development to a complex interaction of white British settlers, Africans, and Caribbeans (Holm, 1989). Some phonological features of Gullah (compared with General American English) include the use of [a] for /æ/, [t] for /θ/, [d] for /ð/, [ʤ] for /z/, and deletion of postvocalic /ɹ/.

Hawaiian Creole arose in the nineteenth century and culminates from the influence of many sources such as Polynesian, European, Asian, and pidgin languages (Holm, 1989). Some phonological features of Hawaiian Creole (compared with General American English) include [t] for /θ/, [d] for /ð/, backing in the environment of [ɹ] (/θɹ/→ [tʃɹ]; /tɹ/ → [tʃɹ]; /str/ → [ʃɹ]), deletion of postvocalic /ɹ/, and deletion of the second member of word-final abutting consonants—for example, /nɛst/ → [nɛs] (Bleile, 1996).

Louisiana French Creole evolved as the native language of descendants of West African slaves brought to southern Louisiana by French colonists (Dubois and Horvath, 2003; Nichols, 1981). The creole has also been influenced by features of Cajun, a variety of regional French brought from Canada (Holm, 1989). It is estimated that there are 60,000 to 80,000 speakers of this creole. The vowel system consists of four front vowels, /i, e, ɛ, a/, four back vowels, /u, o, ɔ, a/, schwa /ə/, and three nasalized vowels /ɛ̃, õ, ã/ (Morgan, 1959; Nichols, 1981; Oetting, 2007). The consonant system contains six oral stops /b, d, g, p, t, k/, three nasal stops /m, n, ɲ/, seven fricatives /f, s, ʃ, v, z, ʒ, h/, two liquids /l, ɹ/, and one glide /j/. There are four common phonological patterns noted by

Nichols (1981). First, abutting consonants across word boundaries are often assimilated to the voicing of the second member of the consonant pair; for example, /pæs ði/ → [pæz ði]. Second, word-final consonants may be deleted. Third, word-final unstressed syllables are often weakened or deleted. Finally, vowel raising may take place in which [i] is substituted for /ɛ/.

Speech-language pathologists might also encounter speakers of *Haitian Creole*. This Caribbean creole, spoken in Haiti, has approximately six million speakers (Muyksen and Veenstra, 1995). There are three dialects of Haitian Creole: northern, central (including the capital Port-au-Prince), and southern. The Haitian Creole vowel system contains seven segments: /i, u, e, o, a/ and two front-rounded vowels /ø/ and /œ/. The creole also contains 17 consonants, six stops /b, d, g, p, t, k/, six fricatives /f, s, ʃ, v, z, ʒ/, three nasals /m, n, ɲ/, and two liquids /l/ and /r/.

Spanish

Spanish has become the second-most common language spoken in the United States, with approximately 28 million speakers, or 10.7 percent of the U.S. population over 5 years of age (U.S. Census Bureau, 2000). According to Hammond (2001), there are two main dialects of American Spanish: Highland Spanish and Coastal Spanish. Dialects are categorized by one of these two types based on the behavior of syllable- and word-final consonants. Dialects in which syllable- and word-final consonants are preserved are known as *conservative dialects;* and those in which final consonants tend to be deleted are known as *radical dialects* (Guitart, 1978, 1996). Mexican Spanish exemplifies a conservative dialect, and Puerto Rican Spanish is emblematic of a radical dialect. In the following sections, we will review Spanish phonology and phonological development in Spanish speakers.

Spanish Phonology

A brief overview of the Spanish consonant and vowel system is presented here (for a more complete description, see Goldstein, 1995, 2007a, and Hammond, 2001). There are five primary vowels in Spanish: the two front vowels /i/ and /e/ and the three back vowels /u/, /o/, and /a/. There are 18 consonants in General Spanish (Núñez-Cedeño and Morales-Front, 1999): the voiceless unaspirated stops /p/, /t/, and /k/; the voiced stops /b/, /d/, and /g/; the voiceless fricatives /f/, /x/, and /s/; the affricate /tʃ/; the glides /w/ and /j/; the lateral /l/; the flap /ɾ/ and trill /r/; and the nasals /m/, /n/, and /ɲ/.

The existence of differences between Spanish dialects further complicates the process of characterizing phonological patterns in Spanish-speaking children. Unlike English, in which dialectal variations are generally defined by variations in vowels, Spanish dialectal differences primarily affect consonant sound classes rather than vowels or a few specific phonemes. The dialect differences primarily affect certain sound classes over others. Fricatives and liquids (in particular /s/, flap /ɾ/, and trill /r/) tend to show more variation than stops, glides, or the affricate. The differences between Spanish dialects make it paramount that SLPs be aware of the dialect the children are speaking. Otherwise, the likelihood of misdiagnosis increases.

Phonological Development in Spanish-Speaking Children

Normative data (summarized in detail in Goldstein, 1995, 2000, 2007a) show that typically developing Spanish-speaking infants will tend to produce CV syllables containing oral and nasal stops with front vowels (e.g., Oller and Eilers, 1982). By the time typically developing Spanish-speaking children reach 3 1/2 years of age, it is likely that they will use the dialect features of the community and will have mastered the vowel system and most of the consonant system (e.g., Anderson and Smith, 1987; Goldstein and Cintron, 2001; Pandolfi and Herrera, 1990). In terms of vowel development in Spanish-speaking children, Oller and Eilers (1982) found that the mean proportion occurrence of vowel-like productions in 12- to 14-month-old English- and Spanish-speaking children was remarkably similar. In general, they noted that the children were likely to produce more anterior-like vowels than posterior-like ones. The rank order of the first 10 vowels in Spanish-speaking infants was: (1) [ε]; (2) [æ]; (3) [e]; (4) [i]; (5) [a]; (6) [ʌ]; (7) [ʊ]; (8) [u]; (9) [ɪ]; and (10) [o] (p. 573). Maez (1981) indicated that by 18 months, the three children in the study had mastered (i.e., produced correctly at least 90 percent of the time) the five basic Spanish vowels, [i], [e], [u], [o], and [a]. Maez's study, however, focused on consonant development, and did not indicate if any vowel errors occurred.

Goldstein and Pollock (2000) examined vowel productions in 23 Spanish-speaking children (10 3-year-olds and 13 4-year-olds) with speech sound disorders. Of the 23 children in the study, 14 exhibited vowel errors. Only 1 child exhibited more than one vowel error (five errors). The other 13 children each exhibited only one vowel error. Across all children, the results indicated that there were only 18 total vowel errors. Almost half the errors were on the vowel /o/.

In terms of consonant production, typically developing children will exhibit some difficulty by the end of preschool with consonant clusters and a few phones, specifically, [ð], [x], [s], [ɲ], [tʃ], [ɾ], [r], and [l] (e.g., Acevedo, 1991; Jimenez, 1987). These children may exhibit low percentages-of-occurrence of the following phonological patterns: cluster reduction, unstressed syllable deletion, stridency deletion, and tap/trill deviation, but will likely have suppressed phonological patterns such as velar and palatal fronting, prevocalic singleton omission, stopping, and assimilation (e.g., Goldstein and Iglesias, 1996a; Stepanof, 1990). For some Spanish-speaking children, phonetic mastery will continue into the early elementary school years when they continue to show some, although infrequent, errors on the fricatives [x] and [s], the affricate [tʃ], the flap [ɾ], the trill [r], the lateral [l], and consonant clusters (e.g., Bailey, 1982; De la Fuente, 1985).

Although there have been quite a number of studies describing phonological patterns in typically developing children, the data remain scarce for Spanish-speaking children with speech sound disorders. Data indicated that the percentage of Spanish-speaking children with speech sound disorders who exhibit specific phonological patterns was similar across studies (e.g., Bichotte, Dunn, Gonzalez, Orpi, and Nye, 1993; Goldstein and Iglesias, 1996b; Meza, 1983). Phonological patterns exhibited by a large percentage of children (>40 percent) included cluster reduction, unstressed syllable deletion, stopping, liquid simplification, and assimilation.

Finally, Goldstein (2007b) found that children speaking the Puerto Rican and Mexican dialects of Spanish show similar error types and error rates on complexity of the phonetic inventory, vowel accuracy, consonant accuracy, sound class accuracy, percentage-of-occurrence of phonological patterns, and frequency and types of substitutions.

Asian Languages

In the year 2000, there were approximately seven million speakers of Asian languages in the United States, 2.7 percent of the total U.S. population over 5 years of age (U.S. Bureau of the Census, 2000). There are three main families of languages spoken in Asia (Crystal, 1997). The first is the over 100 Austro-Asiatic languages, most of the languages spoken in Southeast Asia (the countries between China and Indonesia) including Khmer, Hmong, and Vietnamese. The second is the Tai family centered on Thailand and extending into Laos, North Vietnam, and parts of China. The third branch is Sino-Tibetan containing the languages of China, Tibet, and Burma, including Mandarin (also termed *Putonghua*) and Cantonese. Combined, these families contain over 440 languages spoken by over one billion people. Two other families, Austronesian and Papuan, contain languages spoken in the Pacific Islands (Cheng, 1993). Austronesian contains languages such as Hawaiian, Chamorro, Ilocano, and Tagalog. The Papuan family contains New Guinean.

There are a number of dialectal variations in Asian languages just as there are within English (e.g., Wang, 1990). For example, there are two main dialects of Chinese spoken in the United States: Mandarin and Cantonese (Cheng, 1987). There are also a number of sub-dialects within those two main dialects. Japanese has a few dialects but they are mutually unintelligible; however, Khmer's four dialects are mutually intelligible (Cheng, 1993). In the next two sections, Asian language phonology and phonological development in children speaking Asian languages will be described.

Asian Language Phonology

The phonological structure of Asian languages varies greatly. In general, there are few syllable-final segments and few consonant clusters. For example, (1) the only syllable-final consonants in Mandarin Chinese are /n/ and /ŋ/; (2) there are no labiodental, interdental, or palatal fricatives in Korean; and (3) Hawaiian contains only five vowels and eight consonants. There are, however, segmental systems in Asian languages that are relatively complex. For example, Hmong (the language spoken by dwellers in mountainous areas of Indochina) contains 56 initial consonants, 13 or 14 vowels (depending on dialect), seven tones, and one final consonant /ŋ/ (Cheng, 1993). For segmental information on specific languages and dialects, consult the following sources: Cheng (1987, 1993), Hwa-Froelich, Hodson, and Edwards (2002), Tipton (1975), and Wang (1989).

Syllable structure in Asian languages also shows considerable variation. For example, Laotian contains three syllable types (CVC, CVVC, and CVV). Khmer exhibits eight syllable types (CVC, CCVC, CCCVC, CVVC, CCVVC, CCCVVC, CVV, CCVV); however, there are few polysyllabic words in Khmer (Cheng, 1987). Many Asian languages also show restrictions on the types of segments that may appear in certain syllable positions. Vietnamese has a limited number of final consonants (voiceless stops and nasals); the only final consonant in Hmong is /ŋ/; and in Korean, there are no fricatives or affricates in word-final position. Stress also may be different in Asian languages compared with English.

For example, there is no tonic word stress in Korean so, to native English speakers, native speakers of Korean may sound somewhat "monotone" when speaking English (Cheng, 1993).

Many, but not all, Asian languages are tone languages. For example, Cantonese is a tone language, but Japanese is not. *Tone languages* are ones in which differences in word meaning are signified by differences in pitch. Tone languages are generally composed of register tones (typically two or three in a language) and contour tones (usually two or three per language) (O'Grady, Dobrovolsky, Aranoff, and Rees-Miller, 2004). *Register tones* are level tones, usually signaled by high, mid, and low tones. *Contour tones* are a combination of register tones over a single syllable. For example, in Mandarin Chinese, the phonetic string [ma] takes on different meanings depending on the tone or tone sequence that is applied. If produced with a high, level tone, [ma] means "mother," but if that same phonetic form is produced with a high-fall, register tone (i.e., a high then low tone), it means "scold."

There have been few studies on tone acquisition in Asian languages. Existing studies have illustrated the developmental process of tone (Li and Thompson, 1977; So and Dodd, 1995; Tse, 1978; Zhu and Dodd, 2000a). For example, Tse (1978) found that perceptual discrimination of tone began as early as age 10 months. The results from all four studies found that (1) children acquired the correct tone system relatively quickly (in about eight months), (2) mastery of tone occurred before segmental mastery, (3) high and falling tones were acquired earlier and more easily than rising and contour tones, and (4) substitution errors often exist for rising and contour tones during the two- and three-word stages.

Phonological Development in Speakers of Asian Languages

There are few studies that have investigated phonological patterns in children speaking Asian languages. Existing studies have largely investigated phonological development in children speaking Mandarin (Putonghua) and Cantonese. Zhu and Dodd (2000a) examined the phonological skills of 129 typically developing speakers of Putonghua ages 1;6 to 4;6. Their results indicated that tone was acquired first, followed by syllable-final consonants and vowels and finally syllable-initial consonants. By age 4;6, 90 percent of the children accurately produced all the syllable-initial consonants. Similar to typically developing children acquiring other languages, the Putonghua-speaking children exhibited syllabic and substitution phonological processes such as unstressed syllable deletion, fronting, and gliding. The children also showed language-specific patterns such as deaspiration and triphthong reduction of vowels. So and Dodd (1994, 1995) investigated phonological development in typically developing Cantonese-speaking children and noted similar phoneme acquisition to English but at more rapid rate. In general, anterior consonants were acquired before posterior ones, and oral and nasal stops and glides were acquired before fricatives and affricates. They also noted the presence of phonological processes and found that by age 4, no process was exhibited over 15 percent of the time. Between the ages of 2;0 and 4;0, these children showed processes similar in quantity (>15 percent) and type to English-speaking children: assimilation, cluster reduction, stopping, fronting, affrication, and final consonant deletion.

A few studies have also investigated speakers of Asian languages with speech sound disorders. Zhu and Dodd (2000b) assessed 33 children ages 2;8 to 7;6 with "atypical speech development" (p. 170). The largest subgroup of speakers (18 of 33 children) was characterized with "delayed phonological development" ("use of non-age-appropriate processes and/or restricted phonetic or phonemic inventory" p. 168). Phonological processes exhibited most commonly included fronting and stopping. These children with speech sound disorders had less difficulty with syllable components described as having more "phonological saliency" (p. 180). Phonological saliency, according to the authors, is based on syllable structure and is specific to each ambient language. In the case of Putonghua, tones, vowels, and syllable-final consonants are more salient, and syllable-initial consonants are less salient. As predicted, children with disorders had most difficulty with less salient features (i.e., syllable-initial consonants). So and Dodd (1994, pp. 238–240) outlined and defined four subgroups of children with speech sound disorders: delayed phonological development ("rules or processes used by more than 10% of children acquiring phonology normally"), consistent use of one or more unusual rules ("rules not used by more than 10 percent of children acquiring phonology normally"), articulation disorder ("consistent distortion of a phoneme"), and children who make inconsistent errors ("production of specific words or particular phonological segments"). So and Dodd applied these categories to 17 Cantonese-speaking children with speech sound disorders ages 3;6 to 6;4. Their results revealed that 8 of 17 participants (47 percent) displayed delayed phonological development, 5 of 17 (30 percent) were categorized as consistent users of one or more unusual rules, 2 of 17 (12 percent) had an articulation disorder, and another 2 of 17 (12 percent) were defined as making inconsistent errors.

So and Dodd (1994) further provided increased detail on the phonological patterns exhibited by the 13 children labeled as either "phonological delay" or "consistently disordered." Children with phonological delay tended to exhibit assimilation, cluster reduction, stopping, fronting, deaspiration, affrication, and final consonant deletion. Children with phonological disorder tended to exhibit final consonant deletion, final glide deletion, initial consonant deletion, aspiration, gliding, vowel rule, and backing.

Cheung and Abberton (2000) examined the phonological skills of 251 Cantonese-speaking children (ages 3;6 to 6;0) with speech sound disorders. They found that tones and vowels largely were produced accurately, with consonants being most affected. The children showed most difficulty with /s/, aspirated consonants (e.g., /pʰ/), and labialized consonants (e.g., /kʷ/). Thus, deaspiration was a commonly occurring phonological pattern, as were stopping and fronting of velars.

Tang and Barlow (2006) investigated the phonological skills of four Vietnamese-speaking children (ages 4;4 to 5;5) with speech sound disorders. They found that tone was adult-like for all four children. The four children also produced all vowels and the majority of stops, nasals, and glides in syllable-initial and syllable-final positions. Seven phonological patterns were exhibited by at least two of the children: gliding, fronting, glottal replacement, backing, velar assimilation, stopping, and final consonant deletion. Many of these patterns are common cross-linguistically (e.g., stopping, fronting, and final consonant deletion) although others are not (e.g., glottal replacement). Finally, final consonants were acquired before initial ones.

PHONOLOGICAL DEVELOPMENT IN BILINGUAL CHILDREN

Although there is no doubt that SLPs will be assessing and providing intervention services to monolingual speakers of Spanish and Asian languages, it is more likely that SLPs in the United States will be delivering clinical services to bilingual children acquiring a language in addition to English. Studies of bilingual children indicate that phonological development in these bilingual children is similar, although not identical, to that of monolingual speakers of either language (Goldstein, 2004).

Dodd, So, and Li (1996) examined the phonology of 16 typically developing, Cantonese-speaking children who were acquiring English in preschool. The results indicated that the children differentiated the phonology of each language. They also found that the children's error patterns were atypical for monolingual speakers of either language. However, bilingual children produced a higher number of atypical error patterns (e.g., initial consonant deletion) in an amount usually associated with children evidencing speech sound disorders. Holm and Dodd (2000) examined the phonological skills of two Cantonese-English bilingual children from ages 2;3 to 3;1 and from ages 2;9 to 3;5. They found that the children maintained separate phonological systems of each language; the children's phonetic development was similar to those of monolingual children; and both children exhibited phonological patterns that were not typical for monolingual speakers (e.g., atypical aspiration); however, these patterns were exhibited by Cantonese-English bilingual speakers in other studies (e.g., Dodd et al., 1996).

Gildersleeve, Davis, and Stubbe (1996) examined the English phonological skills of typically developing, bilingual (English-Spanish) 3-year-olds. Their results showed that bilingual children showed an overall lower intelligibility rating, made more consonant and vowel errors, distorted more sounds, and produced more uncommon error patterns than either monolingual English or monolingual Spanish speakers. Gildersleeve-Neumann and Davis (1998), however, demonstrated that although bilingual speakers exhibited different developmental patterns than their monolingual peers and exhibited more errors initially than monolingual speakers, these differences faded over time.

Similarities and differences in phonological skills between monolingual and bilingual speakers are also supported by the work of Goldstein and Washington (2001) and Goldstein, Fabiano, and Washington (2005). These researchers examined the Spanish and English phonological skills in typically developing, 4- and 5-year-old bilingual (Spanish-English) children, respectively. They largely found similarities in phonological skills between bilingual and monolingual children. Differences between groups were relegated to the accuracy of production of sounds in specific sound classes, especially in Spanish. Spirants, flap, and trill in Spanish were produced much less accurately in bilingual children than have been shown for monolingual Spanish-speaking children (Goldstein, 1988).

The results of these studies indicate that bilingual phonological development appears to proceed along the same course as that for monolingual speakers. That trajectory, however, is not the same as it is for monolingual speakers. Bilingual children might exhibit error types that are less common in monolingual speakers, are likely to show cross-linguistic effects, and may be less accurate on some aspects of the phonological system in comparison to their monolingual peers. Those differences seem to diminish over time such that bilingual children are able to achieve adult-like phonological skills in both languages.

The Influence of One Language on Another

When there is contact between speakers of two or more languages, a tendency exists for one language to influence the other (Goldstein, 2007c). This influence is often bi-directional with each language influencing the other. For example, a native Spanish speaker acquiring English will exhibit characteristics of Spanish-influenced English and English-influenced Spanish. In a group of bilingual (Spanish-English) children, Goldstein and Iglesias (1999) found that a few children substituted [tʃ] for /ʃ/; /ʃʌvəl/ *(shovel)* was produced as [tʃʌvəl] (Spanish-influenced English). The children also used the postvocalic "r" of General American English for the Spanish flap; /floɾ/ *(flower)* was produced as [floɚ] (English-influenced Spanish).

For speakers acquiring more than one language, there are many ways that the phonology of one language may have an effect on the phonology of another language (Goldstein, 2007c). First, the specific phonemes and allophones in the inventories of each language will not be the same. For example, the alveo-palatal affricate [tʃ] found in English is not in the inventory of Cantonese (Cheng, 1993). A native Cantonese-speaking individual acquiring English might substitute [ts] for the alveo-palatal affricate because [ts] exists in the inventory of Cantonese and is close to the place of articulation of the English affricate. Second, differences in the distribution of sounds exist across languages. For example, [ŋ] might be the only word-final sound realized in English by a native Hmong speaker because it is the only word-final sound in Hmong (Cheng, 1993). Third, consonants may have different places of articulation in each language. For example, Spanish speakers acquiring English may produce /d/ with a dental place of articulation as is common in Spanish versus an alveolar place of articulation that is typical in English (Perez, 1994). Fourth, phonological rules may be different in each language. For example, the phrase *Cómo se llama su niño?* (What is your child's name?), which would be produced as [komo se jama su niɲo] in Spanish, might be realized as [koʊmoʊ se jama su niɲoʊ] in English-influenced Spanish because the speaker is diphthongizing vowels as is common in English. Finally, how and when pronunciation is acquired may contribute to the influence of one language on another. For some individuals learning English as a second language, their major exposure might be in school where written language is being introduced. The lack of one-to-one correspondence between grapheme and phoneme in English may influence pronunciation (August, Calderón, and Carlo 2002). For example, the grapheme "s" in English is produced as [s] in *basin* and as [ʒ] in *measure* causing a speaker of Spanish-influenced English to produce both as [s].

ASSESSMENT CONSIDERATIONS FOR CHILDREN FROM CULTURALLY AND LINGUISTICALLY DIVERSE POPULATIONS

In assessing the speech and language skills of children from culturally and linguistically diverse populations, the same types of information are gathered as for all children: case history, oral-peripheral examination, hearing screening, language (e.g., syntax, semantics, pragmatics, and the lexicon), voice, fluency, and phonological patterns. The analysis of phonological patterns in children from culturally and linguistically diverse populations requires a determination of whether the child's phonological system is within normal limits for his or her linguistic community (ASHA, 2004). Thus, the assessment must be approached with an understanding of the social, cultural, and linguistic characteristics of that community always guarding against stereotyping (Taylor, Payne, and Anderson, 1987). One cannot assume that any individual from any geographical area or ethnic/racial group is a speaker of a particular dialect. For example, although one African American's production of f/θ in the word *mouth* may be regarded as a dialect feature of AAE, it would be inappropriate to make the same clinical judgment for another African American who also produces f/θ. The first speaker may be an AAE speaker, but the second speaker may not be, and therefore the production would be considered a true error.

Speech-language pathologists must also differentiate dialect differences from speech sound disorders. In ASHA's position papers on social dialects and communication disorders and variations, the association officially acknowledges the distinction between a speech-language difference and a speech-language disorder (ASHA, 1993, 1983). A few investigators have attempted to determine if scoring dialectal features as "errors" would penalize children for patterns that are, in effect, dialect features, thus artificially inflating their severity ratings. In their examination of 10 AAE-speaking children ages 5;11 to 6;11, Cole and Taylor (1990) found that not taking dialect into account resulted in the misdiagnosis of speech sound disorder for half the children, on average, across three phonological assessments. Two other studies, while advocating that dialect should be accounted for in phonological assessment, did not find the same significant results as Cole and Taylor. Fleming and Hartman (1989) examined 72 4-year-old AAE speakers using the *Computer Assessment of Phonological Processes* (*CAPP*; Hodson, 1985). They determined that although some test items are influenced by "Black English phonological rules," the assessment as a whole is not invalidated (p. 28). Moreover, they indicated that no typically developing child was labeled as having a disorder based solely on the factor of dialect. Washington and Craig (1992) examined 28 preschool AAE-speaking children ages 4;6 to 5;3. Their results indicated that dialect scoring changes did "not seem to penalize the BE-speaking preschooler to a degree that is clinically significant" (p. 23). Washington and Craig ascribed the contrast of their results to those of Cole and Taylor on the basis of geographical location. The participants in Cole and Taylor's study were from Mississippi, whereas the children in Washington and Craig's study resided in Detroit. Goldstein and Iglesias (2001) examined 54 typically developing Spanish-speaking children and 54 Spanish-speaking children with speech sound disorders to determine if taking or not taking into account Puerto Rican Spanish dialect features altered the results of the analyses. The results indicated that if dialect features had not been taken into account, almost 75 percent of typically developing children might have been erroneously characterized as exhibiting speech sound disorders. In addition, not taking dialect into account might have resulted in unnecessarily targeting for intervention phonological processes whose percentages-of-occurrence were inflated.

Although the results of these studies reported somewhat different conclusions as to whether scoring dialectal features as "errors" affected the child's severity rating, these researchers all agreed that accounting for dialect features is a prime consideration in the assessment of children from culturally and linguistically diverse populations. Analysis of phonological information must be made taking the child's dialect into account. "Errors" can only be counted as such when they are in conflict with the child's dialect. For example, in the Puerto Rican dialect of Spanish, the production of /dos/ (*"two"*) as [do:] would not be scored as an error because syllable-final /s/ is often deleted. The production of /floɾ/

(*"flower"*) as [flo] would be scored as an error because syllable-final deletion of /r/ is not considered a typical feature of the dialect. Thus, in order to minimize the possibility of misdiagnosis, all phonological analyses should take into account the features of that particular dialect and should not be scored as errors. To account for dialect features in any particular linguistic group, SLPs might (1) become thoroughly familiar with features of the dialects and language, (2) sample the adult speakers in the child's linguistic community, and (3) obtain information from interpreters/support personnel.

In order to minimize the effect that not accounting for dialect features might have on the phonological analysis of speakers from culturally and linguistically diverse populations, Stockman has suggested assessing a minimal competency core (MCC), developed to decrease bias in the assessment of AAE-speaking children (Stockman, 1996b, p. 358). *Minimal competency core* is defined as "the *least* amount of knowledge that one must exhibit to be judged as normal in a given age range" (p. 358, emphasis original). Stockman noted that MCC may best be used as a screening tool on a core subgroup of specific behaviors. The phonological features core includes the following word/syllable initial sounds that are invariable in GAE and AAE: /m, n, p, b, t, d, k, g, f, s, h, w, j, l, ɹ/. Wilcox and Anderson (1998) found that assessing these sounds along with clusters provided enough information to differentiate typical from atypical speech sound development in a group of African American English speakers.

Examiners must be aware of their own dialect and its effect on the assessment process. Seymour and Seymour (1977) noted that the client's perception of the formality of the situation affects dialect density. Casual speaking settings may increase dialect density by encouraging more frequent use of AAE, whereas a more formal setting may result in a decrease in dialect density by inhibiting and stigmatizing speech forms other than General American English. A similar issue may be encountered when a clinician uses Castillian Spanish (i.e., the dialect of Spanish spoken in some areas of Spain and taught in most educational systems in the United States) when conversing with a speaker of any of the other major Spanish dialects. This is not to say that one should force herself or himself to use the client's dialect. One must realize, however, the potential effect that one's particular dialect may have on a client and family.

The assessment of speakers of languages other than or in addition to English presents a challenge to the SLP. The SLP must determine the language or languages of assessment and then choose appropriate assessment tools. Even if the child seems to be a "dominant" English speaker, it is common practice to assess phonological skills in both languages, as the child's phonological knowledge will be distributed across the two languages (Goldstein, 2006). Analyses then should be completed in both languages. The speech-language pathologist must differentiate true speech sound errors from developmental errors from atypical/disordered patterns from cross-linguistic effects (Yavaş and Goldstein, 1998).

A detailed phonological assessment would include both formal measures (instruments standardized on speakers from a particular language group) and informal measures (such as a spontaneous language sample). The formal assessment tool should be designed specifically to assess phonological patterns in that language. Unfortunately, there are few available formal measures covering a variety of languages. Using an assessment tool designed for any other linguistic group other than the one for which it was intended will likely increase bias and lead to over-referral. In the absence of formal measures, the SLP might utilize informal client observations with siblings, peers, and/or parent(s) asking a series of questions designed to determine the adequacy of the child's phonological system (Yavaş and Goldstein, 1998): Does the child sound like other children in his or her peer group (i.e., like other members of their speech community)? What consonants does the child produce (front vs. back, syllable-initial vs. syllable-final)? Does the child make any vowel errors? If appropriate, does the child use tone accurately? What percentage of the time is the child intelligible? Is the child understood by the child's parents, family members, teachers, and friends all, some, or none of the time?

Role of the Monolingual Speech-Language Pathologist

Speech-language pathologists may have difficulty assessing children who speak more than one language because SLPs often are not bilingual themselves (Goldstein, 2001). Clinicians who do not speak the language of the individual they are assessing might consider alternatives such as hiring a bilingual consultant or bilingual diagnostician, training bilingual aides, or using interpreters/translators (I/Ts) (Langdon and Cheng, 2002). If I/Ts are used, SLPs should be sure the I/Ts are trained, have exemplary bilingual/bidialectal communication skills, understand their responsibilities and act professionally, and can relate to members of the cultural group (Kayser; 1995; Langdon and Cheng, 2002). Interpreters/translators should assist the SLP in completing the assessment but not conduct the assessment themselves. It might be tempting for SLPs to use family members as I/Ts. Lynch (2004) advises against this practice because acting in this role may be burdensome to the family member, and family members may be reticent in discussing emotional matters, uncomfortable providing information to older or younger family members or to members of the opposite gender, and leave out information provided by the SLP.

In the absence of a bilingual speech-language pathologist at the site, monolingual SLPs may also play a role in the assessment of non-English-speaking children. If they have knowledge, skills, competencies, and training in providing services to individuals with limited- or non-English proficiency, monolingual SLPs may assess in English, administer an oral-peripheral examination, conduct a hearing screening, and administer nonverbal assessments (ASHA, 1985).

INTERVENTION FOR SPEECH SOUND DISORDERS IN CHILDREN FROM CULTURALLY AND LINGUISTICALLY DIVERSE POPULATIONS

Once the results of an assessment are gathered, SLPs must decide if intervention is warranted. The traditional role of the SLP is to provide clinical services for communication disorders but not for dialectal differences. However, ASHA's position paper on social dialects identifies the following expanded role for SLPs (ASHA, 1983):

> Aside from the traditionally recognized role, the speech-language pathologist may also be available to provide *elective* clinical services to nonstandard English speakers who do not present a disorder. The role of the speech-language pathologist for these individuals is to

prepare the desired competency in Standard English without jeopardizing the integrity of the individual's first dialect. The approach must be functional and based on context-specific appropriateness of the given dialect. (p. 24)

If elective services are to take place, it is important to remember that elective therapy does not mean necessarily that the client wants to eliminate the first dialect (D1). More often, the client prefers to be bidialectal. Taylor (1986) suggested a number of principles for SLPs who seek to guide speakers who want to acquire a second dialect: (1) Develop a positive attitude toward the home dialect of the speaker; (2) compare the features of the home dialect to the one being acquired; (3) select targets based on language acquisition norms, frequency of occurrence of the features, and the speaker's attitude toward the features; (4) know the rules of the speaker's home dialect and the ones to be acquired; (5) take the speaker's learning style into account; and (6) integrate language issues into the larger culture of the speaker. Taylor also proposed a series of steps that must be followed in order to maintain both dialects. First, a positive attitude toward D1 must be established. Second, the client must learn to contrast the features of the first dialect and the second dialect (D2). Finally, the client uses D2 in controlled, structured, and eventually spontaneous situations with a focus on form, content, and use.

Modifying someone's dialect involves more than simply having the person produce consonant and vowels as a native speaker would pronounce them. Learning nonsegmental aspects of speech production such as stress, pitch, and intonation will be equally important. There are likely to be differences between the person's home language/dialect and the variety being acquired as a second language/dialect. For example, stress in English is relatively more complicated than in other languages. Placement of stress depends on a number of factors, including syntactic category and weight of the syllable (i.e., whether the vowel is long or short and the number of consonants that follow the vowel) (Goodluck, 1991). Pitch also differs as a function of language. For example, pitch modulates less in Spanish than it does in English (Hadlich, Holton, and Montes, 1968). Finally, intonational contours for statements, questions, and exclamations may be different in English than in other languages. For example, in English, utterances (statements, questions, and exclamations) may begin at an overall higher pitch than in other languages.

Speech-language pathologists must also recognize how dialectal variation and speech sound disorders interact (Wolfram, 1994). Wolfram has suggested the following guiding principles. He divided impairments into three types. *Type I* impairments were judged to be atypical patterns regardless of the speaker's dialect (e.g., initial consonant deletion (e.g., [it] for /mit/) or velar fronting (e.g., [dot] for /got/)). In *Type II* impairments, there was a cross-dialectal difference in the normative (or underlying) form. For example, the normative form for the word *bathing* would be [beðiŋ] for speakers of General American English but [beviŋ] for AAE speakers even though speakers from both dialect groups might misarticulate that word as [beziŋ]. *Type III* impairments influenced forms that were shared across dialects but were applied with different frequency. For example, syllable-final cluster reduction was exhibited in many dialects. In AAE, this pattern was observed more frequently than in other dialects. Wolfram noted that treating a *Type I* impairment would not necessitate gathering different norms across dialect groups. The treatment of *Type II* and *Type III* impairments, however, would involve taking into account both qualitative and quantitative differences between dialect groups.

Intervention for Bilingual Children with Speech Sound Disorders

Little information is available regarding direct intervention for individuals with speech sound disorders who speak a language other than or in addition to English. Available data indicate that principles guiding intervention choices for these children are both similar to and different from those for monolingual children. As with all children, the intervention process begins with the completion of a comprehensively broad and deep assessment. Once this information is collected, SLPs need to compare those results with the appropriate comparison database. Speech-language pathologists should remember neither to use normative data gathered from English-speaking children to assess children who speak a language other than or in addition to English nor to generalize developmental phonological data from one dialect group to another. That is, phonological skills in the bilingual child being assessed need to be compared to those of other, similar bilingual children.

Once the assessment is completed, the next step should be to determine the intervention goal and the intervention approach (Goldstein, 2006). Choosing the goal and approach will guide the SLP in determining the language of intervention. Kohnert and Derr (2004) and Kohnert, Yim, Nett, Kan, and Duran (2005) have proposed two main approaches for providing intervention to bilingual children. In the *bilingual approach*, they propose that SLPs should improve skills common to both languages. For example, initial goals would be those focusing on constructs common to both languages (e.g., the phoneme /s/, final consonant deletion). To extend that approach, Yavaş and Goldstein (1998) suggested that for a bilingual child with at least a moderate speech sound disorder, SLPs should choose intervention targets based on the error rates in both languages. Initially, error patterns that were exhibited with similar error rates in both languages should be targeted. For example, a pattern such as unstressed syllable deletion would be an initial intervention target because it would likely show similar error rates in both languages and affect intelligibility greatly in both languages. Treating errors that occur frequently in both languages likely will improve intelligibility in both languages, rather than in only one of the bilingual's languages. Using this approach, however, requires frequent monitoring of generalization across both languages, although generalization across languages is not guaranteed. For example, Holm, Dodd, and Ozanne (1997) found that intervention on one sound in English did generalize to Cantonese, but intervention on a phonological pattern did not. Subsequent to treating errors occurring with similar frequency in both languages, error patterns that are exhibited in both languages with unequal frequency should be treated. For example, final consonant deletion is a phonological pattern that is likely to be exhibited in English with a high percentage-of-occurrence but with a low percentage-of-occurrence in Spanish (Goldstein and Iglesias, 1996). Finally, phonological patterns exhibited in only one language should be targeted. For example, final consonant devoicing may be exhibited in English but not in Spanish (Goldstein and Washington, 2001).

In the *cross-linguistic approach*, Kohnert and colleagues suggest that clinicians focus on skills distinct in each constituent language. This approach also will be necessary (likely in conjunction with the bilingual approach) because of the differences in the phonological structures of the two languages. For example, labialized consonants exist in Cantonese, but not in English, and thus can be remediated in only one language. As an adjunct, SLPs might utilize the cross-linguistic approach based on types of errors and/or error rates (Yavaş and Goldstein,

1998). For example, the frequency-of-occurrence of final consonant deletion in Spanish-English bilingual children is higher in their English than in their Spanish (Goldstein et al., 2005). Thus, intervention to decrease the use of final consonant deletion likely will occur in English but not in Spanish. Finally, errors occurring in only one language would be targets for phonological intervention (e.g., final devoicing in Language B but not in Language A).

Adapting Intervention Approaches to Individuals from Culturally and Linguistically Diverse Populations

Although little specific information is available to guide the intervention of speech sound disorders in speakers of languages other than or in addition to English, specific intervention approaches developed for English-speaking children might be adapted for use with those from culturally and linguistically diverse populations. A number of different methods for remediating speech sound errors have been categorized into two main types: phonetic and phonemic (Bauman-Waengler, 2008). *Phonetic approaches*, such as the traditional approach (Van Riper, 1972) and the multiple phoneme approach (Bradley, 1985), and *phonemic approaches*, such as the cycles approach (Hodson and Paden, 1991) and language-based approaches (Hoffman, Norris, and Monjure, 1990), can be adapted for use with individuals from culturally and linguistically diverse populations.

Utilizing a phonetic approach poses several difficulties unless the speech-language pathologist is a speaker of the child's native/home language. First, the SLP must be able to carry out the perceptual training phase of this approach. This includes the ability to produce an auditory model for the child. Second, the SLP must discern the segments in the child's home language, the segments in the child's repertoire, the order of acquisition of the sounds, the ease of production for the sounds, the frequency of occurrence of each phone in the language, and phonetic contexts that may facilitate production of the target sound (Stoel-Gammon and Dunn, 1985).

A phonemic approach also raises several issues for the SLP. First, each specific program would have to be adapted to the child's language and dialect. Second, because this type of approach is based on patterns rather than individual sound segments, the SLP would need to differentiate a series of unrelated errors from a single phonological rule (Williams, 2001). Third, in order to apply this type of approach, the SLP should be able to identify errors most affecting intelligibility, errors that cut across sound classes, and errors that disappear at the earliest age from typically developing children (Stoel-Gammon and Dunn, 1985). Finally, the order of intervention advocated by the approach might need to be altered for a speaker of a language other than English. For example, Hodson and Paden (1991) in their cycles approach suggest treating syllabicity early in the remediation process. That is, if the child does not use two-syllable words, then increasing the child's production of multisyllabic words might be warranted. In a language such as Khmer, for example, which has complex syllable types but few polysyllabic words, this might not be the initial target of choice.

A number of phonemic approaches advocate the use of contrastive word pairs (i.e., minimal opposition pairs, *so/toe*, or maximal opposition pairs, *beet/seat*). Approaches using contrastive word-pairs include the paired stimuli approach (Weston and Irwin, 1985), minimal phonemic contrast approach (Cooper, 1985), minimal "triads" (Nelson, 1995), metaphon (Howell and Dean, 1991), maximal opposition (Gierut, 1989), and multiple oppositions

(Williams, 2000a, 2000b). Contrastive word-pairs, however, may be difficult to adapt to speakers of languages other than English. English, unlike other languages, is replete with minimal pairs. It may be more difficult to apply this methodology to languages other than English if those languages lack a significant number of contrastive word-pairs that are appropriate for children.

SUMMARY

To provide least-biased assessment and evidence-based intervention to linguistically diverse individuals, SLPs must carry out a number of steps. First, they should gather information about the cultural and linguistic norms of the individuals to whom they are providing service. These norms include the phonological rules of the dialects/languages spoken by the client, remembering that not all speakers of a particular dialect will show or use every characteristic of it. Second, SLPs should complete a comprehensive phonological assessment that includes a wide array of independent and relational analyses. For these analyses, they should take into account dialect features that occur in all the client's languages. Finally, extensive information collected from the assessment should be used to plan intervention, remembering that intervention for a dialect difference should not occur, unless elected by the client. For children acquiring more than one language, it is likely that both the bilingual approach and the cross-linguistic approach will be required. Following these steps will aid in providing appropriate services to children from culturally and linguistically diverse populations.

QUESTIONS FOR CHAPTER 8

1. What dialect do you speak? How do you think you acquired your dialect? If your dialect were to change, what dialect would you most/least like to have? Provide reasons for your decisions.

2. Administer a formal assessment to a speaker with a dialect. Score the assessment not taking into account the speaker's dialect features, and then score it taking into account the dialect features. How did the person's score change between each administration? Would the person have been labeled with a speech sound disorder if dialect features had not been taken into account?

3. How would you determine whether the phonological patterns exhibited by someone were characteristic of true errors or dialect features?

4. Design a protocol to use support personnel in the assessment of a preschool child who is bilingual in English and Vietnamese. You might consult the following ASHA papers to aid in your planning:

American Speech-Language-Hearing Association. (2004). Knowledge and skills needed by speech-language pathologists and audiologists to provide culturally and linguistically appropriate services. *ASHA* (Suppl. 24).

American Speech-Language-Hearing Association. (1996, Spring). Guidelines for the training, credentialing, use, and supervision of speech-language pathology assistants. *ASHA, 38* (Suppl. 16), pp. 21–34.

American Speech-Language Hearing Association. (1994, March). ASHA policy regarding support personnel. *ASHA, 36* (Suppl. 13), p. 24.

5. Define *pidgin, creole, dialect*, and *language*. What are the similarities and differences between these language varieties?

6. Take an informal poll about myths and facts about dialect. Ask individuals to give you their opinion on people's dialects and how they feel about certain dialects. You might survey individuals who have a background in languages studies and individuals who do not have such a background to compare their responses. Then write a paper listing those perceptions followed by facts that counter any myths that are mentioned by the people you interview.

7. Create a quick reference guide for phonological development in AAE, Spanish, Cantonese, and Mandarin. You might list sounds in each of their inventories, age of acquisition for segments and tones (if appropriate), and age of suppression for phonological processes. Create a reference guide for a language/dialect not listed here.

8. Design a protocol for modifying the dialect of a native Spanish-speaking woman who wishes to sound "more like a native English speaker." List at least 10 questions you would ask her during the case history, enumerate the ways in which you would assess her speech, and outline your short-term and long-term goals, providing a rationale for each of those goals. What aspects of her speech do you think it will be less difficult and more difficult to modify? Why?

9. Do you think newcomers to the United States who do not speak English should maintain their home language? Provide a rationale for your response. What are the advantages and disadvantages of immigrants to the United States maintaining/losing their native language?

10. Define *dialect, accent*, and *idiolect*. Do you think all children should be given speech therapy in order to speak one type of dialect? Justify your answer.

11. Based on the following productions from an African American–speaking child, age 4:5, indicate if the child's production is a dialect feature of AAE or a true error:

Gloss	Child's Production	AAE Feature	True Error
soap	[top]	No	Yes
mother	[mʌðə]		
mouth	[mɑʊf]		
tell	[tɪl]		
self	[sɛf]		
cool	[ku]		
bell	[bɛ]		
cool	[kũ]		
playing	[pejiŋ]		
fast	[fæs]		
stool	[tul]		

Phonological Awareness: Description, Assessment, and Intervention

LAURA M. JUSTICE
Ohio State University

GAIL T. GILLON
University of Canterbury

C. MELANIE SCHUELE
Vanderbilt University

Running speech consists of varying types of linguistic units that range in size from larger (sentences, words, syllables) to smaller (morphemes, phonemes). Most adult speakers of a language can readily and consciously recognize that speech comprises sentences, words, syllables, morphemes, and phonemes, and that these units are discrete and recurring elements of language. One's ability to consciously analyze the sound structure of speech emerges in early childhood, and this ability is called *phonological awareness*. Young children's phonological awareness is apparent when they successfully perform tasks requiring them to generate rhymes, identify the beginning sounds in words, or segment the individual phonemes comprising words. Children's successful performance on such tasks is consistently associated with performance on reading tasks—particularly those measuring word recognition—indicating that there are integrative linkages between phonological awareness and acquisition of word-level reading skills. Of particular importance to speech-language pathologists is evidence showing that children with speech sound difficulties often show lags in their development of phonological awareness, and that such lags may pose specific risks for their timely development of skilled reading. This chapter provides a framework for understanding phonological awareness, recognizing why children with speech difficulties often have challenges in this area, and considering how such challenges may be addressed through clinical interventions.

WHAT IS PHONOLOGICAL AWARENESS?

Phonological awareness refers to an individual's awareness of the sound (phonological) structure of spoken words. Children exhibiting phonological awareness consciously recognize (or at least are sensitive to) the phonological units comprising a word. Often at relatively young ages (3 to 4 years), children become aware that spoken words contain syllables and that syllables within words contain smaller sound units. With increasing age, children become more aware of the intrasyllabic units of syllables and words, including onsets, rimes, and individual phonemes.

The intrasyllabic structure of a word in the English language can be distinguished on the basis of naturally occurring onset-rime units within a syllable (Anthony and Lonigan, 2004; Treiman, Fowler, Gross, Berch, and Weatherston, 1995). *Onset* refers to the consonant or consonant cluster that precedes the vowel in a syllable, whereas the *rime* encompasses the vowel and any subsequent consonants. For example, the onset of the word *hog* is "h" and the rime is "og." Likewise, the onset of *stripe* is "str" and the rime is "ipe." Studies have shown that the onset and rime compose natural boundaries governing the internal structure of the syllabic unit (Treiman and Zukowski, 1990).

With these terms in mind, *phonological awareness* describes a cluster of skills that includes an individual's awareness of the syllabic structure of words as well as the intrasyllabic structure; the latter includes attending to the onset and rime units within syllables and, at a more advanced level, recognizing that onset and rime units are composed of individual phonemes. This awareness of a word's phonological structure is *sublexical*, meaning that representation of these units occurs at a level distinct from meaning. This awareness is also viewed as being *metalinguistic* in nature, in that it requires an individual to focus on language as an object of thought. Phonological awareness is contingent on and mediated by the child's access to the phonology of his or her language (Wagner and Torgesen, 1987).

Other terms, such as *phonological processing, phonemic* and *phoneme awareness, phonological sensitivity, phonemic analysis, phonetic awareness,* and *linguistic awareness*, have been used more or less interchangeably with the term *phonological awareness*. Some scholars use the term only in reference to awareness at the level of the phoneme. Ball and Blachman (1991), for instance, describe phonological awareness as one's ability to represent spoken words and syllables as discrete sequences of individual sound segments at the level of the phoneme. This restricted use of the term *phonological awareness*, in emphasizing only that level at which conscious, explicit awareness of phonemes is exhibited, does not encompass more implicit levels of sensitivity to the phonological structure of language (e.g., sensitivity to syllables and rime units in words). A more encompassing perspective of phonological awareness includes reference to skills ranging along a continuum of shallow to deep levels of awareness (Anthony, Lonigan, Driscoll, Phillips, and Burgess, 2003; Stanovich, 2000).

Shallow Levels of Awareness

At more shallow levels of phonological awareness, children show sensitivity to the sound patterns that recur across and within words. At these levels, children may recognize, for instance, that the words *bell* and *tell* demonstrate certain phonological similarities (i.e., these words rhyme), and that *bell* can be divided into two components (i.e., its onset and rime: *b* + *ell*).

They are also likely to be able to blend and segment multisyllabic words (e.g., *doorbell, pancake*), and to identify when words share the same singleton onsets (e.g., *me* and *moon*).

Deep Levels of Awareness

At the opposite end of the continuum, representing deeper levels of sensitivity, children demonstrate more conscious levels of awareness regarding a word or syllable's phonological structure. With access to deeper levels of sensitivity, children are able to compare, contrast, and even manipulate phonological segments within and across syllables and words. For example, they can delete phonemes in words to create new words (such as deleting the first sound in the word *track* to create *rack*), and can count the number of sounds in individual words. Phoneme awareness is fully realized when children can recognize that each word or syllable consists of a series of discrete phonemes and can explicitly identify, blend, and segment these phonemes. The terms *phonemic* and *phoneme awareness* have been used by a number of scholars in reference to this sophisticated level of awareness.

A Developmental Perspective

Recognizing that the development of phonological awareness occurs along a continuum is consistent with the perspective that children's attainment of phonological awareness is developmental in nature (Stanovich, 2000). In general, children's development of phonological awareness follows a continuum along which they gain sensitivity first to words followed by syllables, onset/rimes, and then phonemes (Anthony et al., 2003). A considerable body of research supports a developmental trajectory in the growth of phonological awareness in both English and other alphabetic languages (Anthony et al., 2003; Ziegler and Goswami, 2005). Some researchers use the term *quasi-parallel progression* to emphasize how children's sensitivity to words, syllables, onset/rimes, and phonemes emerges in overlapping rather than discrete stages (Anthony et al., 2003). That is, children are developing awareness of onset/rimes simultaneous to developing awareness of phonemes, although they might be closer to mastery for the former. Understanding the quasi-parallel nature of phonological-awareness development suggests that children need not "master" one ability (e.g., rhyming) before another (e.g., identifying initial sounds in words). Children's growth in phonological awareness is highly mediated by both language abilities and experiences (Lonigan, Burgess, Anthony, and Barker, 1998; Stahl and Murray, 1994). In particular, growth in vocabulary development and letter knowledge are considered influential variables on children's early phonological awareness development during the preschool years (Burgess and Lonigan, 1998).

PHONOLOGICAL AWARENESS AS LITERACY DEVELOPMENT

Phonological awareness has often been studied within the context of children's literacy development. Although children's ability to represent and manipulate the phonological structure of words consciously is highly mediated by their linguistic abilities and experiences, the fundamental (and potentially causal) role that phonological awareness plays in reading development has encouraged many scientists and practitioners to study phonological awareness within the framework of literacy development. The term *literacy* is used here in a general sense to describe children's attainment of both emergent and conventional literacy skills; *emergent literacy* refers to skills and knowledge serving as prerequisites to reading and writing, whereas *conventional literacy* refers to fluent and skilled reading and writing.

More specifically, emergent literacy describes precursory reading and writing skills that are acquired by most children within the preschool and kindergarten period. These skills lay the foundation for later skilled and fluent reading (van Kleeck, 1998). The two primary domains of development within this preliterate period are print knowledge (knowledge about forms and functions of written language; Justice and Ezell, 2004) and phonological awareness. Children's development of both print knowledge and phonological awareness are viewed as legitimate and critical elements of literacy development (Whitehurst and Lonigan, 1998) and provide the foundation for their eventual attainment of conventional literacy. To this end, preschool children with sophisticated levels of print knowledge and phonological awareness are more likely to develop into proficient conventional readers and writers as compared to preschoolers with low levels of awareness (Badian, 2000; Christensen, 2000; Storch and Whitehurst, 2002). Conventional literacy is typically acquired within the context of formal instruction, usually beginning in first grade, or at about 6 to 7 years of age.

Historical perspectives of literacy development took the viewpoint—in both theoretical and practical terms—that children's acquisition of literacy skills began only within the context of formal literacy instruction. Relatively recently, scientists began to study literacy development in very young children and found that preschool children, as young as 2 and 3 years of age, possess considerable knowledge about reading and writing. A substantial number of researchers in the last two decades have described what young children know about literacy, as well as determining how this knowledge is mediated by linguistic, cognitive, and environmental influences (e.g., Justice, Pence, Bowles, and Wiggins, 2006; Storch and Whitehurst, 2002). Across numerous studies of literacy development in young children, a single set of variables—those representing phonological awareness—has stood out in terms of its robust value in predicting reading achievement (e.g., Hogan, Catts, and Little, 2005; Torgesen, Wagner, and Rashotte, 1994). Awareness of the phonological structure of spoken language helps children decode printed text, recognize words in print, and spell words (see Gillon, 2004, for review).

THE DEVELOPMENT OF PHONOLOGICAL AWARENESS

Serendipitously, the following conversation between a father and his son (who appeared to be about 4 years old) was overheard by the first author during the preparation of this chapter. The conversation took place in a local bookstore, where father and son were looking at the cover of a magazine.

SON: Is that a butterfly?
DAD: Yes, that's a butterfly.
SON: But-ter-fly. Hey Dad, is *but* a word?

DAD: Yes, *but* is a word.

SON: Is *ter* a word?

DAD: No, *ter* is not a word.

SON: Is *fly* a word?

DAD: Yes, *fly* is a word.

SON: Dad, is *ter* a word?

DAD: Didn't we just go through this?

This dialogue provides a perfect preface to a brief discussion of how young children gradually acquire the ability to analyze words into smaller components. In this particular instance, the child decomposed a multisyllabic word at the level of the syllable; the conversation suggests that the child was trying to make sense of how these smaller units (i.e., the syllables) fit into his existing knowledge of language structure (e.g., Are these smaller units words? Do these smaller units carry meaning?).

As we previously noted, children's development of phonological awareness occurs on a continuum representing a hierarchy of sensitivity to the linguistic units that compose words (Hempenstall, 1997). The order of the linguistic units to which children become increasingly sensitive appears to be based on the size of the unit (Treiman and Zukowski, 1996). Children's early sensitivity to larger units, such as syllables and rime units, represents shallow levels of awareness, whereas later sensitivity to phonemes represents deep or higher levels of awareness (Burgess and Lonigan, 1998). Evidence for this developmental continuum comes from a substantial literature base indicating that sensitivity to syllable structure occurs considerably earlier than sensitivity to phonemes (e.g., Anthony et al., 2003; Lonigan et al., 1998).

Awareness of Rhyme

Sensitivity to rhyme is often viewed as one of the earliest benchmarks in the growth of phonological awareness, given that awareness of rhyme is contingent on one's ability to represent words as discrete units that can be analyzed on a distinctly phonological basis (Bryant, MacLean, and Bradley, 1990). The ability to detect and produce patterns of rhyme across words, observed in children as young as 2 years of age, has been viewed as a critical entry point in the development of phonological awareness (Hempenstall, 1997).

Sensitivity to rhyme begins to emerge in some children not long after they exhibit productive use of oral language. Large-scale laboratory studies of early phonological awareness development suggest that some children can perform above chance level on tasks tapping rhyming knowledge as young as 2 years, and the percentage of children demonstrating rhyming knowledge rapidly increases with age. Laboratory findings have been supported by more naturalistic observations of spontaneous use of rhyme by preschool children. Dowker (1989) elicited poems from 133 children, ages 2 to 6 years. Many of the children's poems exhibited rhyme, even those of the youngest children: 32 percent of the poems produced by children under 3 years of age exhibited rhyming patterns, as compared to 46 percent of 6-year-old children. The majority of children from middle-income backgrounds can show competency on rhyming tasks by age 5. Table 9.1 provides examples of the performance of various age groups on some common tasks used to evaluate young children's awareness of or sensitivity to rhyming words.

■ **TABLE 9.1**   Research Findings Concerning Phonological Awareness Proficiency in Young Children

Task	Example	Age Group	Proficiency by Age Group	Reference
Rhyme oddity	"Which word does not rhyme: *sail, boot, nail?*"	2 years	25% above chance level performance*	Lonigan et al., 1998
		5 years	75% above chance	
Rhyme production	"What rhymes with *boot?*"	3 years	35% could generate at least one rhyming word	Chaney, 1992
Rhyme detection	"Do *boat* and *coat* rhyme?"	3 years	65% accuracy	Chaney, 1992
Alliteration oddity	"Which word does not start the same: *bed, hair, bell?*"	3 years	9% above chance	Lonigan et al., 1998
		5 years	49% above chance	
Alliteration production	"What word starts with the same sound as *bell?*"	3 years	30% could produce at least one word	Chaney, 1992
Blending syllables	"What do you get when you say *sis . . . ter* together?"	3 years	25% above chance	Lonigan et al., 1998
		5 years	89% above chance	
Syllable counting	"How many syllables are in the word *puppy?*"	4 years	50% of children successful	Moats, 2000
		5 years	90% of children successful	
Syllable deletion	"Say *batman* without saying *man.*"	2 years	42% above chance	Lonigan et al., 1998
		4 years	98% above chance	
Phoneme deletion	"Say *heat* without the /t/."	3 years	10% above chance	Lonigan et al., 1998
		5 years	72% above chance	
Phoneme blending	What word is this: /b/ /o/ /n/.	Kindergarten	32% accuracy	Vandervelden & Siegel, 1995
		First grade	75% accuracy	
		Second grade	100% accuracy	
Phoneme segmentation of nonwords	Say the sounds in /fop/	First grade	20% accuracy	Nation & Hulme, 1997
		Third grade	100% accuracy	

*Indicates the percentage of children within that age group whose accurate rate exceeded that which would be expected by chance.

Awareness of Alliteration

Alliteration describes the sharing of a phoneme across two words or syllables, such as *bad* and *big*. Sensitivity to alliteration is also an early indicator of the advent of phonological awareness. By age 3, a few children will begin to show sensitivity to alliteration across words, and by age 5, many children from advantaged backgrounds will demonstrate this level of phonological awareness. Table 9.1 provides examples of growth in alliteration awareness during the preschool years.

The propensity toward alliteration by very young children was described by Dowker (1989) in a naturalistic study of phonological awareness of young children. Examining the elicited poems of children ranging from 2 to 6 years of age, Dowker found that even 2-year-old children used alliteration with some frequency in their poems (27 percent of her 2-year-old sample used alliterative devices). In fact, children who were 2 years of age used alliteration with the same frequency as older children.

Awareness of Syllables

Initially, children begin to recognize that multisyllabic words can be segmented at the level of the syllable (e.g., that *butterfly* can be broken into three parts). Usually around 4 years of age, children begin to exhibit explicit awareness of syllabic distinctions within multi-syllabic words (i.e., that *hotdog* can be readily divided into *hot* and *dog*, or that *baby* can be segmented into *ba-by*) (see Table 9.1). Subsequently, children show increased sensitivity to distinctions within intrasyllabic units. Specific patterns govern children's growth in sensitivity to intrasyllabic units within the syllable. In the early stages of sensitivity to syllable structure (when children are not yet perceiving phonemes as the basic linguistic unit), children show greater facility at segmenting syllables into onsets and rimes when onsets occur as singleton consonants rather than consonant clusters (Treiman, 1983). For instance, children are more likely to be able to segment *tar* into an onset and rime as compared to *star*. They are also more proficient at comparing and contrasting initial phonemes across two words if the words share a common vowel, such as *cup/cut* versus *cup/cat;* the identification of a similarity across the latter pair would be more difficult (Kirtley et al., 1989). In addition, children show substantially greater performance at comparing and contrasting final phonemes across syllables or monosyllabic words if the two words share a common vowel (in other words, the two words share a rime or rhyme; Kirtley et al., 1989). For instance, children are much better at identifying a final phoneme commonality for *map* and *tap* than for *map* and *tip*. Sensitivity to the onset-rime distinction appears to facilitate children's phonemic awareness, providing the framework for word and syllable analyses at the level of the phoneme.

Awareness of Phonemes

Phonemic awareness—the ability to identify phonemes as the units comprising syllables and words—is not exhibited with mastery by many children until about 6 or 7 years of age (Ball, 1993) although Lonigan and colleagues (1998) found that 5-year-old children from advantaged backgrounds performed better than chance level on a phoneme-deletion task (see Table 9.1). Phonemic awareness comprises two areas of growth: phonemic segmentation (or analysis) and phonemic blending (or synthesis) (Torgesen, Morgan, and Davis, 1992). *Phoneme segmentation* is the ability to sequentially isolate all of the individual sounds in a syllable or word, or to segment (elide) a sound from a word or syllable. *Phonemic blending* is the ability to take a sequence of phonemes and build them into a larger linguistic unit. Using the word *pond,* for example, a phonemic segmentation task requires that a child break the word into its component phonemes and express those four phonemes in sequence: /p/ . . . /ɑ/ . . . /n/ . . . /d/. In contrast, a phonemic blending task involves presenting a series of four phonemes to the child (in this case, /p/, /ɑ/, /n/, and /d/) and asking the child to combine the sounds into a word. Skills in both phonemic segmentation and blending are critical requisites for learning to read.

There is a developmental trend in children's performance on phoneme segmentation and blending tasks. In general, performance on phoneme blending tasks is superior to that on segmentation and elision tasks. Table 9.1 shows such skill to begin in kindergarten and rapidly develop following the onset of formal literacy instruction at around 6 years. In contrast, phoneme segmentation and manipulation skills develop much more gradually and performance is highly mediated by the complexity of the linguistic units being analyzed. Segmenting simple consonant-vowel-consonant (CVC) words is much easier that segmenting words with blends (e.g., CCVC words) (Tresman, 1991).

Phonemic awareness requires children to have acquired adequate representations of phonemes as the discrete elements of syllables and words (Nittrouer, 1996); that is, to engage in phonemic awareness tasks, children must have a well-developed phonological system comprising robust representations of the phonemes within their language. In fact, examining children's abilities to manipulate phonemes demonstrates the depth and robustness of their phonemic representations. Calfee, Lindamood, and Lindamood (1973), in their seminal work, examined the attainment of relatively sophisticated levels of phoneme awareness in a study of 660 children from kindergarten through 12th grade. These researchers asked children to manipulate colored blocks representing the phoneme arrangements of nonsense syllables. Although children showed gradual improvement on phoneme manipulation across the grades, 12th-grade students showed only about 60 percent accuracy. Although these students undoubtedly were able to express phonemes with precision (expressive phonology), their receptive performance on phonemic tasks showed that mastery was elusive in more advanced tasks of phonemic awareness. Such findings indicate that although young children gradually increase in their ability to represent words as discrete phonemes, the ability to manipulate words at the level of the phoneme requires more advanced representational abilities. Some children (particularly if they are poor readers) may never acquire proficiency on complex phoneme manipulation tasks.

■ PHONOLOGICAL AWARENESS DEVELOPMENT AND READING

There is considerable overlap between children's development of phonological awareness and learning to read. However, we must note that there is controversy regarding the nature of the relationship between phonological awareness and reading instruction (Johnston,

Anderson, and Holligan, 1996; Morais, Cary, Alegria, and Bertelson, 1979; Vandervelden and Siegel, 1995). Some researchers contend that reading development is driven by phonological awareness, particularly at the phonemic level, a view that asserts a causal relationship between phonemic awareness and reading ability. Research demonstrating that performance on phoneme segmentation and phoneme blending tasks are strong predictors of early reading development supports this position (see Christensen, 1997). Other researchers assert that phonemic awareness and reading skill develop in a reciprocal, rather than causal, manner. Evidence showing that phonological awareness increases reciprocally and concomitantly with reading proficiency provides support for this argument (see Stanovich, 2000). A position representing both perspectives is that a certain level of phonological awareness is required for the development of reading skill, but that subsequently phonemic awareness and reading ability develop in a reciprocal and interrelated manner, as shown in Figure 9.1.

Bradley and Bryant (1983) were among the first researchers to demonstrate a relationship between phonological awareness at preschool and subsequent reading performance. In their seminal work, they tested 403 children ages 4 and 5 in their ability to categorize sounds—that is, their skills in determining which word, of three or four words presented, did not share a common initial phoneme with the other words (e.g., *hill, pig, pen*). This measure of children's sensitivity to alliteration accounted for a significant and substantial proportion of variance in their reading skills three years later. Similar findings were also reported by O'Connor and Jenkins (1999). In their study, measures of phonological awareness (e.g., initial sound identification, rhyme production, phoneme segmentation)

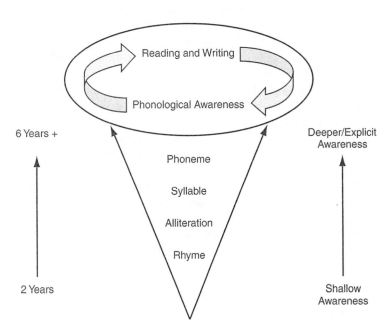

■ **FIGURE 9.1** Developmental model of growth in phonological awareness from early childhood to the years of schooling.

collected at kindergarten predicted differences in reading achievement at the end of first grade and identified children who would later have a reading disability.

The relationship between phonological awareness and reading is best understood by considering the skills that are most critical for the beginning reader. Faced with the task of decoding a novel word, the novice reader must know the distinctive features and names of alphabet letters in the word and must know its phonemic structure. In addition, and most importantly, the novice reader must bridge these two areas of knowledge by recognizing the systematic relationships between letters and phonemes (Hulme, Goetz, Gooch, Adams, and Snowling, 2007). Skill in recognizing and using the systematic correspondence between letters and phonemes is usually referred to as *phonological recoding* (Vandervelden and Siegel, 1995) or *phonological recoding in lexical access* (Wagner and Torgesen, 1987). The successful integration of these two areas of knowledge allows the child to decode novel words. Children with limited awareness of letter names and/or deficits in phonemic awareness are prone to difficulties in reading (Stanovich, 1986).

Stahl and Murray (1994) sought to determine the amount of phonological awareness necessary for a beginning reader to negotiate novel words. These researchers found that the ability to represent onset-rime distinctions and to isolate phonemes at the beginning and end of words were prerequisites for beginning reading. In other words, children who did not have these requisite abilities were unable to achieve or surpass preprimer instructional levels. These findings emphasize the importance of intrasyllabic awareness over word and syllable awareness to reading development (see Gillon, 2004), and converge with reports from other researchers that children's performance on nonrhyming phonological awareness tasks exhibit stronger predictive relationships with reading than with rhyming tasks (Christensen, 1997, 2000; Muter, Hulme, Snowling, and Stevenson, 2004).

For children who are already readers, abilities in phonemic awareness distinguish reliably between children who are proficient at reading and those who are struggling (Catts, Fey, Zhang, and Tomblin, 2001; Muter et al., 2004). In a seminal study, Calfee and colleagues (1973) found that many older and struggling readers show consistent deficits in their ability to represent and manipulate words at the phonemic level. For instance, fifth-grade students who were struggling readers performed phoneme manipulation tasks with about 37 percent accuracy, as compared to about 80 percent accuracy for peers who were above-average readers. Stanovich (2000) referred to this phenomenon as the *Matthew effect*—such that "the poor get poorer and the rich get richer"—in that the gap separating children who are proficient readers from those who are failing steadily gets larger over time.

This contention was supported by Juel (1988), who, in a classic study, followed a group of 54 children from first through fourth grade. Juel found remarkable stability in reading achievement across these grades: "The probability that a child would remain a poor reader at the end of fourth grade, if the child was a poor reader at the end of first grade, was .88" (p. 440). In other words, children who experienced reading failure in first grade continued to experience failure in the next three grades. Deficits in phoneme awareness were important explanatory variables in distinguishing children who failed at reading from those who experienced success. At entry to first grade, children who subsequently experienced reading failure showed no skills in segmenting words into phonemes and analyzing words on the basis of phonemic properties. Such findings implicate the strong and reciprocal relationship between deficits in phonological awareness and the circumstances surrounding reading failure.

PHONOLOGICAL AWARENESS AND DISORDERS OF SPEECH PRODUCTION

Let us now turn to considering the relationship between phonological awareness and disorders of speech production. Among typically developing children, relationships exist between speech production performance and phonological awareness (Foy and Mann, 2001), with more articulation errors associated with lower scores on measures of phonological awareness. It makes sense, then, that research shows children who exhibit clinical disorders of speech production to face increased risks for experiencing difficulty in phonological awareness and subsequent reading and spelling difficulties (for review, see Schuele, 2004). This does not mean, however, that all children who exhibit speech problems will have literacy difficulties. Children with speech production problems specific to deficits in phonological rules are most prone to experiencing difficulties with phonological awareness and reading; we refer to these children as having a *phonological disorder (PD;* Schuele, 2004). Children with PD have multiple speech sound production errors and compromised intelligibility. They may or may not have concomitant language difficulties in other domains (e.g., vocabulary, grammar). The speech sound difficulties of children with PD tend to be more pronounced than the difficulties of children with articulation problems, who may exhibit distortions or substitutions of a relatively small set of sounds (e.g., substituting /w/ for /l/ and /r/ sounds). Phonological disorder is often conceptualized as a cognitive-linguistic disorder rather than an articulatory or motoric disorder, resulting from underspecified or faulty phonological representations. For some children at least, difficulties with phonological development affect both expression (speech sound production problem) and reception (phonological awareness problem).

Children with PD, as a group, face an elevated risk for difficulties in the development of phonological awareness, particularly when these are accompanied by more widespread language difficulties (Bird et al., 1995; Catts et al., 2002; Larrivee and Catts, 1999; Snowling, Bishop, and Stothard, 2000). However, even having a phonological disorder in isolation is linked with early reading difficulties (Nathan, Stackhouse, Goulandris, & Snowling, 2004), and the presence of phonological awareness weakness in preschool children with speech disorders is independent of whether these children have language impairment (Rvachew, Ohberg, Grawburg, and Heyding, 2003). Factors such as genetic risk and low socioeconomic status will further increase these children's risk for reading difficulties (Chatterji, 2006; Lewis et al., 2006; Samuelsson et al., 2007).

Understanding the nature of children's speech difficulties is important for understanding their risk for literacy problems, including difficulties in phonological awareness (Dodd, 2005; Schuele, 2004). Children with speech production problems that are articulatory rather than phonological in nature may not display difficulties in attaining phonological awareness (Bishop and Adams, 1990; Catts, 1993; Levi, Capozzi, Fabrizi, and Sechi, 1982). Catts (1993), for instance, found that first-graders with disorders of articulation performed similarly to a comparison group of typically developing peers on a variety of phonological awareness tasks. Children whose speech production problems are phonological in nature and accompanied by language difficulties (PD + language) face the greatest risks for failing to achieve good phonological awareness and, by extension, skilled reading (Lewis, Freebairn, and Taylor, 2000). By some estimates, nearly 50 percent of these children will fail to be good readers by third or fourth grade. These estimates suggest that growth in phonological awareness and reading achievement needs to be diligently tracked for children with PD, particularly those youngsters who also exhibit comcomitant language problems. An additional group of children who exhibit speech sound problems—those with childhood apraxia of speech—also may demonstrate phonological awareness deficits in syllable rhyme and phoneme awareness and are at high risk for persistent and severe reading and/ or spelling disorder (Gillon and Moriarty, 2007; Marquardt, Sussman, Snow, and Jacks, 2002).

Bird and colleagues (1995) assert that problems in phonological awareness for children with PD can be attributed to their inability to master the phonological system, which translates into difficulties representing the phonological structure of language in both expression (i.e., speech intelligibility) and awareness tasks. These children have particular difficulties perceiving phonemes as the basic phonological building blocks of syllables and are therefore unable to break syllables into phonemic elements (Bird and Bishop, 1992). Research by Sutherland and Gillon (2005) supported this hypothesis, showing that 3- to 5-year-old children with PD performed poorly compared to their typical peers on measures assessing the strength of their phonological representations. As one measure of the strength of phonological representations, children were asked to evaluate whether each word in a series of spoken words was produced in a "good way" or a "not a good way" (e.g., *dunasaur* for *dinosaur*); children with PD performed with about 60 percent accuracy on this task, compared to 76 percent for their typical peers. These early difficulties in phonological awareness appear to be causally associated with the risks for reading failure experienced by children with PD, especially when phonological difficulties are paired with more broadly based language-learning limitations. As Bird and colleagues (1995) explain, "At an age when most children are discovering that letters can represent individual phonemes, children with phonological impairment are still unable to match words that share a common onset or rime" (p. 460).

Collectively, the research on phonological awareness for children with *phonological disorders* suggests several conclusions, although further research on this population is warranted to better understand the impact of speech production difficulties on phonological awareness and literacy.

1. Children with phonological disorder are more likely than their peers with typical development to experience difficulties with phonological awareness and literacy achievement. Children who are most at risk for such problems are those whose speech difficulties are still pronounced at the onset of literacy instruction (e.g., kindergarten and first grade) and who have limited phonemic awareness (Nathan, Stackhouse, Goulandris, and Snowling, 2004).

2. Children with phonological disorder who have concomitant receptive and/or expressive language difficulties are at greater risk than those with phonological disorder alone (Bird et al., 1995; Larrivee and Catts, 1999; Lewis et al., 1998).

3. Some children with phonological disorder may evidence problems in acquiring phonological awareness, but these problems do not present challenges to the early development of literacy. These children may, for example, use strengths in visual memory and semantic or syntactic knowledge to compensate for limited ability to use phonological cues in the reading process (Gillon and Dodd, 2005). However, as demands in the curriculum increase over the elementary period, difficulties in inefficient word decoding as a result of poor phonemic awareness may become evident or more pronounced. Phonological awareness deficits may have their greatest impact on spelling, particularly around third grade and beyond (Clark-Klein and Hodson, 1995).

THE ROLE OF THE SPEECH-LANGUAGE PATHOLOGIST

Speech-language pathologists can and should play a critical role in promoting phonological awareness (and literacy skills in general) for preschool and school-age children who experience communication disorders (ASHA, 2001). We must recognize that language consists of both written and oral dimensions, and that the role of SLPs does not stop with oral language. Moreover, we must also recognize that phonological abilities represent an important bridge between written and oral language because of the alphabetic principle, which relies on systematic relationships between sounds and letters. Children who experience problems with phonology—whether it manifests itself as a speech production problem or not—are more likely than other children to struggle with reading. Consequently, if SLPs are to promote children's success in schooling and in life, we must take a broadened view toward identifying specific goals for treatment so that we expand beyond the traditional dimensions that look at children's production of individual speech sounds or use of specific phonological processes. We must look carefully at children's underlying sensitivities to the way in which spoken language is organized, to ensure that the children are developing phonological awareness in a timely manner.

Within this last decade, SLPs have been encouraged by ASHA (2001) to play a "critical and direct role in the development of literacy for children and adolescents with communication disorders" (p. 3). Primary roles and responsibilities include (1) prevention, (2) identification, (3) assessment, and (4) intervention. An overview of these roles and responsibilities with respect to phonological awareness specifically is presented in Table 9.2. We discuss in further detail the SLP's role in assessment and intervention in the next sections.

TABLE 9.2 Roles and Responsibilities of Speech-Language Pathologies for Addressing Phonological Awareness

Role	Responsibility
Prevention	Encourage development of phonological awareness in young children at risk. Prevention activities focus on preventing problems with phonological awareness before they occur, so necessarily focus on younger children. Primary focus is on high-frequency engagement of children in naturalistic exposure to phonological properties of oral language (e.g., listening to nursery rhymes).
Identification	Locate children who are experiencing difficulties in phonological awareness attainment by (1) observing children in phonological awareness activities and (2) educating other professionals on strategies for identifying early problems with phonological awareness.
Assessment	Adopt a speech-language evaluation protocol that includes assessment of phonological awareness. Preschool assessment includes rhyme and alliteration awareness, and emphasizes informal observation; school-age assessment includes syllable and phonemic awareness and can be accomplished using standardized or criterion-based measures.
Intervention	Implement curriculum-relevant and collaborative interventions that are individualized to target those aspects of phonological awareness that require attention for particular children. Intervention activities are developmentally appropriate, following the normal developmental sequence for phonological awareness (e.g., for preschool and kindergarten children, focus first on awareness of rhyme and alliteration, and only later target analysis at the level of the syllable and phoneme). For elementary students, training in phonological awareness should be combined with explicit alphabetic principle instruction.

Source: Adapted from American Speech-Language-Hearing Association (2001).

■ ASSESSMENT

Phonological awareness should be routinely assessed in children with suspected or identified phonological disorder as part of a comprehensive assessment battery. Assessment materials will vary depending on the developmental stage of the child. The aim of phonological awareness assessment in a 3-year-old child with phonological disorder, for example, is not to diagnose the child with a phonological awareness deficit. The wide variability in phonological awareness development in children with typical development in this young age group would suggest such an assessment aim is inappropriate. Rather, phonological awareness assessment is required in young children with phonological disorder to establish their current levels of awareness and to monitor their growth in phonological awareness over time in response to home and preschool language experiences or specific therapy interventions. In contrast, the assessment aim of a school-age child with phonological disorder is to profile his or her strengths and needs in phonological awareness. Assessment is also used to ascertain whether deficits in phonological awareness, particularly at the phonemic level, are contributing to any current reading or spelling difficulties and whether phonological awareness is sufficiently well developed for the current demands of the child's reading and spelling curriculum. A phonological awareness assessment is also necessary to track the effects of any explicit phonological awareness intervention so that its effects can be documented.

A range of phonological awareness assessment tasks may be implemented, including norm-referenced and criterion-referenced measures as well as dynamic assessment.

Norm-Referenced Measures: Preschool Years

Several norm-referenced measures for assessing phonological awareness in preschool children are available. When considering use of such tools, the clinician needs to consider the normative sample used for developing the instrument and its relevance to the child being assessed. Early language and preschool experiences will influence a child's phonological awareness development. In some early education environments, children may receive extensive and explicit guidance in letter sound knowledge (e.g., the sound /g/ goes with the letter *G*), whereas in other educational facilities the focus may be on rhyme and letter naming with little attention directed at facilitating other levels of phonological awareness or print knowledge. Thus, children's performance on phonological awareness tasks is likely to be influenced by early instructional methods that may vary across differing educational settings. The use of local norms for phonological awareness skill development may be one strategy to help reduce this problem. However, given the general pattern of consistency in phonological awareness development that is evident across countries and across alphabetic languages, norm-referenced assessments with strong psychometric properties will provide a useful guide against which to compare phonological awareness development in preschool and kindergarten children with phonological disorder.

It is also important that the clinician considers the type of assessment task(s) included in measures designed for young children. Many measures were not designed with the child with speech production problems in mind. Consequently, measures that ask children to produce rhyming words, for instance, are nearly impossible to use with children with speech sound problems. For instance, a rhyming production task might ask children to "produce a word that rhymes with *cat*" and a child with a speech disorder says "tat." If this child uses fronting processes, it is hard to know whether the child is saying "tat" or "cat"—for which the latter would not be correct. Likewise, a child with speech production problems who is asked to produce several words that rhyme with *cat* might say "tat, tat, and tat." For a child who represents many initial sounds (e.g., /g/, /k/, /d/, and /t/) with a single phoneme (e.g., /t/), this might be a correct answer, but it is impossible to know. Consequently, measures that rely on receptive tasks (in which the child points, for instance) may provide the most valid approach to assessing phonological awareness in children with speech difficulties. Gillon (2004) provides a comprehensive examination of phonological awareness assessment instruments and their psychometric properties (see also, Schuele, Skibbe, and Rao, 2007).

Norm-Referenced Measures: School-Age Children

Several norm-referenced instruments for evaluating phonological awareness in school-age children have been developed in recent years. Table 9.3 provides a summary of several instruments widely used to assess phonological awareness in school-age children. With one exception (Torgesen and Bryant, 2004), these measures use age norms rather than grade norms; thus, one should be cautious when applying these norms to children who are young or old for their grade, as their experiences may not be similar to that of age-matched peers. In addition, interpretation must consider that educational experiences in the early elementary years can vary widely across schools. Norm-referenced measures such as these may prove useful in delineating the extent to which a child exhibits phonological awareness difficulties compared to a cohort of age-matched peers. They can be particularly useful for identifying children for whom intensive phonological awareness intervention is needed (Heath and Hogben, 2004). With some of these measures, information about potential intervention targets may be gleaned from careful analysis of a child's pattern of performance. However, such targets must also be educationally relevant and developmentally appropriate.

■ **TABLE 9.3** Norm-Referenced Phonological Awareness Measures

Measure Name	Age Range
Comprehensive Test of Phonological Processing (Wagner, Torgesen, & Rashotte, 1999)	5 to 24 years
Phonological Awareness Test 2 (Robertson and Salter, 2007)	5 to 9 years
Pre-Reading Inventory of Phonological Awareness (Dodd, Crosbie, McIntosh, Teitzel, and Ozanne, 2003)	4 to 7 years
Test of Phonological Awareness Skills (Newcomer and Barenbaum, 2003)	5 to 10 years
Test of Phonological Awareness–Second Edition: PLUS (Torgesen and Bryant, 2004)	5 to 8 years

Criterion-Referenced Procedures

Criterion-referenced measures are used to determine a child's performance against a specific criterion (McCauley, 2001). The child's performance is not compared to a cohort of age-matched peers, but rather to a particular local or curriculum-based standard. Several criterion-referenced instruments are available commercially for evaluating phonological awareness (e.g., Lindamood and Lindamood, 1971; Sawyer, 1987). In addition, the research literature also contains several descriptions of useful criterion-referenced tools (e.g., Ball, 1993; Ball and Blachman, 1991; Murray, Smith, and Murray, 2000; Swank and Catts, 1994; Yopp, 1988). These can be used at no cost by clinicians. Dynamic Indicators of Basic Early Literacy Skills (DIBELS; Good and Kaminski, 2002) and Phonological Awareness and Literacy Screening (PALS:K; Invernizzi, Meier, Swank, and Juel, 2001) PALS:1–3; Invernizzi and Meier, 2002–03) are frequently used measures in schools, and include criterion-based measures of phonological awareness. An excellent tool is provided by Catts, Fey, Zhang, and Tomblin (2001), which is reprinted in Table 9.4. This tool was developed by this research team to identify kindergartners who may be at risk for later reading problems. Used in combination with measures of oral language ability, alphabet knowledge, processing speed, and maternal education, researchers were able to identify with a high level of precision those kindergartners most likely to go on to be successful readers.

■ **TABLE 9.4**   Criterion-Referenced Phoneme Deletion Task

The child is shown a picture of a cow and a boy and asked to say "cowboy." After the child responds, the examiner covers the cow and says, "Now say cowboy without the cow." The procedure is repeated with the picture of a tooth and a brush (toothbrush) and a cup and a cake (cupcake). If the child fails a practice item, the examiner provides the appropriate response. After completing the practice items, the examiner asks the child to say each of the test items after deleting the portion that is underlined. In all cases, the portion to be deleted is referred to phonetically (e.g., "say seat without /s/"). No pictures are used for the test items and no feedback is provided. Testing is discontinued following six consecutive errors.

Test Items:

1. baseball	11. baby
2. haircut	12. person
3. Sunday	13. monkey
4. railroad	14. fat
5. sometime	15. seat
6. return	16. shout
7. around	17. tall
8. motel	18. door
9. almost	19. few
10. helpful	20. snail
	21. thread

Source: Catts, Fey, Zhang, and Tomblin (2001). Reprinted with permission.

The goal of criterion-referenced measures is to determine children's competency in a specific area of phonological awareness, and clinicians can devise their own criterion-referenced tasks to use for screening and diagnostic purposes. These more informal tasks can be used to identify children who are deficient relative to an established criterion, describe children's current level of performance (strengths and needs), delineate intervention goals, document treatment progress, and determine when intervention is no longer warranted.

Dynamic Assessment

Dynamic assessment examines children's performance in response to varying types of cues or prompts provided by the clinician; it provides a method for obtaining a clearer picture of children's underlying competencies as well as their potential for learning new skills (Bain and Olswang, 1995). The goal is to determine how much and what type of assistance is required to encourage higher levels of performance by the child (Justice and Ezell, 1999). Knowledge gained from dynamic assessments can identify children's underlying competencies and their short- and long-term propensity for change.

Spector (1992) described the use of dynamic assessment to determine how much assistance children needed to segment words consisting of two or three phonemes. The dynamic assessment procedure was reported as more useful for predicting children's later phonological awareness and reading skills than were normative or criterion-referenced assessments. Table 9.5 describes this procedure. For each word a child is asked to segment, the clinician begins with the first prompt. If the child is not successful, subsequent prompts (2 through 7) are given until the child is successful or all seven prompts have been provided. The clinician records the level of prompt necessary for successful segmentation of each word. To interpret the findings, clinicians would be interested in the extent to which

■ TABLE 9.5   Dynamic Assessment Task

Prompt 1	*Listen while I say the word very slowly.* Model slow pronunciation. *Now can you tell me each sound?*
Prompt 2	*What's the first sound you hear in _____?*
	If first sound is correct: *Now can you tell me each of the sounds?*
	If incorrect or no response: *Try to tell me just a little bit of the word.*
	If child still does not isolate first sound, skip Prompts 3 and 4. Go to Prompt 5.
Prompt 3	If child correctly identified first sound but not next sound(s):
	_____ *is the first sound in _____.*
	What sound comes next?
	Now can you tell me each sound?
Prompt 4	*There are 2 [or 3] sounds in _____. What are they?*
Prompt 5	*Watch me.* Model segmentation of word: Place a token in a square as each sound is spoken. Then repeat word as a whole. After demo say the following: *Try to do what I just did.*
	Score response as correct if child can imitate correct segmentation.
Prompt 6	*Let's try together.* Model segmentation of word with child. Work hand-over-hand with child and ask child to pronounce segments along with you.
	Now try to do it yourself. Do what we just did together.
Prompt 7	Model again with child (as in Prompt 6). *Now try again to do it yourself.*

Source: Spector (1992).

a child who needs strong prompts (e.g., prompts 5 through 7) at the outset of the task becomes successful with weaker prompts (e.g., prompts 1 through 4) on the later presented words. Spector's (1992) prompting procedure can be adapted to assess other aspects of phonological awareness, such as rhyme production or alliteration detection. In addition, children's responses to the various prompts may provide insights into teaching strategies for therapy. Dynamic assessment can be used in conjunction with more static evaluation strategies to derive more sensitive profiles of children's phonological awareness development and to determine therapy goals and strategies.

INTERVENTION

Speech-language pathologists who work with preschool and school-age children ought to include careful attention to phonological awareness in both their assessment and intervention practices; when children show weaknesses in phonological awareness relative to normative or criterion references, phonological awareness targets can be readily integrated into speech-language intervention. Alternatively, SLPs can deliver interventions focused solely on phonological awareness to individual or small groups of children. Several effective practice guidelines for phonological awareness instruction can be gleaned from research over the last two decades (Gillon, 2004; Ehri, 2001; Torgesen and Mathes, 2000). These practice guidelines stem from findings showing only a small percentage of children (less than 5 percent) would struggle with reading if we rigorously supported literacy development from preschool forward (e.g., Moats, 2000). The SLP should play an integral role in promoting effective practice by collaborating with other specialists, including classroom teachers.

1. For preschoolers and kindergartners, clinicians should provide phonological awareness experiences (and literacy experiences in general) as an integral part of therapy. Attention to phonological awareness can be embedded within speech production activities, and clinicians should work collaboratively with classroom teachers and reading specialists to ensure that classroom curricula provide adequate classroom-based phonological awareness experiences.
2. Children who have not attained adequate levels of performance at the end of kindergarten or the beginning of first grade should be provided small-group intensive intervention that includes phonological awareness instruction as a core objective (Torgesen, 1999).
3. Children for whom small-group instructional intervention is not sufficient, intensive one-on-one instruction should be provided; phonological awareness as well as other key reading objectives are addressed (e.g., vocabulary, reading fluency).

Promoting Phonological Awareness in Preschool Children with Phonological Disorders

Speech-language pathologists need to ensure that young children with phonological disorder whose assessment profile suggests that they are at risk for written language difficulties develop strong phonological awareness. Preliminary evidence suggests it is possible to *simultaneously* improve both speech and phonological awareness development in children with speech sound disorders (Gillon, 2000a, 2005; Major & Bernhardt, 1998).

In a longitudinal study, Gillon (2005; Kirk and Gillon, in press) demonstrated significant benefits for later reading and spelling development by facilitating children's phonological awareness and letter knowledge from children as young as 3 years. In this study, 12 children (mean age 3.5 years) with moderate or severe speech disorders commenced school at 5 years of age with strong phoneme awareness and emerging letter knowledge following approximately 25 hours of intervention between the ages of 3 and 5 years. The intervention aimed to improve speech intelligibility, phonemic awareness, and letter knowledge. Results showed that the children accelerated quickly in reading development and 80 percent of the group demonstrated above-average reading ability by the end of the first year. In contrast, 60 percent of children in a control group of children with speech disorder who received intervention to improve speech intelligibility but who did not receive any explicit instruction in phonological awareness showed delayed reading development and poor spelling ability over time.

Other studies have also showed that phonological awareness can be readily facilitated in young children with phonological disorder. Van Kleeck, Gillam, and McFadden (1998) evaluated the effectiveness of a nine-month classroom-based phonological awareness training program for preschool children. Of the 16 children participating in the experimental classrooms, 11 exhibited speech impairment (nine of these children also exhibited language impairment). Over the course of intervention, children participated in approximately 45 minutes of phonological awareness activities daily; for the first 12 weeks of the program, rhyming skills were targeted, and in the final 12 weeks, initial and final phoneme awareness within and across words was targeted. The children in the intervention classrooms made significant gains on measures of phonological awareness (e.g., test scores on rhyme detection and production tasks nearly doubled) when compared to a control group over the nine-month period. However, outcomes for reading and spelling development were not measured in this study.

Intervention Aims

Although a primary goal of intervention for children with phonological disorder is to improve their speech intelligibility, a secondary goal should aim to facilitate these children's phonological awareness, particularly at the phonemic level. Research evidence suggests that to give preschool children with phonological disorder the optimum chance for reading success, intervention should aim to achieve the following prior to formal literacy instruction or at least by the end of the first year of schooling:

- Resolve or significantly improve the child's speech disorder (and any co-occurring language impairment (Nathan et al., 2004).
- Facilitate strong phonological awareness, including early developing awareness of phonemes in words (Gillon, 2005; Kirk and Gillon, in press).
- Facilitate at least some letter sound knowledge and stimulate the child's understanding of the relationship between spoken and written words (Hulme et al., 2007).

Achieving these aims may require relatively intensive periods of intervention during the preschool years, particularly for children with severe speech disorder. If such intervention is successful in preventing reading problems in addition to improving speech intelligibility, the intervention will prove both efficient and cost effective.

Intervention Models

Intervention models that involve collaboration between the SLP, teacher, and parents are considered best practice when attempting to improve the phonological awareness of children with speech or language impairment (Roth and Paul, 2006). Thus, literacy skills are addressed within clinical therapy, within the classroom, and within the home.

Phonological Awareness Experiences Embedded into Therapy

A variety of activities that stimulate phonological awareness along with knowledge of letter sounds can be integrated into therapy for preschool children. There are many relatively inexpensive manuals that can be examined for activity suggestions, as shown in Table 9.6. Also, there are some reputable Internet sites with good ideas, including the University of Virginia PALS website (http://pals.virginia.edu/Virginia/Activities/) and the National Center for

TABLE 9.6 Examples of Published Manualized Programs for Delivering Phonological Awareness Instruction

Program (Author, Year)	Program Overview
Road to the Code (Blachman, Ball, Black, and Tangel, 2000)	44 15–20-minute lessons in spiral-bound book; organized as an 11-week program (4 lessons per week); appropriate for small groups or one-on-one; recommended for kindergartners and first-graders
Phonemic Awareness in Young Children (Adams, Foorman, Lundberg, and Beeler, 1998)	51 15–20-minute lessons in spiral-bound book; organized as an 8-month program for kindergartners or 8-week program for first-graders; appropriate for whole class or small groups; includes pre- and post-test assessment tools
Ladders to Literacy: Preschool (Notari-Syverson, O'Connor, and Vadasy, 1998) and *Ladders to Literacy: Kindergarten* (O'Connor, Notari-Syverson, and Vadasy, 2005)	Available in a preschool and kindergarten version, comprises 50+ 15–20-minute lessons in two spiral-bound books; organized to provide a year of instruction; appropriate for whole classroom or small groups; includes pre- and post-test assessment tools; also includes objectives and activities for language and alphabet skill
The Sounds Abound Program (Lenchner and Podhajski, 1998)	20 lessons and variety of accompanying materials in kit (games, DVD, stickers); organized to provide sequenced classroom-based instruction and supplemental supports for children who struggle; specified for ages preschool to third grade
Sounds Abound: Listening, Rhyming, and Reading (Catts and Olsen, 1993)	Variety of lesson plans for teaching rhyme, alliteration, and phoneme segmenting and blending; appropriate for whole classroom, small groups, or one-on-one; includes pre- and post-test assessment tools

Learning Disabilities Get Ready to Read website (www.getreadytoread.org/). Some practical suggestions include:

1. Write words clearly and in large font underneath stimulus pictures for speech production goals. Specifically draw children's attention to the printed word (rather than the picture) when practicing the speech target words.
2. Regularly employ alliteration activities that ask children to attend to the initial sounds in words; for instance, at the start of therapy, children might have to sort a pile of picture cards into those starting with one sound (e.g., /s/) and those starting with another (/t/).
3. Use an alphabet chart or letter cards to practice target speech sounds and make explicit for the child the link between the letter and the speech sound the letter represents.
4. Model segmentation of target speech words that have two or three phonemes, as in: "Let's break the word *key* into its two sounds: /key/. . ./k/. . ./i/. . . . Now you say it just the way I did, /k/. . ./i/.
5. Read storybooks that feature rhyme and alliteration patterns and explicitly bring the child's attention to these phonological patterns (Justice, Kaderavek, Bowles, and Grimm, 2005; Ukrainetz, Cooney, Dyer, Kysar, and Harris, 2000).
6. Ask children to draw pictures and then write stories to accompany the pictures; as they write, identify and discuss the specific sounds that make up letters (Ukrainetz et al., 2000).

Written letters and words can serve as visual prompts or reminders of particular speech targets for children. For example, if the child is attempting to say sun and says tun, the clinician can point to the written word under a picture of the sun and use the initial letter "s" to cue the child: "Oops. You forgot this /s/ sound at the beginning of the word (pointing to the letter s). Put the /s/ at the beginning." Such activities do not necessarily require that the child understand the alphabetic references in order to produce accurate speech. Rather, the comments clinicians make with reference to print and sound structure are provided alongside the typical cues and prompts used to elicit accurate speech production (e.g., target models, phonetic placement cues). The pairing of letters with their corresponding sounds can provide children extra exposure to the phonological structure of language. Astute clinicians take advantage of teachable moments to scaffold children's attainment of higher levels of phonological awareness.

PHONOLOGICAL AWARENESS EXPERIENCES IN THE CLASSROOM AND AT HOME

The SLP can collaborate with children's teachers and parents to help them identify methods they may use to stimulate phonological awareness across the full range of childhood education settings. Many of the same activities discussed for therapeutic techniques can be used by teachers and parents. For teachers, however, it might be most important for them to adopt a classroom pre-reading curriculum that includes systematic and explicit attention to phonological awareness development over the academic year. Many curricula are available for doing so, and by employing a structured approach, it will be more certain that explicit instruction is systematically employed within the daily classroom curriculum. Parents and teachers can also benefit from understanding other ways to build phonological awareness in less formal ways. Suggestions include encouraging parents and teachers to:

1. Read storybooks with children regularly that include interesting sound patterns (e.g., rhyme, alliteration); draw children's attention to these patterns (Justice et al., 2005; Ukrainetz et al., 2000).
2. Engage children in reciting nursery rhymes together and clap out the beat in the rhymes.
3. Find toys or objects in the house or preschool that start with the same sound and comment on the sounds that are the same. For example: "*Light* and *lid* both start with the /l/ sound. Listen to the /l/ sound at the beginning of these words: *light, lid*. Hear the /l/ sound at the beginning?"
4. Identify the first phoneme in the child's name and family members' names.
5. Clap out the syllables in children's names or segment short names (e.g., *Kim*) into their respective phonemes (e.g., /k/ /I/ /m/)
6. Say words as a series of sounds (e.g., /b/ /I/ /g/) and ask children to guess the word being said.

It is important to remember that the aim of phonological awareness intervention during this preschool period is to facilitate awareness of the sound structure of spoken language, *not to teach skills to mastery level*. The process of learning to read and write following school entry will rapidly develop more advanced levels of phonological awareness and alphabetic knowledge (Perfetti, Beck, Bell, and Hughes, 1987). What is most important for preschool children with phonological disorder is that their phonological awareness is stimulated to a level where they can readily respond to the rigors of formal reading instruction that begins in later kindergarten and early first grade for most children today.

Promoting Phonological Awareness in School-Age Children with Phonological Disorders

School-age children with phonological disorder who are experiencing reading and spelling difficulties may require direct and intensive periods of intervention specifically focused at enhancing phonological awareness, with the greatest attention focused on facilitating phonemic awareness. Numerous studies indicate that intensive small-group or individual phonological awareness intervention results in improved phonological awareness and reading ability for school-age children who are at risk, children experiencing reading difficulties, and children with speech-language impairments (e.g., Ball and Blachman, 1991; Byrne and Fielding-Barnsley, 1991, 1993, 1995; Dayton and Schuele, 1997; Gillon and Dodd, 1995, 1997; Lundberg, Frost, and Peterson, 1988; Schuele, Paul, and Mazzaferri, 1998; van Kleeck et al., 1998; Warrick and Rubin, 1992; Warrick, Rubin, and Rowe-Walsh, 1993). Ehri and colleagues (2001) concluded from a meta-analysis of 52 controlled research studies that phonological awareness has a statistically significant effect on developing reading accuracy and reading comprehension for children with typical development and children at risk. Interventions that focused at the phoneme level and integrate instruction on letter knowledge show the best results for reading development.

Some studies have looked specifically at the effectiveness of phonological awareness intervention for school-age children with phonological disorder. Gillon (2000a) demonstrated that 20 hours of structured phonological awareness intervention (Gillon Phonological Awareness Training Programme for Children at Risk; Gillon, 2000b) was successful in accelerating phonological awareness development in 5- to 7-year-old children with speech disorders to the level of their peers. This intervention resulted in significantly superior reading and spelling development that was maintained over time (Gillon, 2002) compared to a control group of children who received other types of speech and language intervention. The phonological awareness intervention also resulted in improvements in speech production. The intervention was administered by a SLP to the child individually two times weekly for a 10-week period, or until 20 hours of intervention had been implemented. The activities predominantly focused at the phonemic level (e.g., phoneme identification, phoneme segmentation, phoneme blending and manipulation) and used a variety of materials and games to help maintain the child's interest. The link between the spoken and written form of the word was made explicit for the child in each teaching session through the manipulation of letter blocks to form words.

Intervention Aims

The aims of phonological awareness intervention for school age children with phonological disorder are to:

1. Enhance phonological awareness development to that of their peers with typical development.
2. Ensure children have strong phonemic awareness as demonstrated on tasks requiring phoneme segmentation, phoneme blending, and phoneme manipulation.
3. Enable children to use phonological knowledge to help understand the relationship between a spoken and written representation of a word.
4. Enhance transfer of phonological awareness to the reading and spelling process.

Intervention Models

For school-aged children with phonological disorders, the most prevalent models of phonological awareness intervention are small-group intensive intervention, classroom-based intervention, and integration of phonological awareness goals into conventional therapy.

Small-Group Intensive Phonological Awareness Intervention

Increasingly, elementary schools are organizing small-group instruction focused explicitly on phonological awareness for its kindergartners and first-graders who struggle in this area. Led by a SLP, reading specialist, or other member of school, children who are identified as at risk for literacy problems meet in small groups of three to six children one or more times per week for small-group sessions. These sessions may focus exclusively on phonological awareness or may include attention to other literacy goals as needed (e.g., reading fluency, vocabulary).

A number of available curricula exist for organizing small-group intensive phonological awareness programs. One option is to adopt a general instructional sequence (e.g., see Brady et al., 1994, program for classroom-based instruction, as described in Table 9.7),

■ **TABLE 9.7** Example of Classroom-Based Phonological Awareness Training for Kindergartners (5 and 6 Years of Age)

Phase (Weeks)	Major Activities (Example)
I (1–3)	Rhyme awareness (listening to nursery rhymes)
	Rhyme production (generating words rhyming with a target)
	Rhyme detection (selecting words not rhyming with others)
	Syllable deletion (deleting a syllable from a multisyllable word)
II (4–10)	Phoneme isolation (isolating the first sound in words and bringing child's attention to the articulatory features of the word)
	Alliteration detection (selecting words not sharing a target phoneme with others)
	Phoneme deletion (producing words minus a target phoneme)
III (11–18)	Phoneme segmentation and blending (identifying and manipulating the phonemes comprising words)

Source: Adapted from Brady et al. (1994).

and to increase the frequency and intensity of instruction within the highly individualized context provided by small-group instruction. Two commercially available small-group intensive intervention programs that provide explicit guidelines for implementation, and thus can be easily and efficiently implemented, are the following: *Road to the Code* (Blachman, Ball, Black, and Tangel, 2000) and the *Intensive Phonological Awareness Program* (Schuele and Dayton, 2000). Torgesen and Mathes (2000) provide a description and critique of additional programs. These programs are recommended for 5- and 6-year-old children. Small groups of about six children are provided instruction several times weekly for an extended period of time (e.g., four or five months). Instruction can be provided by SLPs, reading specialists, and regular or special educators.

The program *Road to the Code* (Blachman et al., 2000) provides a detailed curriculum for intensive phonological awareness instruction. Lessons are delivered four times weekly in 15-minute sessions for an 11-week period. The program was designed for children who are generally at risk for difficulties in early literacy achievement. The program consists of 44 detailed lesson plans, with scripts to guide implementation. Each lesson includes a phonological awareness (e.g., rhyme production), phonemic segmentation, and letter-sound correspondence activity. Investigators reported on the effectiveness of this program with kindergarten children (e.g., Ball and Blachman, 1988, 1991). They indicated that phonological awareness and word decoding skills improved significantly.

The Intensive Phonological Awareness Program (Schuele and Dayton, 2000) was designed to meet the needs of children with language impairments. Intervention sessions are three times a week (30-minute sessions) for a 12-week period. Skills are targeted in three-week blocks, and include rhyme, initial sounds, final sounds, and phonemic analysis and synthesis. Thirty-six lesson plans describe activities and provide detailed guidance on teaching strategies. Pilot studies (Dayton and Schuele, 1997; Schuele, Justice, Cabell, Knighton, Kingery, and Lee, in press) have suggested that the program is effective in increasing phonological awareness and word decoding skills in children with language impairment and also in a broad sample of kindergartners. However, the efficacy of this program for children with speech impairments still needs to be established.

Classroom-Based Phonological Awareness Instruction

Increasingly, explicit phonological awareness activities are found in the daily activities of preschool, kindergarten, and first-grade classrooms. Providing phonological awareness intervention within the classroom can be an efficient and effective means for promoting these skills in all children, including those with speech difficulties. Service delivery in the classroom is consistent with providing intervention in the least restrictive and most naturalistic environment. Therefore, clinicians should review the school's curriculum to familiarize themselves with how phonological awareness is targeted. They may find that some curricula provide adequate instruction, whereas supplemental activities may be needed with others. Clinicians must work collaboratively with other educators to encourage children's frequent interactions with the sound structure of language.

An example of a successful classroom-based phonological awareness training program was described by Brady, Fowler, Stone, and Winbury (1994). Participants included 96 inner-city kindergarten children (5 to 6 years of age) enrolled in four classrooms (two intervention, two control). Children in the intervention classrooms participated in an 18-week training program (three 20-minute sessions per week) conducted by classroom teachers (the two other classrooms followed the typical curriculum). Children in the intervention classrooms made substantially greater gains than their control group peers on an array of phonological awareness measures, including the ability to generate rhymes and to segment words into phonemes. Follow-up testing at the end of first grade found that children who had received the kindergarten phonological awareness intervention outperformed their peers on a set of early reading measures. An example of a classroom teaching framework for phonological awareness activities based on Brady and colleagues' intervention is presented in Table 9.7.

Speech-language pathologists can partner with classroom teachers to implement classroom-based programs (Hadley, Simmerman, Long, and Luna, 2000). These partnerships can be particularly effective in that they combine the SLPs' strength in knowledge of phonology and teachers' strength in early reading instruction.

Phonological Awareness Integrated into Conventional Therapy

Children with phonological disorder who appear not to have benefited from classroom or small-group phonological awareness programs or for whom these programs are not available for some reason may require explicit phonological awareness instruction embedded into their conventional speech therapy (one on one or small group). Clinicians can include activities in every session to stimulate children's awareness at the phoneme level and also facilitate their generalization of phonological awareness knowledge in reading and in spelling. Twenty hours of intervention (administered by a SLP two times weekly) has proven effective in ensuring long-term gains from phonological awareness to reading and spelling for children with speech impairment (Gillon, 2002). The phonological awareness intervention may be structured to simultaneously target speech goals and phonological awareness knowledge at the phoneme level. An example of integrating speech targets and phonological awareness for a 6-year-old child is provided next (see Gillon, 2004).

Teaching Example

Speech Goal: Reduce speech error pattern of cluster reduction for "st" cluster.

Phonological Awareness Goals: Increase awareness of phonemes in words and make explicit the link between phonemes and graphemes.

Target Speech Words for Lesson: *star, sty, stop, step, Stan*

Stimulus Items: Picture cards of target speech items with the words printed underneath in large clear font (e.g., font size 48).

Prompt: Prompt the correct articulation of the target cluster through integrating phonological awareness and letter knowledge. For example, the child articulates the word *star* as *tar* and the clinician prompts: "When you say *tar* I can't hear the /s/ sound at the beginning (pointing to the letter *s* in the word *star*). Listen to the /s/ sound at the beginning of the word *star*. Let's try again with the /s/ sound at the beginning *star*. (pointing to the letter *s* at the beginning of the word)."

Appendix C provides illustrations of various phonemic awareness activities that can be used to promote children's phonemic awareness. Activities such as these can be readily integrated into conventional therapies focused on speech intelligibility.

Intervention with Older Children

Research suggests that older children can increase their phonological awareness with direct instruction in phonological awareness (Gillon and Dodd, 1995, 1997; Swanson, Hodson, and Schommer-Aikins 2005; Torgesen, Wagner, Rashotte, Alexander, and Conway, 1997). Thus, older children experiencing reading difficulties in combination with phonological disorder may benefit from explicit phonological awareness intervention delivered by the SLP; indeed, deficits in phonological awareness may contribute substantially to many of these children's problems with reading and writing. In addition, some children who have moved beyond the early elementary grades may never have developed an adequate phonological awareness foundation. Other children may have rudimentary skills but fail to develop more complex phonological awareness skills (e.g., phoneme analysis and synthesis). For some children who have histories of phonologic impairment, this weakness may be most evident in poor spelling ability (Clark-Klein and Hodson, 1995). A thorough multidisciplinary evaluation of reading, writing, and phonological awareness will clarify children's needs (Gentry, 1988; Masterson and Crede, 1999). Subsequently, systematic instruction can be provided by clinicians, with specific goals and activities designed to meet these children's individual needs.

We can expect that explicit phonological awareness intervention that facilitates children's awareness of phonemes in words and facilitates understanding of the link between spoken and written words will lead to improved phonological awareness, reading, and spelling for many children with disorders of speech production. However, continued research is necessary to more clearly understand the relationship between phonological disorder, phonological awareness, and reading development. Of greatest need is identifying treatment approaches that are most effective and efficient for addressing speech difficulties simultaneously with phonological awareness challenges. Of particular importance is identifying a sufficient array of approaches so that children who do not respond adequately to one approach can be provided another. In this regard, the educational outcomes and literacy potential of children who exhibit developmental vulnerabilities in both speech and reading can be maximized.

■ QUESTIONS FOR CHAPTER 9

1. What are some key indicators of phonological awareness that emerge during the preschool period?

2. What is the relationship between phonological awareness and reading ability?

3. Why are children with expressive phonological disorders at increased risk for problems with phonological awareness?

4. What is the speech-language pathologist's role with respect to phonological awareness?

5. What are specific strategies that the speech-language pathologist can use to promote phonological awareness for preschool-age children?

6. What might a classroom-based or intensive small-group phonological awareness intervention program look like?

Children's Speech Acquisition

SHARYNNE McLEOD

This compilation of data on typical speech development for English speaking children is designed to be used by speech-language pathologists. It is organised according to children's ages to reflect a typical developmental sequence. However, it should be noted that rates of development vary among typically developing children. Where possible, data from more than one study is presented under each heading at each age to allow for comparison and to encourage consideration of diversity and individuality.

Details of Studies Cited

Authors	Year	Country	No. of Children	Age of Children	Sample Type	Data Collection Method
Anthony, Bogle, Ingram & McIsaac	1971	UK	510	3;0–6;0	Single word (SW)	Cross-sectional
Arlt & Goodban	1976	USA	240	3;0–5;5	SW	Cross-sectional
Chirlian & Sharpley	1982	Australia	1357	2;6–9;0	SW	Cross-sectional
Dodd	1995	UK & Australia	5	1;8–3;0	Connected speech (CS)	Longitudinal
Dodd, Holm, Hua & Crosbie	2003	UK	684	3;0–6;11	SW	Cross-sectional
Donegan	2002	UK & USA	–	–	–	Compilation
Dyson	1988	USA	20	2;0–3;3	CS	Cross-sectional & longitudinal
Flipsen	2006a, b	USA	320	3;1–8;10	CS	Cross-sectional
Grunwell	1987	UK	–	–	–	Compilation
Haelsig & Madison	1986	USA	50	2;10–5;2	SW	Cross-sectional
James	2001	Australia	354	3;0–7;11	SW	Cross-sectional
James, McCormack & Butcher	1999	Australia	240	5;0–7;11	SW	Cross-sectional
James, van Doorn, McLeod	2001	Australia	354	3;0–7;11	SW	Cross-sectional
James, van Doorn, McLeod	2002	Australia	354	3;0–7;11	SW	Cross-sectional

Authors	Year	Country	No. of Children	Age of Children	Sample Type	Data Collection Method
Kehoe	1997	USA	18	1;10–2;10	SW	Cross-sectional
Kehoe	2001	USA	–	1;6–2;10	–	Compilation
Kilminster & Laird	1978	Australia	1756	3;0–9;0	SW	Cross-sectional
Lowe, Knutson & Monson	1985	USA	1048	2;7–4;6	SW	Cross-sectional
McGlaughlin & Grayson	2003	UK	297	0;1–1;0	Crying	Cross-sectional
McLeod, van Doorn & Reed	2001a	Australia	–	–	–	Compilation
McLeod, van Doorn & Reed	2001b	Australia	16	2;0–3;4	CS	Longitudinal
McLeod, van Doorn & Reed	2002	Australia	16	2;0–3;4	CS	Longitudinal
Oller, Eilers, Neal & Schwartz	1999	USA	3400	0;10–1;0	CS; Parent report	Cross-sectional & longitudinal
Otomo & Stoel-Gammon	1992	USA	6	1;10–2;6	SW	Longitudinal
Paynter & Petty	1974	USA	90	2;0–2;6	SW	Cross-sectional
Pollock	2002	USA (Memphis)	162	1;6–6;10	SW & CS	Cross-sectional
Pollock & Berni	2003	USA (Memphis)	165	1;6–6;10	SW & CS	Cross-sectional
Porter & Hodson	2001	USA	520	2;6–8;0	SW	Cross-sectional
Prather, Hedrick & Kern	1975	USA	147	2;0–4;0	SW	Cross-sectional
Preisser, Hodson & Paden	1988	USA	60	1;6–2;5	SW	Cross-sectional
Robb & Bleile	1994	USA	7	0;8–2;1	CS	Longitudinal
Robb & Gillon	2007	New Zealand & USA	20	3;1–3;5 (NZ) 2;11–3;5 (US)	CS	Cross-sectional
Robbins & Klee	1987	USA	90	2;6–6;11	SW	Cross-sectional
Roberts, Burchinal & Footoo	1990	USA	145	2;6–8;0	SW	Cross-sectional & longitudinal
Roulstone, Loader, Northstone, Beveridge & ALSPAC team	2002	UK	1127	2;1	SW; Parent report	Single age group
Selby, Robb & Gilbert	2000	USA	4	1;3–3;0	CS	Longitudinal
Shriberg	1993	USA	–	–	–	Compilation
Smit	1993b	USA	997	3;0–9;0	SW	Cross-sectional
Smit	1993a	USA	997	3;0–9;0	SW	Cross-sectional
Smit, Hand, Frelinger, Bernthal & Bird	1990	USA	997	3;0–9;0	SW	Cross-sectional

Authors	Year	Country	No. of Children	Age of Children	Sample Type	Data Collection Method
Snow	1994	USA	9	1;0–1;8	CS	Longitudinal
Stoel-Gammon	1985	USA	34	1;3–2;0	CS	Longitudinal
Stoel-Gammon	1987	USA	33	2;0	CS	Cross-sectional
Stokes	2005	USA	40	2;1	CS	Single age group
Templin	1957	USA	480	3;0–8;0	SW	Cross-sectional
Ttofari-Eecen, Reilly & Eadie	2007	Australia	1734	1;0	Parent report	Single age group
Waring, Fisher & Aitken	2001	Australia	299	3;5–7;11	SW	Cross-sectional
Watson & Scukanec	1997a, b	USA	12	2;0–3;0	CS	Longitudinal
Wells, Peppé & Goulandris	2004	UK	120	5;6–13;0		

GLOSSARY. Acquired sounds: The age at which a certain percentage (often 75%) of children have acquired a phoneme in initial, medial and final position in single words.
Phonetic inventory: Repertoire of sounds a child can produce, regardless of the adult target. Syllable shape: Structure of a syllable within a word. C = consonant; V = vowel

Developmental Data

0;0 – 1;0 year

"The interaction between infants and their caregivers lays so many foundations for later learning" (McLaughlin, 1998, p. 192)

ORAL MECHANISM

Infant cf. adults

Oral space is smaller. Lower jaw smaller and retracted. Sucking pads are present, teeth emerge. Tongue large compared to size of oral cavity and therefore has more restricted movement. (Moves with jaw) Nose breather. Epiglottis and soft palate are in approximation as a protective mechanism. Newborns breathe/swallow at same time. Larynx is higher in newborns. Eustachian tube lies in horizontal position. (More vertical in adults)

PERCEPTION

"By at least 2 days of age, the neonate has an ability to discriminate language specific acoustic distinctions . . . The 12 month old human has developed the capacity to categorise only those phonemes which are in its native language"   (Ruben, 1997, p. 203)

CRYING

Mean amount of crying/24 hours
1-3 months = 90 mins, mostly in the evening
4-6 months = 64.7 mins, mostly afternoon
7-9 months = 60.5 mins, afternoon/evening
10-12 months = 86.4 mins, mostly evening
Other studies show decrease at 10+ months`

                              (McGlaughlin & Grayson, 2003)

VOCALISATION

0-6 weeks = reflexive vocalisations: cry, fuss
6-16 weeks = coo and laughter: vowel-like
16-30 weeks = syllable-like vocalisations (Stark, Bernstein, & Demorest, 1983)
0–0;2 = phonation, quasivowels & glottals
0;2–0;3 = primitive articulation stage: gooing
0;4–0;5 = expansion stage: full vowels, raspberries, marginal babbling
(Oller, Eilers, Neal & Schwartz, 1999)

BABBLING

" . . . late onset of canonical babbling may be a predictor of disorders . . . [i.e.] smaller production vocabularies at 18, 24 and 36 months" (Oller, Eilers, Neal & Schwartz, 1999, p. 223)
31-50 weeks = reduplicated babbling: series of consonant and vowel-like elements
(Mitchell, 1997; Stark, 1979)
0;6+ = canonical stage: well-formed canonical syllables, reduplicated sequences (e.g., [bababab])
(Oller et al., 1999)
"The sounds babbled most frequently are produced more accurately by English-learning 2-year-olds, and appear more often in the languages of the world, than other sounds." (Locke, 2002, p. 249).

PHONETIC INVENTORY
Consonants

Nasal, plosive, fricative, approximant, labial, lingual (Grunwell, 1981)
1;0 = Mean 4.4 consonants; median 4; range 0–16 (Ttofari-Eecen et al., 2007)
1;0 = /m, d, b, n/ most frequently reported consonants in inventory (Ttofari-Eecen et al., 2007)
0;8 = 5 consonants in initial position (typically / d, t, k, m, h /); 3 consonants in final position (typically / t, m, h/)
0;9 = 5 consonants in initial position (typically / d, m, n, h, w /); 2 consonants in final position (typically / m, h/)
0;10 = 6 consonants in initial position (typically / b, d, t, m, n, h /); 4 consonants in final position (typically t, m, h, s /)
0;11 = 4 consonants in initial position (typically / d, m, n, h /); 2 consonants in final position (typically /m, h/)
1;0 = 5 consonants in initial position (typically / b, d, g, m, h/); 2 consonants in final position (typically /m, h/)(Robb & Bleile, 1994)

Vowels

"Low, non-rounded vowels are favoured in the first year. Front-back vowel differences appear later than height differences." (Donegan, 2002)

PHONOLOGICAL PROCESSES
Present

All phonological processes (Grunwell, 1987)

SYLLABLE STRUCTURE

Primarily mono-syllabic utterances (Bauman-Waengler, 2000, p. 99)

PROSODY

0;10 – 1;0 = Begin with falling contour only. Flat or level contour, usually accompanied by variations such as falsettos or variations in duration of loudness (Marcos, 1987 adapted by Bauman-Waengler, 2000)

1;0 – 2;0 years

"... from 18 to 24 months ... the largest growth within the phonological system takes place ... also ... the child's expressive vocabulary has at least tripled" (Bauman-Waengler, 2000, p. 107)

ORAL MECHANISM
Deciduous teeth continue to emerge

INTELLIGIBILITY
2;0 = 26–50% intelligible   (Weiss, 1982)

ACQUIRED SOUNDS
Consonants (females)
2;0 = /m, n, h, g/   (Chirlian & Sharpley, 1982)

Consonants (males)
2;0 = /m, n/   (Chirlian & Sharpley, 1982)

Consonants (all children)
2;0 = / h, w/   (Paynter & Petty, 1974)
2;0 = /m, n, ŋ, h, p/   (Prather, Hedrick, & Kern, 1975)

Consonant clusters
?

Vowels
?

PERCENT CORRECT
Consonants
2;0 = 69.2 (range 53-91)   (Watson & Scukanec, 1997b)

Consonant clusters
?

Vowels (USA -nonrhotic)
1;6–1;11 = 82% (range = 69–96)   (Pollock & Berni, 2003)

COMMON MISMATCHES
Consonants
?

Consonant clusters
?

PHONOLOGICAL PROCESSES
Present
Final consonant deletion, cluster reduction, fronting of velars, stopping, gliding, context
sensitive voicing   (Grunwell, 1987)

Declining
Reduplication, consonant harmony   (Grunwell, 1987)

PHONETIC INVENTORY

"First words show individual variation in consonants used; phonetic variability in pronunciations"

(Grunwell, 1987)

Consonants

/m, p, b, w, n, t, d/ (Grunwell, 1987)

1;0 = 5 consonants in initial position (typically / b, d, g, m, h/); 2 consonants in final position (typically /m, h/)

1;6 = 6 consonants in initial position (typically / b, d, m, n, h, w /); 3 consonants in final position (typically / t, h, s /)

2;0 = 10 consonants in initial position (typically / b, d, p, t, k, m, n, h, s, w /); 4 consonants in final position (typically / t, k, n, s/) (Robb & Bleile, 1994)

1;0 – Mean = 4.4 consonants; median = 4; range 0-16

1;0 – /m, d, b, n/ most frequently reported consonants in inventory (Ttofari-Eecen et al., 2007)

Vowels (USA)

1;3 = /ɪ, ʊ, ʌ, ɑ/

1;6 = /i, u, ʊ, ʌ, ɔ, ɑ, æ/

1;9 = /i, ɪ, u, ɛ, o, ʌ, ɔ, ɑ

2;0 = /i, ɪ, u, ɛ, e, o, ɔ, ɑ, æ/ (Selby, Robb & Gilbert, 2000)

SYLLABLE STRUCTURE

?

PROSODY

Young children acquire skills that control intonation earlier than final syllable timing skills (Snow, 1994).

1;1 – 1;3 = Rising contour. High falling contour that begins with a high pitch and drops to a lower one prior to 1;6 = high rising and high rising-falling contour

around 1;6 = falling-rising contour. Rising-falling contour (Marcos, 1987 adapted by Bauman-Waengler, 2000)

METALINGUISTIC SKILLS

1;6–2;0 = monitor own utterances: repair spontaneously, adjust speech to different listeners, practice sounds, words, sentences (Clark, adapted by Owens, 1996, p. 386)

2;0 – 3;0 years

"Unlike toddlers, preschoolers develop more freedom of movement and therefore, soon become trailblazers in every sense of the word" (McLaughlin, 1998, p. 271)

ORAL MECHANISM

During first 3 years of life:

Oral space enlarges. Growth of lower jaw + other bony structures. Disappearance of sucking pads. Increased muscle tone and "skilled" tongue movement. (Tongue movement becomes dissociated from jaw movement. Important for feeding & speech) Lowering & more sophisticated movement of larynx. Separation of epiglottis & soft palate.

DDK (2;6 – 2;11)
/pʌ/ = 3.7 per second; /tʌ/ = 3.7 per second
/kʌ/ = 3.65 per second; patticake = 1.26/sec   (Robbins & Klee, 1987)

Maximum phonation time
2;6 – 2;11 = 5.55 sec   (Robbins & Klee, 1987)

INTELLIGIBILITY

2;1 = ". . . children were mostly intelligible to their parents with 12.7% parents finding their child difficult to understand and only 2.1% of parents reporting that they could rarely understand their child"   (Roulstone et al., 2002, p. 264)
3;0 = 95.68% (88.89–100.00)% of words that could be reliably understood by the transcriber
(Flipsen, 2006b)

2;0 = 26-50% intelligible
2;6 = 51-70% intelligible
3;0 = 71-80% intelligible   (Weiss, 1982)
3;0 = 73% (50-80%) intelligible judged by three unfamiliar listeners. The children who used more complex sentences were more difficult to understand   (Vihman, 1988)

ACQUIRED SOUNDS
Consonants (females)
≤3;0 = / m, n, h, w, p, b, t, d, k, g, f/
3;0 = + / s/   (Smit, et al., 1990)
2;0 = /m, n, h, g/
2;6 = + /p, ŋ, w, t, d, k/
3;0 = + / j, f/   (Chirlian & Sharpley, 1982)
3;0 = /h, ŋ, p, m, w, b, n, d, t, k, ʒ, f/   (Kilminster & Laird, 1978)

Consonants (males)
≤3;0 & 3;0 = /m, n, h, w, p, b, t, d, k, g/   (Smit, et al., 1990)
2;0 = /m, n/
2;6 = + / ŋ, d/
3;0 = + / p, b, h, w, k, g/   (Chirlian & Sharpley, 1982)
3;0 = /h, ŋ, p, m, w, b, n, d, j, g, ʒ   (Kilminster & Laird, 1978)

Consonants (all children)
2;0 = /h, w/
2;6 = + /p, b, t, m/   (Paynter & Petty, 1974)
2;0 = /m, n, ŋ, h, p/
2;4 = +/j, d, k, f/
2;8 = +/w, b, t/
3;0 = +/g, s/   (Prather, Hedrick, & Kern, 1975)
3;0 = / p, b, t, d, k, g, m, n, ŋ, h, f, w /   (Arlt & Goodban, 1976)
3;0 = / p, b, t, d, k, g, m, n, ŋ, f, v, s, z, h, w, l, j /   (Dodd et al., 2003)

Consonant clusters
"Two-year-old children can produce consonant clusters, but these may not be of the same form as the ambient language"   (McLeod, van Doorn & Reed, 2001a)

Vowels
"The literature on vowel development suggests that vowels are acquired early, both in production and perception. There is considerable variability in their production, but most studies suggest

that vowel production is reasonably accurate by age 3, although some studies call this into question."   (Donegan, 2002, p. 2)

1;10-2;6= /i, ɑ/ mastered early, /e, æ/ next, /ɪ, ɛ/ least accurate   (Otomo & Stoel-Gammon, 1992)

PERCENT CORRECT

Consonants

PCC = 70%   (Stoel-Gammon, 1987)

2;0 = 69.2% (range 53-91)

2;3 = 69.9% (range 51-91)

2;6 = 75.1% (range 61-94)

2;9 = 82.1% (range 63-96)

3;0 = 86.2% (range 73-99)   (Watson & Scukanec, 1997b)

3;0–3;11 = 82.11%   (Dodd et al., 2003)

Consonant clusters

2;0-3;4 = 29.5% (mean); 0.0 - 79.1% (range) in conversational speech

                                                                                        (McLeod, van Doorn & Reed, 2001b)

Vowels (UK)

3;0–3;11 = 97.39%   (Dodd et al., 2003)

Vowels (USA - nonrhotic)

2;0–2;5 = 92.4% (range = 78–100)

2;6–2;11 = 93.9% (range = 78–100)   (Pollock, 2002; Pollock & Berni, 2003)

Vowels (USA - rhotic)

2;0–2;5 = 37.5% (range = 0–87)

2;6–2;11 = 62.5% (range = 0–100)   (Pollock, 2002)

PERCENT ERROR

Consonants

2;7 = mean error rate for velars = 31%

2;7 = mean error rate for fricatives = 38%

2;7 = mean error rate for liquids = 57%   (Roulstone et al., 2002)

Consonant clusters

2;7 = mean error rate 72%   (Roulstone et al., 2002)

COMMON MISMATCHES

Consonants (>15%)

ŋ → n; j → Ø; l → w; r → w; r → w; v → b; θ → f; ð → d; s → dentalised; z → d; ʃ → s; tʃ → t/d; ʒ → d   (Smit, 1993a)

Consonant clusters (>15%)

pr → p, pw; br → b, bw; tr → t, tw; dr → d, dw; kr → k, kw; gr → g, gw; fr → f, fw; θr → f, θw; sw → w; sm → m; sn → n; sp → p, b; st → t, d; sk → k, skw → k, t, kw, gw; spl → p, b, pl, pw; spr → p, pw, pr, sp; str → t, d, st, tw, sw; skr → k, w, kw, gw, fw   (Smit, 1993b)

PHONOLOGICAL PROCESSES

Present

Cluster reduction, fronting of velars, fronting /ʃ/, stopping /v, θ, ð, tʃ, ʤ/, gliding, context sensitive voicing   (Grunwell, 1987)

Most prevalent = cluster reduction & liquid deviations (gliding) (Preisser et al., 1988)

2;0 = final consonant deletion, liquid simplification, later stopping, cluster reduction, vowelisation

3;0 = later stopping, cluster simplification (Watson & Scukanec, 1997b)

2;7–3;0 = 23% fronting (Lowe, Knutson & Monson, 1985)

Declining

Final consonant deletion (Grunwell, 1987)

Affrication, depalatisation, gliding, meathesis, prevocalic voicing, vowel changes (James, 2001)

PHONETIC INVENTORY

Consonants (word-initial)

9-10 consonants (Stoel-Gammon, 1987)

2;0 = /p, b, t, d, k, m, n, s, f, h, w, j/

2;3 = /p, b, t, d, k, g, m, n, s, f, h, w, j, l/

2;6 = /p, b, t, d, k, g, m, n, s, f, h, tʃ, w, j, l/

2;9 = /p, b, t, d, k, g, m, n, s, f, h, tʃ, w, j, l/

3;0 = /p, b, t, d, k, g, m, n, s, f, h, tʃ, ð, w, j, l/ (Watson & Scukanec, 1997b)

/m, p, b, w, n, t, d, (ŋ), (k), (g), h/ (Grunwell, 1987)

2;0, 2;5, 2;9 = /p, b, t, d, k, g, f, s, h, m, n, w, j, l/ (Dyson, 1988)

Consonants (word-final)

5-6 final consonants (Stoel-Gammon, 1987)

2;0 = /p, t, k, m, n, s, z/

2;3 = /p, t, d, m, n, s, z/

2;6, 2;9, 3;0 = /p, t, d, k, m, n, s, z, l, r/ (Watson & Scukanec, 1997b)

2;0 = /p, t, d, k, tʃ, ʔ, f, s, ʃ, m, n/

2;5 = /p, t, d, k, tʃ, ʔ, f, s, ʃ, m, n, ŋ, ɚ/

2;9 = /p, t, k, ʔ, f, s, ʃ, m, n, ɚ/ (Dyson, 1988)

Consonant clusters

"A few clusters" (Stoel-Gammon, 1987)

2;6 = /pw, bw, -nd, -ts/

2;9 = /pw, bw, bl, -nd, -ts, -nt, -nz/

3;0 = /st, sp, pl, -nd, -ts, -nt, -nz, -st, -rŋk/ (Watson & Scukanec, 1997b)

2;0 = /fw, -ts (-ŋk)/

2;5 = (/fw), (bw), -ts, (-ps), (ntŋ), (ŋk)//

2;9 = (/fw), (kw), (-ps), (-ts), (-nts), (-ŋk)/ (Dyson, 1988)

2;0 = predominantly word-initial consonant clusters containing /w/ (e.g., [bw, kw])

3;0 = range of word-initial clusters predominantly containing /l/, /w/ or /s/.

Common word-final clusters contained nasals (e.g., [-nd, -nt, -ŋk]).

(McLeod, van Doorn & Reed, 2001b)

Vowels

2;0 = /i, ɛ, u, ɛ, e, o, ɔ, ɑ, æ/

3;0 = /i, ɛ, u, ʊ, ɛ, e, o, ʌ, ɔ, ɜ , ɑ, æ/ (Selby, Robb & Gilbert, 2000)

SYLLABLE STRUCTURE

Syllable shapes

CV, CVC, CVCV, CVCVC (Stoel-Gammon, 1987)

CV, VC, CVC, 2-syllable (Shriberg, 1993)

Monosyllabic words - V, CV, VC, CVC,

CCVC, CVCC, CCVCC,
CCVCCC, CCCCVC
Polysyllabic words - V, CV, VC, CVC, CCVC   (Dodd, 1995; Watson & Skucanec, 1997)

PROSODY

"Significantly greater number of stress errors in SWS words (S = strong; W = weak). Tendency for greater number of stress errors in SWSW words. Stress errors were more frequent in imitated than spontaneous productions." (Kehoe, 1997)

"An analysis of children's truncation error syllable deletion patterns revealed the following robust findings:

(a) Stressed and word-final unstressed syllables are preserved more frequently than nonfinal unstressed syllables,

(b) word-internal unstressed syllables with obstruent onsets are preserved more frequently than word-internal syllables with sonorant onsets,

(c) unstressed syllables with non-reduced vowels are preserved more frequently than unstressed syllables with reduced vowels,

(d) right-sided stressed syllables are preserved more frequently than left-sided stressed syllables. An analysis of children's stress patterns revealed that children made greater numbers of stress errors in target words with irregular stress."   (Kehoe, 2001, p. 284)

METALINGUISTIC SKILLS

1;6–2;0 = monitor own utterances: repair spontaneously, adjust speech to different listeners, practice sounds, words, sentences   (Clark, adapted by Owens, 1996, p. 386)

3;0 – 4;0 years

"A client 3 years of age or older who is unintelligible is a candidate for treatment" (Bernthal & Bankson, 1998, p. 272)

ORAL MECHANISM

3 yrs = adult-like swallow

DDK (3;0–3;5/ 3;6–3;11)
/pʌ = 4.66/ 4.81 per second
/tʌ = 4.56/ 4.78 per second
/kʌ/ = 3.82/ 4.83 per second
patticake = 1.36/ 1.75 per second   (Robbins & Klee, 1987)

Maximum phonation time
/a/ = 5.51/ 7.79 sec   (Robbins & Klee, 1987)

INTELLIGIBILITY

3;0 = 95.68% (88.89–100.00)
4;0 = 96.82% (88.42–100.00)
% of words that could be reliably understood by the transcriber   (Flipsen, 2006b)
3;0 = 71–80% intelligible   (Weiss, 1982)
3;0 = 73% (50-80%) intelligible judged by three unfamiliar listeners   (Vihman, 1988)
"A client 3 years of age or older who is unintelligible is a candidate for treatment"
                    (Bernthal & Bankson, 1998, p. 272)

ACQUIRED SOUNDS

"3-year-olds had acquired all major phoneme classes, except liquids . . . sibilant lisps were still common until the age of 7 years"   (Porter & Hodson, 2001, p.165)

Consonants (females)

3;0 = /m, n, h, w, p, b, t, d, k, g, f, s/
3;6 = + /j/
4;0 = +/ v, ð, ʃ, tʃ/   (Smit, et al., 1990)
3;0 = /m, n, h, g, p, ŋ, w, t, d, k, j, f/
3;6 = + /b, ʃ, tʃ, s/
4;0 = +/ l, ʒ, ʤ/   (Chirlian & Sharpley, 1982)
3;0 = /h, ŋ, p, m, w, b, n, d, t, k, ʒ, f/
3;6 = + /j, g, l/
4;0 = +/ʃ, tʃ, ʤ/   (Kilminster & Laird, 1978)

Consonants (males)

3;0 = /m, n, h, w, p, b, t, d, k, g/
3;6 = + /j, f/
4;0 = +/ʤ/   (Smit, et al., 1990)
3;0 = /m, n, ŋ, d, p, b, h, w, k, g/
3;6 = + /j, t, f, l, ʃ, tʃ, ʤ/
4;0 = + /s/   (Chirlian & Sharpley, 1982)
3;0 = /h, ŋ, p, m, w, b, n, d, j, g, ʒ/
3;6 = + /k, f/
4;0 = as above   (Kilminster & Laird, 1978)

Consonants (all children)

3;0 = / p, b, t, d, k, g, m, n, ŋ, h, f, w/
3;6 = +/v/
4;0 = +/s, z, ʒ, tʃ, ʤ, l/   (Arlt & Goodban, 1976)
3;0 = /m, n, ŋ, h, p, j, d, k, f, w, b, t, g, s/
3;4 = +/l, r/
3;8 = +/ʃ, tʃ/
4;0 = +/ð, ʒ/   (Prather, Hedrick, & Kern, 1975)
3;0 = / p, b, t, d, k, g, m, n, ŋ, f, v, s, z, h, w, l, j/
3;6 = +/tʃ/
4;0 = +/ʒ, ʤ/   (Dodd et al., 2003)

Consonant clusters

3;6 (males & females)= /tw, kw/
4;0 (females) = /tw, kw, pl, bl, kl/
4;0 (males) = /tw, kw/   (Smit, et al., 1990)
4;0 = /tw, kw, sp, st, sk, sm, sn, pl, bl, kl, gl, pr, br, tr, dr, kr, gr/   (Templin, 1957)
4;0 = /kw/   (Anthony et al., 1971)

Vowels

Paradigmatic production (ie production of individual vowels) is generally mastered by 3 years. However, syntagmatic production (production of vowels in context such as polysyllabic words) takes up to at least 6 years   (James, van Doorn & McLeod, 2001)

PERCENT CORRECT

Consonants

3;0-3;11 = 76.77% in monosyllabic words

3;0-3;11 = 76.41% in polysyllabic words　　　　　　　　　　(James, van Doorn & McLeod, 2002)
3;5-3;11 = 85.2%　　　　　　　　　　　　　　　　　　　　　(Waring, Fisher, Atkin, 2001)
3;0-3;11 = 82.11%　　　　　　　　　　　　　　　　　　　　　　　　　(Dodd et al., 2003)

Consonant clusters
3;5–3;11 = 86.4%　　　　　　　　　　　　　　　　　　　　　(Waring, Fisher, Atkin, 2001)

Vowels (Australian)
3;0-3;11 = 94.9% in monosyllabic words
3;0-3;11 = 88.28% in polysyllabic words　　　　　　　　　　(James, van Doorn & McLeod, 2001)

Vowels (UK)
3;0-3;11 = 97.39% (Dodd et al., 2003)

Vowels (USA - nonrhotic)
3;0-3;5 = 97.3% (range) = 89-100)
3;6-3;11 = 97.2% (range = 91-100)　　　　　　　　(Pollock, 2002; Pollock & Berni, 2003)

Vowels (USA - rhotic)
3;0-3;5 = 79.2% (range = 4-100)
3;6-3;11 = 76.5% (range = 4-100)　　　　　　　　　　　　　　　　　　　　(Pollock, 2002)

COMMON MISMATCHES

Consonants (>15%)
ŋ → n; r → w; v→ b; θ → f; ð → d; s → dentalised　　　　　　　　　　　　　(Smit, 1993a)

Consonant clusters (>15%)
pr → pw; br → bw; tr → tw; dr → dw; kr → kw;
gr → gw; fr → fw; θr → fr; st → θt;
skw → θkw; spl → θpl, spw; spr → θpr, spw;
str → θtr, stw; skr → θkr, skw　　　　　　　　　　　　　　　　　　　　　(Smit, 1993b)

PHONOLOGICAL PROCESSES

Present
Stopping /v, θ, ð/, fronting /ʃ, tʃ, ʤ/, gliding,　　　　　　　　　　　　　(Grunwell, 1987)
3;0-3;6 Gliding of liquids, weak syllable deletion, glottal replacement, alveolar & labial assimilation,
cluster reduction, stopping, vocalization, final consonant deletion　　　　(Haelsig & Madison, 1986)
3;0-3;11 gliding, deaffrication, cluster reduction, fronting, weak syllable deletion, (stopping – only
used by 3;0-3;5)　　　　　　　　　　　　　　　　　　　　　　　　　(Dodd et al., 2003)

Declining
Cluster reduction　　　　　　　　　　　　　　　　　　　　　　　　　(Grunwell, 1987)
Backing, cluster reduction, deaffrication, final consonant deletion, final devoicing, initial consonant
deletion, labial assimilation, palatalisation, stopping, unstressed syllable deletion, fricative
simplification　　　　　　　　　　　　　　　　　　　　　　　　　　　　　(James, 2001)

PHONETIC INVENTORY

Consonants
/m, p, b, w, n, t, d, ŋ, k, g, h, f, w, s, (l), j, h/　　　　　　　　　　　　　(Grunwell, 1987)
initial = /p, b, t, d, k, g, f, s, h, m, n, w, j, l, r/;
final = /p, t, d, k, ʔ, f, v, s, z, ʃ, m, n, ŋ, r, ɚ/　　　　　　　　　　　　　　(Dyson, 1988)

Consonant clusters
3;3 = /-ts, (fw), (kw), (tr), (sp), (st), (sn), (sl), (bw), (-ps), (-ns), (-ntʃ), (-ŋk)/　　　(Dyson, 1988)

Obstruent + approximant used, /s/ clusters may occur (Grunwell, 1987)
3;0 = range of word-initial clusters predominantly containing /l/, /w/ or /s/.
Common word-final clusters contained nasals (e.g., [-nd, -nt, -ŋk]).

(McLeod, van Doorn & Reed, 2001b)

Vowels
N.Zealand /i, e, u, o, ɒ, ɪ, ɛ, æ , ə, ʌ, ɔ, ʊ/
USA /i, e, u, o, ɒ, ɪ, ɛ, æ , ə, ʌ, ɔ, ʊ, ɝ, ɚ/ (Robb & Gillon, 2007)

SYLLABLE STRUCTURE

CV, VC, CVC, Cn_ or _Cn, 2-syllable (Shriberg, 1993)
Average number of syllables/words
3;0 = 1.26
4;0 = 1.27 (Flipsen, 2006a)

PROSODY

Speaking rate
New Zealand = 182 syllables per minute; 7.15 phones per second
USA = 208 syllables per minute; 8.17 phones per second (Robb & Gillon, 2007)
Stress
". . . after 2 years of age, deletion of stressed syllables is relatively infrequent, and after 3 years of age, deletion of unstressed syllables is less frequent" (Kehoe, 2001, 291)

PHONOLOGICAL AWARENESS

Emerging skills (Dodd & Gillon, 2001)
"The majority of 4-year-old children . . . will not exhibit phonological awareness other than syllable segmentation and the emergence of rhyme awareness" (Dodd & Gillon, 2001, 142)

4;0 – 5;0 years

"Five-year-old children are producing long, complex sentences . . . and maintaining a topic for several turns. In a few short years, children move much closer to the adult level of linguistic and communicative competence." (James, 1990, p. 74)

ORAL MECHANISM

DDK (4;0 - 4;5/ 4;6 - 4;11)
/pʌ/ = 4.89/ 4.64 per second
/tʌ/ = 4.77/ 4.46 per second
/kʌ/ = 4.58/ 4.29 per second
patticake = 1.56/ 1.33 per second (Robbins & Klee, 1987)

Maximum phonation time
/a/ = 8.01/ 9.22 sec (Robbins & Klee, 1987)

INTELLIGIBILITY

"A client 3 years of age or older who is unintelligible is a candidate for treatment"
(Bernthal & Bankson, 1998, p. 272)

3;0 = 95.68% (88.89 – 100.00)
4;0 = 96.82% (88.42 – 100.00)
5;0 = 98.05% (89.84 – 100.00)
% of words reliably understood by the transcriber   (Flipsen, 2006b)
4;0 = 93% (73-100%) intelligible in conversational speech with unfamiliar listeners (Gordon-Brannan, 1993 cited in Gordon-Brannan, 1994).

ACQUIRED SOUNDS

Consonants (females)
4;0 = /m, n, h, w, p, b, t, d, k, g, f, s, j, v, ð, ʃ, tʃ/
4;6 = + /ʤ, l/ 5;0 = + /z/   (Smit, et al., 1990)
4;0 = /m, n, h, g, p, ŋ, w, t, d, k, j, f, b, ʃ, tʃ, s, l, ʒ, ʤ/
5;0 = + /r, v /   (Chirlian & Sharpley, 1982)
4;0 = /h, ŋ, p, m, w, b, n, d, t, k, ʒ, f, j, g, l, ʃ, tʃ, ʤ/
4;6 = + /s, z/ 5;0 = + /r/   (Kilminster & Laird, 1978)

Consonant (males)
4;0 = /m, n, h, w, p, b, t, d, k, g, j, f , ʤ/
4;6 = + v, z/ 5;0 = + /s, ʃ, tʃ/   (Smit, et al., 1990)
4;0 = /m, n, ŋ, d, p, b, h, w, k, g, j, t, f, l, ʃ, tʃ, ʤ, s/
4;6 = + /ʒ/ 5;0 = + /r/   (Chirlian & Sharpley, 1982)
4;0 = /h, ŋ, p, m, w, b, n, d, j, g, ʒ, k, f /
4;6 = /t, l, ʃ, tʃ, ʤ/
5;0 = /r/   (Kilminster & Laird, 1978)

Consonants (all children)
4;0 = / p, b, t, d, k, g, m, n, ŋ, h, f, w, v, s, z, ʒ, tʃ, ʤ, l/
4;6 = + /ʃ/
5;0 = + /θ, ð, r /   (Arlt & Goodban, 1976)
4;0 = /m, n, ŋ, h, p, j, d, k, f, w, b, t, g, s, l, r, ʃ, tʃ, ð, ʒ/
>4;0 = + /v, θ, z, ʤ/   (Prather, Hedrick, & Kern, 1975)
4;0 = / p, b, t, d, k, g, m, n, ŋ, f, v, s, z, h, w, l, j, tʃ, ʒ, ʤ/
5;0 = +/ʃ/   (Dodd et al., 2003)

Consonant clusters (all children)
4;0 = /tw, kw, sp, st, sk, sm, sn, pl, bl, kl, gl, pr, br, tr, dr, kr/
4;6 = /tw, kw, sp, st, sk, sm, sn, pl, bl, kl, gl, pr, br, tr, dr, kr, gr, fr/
5;0 = /tw, kw, sp, st, sk, sm, sn, pl, bl, kl, gl, fl, pr, br, tr, dr, kr, gr, fr, str/   (Templin, 1957)
4;0 = /kw/
4;6 = + /kr, fl/
5;0 = + /gl, tr, kl, br/   (Anthony et al., 1971)

Consonant clusters (females)
4;0 = /tw, kw, pl, bl, kl/
4;6 = /tw, kw, sp, st, sk, sw, pl, bl, kl, gl, fl, kr, skw/
5;0 = same as for 4;6   (Smit, et al., 1990)

Consonant clusters (males)
4;0 = /tw, kw/
4;6 = /tw, kw, gl/
5;0 = /tw, kw, sp, st, sn, bl, gl, dr/   (Smit, et al., 1990)

Vowels
Paradigmatic production (ie production of individual vowels) is generally mastered by 3 years. However, syntagmatic production (production of vowels in context such as polysyllabic words) takes up to at least 6 years of age. (James, van Doorn & McLeod, 2001)

PERCENT CORRECT
Consonants
4;0-4;11 = 83.97% in monosyllabic words
4;0-4;11 = 82.45% in polysyllabic words (James van Doorn & McLeod, 2002)
4;0-4;11 = 88.5% (Waring, Fisher, Atkin, 2001)
4;0-5;5 = 90.37% (Dodd et al., 2003)

Consonant clusters
4;0-4;11 = 88.1% (Waring, Fisher, Atkin, 2001)

Vowels (UK)
4;0-5;5 = 98.93% (Dodd et al., 2003)

Vowels (Australian)
4;0-4;11 = 95.2% in monosyllabic words
4;0-4;11 = 92.08% in polysyllabic words (James van Doorn & McLeod, 2001)

Vowels (USA - nonrhotic)
4;0-4;5 = 98% (range = 91-100)
4;6-4;11 = 99% (range = 94-100) (Pollock, 2002; Pollock & Berni, 2003)

Vowels (USA - rhotic)
4;0-4;5 = 90.1% (range = 37-100)
4;6-4;11 = 86.8% (0-100) (Pollock, 2002)

COMMON MISMATCHES
Consonants (>15%)
θ → f; s → dentalised (Smit, 1993a)

Consonants clusters (>15%)
pr → pw; br → bw; tr → tw; dr → dw; kr → kw;
gr → gw; fr → fw; θr → fr; st → θt; skw → θkw; spl → θpl, spw; spr → θpr, spw; str → θtr, stw;
skr → θkr, skw (Smit, 1993b)

PHONOLOGICAL PROCESSES
Present
/θ/ ð -> [ŋ], /ð/ -> d, v], palatisation of /ʃ, tʃ, ʤ/, gliding (Grunwell, 1987)
4;0-4;6 Weak syllable deletion, vocalization, gliding of liquids (20% criterion) (Haelsig & Madison, 1986)
4;0-4;11 Gliding, deaffrication, cluster reduction (3 element clusters only) (Dodd et al., 2003)

Declining
Cluster reduction (Grunwell, 1987)
Depalatalisation, gliding, glottal replacement (James, 2001)

PHONETIC INVENTORY
Consonants
/m, p, b, w, n, t, d, ŋ, k, g, h, f, v, w, s, z, ʃ, tʃ, ʤ, l, r, j, h/   (Grunwell, 1987)

Consonant clusters
obstruent + approximant; /s/ clusters (may be "immature")   (Grunwell, 1987)

SYLLABLE STRUCTURE
CV, VC, CVC, Cn_, _Cn, Cn_Cn, 2-syllable, 3-syllable   (Shriberg, 1993)
Average number of syllables/words
4;0 = 1.27; 5;0 = 1.29   (Flipsen, 2006a)

5;0–6;0 years

"By the time children enter school, their phonological development has progressed considerably"
(Bauman-Waengler, 2000, p. 118)

ORAL MECHANISM
DDK (5;0–5;5/ 5;6–5;11)
/pʌ/ = 4.76/ 5.09 per second
/tʌ/ = 4.82/ 5.22 per second
/kʌ/ = 4.56/ 4.91 per second
patticake = 1.58/ 1.65 per second   (Robbins & Klee, 1987)

Maximum phonation time
/a/ = 8.06/ 9.42sec   (Robbins & Klee, 1987)

INTELLIGIBILITY
5;0 = 98.05% (89.84–100.00)
6;0 = 98.43% (91.67–100.00)
% of words that could be reliably understood by the transcriber   (Flipsen, 2006b)
Intelligible   (Gordon-Brannan, 1994)

ACQUIRED SOUNDS
Consonants
"By age 5, /l/ was acquired (93.4%) and /r/ was almost at criterion (84.8%). By age 6, all of the
phonological deviation means, including liquids, were less than 5%."
                    (Porter & Hodson, 2001, p. 169)

Consonants (females)
5;0 = /m, n, h, w, p, b, t, d, k, g, f, s, j, v, ð, ʃ, tʃ, ʤ, I, z/
5;6 = + /ŋ, θ/
6;0 = + /r/   (Smit, et al., 1990)
5;0 = / m, n, h, g, p, ŋ, w, t, d, k, j, f, b, ʃ, tʃ, s, l, ʒ, ʤ r, v/
No more at 5;6 or 6;0   (Chirlian & Sharpley, 1982)
5;0 = /h, ŋ, p, m, w, b, n, d, t, k, j, f, j, g, l, ʃ, tʃ, ʤ, s, z, r/
5;6 = + /v/   (Kilminster & Laird, 1978)

Consonants (males)
5;0 = /m, n, h, w, p, b, t, d, k, g, j, f, ʤ, v, z, s, ʃ, tʃ/

5;6 = /ð, r/
6;0 = /ŋ, θ, z, l/ (Smit, et al., 1990)
5;0 = / m, n, ŋ, d, p, b, h, w, k, g, j, t, f, l, ʃ, tʃ, ʤ, s, ʒ, r/
No more at 5;6 or 6;0 (Chirlian & Sharpley, 1982)
5;0 = /h, ŋ, p, m, w, b, n, d, j, g, ʒ, k, f, t, l, ʃ, tʃ, ʤ, r/
No more 5;6 or 6;0 (Kilminster & Laird, 1978)

Consonants (all children)
5;0 = / p, b, t, d, k, g, m, n, ŋ, h, f, w, v, s, z, ʒ, tʃ, ʤ, l, ʃ, θ, ð, r/ (Arlt & Goodban, 1976)
5;0 = / p, b, t, d, k, g, m, n, ŋ, f, v, s, z, h, w, l, j, tʃ, ʒ, ʤ, ʃ/
6;0 = + /r/ (Dodd et al., 2003)

Consonant clusters (all children)
5;0 = /tw, kw, sp, st, sk, sm, sn, pl, bl, kl, gl, fl, pr, br, tr, dr, kr, gr, fr, str/
6;0 = /tw, kw, sp, st, sk, sm, sn, pl, bl, kl, gl, fl, pr, br, tr, dr, kr, gr, fr, skw, str/ (Templin, 1957)
5;0 = /kw, kr, fl, gl, tr, kl, br/
5;6 = +/sl/
>5;6 = +/θ r, sm, st, str, sp/ (Anthony et al., 1971)

Consonant clusters (females)
5;0 = /tw, kw, sp, st, sk, sw, pl, bl, kl, gl, fl, kr, skw/
5;6 = /tw, kw, sp, st, sk, sm, sn, sw, pl, bl, kl, gl, fl, kr, skw/
6;0 = /tw, kw, sp, st, sk, sm, sn, sw, sl, pl, bl, kl, gl, fl, pr, br, tr, dr, kr, gr, fr, skw, spl/
(Smit, et al., 1990)

Consonant clusters (males)
5;0 = /tw, kw, sp, st, sn, bl, gl, dr/
5;6 = /tw, kw, sp, st, sn, pl, bl, kl, gl, fl, pr, tr, kr, gr, fr, dr/
6;0 = /tw, kw, sp, st, sk, sn, sw, pl, bl, kl, gl, fl, pr, br, tr, kr, gr, fr, dr/ (Smit, et al., 1990)

Vowels
Paradigmatic production (i.e., production of individual vowels) is generally mastered by 3 years. However syntagmatic production (production of vowels in context such as polysyllabic words) takes up to at least 6 years of age. (James et al., 2001)

PERCENT CORRECT

Consonants
5;0-5;11 = 89.54% in monosyllabic words
5;0-5;11 = 88.36% in polysyllabic words (James van Doorn & McLeod, 2002)
5;0-5;11 = 93.4% (Waring, Fisher, Atkin, 2001)
4;0-5;5 = 90.37%
5;6-7;0 = 95.86% (Dodd et al., 2003)

Consonant clusters
5;0-5;11 = 94.9% (Waring, Fisher, Atkin, 2001)

Vowels (UK)
4;0-5;5 = 98.93% (Dodd et al., 2003)
5;6-7;0 = 99.19% (Dodd et al., 2003)

Vowels (Australian)
5;0-5;11 = 94.8% in monosyllabic words
5;0-5;11 = 94.3% in polysyllabic words (James van Doorn & McLeod, 2001)

Vowels (USA - nonrhotic)
5;0-5;5 = 99% (range = 98-100)
5;6-5;11 = 99% (range = 98-100) (Pollock, 2002; Pollock & Berni, 2003)

Vowels (USA - rhotic)
5;0-5;5 = 88.2% (range = 0-100)
5;6-5;11 = 80.31% (range = 0-100) (Pollock, 2002)

COMMON MISMATCHES

Consonants (>15%)
Nil (Smit, 1993a)
Consonant clusters (>15%)
>5;6 = pr → pw; br → bw; tr → tw; dr → dw; kr → kw; gr → gw; skw → θkw; spl → θpl, spw; spr → θpr, spw; str → θtr, stw; skr → θkr, skw (Smit, 1993b)

PHONOLOGICAL PROCESSES

Declining
Deaffrication, epenthesis, metathesis, fricative simplification (v/ð) (James, 2001)
5;0-5;11 Gliding (Dodd et al., 2003)

SYLLABLE STRUCTURE

CV, VC, CVC, Cn_, _Cn, Cv_Cn, 2 syllable, 3+ syllable (Shriberg, 1993)
Average number of syllables/words
5;0 = 1.29
6;0 = 1.30 (Flipsen, 2006a)

PHONETIC INVENTORY

Consonants
/m, p, b, w, n, t, d, ŋ, k, g, h, f, v, θ, ð, w, s, z, ʃ, ʒ, tʃ, ʤ, l, r, j, h/ (Grunwell, 1987)

PROSODY

Significant differences were found between children with language impairment and normally developing peers on: form (chunking input, chunking output) and function (focus input, interaction input, interaction output) (Wells & Peppé, 2003)

PHONOLOGICAL AWARENESS

5;0 – 5;5 = syllable segmentation, rhyme awareness, alliteration awareness, phoneme isolation (+ letter knowledge, UK)
5;6 – 5;11 = phoneme segmentation (Dodd & Gillon, 2001)

6;0 + years

"As time goes on, it becomes more difficult to clearly number the individual developments. Major changes may be less specific . . . " (McLaughlin, 1998, p. 353)

ORAL MECHANISM

6 yrs = skull reaches adult size
6 yrs = permanent teeth emerge
7-10yrs = lower face "growth spurt"
9-13 = tongue and lips "growth spurt"

Mandible + tongue + lips continue to grow
until 16 yrs (girls) and 18 yrs (boys)
(Bauman-Waengler, 2000)

DDK (6;0 – 6;5/ 6;6 – 6;11)
/pʌ/ = 5.36/ 5.51 / sec /tʌ/ = 5.32/ 5.37 /sec
/kʌ/ = 4.94/ 4.85 /sec patticake = 1.61/ 1.64   (Robbins & Klee, 1987)

Maximum phonation time
/a/ = 10.99/11.47 sec   (Robbins & Klee, 1987)

INTELLIGIBILITY

6;0 = 98.43% (91.67 – 100.00)
7;0 = 99.51% (97.36 – 100.00)
8;0 = 99.01% (97.07 – 100.00)
% of words that could be reliably understood by the transcriber   (Flipsen, 2006b)
Intelligible   (Gordon-Brannan, 1994).

ACQUIRED SOUNDS

Consonants (all children)
6;0 = / p, b, t, d, k, g, m, n, ŋ, f, v, s, z, h, w, l, j, tʃ, ʒ, ʤ, ʃ, r/
>6;6 = +/θ, ð/   (Dodd et al., 2003)

Consonants (females)
6;0 = ALL = /m, n, h, w, p, b, t, d, k, g, f, s, j, v, ð, ʃ, tʃ, ʤ, l, z, ŋ, θ, r/   (Smit, et al., 1990)
6;0 = / m, n, h, g, p, ŋ, w, t, d, k, j, f, b, ʃ, tʃ, s, l, ʒ, ʤ r, v/
7;6 = + /θ, ð/   (Chirlian & Sharpley, 1982)
6;0 = /h, ŋ, p, m, w, b, n, d, t, k, ʒ, f, j, g, l, ʃ, tʃ, ʤ, s, z, r, v/
7;6 = + /θ, ð/   (Kilminster & Laird, 1978)

Consonants (males)
6;0 = / m, n, ŋ, d, p, b, h, w, k, g, j, t, f, l, ʃ, tʃ, ʤ, s, ʒ, r/
7;6 = +/ð/ 8;0 = + /θ/
9;0 = + /v/ (/z/ not achieved)   (Chirlian & Sharpley, 1982)
6;0 = ALL = /m, n, h, w, p, b, t, d, k, g, j, f, ʤ, v, z, s, ʃ, tʃ, ð, r, ŋ, θ, z, l/   (Smit, et al., 1990)
6;0 = /h, ŋ, p, m, w, b, n, d, j, g, ʒ, k, f, t, l, ʃ, tʃ, ʤ, r/
6;6 = + /s, z, v/ (/θ, ð/ not achieved by 9;0)   (Kilminster & Laird, 1978)

Consonant clusters (all children)
6;0 = /tw, kw, sp, st, sk, sm, sn, pl, bl, kl, gl, fl, pr, br, tr, dr, kr, gr, fr, skw, str/
7;0 = /tw, kw, sp, st, sk, sm, sn, sw, sl, pl, bl, kl, gl, fl, pr, br, tr, dr, kr, gr, fr, θr, skw, spl, spr, str, skr/   (Templin, 1957)

Consonant clusters (females)
6;0 = /tw, kw, sp, st, sk, sm, sn, sw, sl, pl, bl, kl, gl, fl, pr, br, tr, dr, kr, gr, fr, skw, spl/
7;0 = /tw, kw, sp, st, sk, sm, sn, sw, sl, pl, bl, kl, gl, fl, pr, br, tr, dr, kr, gr, fr, θr, skw, spl/
8;0 = /tw, kw, sp, st, sk, sm, sn, sw, sl, pl, bl, kl, gl, fl, pr, br, tr, dr, kr, gr, fr, θr, skw, spl, spr, str, skr/   (Smit, et al., 1990)

Consonant clusters (males)
6;0 = /tw, kw, sp, st, sk, sn, sw, pl, bl, kl, gl, fl, pr, br, tr, kr, gr, fr, dr/
7;0 = + / sm, sl, θr, skw, spl/
8;0 = + / spr, str, skr/   (Smit, et al., 1990)

Vowels
Paradigmatic production (ie production of individual vowels) is generally mastered by 3 years. However syntagmatic production (production of vowels in context such as polysyllabic words) takes up to at least 6 years of age.   (James et al., 2001)

PERCENT CORRECT

Consonants
6;0-6;11 = 93.74% in monosyllabic words
6;0-6;11 = 90.76% in polysyllabic words
7;0-7;11 = 93.93% in monosyllabic words
7;0-7;11 = 90.99% in polysyllabic words   (James van Doorn & McLeod, 2002)
6;0-6;11 = 95.1%
7;0-7;11 = 98.4%   (Waring, Fisher, Atkin, 2001)
5;6-7;0 = 95.86%   (Dodd et al., 2003)

Consonant clusters
6;0-6;11 = 96.6%
7;0-7;11 = 98.3%   (Waring, Fisher, Atkin, 2001)

Vowels (UK)
5;6-7;0 = 99.19%   (Dodd et al., 2003)

Vowels (Australian)
6;0-6;11 = 95.39% in monosyllabic words
6;0-6;11 = 94.86% in polysyllabic words
7;0-7;11 = 95.10% in monosyllabic words
7;0-7;11 = 95.44% in polysyllabic words   (James van Doorn & McLeod, 2001)

Vowels (USA - nonrhotic)
6;0-6;5 = 98.5% (range = 94-100)
6;6-6;10 = 99.2% (range = n/a)   (Pollock, 2002; Pollock & Berni, 2003)

Vowels (USA - rhotic)
6;0-6;5 = 80.3% (range = 0-100)
6;6-6;10 = 77.2% (range = 2-100)   (Pollock, 2002)

COMMON MISMATCHES

Consonants (>15%)
Nil   (Smit, 1993a)

Consonant clusters (>15%)
tr → tw; skw → θkw; spl → θpl; spr → θpr, spw; str → θtr, stw; skr → θkr, skw   (Smit, 1993b)

SYLLABLE STRUCTURE

All   (Shriberg, 1993)
Average number of syllables/words
6;0 = 1.30
7;0 = 1.32
8;0 = 1.33   (Flipsen, 2006a)

PHONETIC INVENTORY

Consonants
ALL - /m, p, b, w, n, t, d, ŋ, k, g, h, f, v, θ, ð, w, s, z, ʃ, ʒ, tʃ, ʤ, l, r, j, h/   (Grunwell, 1987)

PROSODY

"Intonation production continues to be mastered until 8;7. Intonation comprehension continues to develop up to 10;10."   (Wells, Peppé, & Goulandris, 2004)

PHONOLOGICAL AWARENESS

Established skills (Australia)

6;0 – 6;5 = syllable segmentation, rhyme awareness, alliteration awareness, phoneme isolation
6;6 – 6;11 = phoneme segmentation   (Dodd & Gillon, 2001)

Established skills (UK)

6;0 – 6;11 = syllable segmentation, rhyme awareness, alliteration awareness, phoneme isolation, letter knowledge,phoneme segmentation   (Dodd & Gillon, 2001)

Procedures for Teaching Sounds

◾ SPECIFIC INSTRUCTIONAL TECHNIQUES

As a supplement to the establishment procedures presented in Chapter 7, the following methods for teaching sounds are presented. Clinicians must be familiar not only with general approaches to the establishment of phonemes but also with specific suggestions for teaching sounds. Material presented on the following pages represents a potpourri of ideas that may be helpful to those who are beginning to develop a repertoire of techniques for evoking and establishing consonant sounds frequently in error. Sources such as Nemoy and Davis (1954) and Bosley (1981) include more extensive instruction for phonetic placement and successive approximation approaches to sound teaching. Clinicians who need word lists, pictures, and/or treatment materials are referred to CD-Rom productions such as *Articulation I: Consonant Phonemes* (Scarry-Larkin, 2001) and materials available from commercial vendors: *Target Words for Contextual Training* (Secord and Shine, 1997); *Contrasts: The Use of Minimal Pairs in Articulation Training* (Elbert, Rockman, and Saltzman, 1980); *Phonetic Context Drill Book* (Griffith and Miner, 1979); *Articulation* (Lanza and Flahive, 2000); *Phonological Processing* (Flahive and Lanza, 1998); and *Manual of Articulation and Phonological Disorders* (Bleile, 1995).

Instructions for Correction of an Interdental Lisp

It is important to remember that /s/ may be taught by having the client place his or her tongue behind either the upper teeth or the lower teeth.

1. Instruct the client to protrude the tongue between the teeth and produce a /θ/, and then push the tip of his or her tongue inward with a thin instrument, such as a tongue blade. As a variation, instruct the client to slowly and gradually withdraw the tongue while saying /θ/ and, while still attempting to make /θ/, scrape the tongue tip along the back of the front teeth and upward.
2. Instruct the client to produce /t/ in a word like *tea*. Have him or her pronounce it with a strong aspiration after release of the /t/ prior to the vowel. Instruct the client to slowly slide the tip of the tongue backward from the alveolar ridge following a prolonged release. The result should be [ts]. Then prolong the [s] portion of [ts].
3. Instruct the client to say the following word-pairs, pointing out that the tongue is in a similar position for /t/ and /s/.

| tea—sea | teal—seal | tell—sell | told—sold | tame—same | tip—sip |
| top—sop | tight—sight | too—Sue | tub—sub | turf—surf | till—sill |

4. Instruct the client to open his or her mouth, put the tongue in position for /t/, drop the tip of the tongue slightly, and send the airstream through the passage. The client can sometimes feel the emission of air by placing a finger in front of his or her mouth.

5. Instruct the client to produce /ʃ/ and then retract his or her lips (smile) and push the tongue slightly forward.

6. Instruct the client to say /i/ and blow through the teeth to produce /s/.

7. Insert a straw in the groove of the tongue and have the client blow to produce /s/.

8. Instruct the client to use the following phonetic placement cues:
   a. Raise the tongue so that the sides are firmly in contact with the inner surface of the upper back teeth.
   b. Groove the tongue slightly along the midline.
   c. Place the tip of the tongue about a quarter of an inch behind the upper teeth.
   d. Bring the teeth together.
   e. Direct the airstream along the groove of the tongue toward the cutting edges of the lower teeth.

Instructions for Correction of a Lateral Lisp

1. Position a straw so that it protrudes from the side of the mouth. When a lateral [s] is made, the straw should resonate on the side of the mouth where the air stream is directed. When the straw is inserted into the front of the mouth and a correct /s/ is made, the straw will resonate in the front of the mouth.

2. Direct attention to a central emission of the air stream by holding a feather, a strip of paper, or a finger in front of the center of the mouth, or have the client tap the incisor gently with his or her forefinger while [s] is being produced. If the sound is being emitted through a central aperture, a break in continuity of the outflow of the breath will be noted. If the sound is being emitted laterally, no break in the continuity of the air stream will be noted. An awareness of central emission may also be developed by instructing the client to inhale air and directing his or her attention to the cool sensation from the intake of air. Then instruct the client to exhale the air through the same aperture by which air entered upon inhalation.

3. Instruct the client to put a tongue blade down the midline of the tongue in order to establish a groove for the air stream.

4. Instruct the client to retract the lips sharply and push the tongue forward, attempting to say /s/.

5. Instruct the client to make /t/, holding the release position for a relatively long time, then retract the lips and drop the jaw slightly. A [ts] should be heard if grooving was maintained properly. Then extend the duration of the [ts], gradually decreasing the release phase of [t] until /s/ is approximated. Saying a word that ends with /ts/, such as /kæts/ or /lɛts/ might be useful.

Instructions for Production of the /ɝ/

1. Instruct the client to growl like a tiger (*grrr*), crow like a rooster (*r-rr-rr*) or sound like a race car (*rrr*).
2. Instruct the client to lower the jaw, say /l/, and push the tongue back until [ɝ] is produced. One can also move from [n] to [nɝ] or [d] to [dɝ].
3. Instruct the client to produce /l/. Then, using a tongue blade, gently push the tip of the tongue back until the depressor can be inserted between the tongue tip and teeth ridge so that an /ɝ/ is produced.
4. Instruct the client to imitate a trilled tongue plus /ɝ/ sound with the tongue tip on the alveolar ridge. Stop the trill but continue producing /ɝ/.
5. Instruct the client to produce /a/ as in the word *father*. As he or she produces the [a], instruct him or her to raise the tongue tip and blade, arching the tongue toward the palate but not touching the palate.
6. Instruct the client to produce /i/ and then lift and retract the tongue tip to produce /ɝ/.
7. Instruct the client to place the tongue lightly between the incisors as in /θ/ and then retract the tip quickly into the /ɝ/. Instruct the client to keep the tip of the tongue near the alveolar ridge to avoid the intrusion of a vowel sound.
8. Instruct the client to say /z/ and to continue to do so while dropping the jaw and saying /ɝ/.
9. Instruct the client to position the tongue for /d/ and then retract it slightly, at the same time dropping the tongue tip and saying /ɝ/. Other clusters such as /tr/, /θr/, and /gr/ may also be used.
10. Spread the sides of the child's mouth with his or her finger, then ask him or her to produce a prolonged /n/ and then curl the tongue backward, continuing to make the sound.
11. Contrast pairs of words beginning with /w/ and /r/. This task may make the distinction between these two sounds more obvious for the client who substitutes /w/ for /r/. Practice word-pairs might include:

    wipe—ripe　*woo—rue*　*wing—ring*　*way—ray*　*wake—rake*
    wag—rag　　*wail—rail*　*woe—roe*　　*weep—reap*　*wed—red*

Instructions for Production of /l/

1. Instruct the client to produce /l/ with the mouth open in front of a mirror.
2. Instruct the client to position the tongue for /l/ and then lower it to produce /a/. Alternate these movements. The result should be [la], [la], [la]. This procedure can be varied by using /i/ and /u/ instead of /a/.
3. Instruct the client to imitate the clinician's singing of the nonsense syllables [leɪ], [li], [laɪ].
4. Using a lollipop, peanut butter, or tongue blade, touch the place on the client's alveolar ridge where the tongue tip makes contact to produce a correct /l/. Then tell the client to place the tongue at that point and say /l/.
5. Instruct the client to pretend that the tongue is one part of a bird's beak and the roof of the mouth is the other part of the beak. Tell him or her to put the tongue directly

behind the teeth and move it up and down quickly, as a bird's beak might move when it is chirping, and say /a/.

Instructions for Production of /f/ and /v/

1. Instruct the client to touch the lower lip with the upper front teeth and blow. The breath stream may be directed by placing a feather or strip of paper in front of his or her mouth while /f/ or /v/ is being produced.
2. Instruct the client to say [a], place the lower lip under the edge of the upper teeth, and blow the breath stream between the lip and teeth so that frication is audible.

Instructions for Production of /k/ and /g/

1. Press underneath the posterior portion of the child's chin and ask him or her to say [kʌ] in a whisper as the pressure is suddenly released.
2. Hold the tongue tip behind the lower teeth, using a tongue blade if necessary. Instruct the client to hump the back of the tongue and build up oral pressure. The tongue contact should be released quickly, thus releasing the pressure built up behind the constriction.
3. Instruct the client to imitate the clinician as the clinician pretends to shoot a gun, producing a lingua-fricative, as in [ka].
4. Instruct the client to alternate the raising of the back and front of the tongue in a rocking movement from [k] to [t].

Instructions for Production of /t/ and /d/

1. Instruct the client to press the tongue tip firmly against the upper dental ridge in front of a mirror. Then have him or her quickly lower the tongue; air pressure will be released, producing approximations of /t/ or /d/.
2. Instruct the client to make a /p/. Then ask him or her to place the tongue tip between the lips and again to try to say /p/. This gives the tactual sensation of a stop made with the tip of the tongue but is not the correct position for /t/ or /d/. Finally, instruct the client to make a similar sound with the tongue tip in contact with the upper lip only. Repeat with the tongue tip touching the alveolar ridge.

Activities for Facilitating Phonemic Awareness in School-Age Children

PHONEME IDENTITY

Teach the child to identify the initial sounds in words. Find pictures (with words written clearly underneath) that start with /s/. Prompt the child as necessary to articulate each word by "reading" the word under the picture. Ask the child to identify those words that begin with the sound /s/. Initially, introduce distracter items that have wide initial phonological and visual contrasts. An initial set of words might include *star, moon, step, box, Stan, Carl, stop, go, sty,* and *barn.*

After several experiences with the above, repeat the activity but remove the picture stimuli and focus the child's attention on the print. Place words written in large clear font in front of the child or on a computer screen and ask the child to find the words that start with /s/. A fun alternative is by putting the words on the floor (as below) and asking the child to jump onto the words that start with /s/. As the child read the words aloud, prompt for the correct articulation of the /s/ cluster.

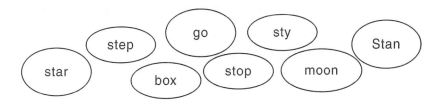

Use the same activity to teach any other initial sounds in words.

PHONEME SEGMENTATION

Teach the child that words can be segmented into phonemes. Use differing colored blocks to represent each sound in a word to help the child understand the concept of segmentation. Require the child to articulate each phoneme using colored blocks, for which one block represents each color.

Red	Blue	Green	Black
/s/	/t/	/ɛ/	/p/ = step

The child moves a colored block as he or she produces each sound in a word. This can be repeated for many different words, as in:

Stop:	s-t-o-p	(4 different colored blocks)
Star:	s-t-ar	(3 different colored blocks)
Stan:	s-t-a-n	(4 different colored blocks)
Sty:	s-t-y	(3 different colored blocks)

PHONEME MANIPULATION

Similar to the above activity, here the child is taught that the phonemes in words can be re-arranged to make new words. Colored blocks or cards featuring individual letters can serve this purpose. The child is asked to manipulate phonemes in words to form new words using blocks or cards; encourage the child to articulate each new word and to reflect on the sound change that is being made. Prompt the child as necessary to ensure success and gradually reduce the prompts. Here is an example:

THERAPIST: "If this word says "top" show me "stop.""

The child adds a new block to the beginning of the word and says "stop."

THERAPIST: "Now, then, turn "stop" into "tops.""

The child moves the initial block to the end of the word and says "tops."

SPELLING

Practice spelling target speech words by putting letters into boxes that represent the number of phonemes in the word. Begin by modeling the activity for the child and articulate the phonemes as you write each letter into a box for the child. Repeat the activity and encourage the child to write the letters in each box as she or he segments the word and articulates the phonemes. If the child is unable to write the letters easily, use letter cards or letter blocks to spell the word. Prompt as necessary to ensure success.

s	t	ar

References

Aase, D., C. Hovre, K. Krause, S. Schelfhout, J. Smith, and L. Carpenter, *Contextual Test of Articulation.* Eau Clair, WI: Thinking Publications, 2000.

Acevedo, M., "Spanish consonants among two groups of Head Start children." Paper presented at the convention of the American Speech-Language-Hearing Association, Atlanta, GA, 1991.

Acevedo, M. A., "Development of Spanish consonants in preschool children." *Journal of Childhood Communication Disorders, 15* (1993): 9–15.

Ackerman, J. L., A. L. Ackerman, and A. B. Ackerman, "Taurodont, pyramidal and fused molar roots associated with other anomalies in a kindred." *American Journal of Physical Anthropology, 38* (1973): 681–694.

Adams, M. J., B. R. Foorman, I. Lunberg, and T. Beeler, "Phonemic awareness in young children." Baltimore, MD: Brookes, 1998.

Adams, P. F., and V. Benson, "Current estimates from the National Health Interview Survey." Hyattsville, MD: National Center for Health Statistics. *Vital Health Statistics, 10,* 181 (1991).

Adams, S. G., "Rate and clarity of speech: An x-ray microbeam study." Ph.D. dissertation, University of Wisconsin-Madison, 1990.

Adams, S. G., G. Weismer, and R. D. Kent, "Speaking rate and speech movement velocity profiles." *Journal of Speech and Hearing Research, 36* (1993): 41–54.

Adler, S., "*Cultural Language Differences: Their Educational and Clinical-Professional Implications.*" Springfield, IL: Charles Thomas, 1984.

Allen, G., and S. Hawkins, "Phonological rhythm: definition and development." In G. Yeni-Komshian, J. Kavanagh, and C. Ferguson (Eds.), *Child Phonology*, Volume 1 (pp. 227–256). New York: Academic Press, 1980.

Allen, M. C., T. P. Nikolopoulos, and G. M. O'Donoghue, "Speech intelligibility in children after cochlear implantation." *The American Journal of Otology, 19* (1998): 742–746.

Amayreh, M., and A. Dyson, "The acquisition of Arabic consonants." *Journal of Speech, Language, and Hearing Research, 41* (1998): 642–653.

Amayreh, M., and A. Dyson, "Phonetic inventories of young Arabic-speaking children." *Clinical Linguistics and Phonetics, 14* (2000): 193–215.

American Speech-Language Hearing Association, "Social dialects: A position paper." *Asha* (1983): 23–27.

American Speech-Language Hearing Association, "Clinical management of communicatively handicapped minority language populations." *ASHA* (1985): 29–32.

American Speech-Language-Hearing Association, "Report of ad hoc committee on labial-lingual posturing function." *ASHA, 31* (1989): 92–94.

American Speech-Language-Hearing Association, "The role of the speech-language pathologist in management of oral myofunctional disorders." *ASHA, 33,* Suppl. 5 (1991): 7.

American Speech-Language Hearing Association, "Definitions of communication disorders and variations." *ASHA,* Suppl. 10 (1993): 40–41.

American Speech-Language-Hearing Association, "Roles and responsibilities of speech-language pathologists with respect to reading and writing in children and adolescents (position statement, executive summary of guidelines, technical report)." *ASHA,* Suppl 21 (2001): 17–27.

American Speech-Language Hearing Association, "Knowledge and skills needed by speech-language pathologists and audiologists to provide culturally and linguistically appropriate services." Rockville, MD: ASHA, 2004.

American Speech-Language-Hearing Association, "Background Information and Standards and Implementation for the Certificate of Clinical Competence in Speech-Language Pathology [Standards/Quality Indicators]." Available from www.asha.org/policy, 2005.

American Speech-Language-Hearing Association, "Childhood apraxia of speech [Position Statement]." Rockville, MD: ASHA, 2007a.

413

American Speech-Language-Hearing Association, "Childhood apraxia of speech [Technical Report]." Rockville, MD: ASHA, 2007b.

Anderson, R., "Onset clusters and the sonority sequencing principle in Spanish: A treatment efficacy study." Poster presented at the VIIIth International Clinical Phonetics and Linguistics Association Conference, Edinburgh, 2000.

Anderson, R. T., "Phonological acquisition in preschoolers learning a second language via immersion: A longitudinal study." *Clinical Linguistics and Phonetics, 18* (2004): 183–210.

Anderson, R., and B. Smith, "Phonological development of two-year-old monolingual Puerto Rican Spanish-speaking children." *Journal of Child Language, 14* (1987): 57–78.

Anthony, A., D. Bogle, T. T. S. Ingram, and M. W. McIsaac, *The Edinburgh Articulation Test.* Edinburgh, UK: E. and S. Livingstone, 1971.

Anthony, J., and C. Lonigan," The nature of phonological awareness: Converging evidence from four studies of preschool and early grade school children." *Journal of Educational Psychology 96* (2004): 43–55.

Anthony, J. L., C. J. Lonigan, K. Driscoll, B. M. Phillips, and S. R. Burgess, "Phonological sensitivity: A quasi-parallel progression of word structure units and cognitive operations." *Reading Research Quarterly 38* (2003): 470–487.

Arlt, P. B., and M. T. Goodban, "A comparative study of articulation acquisition as based on a study of 240 normals, aged three to six." *Language, Speech, and Hearing Services in Schools, 7* (1976): 173–180.

Arndt, W., M. Elbert, and R. Shelton, "Standardization of a test of oral stereognosis." In J. Bosman (Ed.), *Second Symposium on Oral Sensation and Perception.* Springfield, IL: Charles Thomas, 1970.

Arnst, D., and D. Fucci, "Vibrotactile sensitivity of the tongue in hearing impaired subjects." *Journal of Auditory Research, 15* (1975): 115–118.

Aslin, R. N., D. B. Pisoni, and P. W. Jusczyk, "Auditory development and speech perception in infancy." In M. M. Haith and J. J. Campos (Eds.), *Infancy and Psychobiology* (pp. 573–687). New York: Wiley, 1983.

August, D., M. Calderón, and M. Carlo, "Transfer of skills from Spanish to English: A study of young learners." Washington, DC: Center for Applied Linguistics, 2002.

Augustyn, M., and B. Zuckerman, "From mother's mouth to infant's brain." *Archives of Disease in Childhood: Fetal and Neonatal Edition, 92, 2* (2007): F82.

Aungst, L., and J. Frick, "Auditory discrimination ability and consistency of articulation of /r/." *Journal of Speech and Hearing Disorders, 29* (1964): 76–85.

Backus, O., "Speech rehabilitation following excision of tip of the tongue." *American Journal of the Disabled Child, 60* (1940): 368–370.

Badian, N. A., "Do preschool orthographic skills contribute to prediction of reading?" In N. A. Badian (Ed.), *Prediction and Prevention of Reading Failure* (pp. 31–56). Timonium, MD: York, 2000.

Bailey, G., and E. Thomas, "Some aspects of African-American Vernacular English phonology." In S. Mufwene, J. Rickford, G. Bailey, and J. Baugh (Eds.), *African American English: History and Use* (pp. 85–109). London: Routledge, 1998.

Bailey, S., "Normative data for Spanish articulatory skills of Mexican children between the ages of six and seven." Unpublished master's thesis, San Diego State University, San Diego, CA, 1982.

Bain, B., and L. Olswang, "Examining readiness for learning two-word utterances by children with specific expressive language impairment: Dynamic assessment validation." *American Journal of Speech-Language Pathology, 4, 1* (1995): 81–91.

Baker, E., "Changing nail to snail: A treatment efficacy study of phonological impairment in children." Unpublished doctoral thesis, Sydney, Australia: The University of Sydney, 2000.

Baker, E., K. Croot, S. McLeod, and R. Paul, "Psycholinguistic models of speech development and their application to clinical practice." *Journal of Speech, Language, and Hearing Research, 44* (2001): 685–702.

Ball, E., "Assessing phoneme awareness." *Language, Speech, and Hearing Services in Schools, 24* (1993): 130–139.

Ball, E., and B. Blachman, "Phoneme segmentation training: Effect on reading readiness." *Annals of Dyslexia, 38* (1988): 208–225.

Ball, E., and B. Blachman, "Does phoneme awareness training in kindergarten make a difference in early word recognition and developmental spelling?" *Reading Research Quarterly, 26* (1991): 49–66.

Ball, L., "Communication characteristics of children with developmental apraxia of speech." Unpublished Doctoral Dissertation, University of Nebraska–Lincoln, 1999.

Ball, L., D. Beukelman, and J. Bernthal, "Profiling communication characteristics of children with developmental apraxia of speech." *Journal of Medical Speech-Language Pathology, 10* (2002): 221–229.

Ball, M. J., and F. Gibbon (Eds.), *Vowel Disorders.* Woburn, MA: Butterworth Heineman, 2001.

Ball, M. J., and R. D. Kent (Eds.), *The New Phonologies: Developments in Clinical Linguistics.* San Diego, CA: Singular Publishing, 1997.

Ball, M. J., and N. Müller, "Sonority as an explanation in clinical phonology." Paper presented at the 9th meeting of the International Clinical Phonetics and Linguistics Association, 2002.

Bankson, N. W., and J. E. Bernthal, *Quick Screen of Phonology.* Chicago: Riverside Press, 1990a.

Bankson, N. W., and J. E. Bernthal, *Bankson-Bernthal Test of Phonology.* San Antonio, TX: Special Press, 1990b.

Bankson, N. W., and M. Byrne, "The relationship between missing teeth and selected consonant sounds." *Journal of Speech and Hearing Disorders, 24* (1962): 341–348.

Bankson, N. W., and M. C. Byrne, "The effect of a timed correct sound production task on carryover." *Journal of Speech and Hearing Research, 15* (1972): 160–168.

Barkovich, A. J., B. O Kjos, D. E. Jackson Jr., and D. Norman, "Normal maturation of the neonatal and infant brain: MR imaging at 1.5 T." *Radiology, 166* (1988): 173–180.

Barlow, J. A., "Variability and phonological knowledge." In T. W. Powell (Ed.), *Pathologies of Speech and Language: Contributions of Clinical Phonetics and Linguistics* (pp. 125–133) New Orleans, LA: International Clinical Phonetics and Linguistics Association, 1996.

Barlow, J. A., "The structure of /s/-sequences: Evidence from a disordered system." *Journal of Child Language, 28* (2001): 291–324.

Barlow, J. A., and J. A. Gierut, "Optimality theory in phonological acquisition." *Journal of Speech, Language, and Hearing Research, 42* (1999): 1482–1498.

Barton, D., "The role of perception in the acquisition of phonology." Ph.D. Dissertation, London, University of London, 1976.

Bashir, A., F. Grahamjones, and R. Bostwick, "A touch-cue method of therapy for developmental apraxia." *Seminars in Speech and Language, 5* (1984): 127–137.

Bates, E., P. S. Dale, and D. Thal, "Individual differences and their implications for theories of language development." In P. Fletcher and B. MacWhinney (Eds.), *The Handbook of Child Language* (pp. 96–151) Oxford, UK: Blackwell, 1995.

Bauman-Waengler, J., *Articulatory and phonological impairments: A clinical focus* (2nd ed.). Boston: Allyn and Bacon, 2004.

Bauman-Waengler, J., *Articulatory and phonological impairments: A clinical focus* (3rd ed.). Boston: Allyn and Bacon, 2008.

Behne, D., "Acoustic effects of focus and sentence position on stress in English and French." Ph.D. dissertation, University of Wisconsin–Madison, 1989.

Bennett, B., C. Bennett, and C. James, "Phonological development from concept to classroom." Paper presented at the Speech-Language-Hearing Association of Virginia Annual Conference, Roanoke, VA, 1996.

Berg, T., "Sound change in child language: A study of inter-word variation." *Language and Speech, 38* (1995): 331–363.

Bernhardt, B., "Application of nonlinear phonology to intervention with six phonologically disordered children." Unpublished Ph.D. thesis, University of British Columbia, Vancouver, B.C., Canada, 1990.

Bernhardt, B., "Developmental implications of nonlinear phonological theory." *Clinical Linguistics and Phonetics, 6* (1992a): 259–281.

Bernhardt, B., "The application of nonlinear phonological theory to intervention with one phonologically disordered child." *Clinical Linguistics and Phonetics, 6* (1992b): 283–316.

Bernhardt, B. H., and J. Stemberger, *Handbook of Phonological Development from the Perspective of Constraint-Based Nonlinear Phonology.* San Diego, CA: Academic Press, 1998.

Bernhardt, B. H., and J. P. Stemberger, *Workbook in Nonlinear Phonology for Clinical Application.* Austin, TX: ProEd, 2000.

Bernhardt, B. H., J. P. Stemberger, and E. Major, "General and nonlinear phonological intervention perspectives for a child with a resistant phonological impairment." *Advances in Speech-Language Pathology, 8,* 3 (2006): 190–206.

Bernhardt, B. H., and C. Stoel-Gammon, "Nonlinear phonology: Introduction and clinical application." *Journal of Speech and Hearing Research, 37* (1994): 123–143.

Bernstein, M., "The relation of speech defects and malocclusion." *American Journal of Orthodontia, 40* (1954): 149–150.

Bernstein-Ratner, N., "Interactive influences on phonological behaviour: A case study." *Journal of Child Language, 20* (1993): 191–197.

Bernthal, J. E., and N. W. Bankson (Eds.), *Articulation and Phonological Disorders* (4th ed.). Boston: Allyn and Bacon, 1998.

Bernthal, J. E., and D. R. Beukelman, "Intraoral air pressures during the production of *p* and *b* by children, youths, and adults." *Journal of Speech and Hearing Research, 21* (1978): 361–371.

Bertoncini, J., and J. Mehler, "Syllables as units in infant speech perception." *Infant Behavior and Development, 4* (1981): 247–260.

Bichotte, M., B. Dunn, L. Gonzalez, J. Orpi, and C. Nye, "Assessing phonological performance of bilingual school-age Puerto Rican children." Paper presented at the annual convention of the American Speech-Language-Hearing Association, Anaheim, CA, 1993.

Biever, A., and D. Kelsall. "Impact of bilateral pediatric cochlear implantation on speech perception abilities in quiet and noise." Paper presented at the 11th International Conference on Cochlear Implants in Children, Charlotte, NC, 2007.

Bird, A., and A. Higgins. *Minimal Pair Cards*. Austin, TX: Pro-Ed, 1990.

Bird, J., and D. Bishop, "Perception and awareness of phonemes in phonologically impaired children." *European Journal of Disorders of Communication, 27* (1992): 289–311.

Bird, J., D. Bishop, and N. H. Freeman, "Phonological awareness and literacy development in children with excessive phonological impairments." *Journal of Speech and Hearing Research, 38* (1995): 446–462.

Bishop, D., and C. Adams, "A prospective study of the relationship between specific language impairment, phonological disorders and reading retardation." *Journal of Child Psychology and Psychiatry, 31* (1990): 1027–1050.

Bishop, M., R. Ringel, and H. House, "Orosensory perception, speech production and deafness." *Journal of Speech and Hearing Research, 16* (1973): 257–266.

Blache, S. E., "A distinctive feature approach." In N. Creaghead, P. Newman, and W. Secord (Eds.), *Assessment and Remediation of Articulatory and Phonological Disorders* (2nd ed.). Columbus, OH: Merrill, 1989.

Blachman, B., E. Ball, R. Black, and D. Tangel, *Road to the Code: A Phonological Awareness Program for Young Children*. Baltimore, MD: Brookes, 2000.

Blakely, R., *Screening Test for Developmental Apraxia of Speech* (2nd ed.). Austin, TX: Pro-Ed, 2001.

Bleile, K., "Consonant ordering in Down's Syndrome," *Journal of Communicative Disorders, 15* (1982): 275–285.

Bleile, K. M., "Individual differences." In K. M. Bleile (Ed.), *Child Phonology: A Book of Exercises for Students* (pp. 57–71). San Diego, CA: Singular Publishing, 1991.

Bleile, K. M., *Manual of Articulation and Phonological Disorders*. San Diego, CA: Singular Publishing, 1995.

Bleile, K. M., *Articulation and Phonological Disorders: A Book of Exercises* (2nd ed.). San Diego, CA: Singular Publishing, 1996.

Bleile, K. M., *Manual of Articulation and Phonological Disorders: Infancy Through Adulthood* (2nd ed.). Clifton Park, NY: Thomson Delmar Learning, 2004.

Bleile, K. M., *The Late Eight*. San Diego, CA: Plural Publishing, 2006.

Bleile, K. M., "Neurological foundations of speech acquisition." In S. McLeod (Ed.), *The International Guide to Speech Acquisition* (pp. 14–18). Clifton Park, NY: Thomson Delmar Learning, 2007.

Bleile, K. M., and H. Wallach, "A sociolinguistic investigation of the speech of African-American preschoolers," *American Journal of Speech-Language Pathology, 1* (1992): 44–52.

Bloch, R., and L. Goodstein, "Functional speech disorders and personality: A decade of research," *Journal of Speech and Hearing Disorders, 36* (1971): 295–314.

Bloomer, H., and A. Hawk, "Speech considerations: Speech disorders associated with ablative surgery of the face, mouth and pharynx—Ablative approaches to learning." In ASHA Report #8: Orofacial Anomalies. Washington, DC: ASHA, 1973.

Bock, J. K., "Toward a cognitive psychology of syntax: Information processing contributions to sentence formulation." *Psychological Review, 89* (1982): 1–47.

Bonvillian, J. D., V. P. Raeburn, and E. A. Horan, "Talking to children: The effects of rate, intonation, and length on children's sentence imitation." *Journal of Child Language, 6* (1979): 459–467.

Bordon, G., "Consideration of motor-sensory targets and a problem of perception." In H. Winitz (Ed.), *Treating Articulation Disorders: For Clinicians by Clinicians*. Austin, TX: Pro-Ed, 1984.

Bosley, E., *Techniques for Articulatory Disorders*. Springfield, IL: Charles Thomas, 1981.

Bowen, C., personal communication, 2002.

Bowen, C., and L. Cupples, and children together (PACT), "A collaborative approach to phonological therapy." *International Journal of Language and Communication Disorders, 34* (1999): 35–55.

Bradford, A., B. Murdoch, E. Thompson, and P. Stokes. "Lip and tongue function in children with developmental speech disorders: A preliminary investigation." *Clinical Linguistics and Phonetics, 11* (1997): 363–387.

Bradley, D., "A systematic multiple-phoneme approach to articulation treatment." In P. Newman, N. Creaghead, and W. Secord (Eds.), *Assessment and Remediation of Articulatory and Phonological Disorders* (pp. 315–335). Columbus, OH: Merrill, 1985.

Bradley, L., and P. E. Bryant, "Categorizing sounds and learning to read—A causal connection." *Nature, 301* (1983): 419–421.

Brady, S., A. Fowler, B. Stone, and N. Winbury, "Training phonological awareness: A study with inner-city kindergarten children." *Annals of Dyslexia, 44* (1994): 26–59.

Braine, M. D. S., *On What Might Constitute Learnable Phonology.* San Diego, CA: College Hill, 1979.

Branigan, G., "Syllabic structure and the acquisition of consonants: The great conspiracy in word formation." *Journal of Psycholinguistic Research, 5* (1976): 117–133.

Branigan, G., "Some reasons why successive single word utterances are not." *Journal of Child Language, 6* (1979): 411–421.

Bressmann, T., R. Sader, T. L. Whitehill, and N. Samman, "Consonant intelligibility and tongue mobility in patients with partial glossectomy." *Journal of Oral and Maxillofacial Surgery, 62* (2004): 298–303.

Broomfield, J., and B. Dodd, "The nature of referred subtypes of primary speech disability." *Child Language Teaching and Therapy, 20* (2004): 135–151.

Bryan, A., and D. Howard, "Frozen phonology thawed: The analysis and remediation of a developmental disorder of real word phonology." *European Journal of Disorders of Communication, 27* (1992): 343–365.

Bryant, P., M. MacLean, and L. Bradley, "Rhyme, language, and children's reading." *Applied Psycholinguistics, 11* (1990): 237–252.

Bryant, T., S. Velleman, L. Abdualkarim, and H. Seymour, "A sonority account of consonant cluster reduction in AAE." Paper presented at the Child Phonology Conference, Boston, 2001.

Burgess, S. R., and C. J. Lonigan, "Bidirectional relations of phonological sensitivity and prereading abilities: Evidence from a preschool sample." *Journal of Experimental Child Psychology, 70* (1998): 117–141.

Burt, L., A. Holm, and B. Dodd, "Phonological awareness skills of 4-year-old British children: An assessment and developmental data." *International Journal of Language and Communication Disorders, 34*, 3 (1999): 311–335.

Butterfield, E., and G. Cairns, "Discussion-summary of infant reception research." In R. Schiefulbusch and L. Lloyd (Eds.), *Language Perspectives: Acquisition, Retardation and Intervention.* Baltimore, MD: University Park Press, 1974.

Byrne, B., and R. Fielding-Barnsley, "Evaluation of a program to teach phonemic awareness to young children." *Journal of Educational Psychology, 83* (1991): 451–455.

Byrne, B., and R. Fielding-Barnsley, "Evaluation of a program to teach phonemic awareness to young children: A 1-year follow-up." *Journal of Educational Psychology, 85* (1993): 104–111.

Byrne, B., and R. Fielding-Barnsley, "Evaluation of a program to teach phonemic awareness to young children: A 2- and 3-year follow-up and a new preschool trial." *Journal of Educational Psychology, 87* (1995): 488–503.

Bzoch, K. R., *Communicative Disorders Related to Cleft Lip and Palate* (5th ed.). Austin, TX: Pro-Ed, 2004.

Calfee, R. C., P. Lindamood, and C. Lindamood, "Acoustic-phonetic skills and reading—Kindergarten through twelfth grade." *Journal of Educational Psychology, 64* (1973): 293–298.

Calvert, D., "Articulation and hearing impairments." In L. Lass, J. Northern, D. Yoder, and L. McReynolds (Eds.), *Speech, Language and Hearing,* Volume 2. Philadelphia: Saunders, 1982.

Camarata, S., "Final consonant repetition: A linguistic perspective." *Journal of Speech and Hearing Disorders, 54* (1989): 159–162.

Camarata, S., and J. Gandour, "Rule invention in the acquisition of morphology by a language-impaired child." *Journal of Speech and Hearing Disorders, 50* (1985): 40–45.

Camarata, S., and R. Schwartz, "Production of object words and action words: Evidence for a relationship between phonology and semantics." *Journal of Speech and Hearing Research, 26* (1985): 50–53.

Campbell, T. F., C. A. Dollaghan, H. E. Rockette, J. L. Paradise, H. M. Feldman, L. D. Shriberg, et al.,

"Risk factors for speech delay of unknown origin in 3-year-old children." *Child Development, 74* (2003): 346–357.

Canning, B., and M. Rose, "Clinical measurements of the speech, tongue and lip movements in British children with normal speech." *British Journal of Disorders of Communication, 9* (1974): 45–50.

Canoy, D., J. Pekkanen, P. Elliott, A. Pouta, J. Laitinen, A.-L. Hartikainen, P. Zitting, S. Patel, M. P. Little, and M.-R. Jarvelin, "Early growth and adult respiratory function in men and women followed from the fetal period to adulthood." *Thorax, 62*, 5 (2007): 396–402.

Carrell, J., and K. Pendergast, "An experimental study of the possible relation between errors of speech and spelling." *Journal of Speech and Hearing Disorders, 19* (1954): 327–334.

Carrier, J. K., "A program of articulation therapy administered by mothers." *Journal of Speech and Hearing Disorders, 33* (1970): 344–353.

Carroll, J. M., M. J. Snowling, C. Hulme, and J. Stevenson, "The development of phonological awareness in preschool children." *Developmental Psychology, 39* (2003): 913–923.

Carter, E., and M. Buck, "Prognostic testing for functional articulation disorders among children in the first grade." *Journal of Speech and Hearing Disorders, 23* (1958): 124–133.

Catts, H. W., "Speech, production/phonological deficits in reading-disordered children." *Learning Disabilities, 19* (1986): 504–508.

Catts, H. W., "Facilitating phonological awareness: Role of speech-language pathologists." *Language, Speech, and Hearing Services in Schools, 22* (1991): 196–203.

Catts, H. W., "The relationship between speech-language impairments and reading disabilities." *Journal of Speech and Hearing Research, 36* (1993): 948–958.

Catts, H. W., M. E. Fey, J. B. Tomblin, and X. Y. Zhang, "A longitudinal investigation of reading outcomes in children with language impairments." *Journal of Speech Language and Hearing Research, 45* (2002): 1142–1157.

Catts, H. W., M. E. Fey, X. Zhang, and J. B. Tomblin, "Estimating the risk of future reading difficulties in kindergarten children: A research-based model and its clinical implementation." *Language, Speech, and Hearing Services in Schools, 32* (2001): 38–50.

Catts, H. W., and T. Olsen, *Sounds Abound: Listening, Rhyming, and Reading*. East Moline, IL: Linguisystems, 1993.

Cavagna, G. A., and R. Margaria, "Airflow rates and efficiency changes during phonation: Sound production in man." *Annals of the New York Academy of Sciences, 155* (1968): 152–164.

Chaney, C., "Language development, metalinguistic skills, and print awareness in 3-year-old children." *Applied Psycholinguistics, 13* (1992): 485–514.

Chaney, C., and P. Menyuk, "Production and identification of /w, l, r/ in normal and articulation-impaired children." Paper presented at the convention of the American Speech and Hearing Association, Washington, DC, 1975.

Chatterji, M. "Reading achievement gaps, correlates, and moderators of early reading achievement: Evidence from the Early Childhood Longitudinal Study (ECLS) kindergarten to first grade sample." *Journal of Educational Psychology 98* (2006): 489–507.

Cheng, H. Y., B. E. Murdoch, and J. V. Goozee, "Temporal features of articulation from childhood to adolescence: An electropalatographic investigation." *Clinical Linguistics and Phonetics, 21*, 6 (2007): 481–499.

Cheng, H. Y., B. E. Murdoch, J. V. Goozee, and D. Scott, "Electropalatographic assessment of tongue-to-palate contact patterns and variability in children, adolescents, and adults." *Journal of Speech, Language, and Hearing Research, 50*, 2 (2007a): 375–392.

Cheng, H. Y., B. E. Murdoch, J. V. Goozee, and D. Scott, "Physiologic development of tongue-jaw coordination from childhood to adulthood." *Journal of Speech, Language, and Hearing Research, 50*, 2 (2007b): 352–360.

Cheng, L. R. L. (1987). *Assessing Asian Language Performance: Guidelines for Evaluating Limited-English-Proficient Students*. Rockville, MD: Aspen.

Cheng, L. R. L., "Asian-American cultures." In D. Battle (Ed.), *Communication Disorders in Multicultural Populations* (pp. 38–77). Boston: Andover Medical Publishers, 1993.

Chervela, N., "Medial consonant cluster acquisition by Telugu children." *Journal of Child Language, 8* (1981): 63–73.

Cheung, P., and Abberton, E., "Patterns of phonological disability in Cantonese-speaking children in Hong Kong." *International Journal of Language and Communication Disorders, 35* (2000): 451–473.

Chiat, S., "The relation between prosodic structure, syllabification and segmental realization: Evidence from a child with fricative stopping." *Clinical Linguistics and Phonetics, 3* (1989): 223–242.

Chiat, S., "From lexical access to lexical output: What is the problem for children with impaired phonology?" In M. Yavaş (Ed.), *First and Second Language Pathology* (pp. 107–133). San Diego, CA: Singular Publishing, 1994.

Chin, S. B., "The role of the sonority hierarchy in delayed phonological systems." In T. Powell (Ed.), *Pathologies of Speech and Language: Contributions of Clinical Phonetics and Linguistics* (pp. 109–117). New Orleans, LA: International Clinical Phonetics and Linguistics Association, 1996.

Chin, S. B., and D. A. Dinnsen, "Feature geometry in disordered phonologies." *Clinical Linguistics and Phonetics, 5* (1991): 329–337.

Chin, S. B., and D. B. Pisoni, "A phonological system at 2 years after cochlear implantation." *Clinical Linguistics and Phonetics, 14* (2000): 53–73.

Ching, T. Y. C., P. Incerti, M. Hill, and E. van Wanrooy. "An overview of binaural advantages for children and adults who use binaural/bimodal hearing devices." *Audiology and Neurotology, 11*, Supplement 1 (2006): 6–11.

Chirlian, N. S., and C. F. Sharpley, "Children's articulation development: Some regional differences." *Australian Journal of Human Communication Disorders, 10* (1982): 23–30.

Chomsky, N., and M. Hallé, *The Sound Pattern of English*. New York: Harper & Row, 1968.

Christian, D., W. Wolfram, and N. Nube, *Variation and Change in Geographically Isolated Communities: Appalachian English and Ozark English*. Tuscaloosa, AL: The University of Alabama Press, 1988.

Christensen, C. A., "Onset, rhymes, and phonemes in learning to read." *Scientific Studies of Reading, 1* (1997): 341–358.

Christensen, C. A., "Preschool phonological awareness and success in reading." In N. A. Badian (Ed.), *Prediction and Prevention of Reading Failure* (pp. 153–178). Timonium, MD: York, 2000.

Chumpelik, D., "The prompt system of therapy: Theoretical framework and applications for developmental apraxia of speech." *Seminars in Speech and Language, 5* (1984): 139–155.

Clark, R. "Maturation and speech development." *Logos, 2* (1959): 49–54.

Clark-Klein, S., and B. Hodson, "A phonologically based analysis of misspellings by third graders with

disordered-phonology histories." *Journal of Speech and Hearing Research, 38* (1995): 839–849.

Clements, G. N., "The role of the sonority cycle in core syllabification." In J. Kingston and M. Beckman (Eds.), *Papers in Laboratory Phonology 1: Between the Grammar and Physics of Speech.* (pp. 283–333). Cambridge: Cambridge University Press, 1990.

Clements, G. N., and S. J. Keyser, *CV Phonology.* Cambridge, MA: M.I.T. Press, 1983.

Cohen, A., R. Collier, and J. t'Hart, "Declination: Construct or intrinsic feature of speech pitch?" *Phonetica, 39* (1982): 254–273.

Cole, P., and Taylor, O., "Performance of working class African-American children on three tests of articulation. " *Language, Speech, and Hearing Services in Schools, 21* (1990): 171–176.

Cooper, R., "The method of meaningful minimal contrasts." In P. Newman, N. Creaghead, and W. Secord (Eds.), *Assessment and Remediation of Articulatory and Phonological Disorders* (pp. 369–382). Columbus, OH: Merrill, 1985.

Cooper, R. P., and R. N. Aslin, "Preference for infant-directed speech in the first month after birth." *Child Development, 61* (1990): 1584–1595.

Coplan, J., and J. R. Gleason, "Unclear speech: Recognition and significance of unintelligible speech in preschool children." *Pediatrics, 82* (1988): 447–452.

Costello, J., and C. Bosler, "Generalization and articulation instruction." *Journal of Speech and Hearing Disorders, 41* (1976): 359–373.

Costello, J., and J. Onstein, "The modification of multiple articulation errors based on distinctive feature theory." *Journal of Speech and Hearing Disorders, 41* (1976): 199–215.

Courchesne, E., H. J. Chisum, J. Townsend, A. Cowles, J. Covington, B. Egaas, M. Harwood, S. Hinds, and G. A. Press, "Normal brain development and aging: Quantitative analysis at in vivo MR imaging in healthy volunteers." *Radiology, 216* (2000): 672–682.

Crosbie, S., A. Holm, and B. Dodd, "Intervention for children with severe speech disorder: A comparison of two approaches." *International Journal of Language and Communication Disorders, 40* (2005): 467–491.

Crosbie, S., C. Pine, A. Holm, and B. Dodd, "Treating Jarrod: A core vocabulary approach." *Advances in Speech-Language Pathology, 8*, 3 (2006): 316–321.

Crowe-Hall, B. J., "Attitudes of fourth and sixth graders toward peers with mild articulation disorders."

Language, Speech, and Hearing Services in Schools, 22 (1991): 334–340.

Crystal, D., *Prosodic Systems and Intonation in English.* Cambridge: Cambridge University Press, 1969.

Crystal, D., "Non-segmental phonology in language acquisition: A review of the issues." *Lingua, 32* (1973): 145.

Crystal, D., *Profiling Linguistic Disability.* London: Edward Arnold, 1982.

Crystal, D., "Prosodic development." In P. J. Fletcher and M. Garman (Eds.), *Studies in First Language Development* (pp. 174–197) New York: Cambridge University Press, 1986.

Crystal, D., "Towards a 'bucket' theory of language disability: Taking account of interaction between linguistic levels." *Clinical Linguistics and Phonetics, 1* (1987): 7–22.

Crystal, D. *The Cambridge Encyclopedia of Language* (2nd ed.) Cambridge: Cambridge University Press, 1997.

Cunningham, I., *A Syntactic Analysis of Sea Island Creole.* Tuscaloosa: The University of Alabama Press, 1992.

Curtis, J., and J. Hardy, "A phonetic study of misarticulations of /r/." *Journal of Speech and Hearing Research, 2* (1959): 224–257.

Daniloff, R. G., and K. L. Moll, "Coarticulation of lip rounding." *Journal of Speech and Hearing Research, 11* (1968): 707–721.

Darley, F., A. Aronson, and J. Brown, *Motor Speech Disorders.* Philadelphia: Saunders, 1975.

Davis, B. L., "Goal and target selection for developmental speech disorders." In K. E. Pollock and A. G. Kamhi (Eds.), *Phonological Disorders in Children: Clinical Decision Making in Assessment and Intervention* (pp. 89–100) Baltimore, MD: Brookes, 2005.

Davis, B. L., K. J. Jakielski, and T. P. Marquardt, "Developmental apraxia of speech: Determiners of differential diagnosis." *Clinical Linguistics and Phonetics, 12* (1998): 25–45.

Davis, B. L., and P. F. MacNeilage, "The articulatory basis of babbling." *Journal of Speech and Hearing Research, 38* (1995): 1199–1211.

Davis, E., "The development of linguistic skills in twins, singletons with siblings, and only children from age five to ten years." *Institute of Child Welfare Monograph Series 14.* Minneapolis: University of Minnesota Press, 1937.

Dawson, J. I., and P. J. Tattersall, *Structured Photographic Articulation Test–II.* DeKalb, IL: Janelle Publications, 2001.

Dawson, L., "A study of the development of the rate of articulation." *Elementary School Journal, 29* (1929): 610–615.

Dayton, N., and C. Schuele, "Effects of phonological awareness training on young children with specific language impairment." Paper presented at the annual convention of the American Speech-Language-Hearing Association, Boston, 1997.

DeCasper, A. J., and W. P. Fifer, "Of human bonding: Newborns prefer their mothers' voices." *Science, 208* (1980): 1174–1176.

DeCasper, A. J., J.-P. LeCanuet, M.-C. Busnel, C. Granier-Deferre, and R. Maugeais, "Fetal reactions to recurrent maternal speech." *Infant Behavior and Development, 17* (1994): 159–164.

De la Fuente, M. T., "The order of acquisition of Spanish consonant phonemes by monolingual Spanish speaking children between the ages of 2.0 and 6.5." Unpublished doctoral dissertation, Georgetown University, Washington, DC, 1985.

Dewey, G., *Relative Frequency of English Speech Sounds.* Cambridge, MA: Harvard University Press, 1923.

Diedrich, W. M., "Procedures for counting and charting a target phoneme." *Language, Speech, and Hearing Services in Schools, 2* (1971): 18–32.

Diedrich, W. M., "Stimulability and articulation disorders." In J. Locke (Ed.), *Assessing and Treating Phonological Disorders: Current Approaches. Seminars in Speech and Language, 4.* New York: Thieme-Stratton, 1983.

Diedrich, W. M., and J. Bangert, "Training and speech clinicians in recording and analysis of articulatory behavior." Washington, D.C.: U.S. Office of Education Grant No. OEG-0-70-1689 and OEG-0-71-1689, 1976.

Dinnsen, D. A., J. A. Barlow, and M. L. Morrisette, "Long-distance place assimilation with an interacting error pattern in phonological acquisition." *Clinical Linguistics and Phonetics, 11* (1997): 319–338.

Dinnsen, D. A., S. B. Chin, M. Elbert, and T. Powell, "Some constraints on functionally disordered phonologies: Phonetic inventories and phonotactics." *Journal of Speech and Hearing Research, 33* (1990): 28–37.

Dinnsen, D., and M. Elbert, "On the relationship between phonology and learning." In M. Elbert, D. Dinnsen, and G. Weismer (Eds.), *Phonological Theory and the Misarticulating Child, ASHA Monographs, 22.* Rockville, MD: ASHA, 1984.

Dodd, B., "Children's acquisition of phonology." In B. Dodd (Ed.), *Differential Diagnosis and Treatment of Children with Speech Disorder* (pp. 21–48) San Diego, CA: Singular Publishing, 1995a.

Dodd, B., "Procedures for classification of sub groups of speech disorder." In B. Dodd (Ed.), *Differential Diagnosis and Treatment of Children with Speech Disorder* (pp. 49–64) San Diego, CA: Singular Publishing, 1995b.

Dodd, B., *Differential Diagnosis and Treatment of Children with Speech Disorder* (2nd ed.). London: Whurr Publishers, 2005.

Dodd, B., and A. Bradford, "A comparison of three therapy methods for children with different types of developmental phonological disorder." *International Journal of Language and Communication Disorders, 35* (2000): 189–209.

Dodd, B., S. Crosbie, and A. Holm, *Core Vocabulary Therapy: An Intervention for Children with Inconsistent Speech Disorders.* Brisbane, Australia: Perinatal Research Centre, Royal Brisbane & Women's Hospital, University of Queensland, 2004.

Dodd, B., S. Crosbie, B. McIntosh, T. Teitzel, and A. Ozanne. *Pre-Reading Inventory of Phonological Awareness.* San Antonio, TX: Harcourt, 2003.

Dodd, B., and G. Gillon, "Exploring the relationship between phonological awareness, speech impairment, and literacy." *Advances in Speech-Language Pathology, 3* (2001): 139–147.

Dodd, B., A. Holm, S. Crosbie, and P. McCormack, "Differential diagnosis of phonological disorders." In B. Dodd (Ed.), *Differential Diagnosis and Treatment of Children with Speech Disorder* (2nd ed., p. 70). London: Whurr Publishers, 2005.

Dodd, B., A. Holm, Z. Hua, and S. Crosbie, "Phonological development: A normative study of British English-speaking children." *Clinical Linguistics and Phonetics, 17* (2003): 617–643.

Dodd, B., Z. Hua, S. Crosbie, A. Holm, and A. Ozanne, *Diagnostic Evaluation of Articulation and Phonology (DEAP).* London: Psychological Corporation, 2002.

Dodd, B., Z. Hua, S. Crosbie, A. Holm, and A. Ozanne. *Diagnostic Evaluation of Articulation and Phonology (DEAP).* San Antonio, TX: Harcourt Assessment, 2006.

Dodd, B., L. So., and W. Li, "Symptoms of disorder without impairment: The written and spoken errors of bilinguals." In B. Dodd, R. Campbell, and L. Worrall (Eds.), *Evaluating Theories of Language: Evidence From Disorder* (pp. 119–136). London: Whurr Publishers, 1996.

Donegan, P., "Normal vowel development." In M. J. Ball and F. E. Gibbon (Eds.), *Vowel Disorders* (pp. 1–35). Woburn, MA: Butterworth-Heinemann, 2002.

Dore, J., "Holophrases, speech acts and language universals." *Journal of Child Language, 2,* 1 (1975): 21–40.

Dowker, A. "Rhyme and Alliteration in Poems Elicited from Young Children." *Journal of Child Language 16* (1989): 181–202.

Drumwright, A., *The Denver Articulation Examination.* Denver: Ladoca Project and Publishing Foundation, 1971.

Dubois, E., and J. Bernthal, "A comparison of three methods for obtaining articulatory responses." *Journal of Speech and Hearing Disorders, 43* (1978): 295–305.

Dubois, S., and B. Horvath, "The English vernaculars of the Creoles of Louisiana." *Language Variation and Change, 15* (2003): 255–288.

Duffy, J. R. *Motor Speech Disorders. Substrates, Differential Diagnosis, and Management* (2nd ed.). St. Louis, MO: Elsevier Mosby, 2005.

Dunn, C., and L. Newton, "A comprehensive model for speech development in hearing-impaired children." *Topics in Language Disorders, 6* (1986): 25–46.

Dworkin, J., "Protrusive lingual force and lingual diadochokinetic rates: A comparative analysis between normal and lisping speakers." *Language, Speech, and Hearing Services in Schools, 9* (1978): 8–16.

Dworkin, J., and R. Culatta, "Tongue strength: Its relationship to tongue thrusting, open-bite, and articulatory proficiency." *Journal of Speech and Hearing Disorders, 45* (1980): 227–282.

Dworkin, J. P., and R. A. Culatta, "Oral structural and neuromuscular characteristics in children with normal and disordered articulation." *Journal of Speech and Hearing Disorders, 50* (1985): 150–156.

Dyson, A. T., "Development of velar consonants among normal two-year-olds." *Journal of Speech and Hearing Research, 29* (1986): 493–498.

Dyson, A. T., "Phonetic inventories of 2- and 3- year old children." *Journal of Speech and Hearing Disorders, 53* (1988): 89–93.

Dyson, A. T., and M. Amayreh, "Phonological errors and sound changes in Arabic-speaking children." *Clinical Linguistics and Phonetics, 14* (2000): 79–109.

Dyson, A. T., and E. P. Paden, "Some phonological acquisition strategies used by two-year-olds." *Journal of Childhood Communication Disorders, 7* (1983): 6–18.

Edwards, M. L., "Issues in phonological assessment." In J. Locke (Ed.), *Assessing and Treating Phonological Disorders: Current Approaches. Seminars in Speech and Language, 4*. New York: Thieme-Stratton, 1983.

Edwards, M. L., "Issues in phonological assessment." *Seminars in Speech and Language, 4* (1983): 351–374.

Edwards, M. L., "Phonological theories." In B. W. Hodson (Ed.), *Evaluating and Enhancing Children's Phonological Systems* (pp. 145–170). Greenville, SC: Thinking Publications, 2007.

Edwards, M. L., and L. D. Shriberg, *Phonology. Applications in Communicative Disorders.* San Diego, CA: College-Hill Press, 1983.

Eguchi, S., and I. J. Hirsh, "Development of speech sounds in children." *Acta Orolaryngologica, Supplement No. 257* (1969).

Ehri, L. C., S. R. Nunes, D. M. Willows, B. V. Schuster, Z. Yaghoub-Zadeh, and T. Shanahan, "Phonemic awareness instruction helps children learn to read: Evidence from the National Reading Panel's meta-analysis." *Reading Research Quarterly 36* (2001): 250–287.

Eilers, R. E., and D. K. Oller, "The role of speech discrimination in developmental sound substitutions." *Journal of Child Language, 3* (1976): 319–329.

Eilers, R. E., W. R. Wilson, and J. M. Moore, "Developmental changes in speech discrimination in infants." *Journal of Speech and Hearing Research, 20* (1977): 766–780.

Eimas, P., "Linguistic processing of speech by young infants." In R. Schiefelbusch and L. Lloyd (Eds.), *Language Perspectives: Acquisition, Retardation and Intervention* (pp. 55–73) Baltimore, MD: University Park Press, 1974a.

Eimas, P., "Auditory and linguistic units of processing of cues for place of articulation by infants." *Perception and Psychophysics, 16* (1974b): 341–347.

Eimas, P., E. Siqueland, P. Jusczyk, and J. Vigorito, "Speech perception in infants." *Science, 171* (1971): 303–306.

Elbers, L., and J. Ton, "Play pen monologues: The interplay of words and babbles in the first words period." *Journal of Child Language, 12* (1985): 551–565.

Elbert, M., "Dismissal criteria from therapy." Unpublished Manuscript, 1967.

Elbert, M., D. A. Dinnsen, P. Swartzlander, and S. B. Chin, "Generalization to conversational speech." *Journal of Speech and Hearing Disorders, 55* (1990): 694–699.

Elbert, M., and J. Gierut, *Handbook of Clinical Phonology: Approaches to Assessment and Treatment*. San Diego, CA: College-Hill Press, 1986.

Elbert, M., and L. V. McReynolds, "Transfer of /r/ across contexts." *Journal of Speech and Hearing Disorders, 40* (1975): 380–387.

Elbert, M., and L. V. McReynolds, "An experimental analysis of misarticulating children's generalization." *Journal of Speech and Hearing Research, 21* (1978): 136–149.

Elbert, M., T. W. Powell, and P. Swartzlander, "Toward a technology of generalization: How many exemplars are sufficient?" *Journal of Speech and Hearing Research, 34* (1991): 81–87.

Elbert, M., B. Rockman, and D. Saltzman, *Contrasts: The Use of Minimal Pairs in Articulation Training.* Austin, TX: Exceptional Resources, 1980.

Elbert, M., R. L. Shelton, and W. B. Arndt, "A task for education of articulation change." *Journal of Speech and Hearing Research, 10* (1967): 281–288.

Engel, D. C., and L. R. Groth, "Case studies of the effect on carry-over of reinforcing postarticulation responses based on feedback." *Language, Speech, and Hearing Services in Schools, 7* (1976): 93–101.

Eski, M., M. Nisanci, A. Aktas, and M. Sengezer, "Congenital double lip: Review of 5 cases." *British Journal of Oral and Maxillofacial Surgery, 45* (2007): 68–70.

Everhart, R., "The relationship between articulation and other developmental factors in children." *Journal of Speech and Hearing Disorders, 18* (1953): 332–338.

Everhart, R., "Paternal occupational classification and the maturation of articulation." *Speech Monographs, 23* (1956): 75–77.

Everhart, R., "Literature survey of growth and developmental factors in articulation maturation." *Journal of Speech and Hearing Disorders, 25* (1960): 59–69.

Fairbanks, G., and E. Green, "A study of minor organic deviations in 'functional' disorders of articulation; 2. Dimension and relationships of the lips." *Journal of Speech and Hearing Disorders, 15* (1950): 165–168.

Fairbanks, G., and M. Lintner, "A study of minor organic deviations in functional disorders of articulation."

Journal of Speech and Hearing Disorders, 16 (1951): 273–279.

Farquhar, M. S., "Prognostic value of imitative and auditory discrimination tests." *Journal of Speech and Hearing Disorders, 26* (1961): 342–347.

Fee, J., and D. Ingram, "Reproduction as a strategy of phonological development." *Journal of Child Language, 9* (1982): 41–54.

Fee, E. J., "Segments and syllables in early language acquisition." In J. Archibald (Ed.), *Phonological Acquisition and Phonological Theory* (pp. 43–61) Hillsdale, NJ: Erlbaum, 1995.

Felsenfeld, S., M. McGue, and P. A. Broen, "Familial aggregation of phonological disorders: Results from a 28-year follow-up." *Journal of Speech and Hearing Research, 38* (1995): 1091–1107.

Ferguson, C. A., "Learning to pronounce: The earliest stages of phonological development." In F. D. Minifie and L. L. Lloyd (Eds.), *Communicative and Cognitive Abilities: Early Behavioral Assessment* (pp. 273–297) Baltimore, MD: University Park Press, 1978.

Ferguson, C. A., and C. B. Farwell, "Words and sounds in early language acquisition." *Language, 51* (1975): 419–439.

Ferrier, L., and M. Davis, "A lexical approach to the remediation of final sound omission." *Journal of Speech and Hearing Disorders, 38* (1973): 126–130.

Fey, M. E., *Language Intervention with Young Children.* San Diego, CA: College Hill Press/Little Brown, 1986.

Fey, M. E., "Articulation and phonology: Inextricable constructs in speech pathology." *Language, Speech, and Hearing Services in Schools, 23* (1992): 225–232.

Fey, M. E., P. L. Cleave, A. I. Ravida, S. H. Long, A. E. Dejmal, and D. L. Easton, "Effects of grammar facilitation on the phonological performance of children with speech and language impairments." *Journal of Speech and Hearing Research, 37* (1994): 594–607.

Fey, M. E., and J. Gandour, "Rule discovery in phonological acquisition." *Journal of Child Language, 9* (1982): 71–81.

Field, T. M., R. Woodson, R. Greenberg, and D. Cohen, "Discrimination and imitation of facial expression by neonates." *Science, 218,* 4568 (1982): 179–181.

Fitch, W. T., and J. Giedd, "Morphology and development of the human vocal tract: A study using magnetic resonance imaging." *The Journal of the Acoustical Society of America, 106,* 3 (1999): 1511–1522.

Fitzsimons, R., "Developmental, psychosocial and educational factors in children with nonorganic articulation problems." *Child Development, 29* (1958): 481–489.

Flahive, L. K., and J. R. Lanza, *Phonological Processing.* East Moline, IL: LinguiSystems, 1998.

Fleming, K., and J. Hartman, "Establishing cultural validity of the computer analysis of phonological processes." *Florida Educational Research Council Bulletin, 22* (1989): 8–32.

Fletcher, S., "Time-by-count measurement of diadochokinetic syllable rate." *Journal of Speech and Hearing Research, 15* (1972): 763–780.

Fletcher, S., R. Casteel, and D. Bradley, "Tongue thrust swallow, speech articulation and age." *Journal of Speech and Hearing Disorders, 26* (1961): 201–208.

Fletcher, S., and J. Meldrum, "Lingual function and relative length of the lingual frenulum." *Journal of Speech and Hearing Research, 11* (1968): 382–399.

Flipsen, P., Jr., "Speaker-listener familiarity: Parents as judges of delayed speech intelligibility." *Journal of Communication Disorders, 28* (1995): 3–19.

Flipsen, P., Jr., "Longitudinal changes in articulation rate and phonetic phrase length in children with speech delay." *Journal of Speech, Language, and Hearing Research, 45,* 1 (2002a): 100–110.

Flipsen, P., Jr. "Causes and speech sound disorders. Why worry?" Paper presented at the Speech Pathology Australia National Conference, Alice Springs, Australia, 2002b.

Flipsen, P., Jr., "Syllables per word in typical and delayed speech acquisition." *Clinical Linguistics and Phonetics, 20,* 4 (2006a): 293–301.

Flipsen, P., Jr., "Measuring the intelligibility of conversational speech in children." *Clinical Linguistics and Phonetics, 20,* 4 (2006b): 303–312.

Flipsen, P., Jr. (2007). "Appalachian English speech acquisition." In S. McLeod (Ed.), *The international guide to speech acquisition* (pp. 161–168). Clifton Park, NY: Thomson Delmar Learning.

Flipsen, P., Jr., and Colvard, L. G., "Intelligibility of conversational speech produced by children with cochlear implants." *Journal of Communication Disorders, 39* (2006): 93–108.

Flipsen, P., Jr., J. B. Hammer, and K. M. Yost, "Measuring severity of involvement in speech delay: Segmental and whole-word measures." *American Journal of Speech-Language Pathology, 14* (2005): 298–312.

Flipsen, P., Jr., and R. G. Parker, "Phonological patterns in the speech of children with cochlear implants." *Journal of Communication Disorders*. Manuscript in press (2007).

Fluharty, N., *Fluharty Preschool Speech and Language Screening Test–Second Edition*. Austin, TX: Pro-Ed, 2000.

Flynn, P., and M. Byrne, "Relationship between reading and selected auditory abilities of third-grade children." *Journal of Speech and Hearing Research, 13* (1970): 731–740.

Forrest, K. "Are oral-motor exercises useful in the treatment of phonological/articulatory disorders?" *Seminars in Speech and Language, 23 (2002):* 15–25.

Foster, D., K. Riley, and F. Parker, "Some problems in the clinical applications of phonological theory." *Journal of Speech and Hearing Disorders, 50* (1985): 294–297.

Foy, J. G., and V. Mann, "Does strength of phonological representations predict phonological awareness?" *Applied Psycholinguistics, 22* (2001): 301–325.

French, A., "The systematic acquisition of word forms by a child during the first fifty word stage." *Journal of Child Language, 16* (1989): 69–90.

Fry, D., "Duration and intensity as physical correlates of linguistic stress." *Journal of the Acoustical Society of America, 27* (1955): 765–768.

Fucci, D., "Oral vibrotactile sensation: An evaluation of normal and defective speakers." *Journal of Speech and Hearing Research, 15* (1972): 179–184.

Fudala, J. B., and W. M. Reynolds, *Arizona Articulation Proficiency Scale* (2nd ed.). Los Angeles: Western Psychological Services, 1986.

Gable, T. O., A. W. Kummer, L. Lee, N. A. Creaghead, and L. J. Moore, "Premature loss of the maxillary incisors: Effect on speech production." *Journal of Dentistry for Children, 62* (1995): 173–179.

Gallagher, R., and T. Shriner, "Contextual variables related to inconsistent /s/ and /z/ production in the spontaneous speech of children." *Journal of Speech and Hearing Research, 18* (1975): 623–633.

Galvin, K., M. Mok, and R. Dowell, "Sequential bilateral implants for young children: Subjective outcomes, left versus right localization and speech detection results." Paper presented at the 11th International Conference on Cochlear Implants in Children, Charlotte, NC, 2007.

Gammon, S., P. Smith, R. Daniloff, and C. Kim, "Articulation and stress juncture production under oral anesthetization and masking." *Journal of Speech and Hearing Research, 14* (1971): 271–282.

Gandour, J., "The nondeviant nature of deviant phonological systems." *Journal of Communication Disorders, 14* (1981): 11–29.

Garrett, R., "A study of children's discrimination of phonetic variations of the /s/ phoneme." Ph.D. dissertation, Ohio University, 1969.

Geers, A. E., "Factors influencing spoken language outcomes in children following early cochlear implantation." *Advances in Otorhinolaryngology, 64* (2006): 50–65.

Gentry, J., "Developmental spelling and the speech-language pathologist." *National Student Speech-Language-Hearing Association, XX* (1988): 50–60.

Gerken, L., and K. McGregor, "An overview of prosody and its role in normal and disordered child language." *American Journal of Speech-Language Pathology, 7* (1998): 38–48.

Gierut, J., "Maximal opposition approach to phonological treatment." *Journal of Speech and Hearing Disorders, 54* (1989): 9–19.

Gierut, J. A., "Differential learning of phonological oppositions." *Journal of Speech and Hearing Research, 33* (1990): 540–549.

Gierut, J. A., "Homonymy in phonological changes." *Clinical Linguistics and Phonetics, 5* (1991): 119–137.

Gierut, J. A., "The conditions and courses of clinically-induced phonological changes." *Journal of Speech and Hearing Research, 35* (1992): 1049–1063.

Gierut, J. A., "Natural domains of cyclicity in phonological acquisition." *Clinical Linguistics and Phonetics, 12* (1998): 481–499.

Gierut, J. A., "Syllable onsets: Clusters and adjuncts in acquisition." *Journal of Speech, Language, and Hearing Research, 42* (1999): 708–726.

Gierut, J. A., "Complexity in phonological treatment: Clinical factors." *Language, Speech, and Hearing Services in Schools, 32* (2001): 229–241.

Gierut, J. A., and A. Champion, "Syllable onsets II: Three-element clusters in phonological treatment." *Journal of Speech, Language, and Hearing Research, 44* (2001): 886–904.

Gierut, J. A., M. Elbert, and D. A. Dinnsen, "A functional analysis of phonological knowledge and generalization learning in misarticulating children." *Journal of Speech and Hearing Research, 30* (1987): 462–479.

Gierut, J. A., M. L. Morrisette, M. T. Hughes, and S. Rowland, "Phonological treatment efficacy and developmental norms." *Language, Speech, and Hearing Services in Schools, 27* (1996): 215–230.

Gierut, J. A., and H. J. Neumann, "Teaching and learning /θ/: A nonconfound." *Clinical Linguistics and Phonetics, 6* (1992): 191–200.

Gildersleeve, C., B. Davis, and E. Stubbe, "When monolingual rules don't apply: Speech development in a bilingual environment." Paper presented at the annual convention of the American Speech-Language-Hearing Association, Seattle, WA, 1996.

Gildersleeve-Neumann, C., and B. Davis, "Learning English in a bilingual preschool environment: Change over time." Paper presented at the annual convention of the American Speech-Language-Hearing Association, San Antonio, TX, 1998.

Giles, S. B., "A study of articulatory characteristics of /l/ allophones in English." Ph.D. dissertation, University of Iowa, 1971.

Gillon, G. T., "The efficacy of phonological awareness intervention for children with spoken language impairment." *Language, Speech, and Hearing Services in Schools, 31* (2000a): 126–141.

Gillon, G. T., *The Gillon Phonological Awareness Training Programme* (2nd ed.). Christchurch, New Zealand: Canterprise, University of Canterbury. www.cmds.canterbury.ac.nz/people/gillon.shtml, 2000b.

Gillon, G. T., "Follow-up study investigating benefits of phonological awareness intervention for children with spoken language impairment." *International Journal of Language and Communication Disorders, 37* (2002c): 381–400.

Gillon, G. T., *Phonological Awareness: From Research to Practice.* New York: Guilford Press, 2004.

Gillon, G. T., "Facilitating phoneme awareness development in 3- and 4-year-old children with speech impairment." *Language Speech and Hearing Services in Schools, 36* (2005): 308–324.

Gillon, G. T., and B. Dodd, "Enhancing the phonological processing skills of children with specific reading disability." *European Journal of Disorders of Communication, 32* (1997): 67–90.

Gillon, G. T., and B. Dodd, "The effects of training phonological, semantic, and syntactic processing skills in spoken language on reading ability." *Language, Speech, and Hearing Services in Schools, 26* (1995): 58–68.

Gillon, G. T., and B. Dodd, "Understanding the relationship between speech-language impairment and literacy difficulties: The central role of phonology." In B. Dodd (Ed.), *Differential Diagnosis and Treatment of Children with Speech Disorder* (2nd ed., pp. 289–304). London: Whurr Publishers, 2005.

Gillon, G. T., and B. C. Moriarty, "Childhood apraxia of speech: Children at risk for persistent reading and spelling disorder." *Seminars in Speech and Language, 28* (2007): 48–57.

Gillon, G. T., and Schwarz, I. E. "Screening New Zealand children's spoken language skills for academic success." In L. Wilson and S. Hewat (Eds.), *Proceedings of the 2001 Speech Pathology Australia National Conference* (pp. 207–214). Melbourne: Speech Pathology Australia, 2001.

Glaspey, A., and C. Stoel-Gammon, "Dynamic assessment in phonological disorders." *Topics in Language Disorders, 25* (2005): 220–230.

Gold, T. "Speech production in hearing-impaired children." *Journal of Communication Disorders, 13* (1980): 397–418.

Goldman, R., and M. Fristoe, *Goldman-Fristoe Test of Articulation.* Circle Pines, MN: American Guidance Service, 1986, 2000.

Goldman, R., M. Fristoe, and R. Woodcock, *The Goldman-Fristoe-Woodcock Test of Auditory Discrimination.* Circle Pines, MN: American Guidance Service, 1970.

Goldsmith, J., "Autosegmental phonology." Ph.D. dissertation, Massachusetts Institute of Technology, 1976 (published by Garland Press, 1979).

Goldsmith, J. A., *Autosegmental and Metrical Phonology.* Oxford: Blackwell, 1990.

Goldstein, B., "The evidence of phonological processes of 3- and 4-year-old Spanish speakers." Unpublished master's thesis, Temple University, Philadelphia, PA, 1988.

Goldstein, B., "Spanish phonological development." In H. Kayser (Ed.), *Bilingual Speech-Language Pathology: An Hispanic focus* (pp. 17–38). San Diego, CA: Singular Publishing, 1995.

Goldstein, B., *Cultural and Linguistic Diversity Resource Guide for Speech-Language Pathology.* San Diego, CA: Singular Publishing, 2000.

Goldstein, B., "Assessing phonological skills in Hispanic/Latino children." *Seminars in Speech and Language, 22* (2001): 39–49.

Goldstein, B., "Phonological development and disorders in bilingual children." In B. Goldstein (Ed.), *Bilingual Language Development and Disorders in*

Spanish-English Speakers (pp. 257–286). Baltimore, MD: Brookes, 2004.

Goldstein, B., "Clinical implications of research on language development and disorders in bilingual children." *Topics in Language Disorders, 26* (2006): 318–334.

Goldstein, B., "Spanish speech acquisition." In S. McLeod (Ed.), *The International Guide to Speech Acquisition* (pp. 539–553). Clifton Park, NY: Thomson Delmar Learning, 2007a.

Goldstein, B., "Phonological skills in Puerto Rican- and Mexican-Spanish speaking children with phonological disorders." *Clinical Linguistics and Phonetics, 21* (2007b): 93–109.

Goldstein, B., "Speech acquisition across the world: Spanish Influenced English." In S. McLeod (Ed.), *The International Guide to Speech Acquisition* (pp. 345–356). Clifton Park, NY: Thomson Delmar Learning, 2007c.

Goldstein, B., and P. Cintron, "An investigation of phonological skills in Puerto Rican Spanish-speaking 2-year-olds." *Clinical Linguistics and Phonetics, 15* (2001): 343–361.

Goldstein, B., L. Fabiano, and P. Washington, "Phonological skills in predominantly English, predominantly Spanish, and Spanish-English bilingual children." *Language, Speech, and Hearing Services in Schools, 36* (2005): 201–218.

Goldstein, B., and A. Iglesias, "Phonological patterns in normally developing Spanish-speaking 3- and 4-year-olds of Puerto Rican descent. *Language, Speech, and Hearing Services in Schools, 27* (1996a): 82–90.

Goldstein, B., and A. Iglesias, "Phonological patterns in Puerto Rican Spanish-speaking children with phonological disorders." *Journal of Communication Disorders, 29* (1996b): 367–387.

Goldstein, B., and A. Iglesias, "Phonological patterns in bilingual (Spanish-English) children." Seminar presented at the 1999 Texas Research Symposium on Language Diversity, Austin, TX, 1999.

Goldstein, B., and A. Iglesias, "The effect of dialect on phonological analysis: Evidence from Spanish-speaking children." *American Journal of Speech-Language Pathology, 10* (2001): 394–406.

Goldstein, B., and K. Pollock, "Vowel errors in Spanish-speaking children with phonological disorders: A retrospective, comparative study." *Clinical Linguistics and Phonetics, 14* (2000): 217–234.

Goldstein, B., and P. Washington, "An initial investigation of phonological patterns in 4-year-old typically developing Spanish-English bilingual children." *Language, Speech, and Hearing Services in Schools, 10* (2001): 153–164.

Good, R., and R. Kaminski, *Dynamic indicators of basic early literacy skills* (6th ed.). Eugene OR: Institute for the Development of Educational Achievement.

Goodluck, H., *Language Acquisition: A Linguistic Introduction*. Oxford: Blackwell, 1991.

Goodsitt, J., P. Morse, and J. Ver Hoeve, "Infant speech recognition in multisyllabic contexts." *Child Development, 55* (1984): 903–910.

Gordon-Brannan, M., "Assessing intelligibility: Children's expressive phonologies." *Topics in Language Disorders, 14* (1994): 17–25.

Gordon-Brannan, M., B. Hodson, and M. Wynne, "Remediating unintelligible utterances of a child with a mild hearing loss." *American Journal of Speech-Language Pathology, 1,* 4 (1992): 28–38.

Goswami, U., and P. E. Bryant, *Phonological Skills and Learning to Read*. Hove, East Sussex: Psychology Press, 1990.

Gray, B., "A field study on programmed articulation therapy." *Language, Speech, and Hearing Services in Schools, 5* (1974): 119–131.

Gray, B., and B. Ryan, *A Language Program for the Non-language Child*. Champaign, IL: Research Press, 1973.

Gray, S. I., and R. L. Shelton, "Self-monitoring effects on articulation carryover in school-age children." *Language, Speech, and Hearing Services in Schools, 23* (1992): 334–342.

Green, J. R., C. A. Moore, and K. J. Reilly, "The sequential development of jaw and lip control for speech." *Journal of Speech, Language, and Hearing Research, 45* (2002): 66–79.

Greenlee, M., "Interacting processes in the child's acquisition of stop-liquid clusters." *Papers and Reports on Child Language Disorders, Stanford University, 7* (1974): 85–100.

Griffith, J., and L. E. Miner, *Phonetic Context Drill Book*. Englewood Cliffs, NJ: Prentice-Hall, 1979.

Grogan, M. L., E. J. Barker, S. J. Dettman, and P. J. Blamey, "Phonetic and phonologic changes in the connected speech of children using a cochlear implant." *Annals of Otology, Rhinology, and Laryngology, Supplement 166* (1995): 390–393.

Gruber, F. A., S. D. Lowery, H-K. Seung, and R. E. Deal, "Approaches to speech-language intervention and the true believer." *Journal of Medical Speech-Language Pathology, 11* (2003): 95–104.

Grunwell, P., "The development of phonology: A descriptive profile." *First Language, 3* (1981): 161–191.

Grunwell, P., *Clinical Phonology*. Rockville, MD: Aspen, 1982.

Grunwell, P., *Phonological Assessment of Child Speech (PACS)*. Windsor, UK: NFER-Nelson, 1985.

Grunwell, P., *Clinical Phonology* (2nd ed.). London: Croom Helm, 1987.

Grunwell, P., and M. Yavaş, "Phonotactic restrictions in disordered child phonology: A case study." *Clinical Linguistics and Phonetics, 2* (1988): 1–16.

Guitart, J., "Conservative versus radical dialects in American Spanish: Implications for language instruction." *Bilingual Review, 5* (1978): 57–64.

Guitart, J., "Spanish in contact with itself and the phonological characterization of conservative and radical styles." In A. Roca and J. Jensen (Eds.), *Spanish in Contact: Issues in Bilingualism* (pp. 151–157). Somerville, MA: Cascadilla, Press, 1996.

Hadley, P., A. Simmerman, M. Long, and M. Luna, "Facilitating language development for inner-city children: Experimental evaluation of a collaborative, classroom-based intervention." *Language, Speech, and Hearing Services in Schools, 31* (2000): 280–295.

Hadlich, R., Holton, J., and Montes, M., *A Drillbook of SpanishPpronunciation*. New York: Harper & Row, 1968.

Haelsig, P. C., and C. L. Madison, "A study of phonological processes exhibited by 3, 4, and 5-year-old children." *Language, Speech, and Hearing Services in Schools, 17* (1986): 107–114.

Hall, M., "Auditory factors in functional articulatory speech defects." *Journal of Experimental Education, 7* (1938): 110–132.

Hammond, R., *The Sounds of Spanish: Analysis and Application (with special reference to American English)*. Somerville, MA: Cascadilla Press, 2001.

Hansen, B., "The application of sound discrimination tests to functional articulatory defectives with normal hearing." *Journal of Speech Disorders, 9* (1944): 347–355.

Hanson, M. L., "Orofacial myofunctional disorders: Guidelines for assessment and treatment." *International Journal of Orofacial Myology, 14* (1988a): 27–32.

Hanson, M. L., "Orofacial myofunctional therapy: Historical and philosophical considerations." *International Journal of Orofacial Myology, 14* (1988b): 3–10.

Hanson, M. L., "Oral myofunctional disorders and articulatory patterns." In J. Bernthal and N. Bankson (Eds.), *Child Phonology: Characteristics, Assessment, and Intervention with Special Populations* (pp. 29–53). New York: Thieme Medical Publishers, 1994.

Hardcastle, W. J., *Physiology of Speech Production*. London: Academic Press, 1976.

Harrington, J., I. Lux, and R. Higgins, "Identification of error types as related to stimuli in articulation tests." Paper presented at the annual convention of the American Speech-Language-Hearing Association, San Francisco, 1984.

Hauner, K. K. Y., L. D. Shriberg, J. Kwiatkowski, and C. T. Allen, "A subtype of speech delay associated with developmental psychosocial involvement." *Journal of Speech, Language, and Hearing Research, 48* (2005): 635–650.

Hayes, B., "Metrics and phonological theory." In F. Newmeyer (Ed.), Linguistics: *The Cambridge Survey. II. Linguistic Theory: Extensions and Implications* (pp. 220–249). Cambridge: Cambridge University Press, 1988.

Haynes, W., and M. Moran, "A cross-sectional developmental study of final consonant production in Southern Black children from preschool through third grade." *Language, Speech, and Hearing Services in Schools, 20* (1989): 400–406.

Hazan, V., and S. Barrett, "The development of phonemic categorization in children aged 6–12." *Journal of Phonetics, 28* (2000): 377–396.

Heath, S. M., and J. H. Hogben, "Cost-effective prediction of reading difficulties." *Journal of Speech, Language, and Hearing Research, 47* (2004): 751–765.

Hedrick, D., E. Prather, and A. Tobin, *Sequenced Inventory of Consonant Development*. Seattle: University of Washington Press, 1975.

Helfrich-Miller, K., "Melodic intonation therapy with developmentally apraxic children." *Seminars in Speech and Language, 5* (1984): 119–126.

Heller, J., J. Gabbay, C. O'Hara, M. Heller, and J. P. Bradley, "Improved ankyloglossia correction with four-flap z-frenuloplasty." *Annals of Plastic Surgery, 54* (2005): 623–628.

Hempenstall, K., "The role of phonemic awareness in beginning reading: A review." *Behaviour Change 14* (1997): 201–214.

Hepper, P. G., and S. Shahidullah, "Development of fetal hearing." *Archives of Disease in Childhood, 71*, 2 (1994): F81–F87.

Hesketh, A., E. Dima, and V. Nelson, "Teaching phoneme awareness to pre-literate children with speech disorder: A randomized controlled trial." *International Journal of Language and Communication Disorders, 42* (2007): 251–271.

Hetrick, R. D., and R. K. Sommers, "Unisensory and bisensory processing skills of children having misarticulations and normally speaking peers." *Journal of Speech and Hearing Research, 31* (1988): 575–581.

Hewlett, N., "Processes of development and production." In P. Grunwell (Ed.), *Developmental Speech Disorders* (pp. 15–38) Edinburgh, UK: Churchill Livingstone, 1990.

Hewlett, N., F. Gibbon, and W. Cohen-McKenzie, "When is a velar an alveolar? Evidence supporting a revised psycholinguistic model of speech production in children." *International Journal of Language and Communication Disorders, 33* (1998): 161–176.

Hickman, L., *The Apraxia Profile*. San Antonio, TX: Psychological Corporation, 1997.

Higgs, J. A. W., "The phonetic development of word initial /s/ plus stop clusters in a group of young children." *British Journal of Disorders of Communication, 3* (1968): 130–138.

Hilton, L., "Treatment of deviant phonologic systems: Tongue thrust." In W. Perkins (Ed.), *Phonological-articulatory Disorders*. New York: Thieme-Stratton, 1984.

Hinton, L., and K. Pollock, "Regional variations in the phonological characteristics of African American Vernacular English (AAVE) speakers." Paper presented at the Texas Research Symposium on Language Diversity, Austin, TX, 1999.

Hixon, T. J., "Mechanical aspects of speech production." Paper read at Annual Convention of the American Speech and Hearing Association, Chicago, 1971.

Hockett, C. F., "A manual of phonology." *International Journal of American Linguistics (Memoir II)*. Baltimore, MD: Waverly Press, 1955.

Hodson, B., *Computer Analysis of Phonological Processes (CAPP)*. Stonington, IL: Phonocomp, 1985.

Hodson, B., "Phonological remediation: A cycles approach." In N. Creaghead, P. Newman, and W. Secord (Eds.), *Assessment and Remediation of Articulatory and Phonological Disorders*. Columbus, OH: Merrill, 1989.

Hodson, B. W., *Computerized Analysis of Phonological Patterns (HCAPP)*. Wichita, KS: Phonomp Software, 2003.

Hodson, B. W., *Hodson Assessment of Phonological Patterns* (3rd ed.). Austin, TX: Pro-Ed, 2004.

Hodson, B. W., *Evaluating and Enhancing Children's Phonological Systems*. Greenville, SC: Thinking Publications, 2007a.

Hodson, B. W., "Overview of the diagnostic evaluation process for children with highly unintelligible speech." In B. W. Hodson (Ed.), *Evaluating and Enhancing Children's Phonological Systems* (pp. 45–64) Greenville, SC: Thinking Publications, 2007b.

Hodson, B. W., L. Chin, B. Redmond, and R. Simpson, "Phonological evaluation and remediation of speech deviations of a child with a repaired cleft palate: A case study." *Journal of Speech and Hearing Disorders, 48* (1983): 93–98.

Hodson, B. W., and E. P. Paden, "Phonological processes which characterize unintelligible and intelligible speech in early childhood." *Journal of Speech and Hearing Disorders, 46* (1981): 369–373.

Hodson, B. W., and E. P. Paden, *Targeting Intelligible Speech: A Phonological Approach to Remediation* (2nd ed.). Austin, TX: Pro-Ed, 1991.

Hoffman, P., "Spelling, phonology, and the speech pathologist: A whole language perspective." *Language, Speech, and Hearing Services in Schools, 21* (1990): 238–243.

Hoffman, P., and J. Norris, "On the nature of phonological development: Evidence from normal children's spelling errors." *Journal of Speech and Hearing Research, 32* (1989): 787–794.

Hoffman, P., J. Norris, and J. Monjure, "Comparison of process targeting and whole language treatments of phonologically delayed children." *Language, Speech, and Hearing Services in Schools, 21* (1990): 102–109.

Hoffman, P., and G. H. Schuckers, "Articulation remediation treatment models." In R. G. Daniloff (Ed.), *Articulation Assessment and Treatment Issues*. San Diego: College-Hill Press, 1984.

Hoffman, P., G. Schuckers, and R. Daniloff, *Children's Phonetic Disorders: Theory and Treatment*. Boston: Little, Brown, 1989.

Hoffman, P., G. Schuckers, and D. Ratusnik, "Contextual-coarticulatory inconsistency of /r/ misarticulations." *Journal of Speech and Hearing Research, 20* (1977): 631–643.

Hoffman, P., S. Stager, and R. Daniloff, "Perception and production of misarticulated /r/." *Journal of Speech and Hearing Disorders, 48* (1983): 210–214.

Hoffmann, K. A., "Speech sound acquisition and natural process occurrence in the continuous speech of three- to six-year-old children." Unpublished master's thesis, University of Wisconsin–Madison, 1982.

Hogan, T., H. Catts, and T. Little, "The relationship between phonological awareness and reading: Implications for the assessment of phonological awareness." *Language, Speech, and Hearing Services in Schools, 36* (2005): 285–293.

Holland, A., "Training speech sound discrimination in children who misarticulate. A demonstration of teaching machine technique in speech correction." Project No. 5007. Washington, DC: U.S. Department of Health, Education and Welfare, 1967.

Holm, A., and B. Dodd, "A longitudinal study of the phonological development of two Cantonese-English bilingual children." *Applied Psycholinguistics, 20* (2000): 349–376.

Holm, A., B. Dodd, and A. Ozanne, "Efficacy of intervention for a bilingual childmaking articulation and phonological errors." *International Journal of Bilingualism, 1* (1997): 55–69.

Holm, A., F. Farrier, and B. Dodd, "Phonological awareness, reading accuracy and spelling ability of children with inconsistent phonological disorder." *International Journal of Language and Communication Disorders*, (2007).

Holm, A., S. Crosbie, and B. Dodd, "Differentiating normal variability from inconsistency in children's speech: Normative data." *International Journal of Language and Communication Disorders, 42*(4) (2007): 467–486.

Holm, J., *Pidgins and Creoles, Volume I: Theory and Structure*. Cambridge: Cambridge University Press, 1988.

Holm, J., *Pidgins and Creoles, Volume II: Reference Survey*. Cambridge: Cambridge University Press, 1989.

Howard, S., "English speech acquisition." In S. McLeod (Ed.), *The International Guide to Speech Acquisition* (pp. 188–203) Clifton Park, NY: Thomson Delmar Learning, 2007.

Howard, S. J., and B. C. Heselwood, "The contribution of phonetics to the study of vowel development and disorders." In M. J. Ball and F. E. Gibbon (Eds.), *Vowel Disorders* (pp. 37–82) New York: Butterworth-Heinemann, 2002.

Howell, J., and E. Dean, *Treating Phonological Disorders in Children: Metaphon—Theory to Practice*. San Diego: Singular Publishing, 1991.

Hull, F., P. Mielke, R. Timmons, and J. Willeford, "The national speech and hearing survey: Preliminary results." *ASHA, 13* (1971): 501–509.

Hulme, C., K. Goetz, D. Gooch, J. Adams, and M. J. Snowling, "Paired-associate learning, phoneme awareness, and learning to read." *Journal of Experimental Child Psychology, 96* (2007): 150–166.

Humphreys, M., "A contribution to infantile linguistics." *Transactions of the American Philological Association, 11* (1880): 5–17.

Hwa-Froelich, D., B. Hodson, and H. Edwards, "Characteristics of Vietnamese phonology." *American Journal of Speech-Language Pathology, 11* (2002): 264–273.

Hyman, L. M., *Phonology: Theory and Analysis*. New York: Holt, Rinehart and Winston, 1975.

Hyter, Y., "Ties that bind: The sounds of African American English." *ASHA Special Interest Division 14 Newsletter, 2*, (1996): 3–6.

Individuals with Disabilities Education Act Amendments of 2004, PL No. 108–446, 20 U.S.C. Section 1400 et seq.

Ingram, D., *Phonological Disability in Children*. London: Edward Arnold, 1976.

Ingram, D., "Phonological patterns in the speech of young children." In P. Fletcher and M. Garman (Eds.), *Language Acquisition*. Cambridge: Cambridge University Press, 1979.

Ingram, D., *Procedures for the Phonological Analysis of Children's Language*. Baltimore, MD: University Park Press, 1981.

Ingram, D., "On children's homonyms." *Journal of Child Language, 12* (1985): 671–680.

Ingram, D., *Phonological Disability in Children* (2nd ed.). London: Cole and Whurr, 1989a.

Ingram, D., *First Language Acquisition: Method, Description and Explanation*. Cambridge: Cambridge University Press, 1989b.

Ingram, D., L. Christensen, S. Veach, and B. Webster, "The acquisition of word-initial fricatives and affricates in English by children between 2 and 6 years." In G. H. Yeni-Komshian, J. F. Kavanagh, and C. A. Ferguson (Eds.), *Child Phonology. Vol 1: Production* (pp. 169–192) New York: Academic Press, 1980.

Ingram, D., and K. D. Ingram, "A whole-word approach to phonological analysis and intervention." *Language, Speech, and Hearing Services in Schools, 32* (2001): 271–283.

Ingram, J., "Connected speech processes in Australian English." *Australian Journal of Linguistics, 9* (1989): 21–49.

Ingram, J., J. Pittman, and D. Newman, "Developmental and socio-linguistic variation in the speech of Brisbane school children." *Australian Journal of Linguistics, 5* (1985): 233–246.

Inscoe, J., "Communication outcomes after paediatric cochlear implantation." *International Journal of Pediatric Otorhinolaryngology, 47* (1999): 195–200.

Invernizzi, M., and J. Meier, *Phonological awareness literacy screening (PALS: 1–3).* Charlottesville: The Virginia State Department of Education and The University of Virginia.

Invernizzi, M., J. Meier, L. Swank, and C. Juel, *Phonological awareness literacy screening (PALS-K).* Charlottesville: The Virginia State Department of Education and The University of Virginia.

Irwin, J. V., and S. P. Wong (Eds.), *Phonological Development in Children 18 to 72 Months.* Carbondale, IL: Southern Illinois University Press, 1983.

Irwin, R. B., J. F. West, and M. A. Trombetta, "Effectiveness of speech therapy for second grade children with misarticulations: Predictive factors." *Exceptional Children, 32* (1966): 471–479.

Itoh, M., and S. Sasanuma, "Articulatory movements in apraxia of speech." In J. Rosenbek, M. McNeil, and A. Aronson (Eds.), *Apraxia of Speech: Physiology, Acoustics, Linguistics, Management.* San Diego: College-Hill Press, 1984.

Jakobson, R., *Child Language Aphasia and Phonological Universals.* The Hague: Mouton, 1968.

James, D., "Hippopotamus is so hard to say: Children's acquisition of polysyllabic words." Unpublished doctoral dissertation, The University of Sydney, Australia, 2007.

James, D., "The use of phonological processes in Australian children aged 2 to 7:11 years." *Advances in Speech-Language Pathology, 3* (2001): 109–128.

James, D., "Part II: On assessing normal speech development." *ACQuiring Knowledge in Speech, Language and Hearing, 4* (2002): 147–150.

James, D., P. McCormack, and A. Butcher, "Children's use of phonological processes in the age range of five to seven years." In S. McLeod and L. McAllister (Eds.), *Proceedings of the 1999 Speech Pathology Australia National Conference* (pp. 48–57). Melbourne: Speech Pathology Australia, 1999.

James, D., J. van Doorn, and S. McLeod, "Vowel production in mono-, di- and poly-syllabic words in children 3;0 to 7;11 years." In L. Wilson and S. Hewat (Eds.), *Proceedings of the Speech Pathology Australia Conference* (pp. 127–136). Melbourne: Speech Pathology Australia, 2001.

James, D., J. van Doorn, and S. McLeod, "Segment production in mono-, di- and polysyllabic words in children aged 3–7 years." In F. Windsor, L. Kelly, and N. Hewlett (Eds.), *Themes in Clinical Phonetics and Linguistics* (pp. 287–298). Hillsdale, NJ: Erlbaum, 2002.

James, D., J. van Doorn, and S. McLeod, "The contribution of polysyllabic words in clinical decision making about children's speech." *Clinical Linguistics and Phonetics, 22*(4) (2008): 345–353.

James, S. L., *Normal Language Acquisition.* Boston: Allyn and Bacon, 1990.

Jann, G., M. Ward, and H. Jann, "A longitudinal study of articulation, deglutition and malocclusion." *Journal of Speech and Hearing Disorders, 29* (1964): 424–435.

Jimenez, B. C., "Acquisition of Spanish consonants in children aged 3–5 years, 7 months." *Language, Speech, and Hearing Services in Schools, 18* (1987): 357–363.

Johns, D., and F. Darley, "Phonemic variability in apraxia of speech." *Journal of Speech and Hearing Research, 13* (1970): 556–583.

Johns, D., and K. Salyer, "Surgical and prosthetic management of neurogenic speech disorders." In D. Johns (Ed.), *Clinical Management of Neurogenic Communicative Disorders.* Boston: Little, Brown, 1978.

Johnson, C. A., A. D. Weston, and B. A. Bain, "An objective and time efficient method for determining severity of childhood speech delay." *American Journal of Speech-Language Pathology, 13* (2004): 55–65.

Johnston, R. S., M. Anderson, and C. Holligan, "Knowledge of the alphabet and explicit awareness of phonemes in pre-readers: The nature of the relationship." *Reading and Writing: An Interdisciplinary Journal, 8* (1996): 217–234.

Jong, K. J. de, "The oral articulation of English stress accent." Ph.D. dissertation, Ohio State University, Columbus, 1991.

Jordan, L., J. Hardy, and H. Morris, "Performance of children with good and poor articulation on tasks of tongue placement." *Journal of Speech and Hearing Research, 21* (1978): 429–439.

Juel, C., "Learning to read and write: A longitudinal study of 54 children from first through fourth grades." *Journal of Educational Psychology, 80* (1988): 437–447.

Jusczyk, P., and P. A. Luce, "Speech perception and spoken word recognition: Past and present." *Ear & Hearing, 23* (2002): 2–40.

Jusczyk, P., and E. Thompson, "Perception of phonetic contrasts in multisyllabic utterances by 2 month old infants." *Perception and Psychophysics, 23* (1978): 105–109.

Justice, L., J. Kaderavek, R. Bowles, and K. Grim, "Language impairment, parent-child shared reading, and phonological awareness: A feasibility study." *Topics in Early Childhood Special Education, 25*(2005): 143–156.

Justice, L. M., and H. K. Ezell, "Vygotskian theory and its application to language assessment: An overview for speech-language pathologists." *Contemporary Issues in Communication Science and Disorders, 26* (1999): 111–118.

Justice, L. M., and H. K. Ezell, "Print referencing: An emergent literacy enhancement strategy and its clinical applications." *Language Speech and Hearing Services in Schools 35* (2004): 185–193.

Justice, L. M., K. Pence, R. B. Bowles, and A. Wiggins, "An investigation of four hypotheses concerning the order by which 4-year-old children learn the alphabet letters." *Early Childhood Research Quarterly 21* (2006): 374–389.

Kager, R., *Optimality Theory.* Cambridge: Cambridge University Press, 1999.

Kamhi, A. G., R. Friemoth-Lee, and L. Nelson, "Word, syllable and sound awareness in language disordered children." *Journal of Speech and Hearing Disorders, 50* (1985): 207–212.

Kantner, C. E., and R. West, *Phonetics.* New York: Harper & Row, 1960.

Karlsson, H. B., L. D. Shriberg, P. Flipsen Jr., and J. L. McSweeny, "Acoustic phenotypes for speech-genetics studies: Toward an acoustic marker for residual /s/ distortions." *Clinical Linguistics and Phonetics, 16* (2002): 403–424.

Kaufman, N., *Kaufman Speech Praxis Test for Children.* Detroit, MI: Wayne State University Press, 1995.

Kayser, H. "Interpreters." In H. Kayser (Ed.), *Bilingual Speech-Language Pathology: An Hispanic Focus* (pp. 207–221). San Diego, CA: Singular Publishing, 1995.

Kehoe, M., "Stress error patterns in English-speaking children's word productions." *Clinical Linguistics and Phonetics, 11* (1997): 389–409.

Kehoe, M. M., "Prosodic patterns in children's multisyllabic word productions." *Language, Speech, and Hearing Services in Schools, 32* (2001): 284–294.

Kemaloglu, Y. K., T. Kobayashi, and T. Nakajima, "Analysis of the craniofacial skeleton in cleft children with otitis media with effusion." *International Journal of Pediatric Otorhinolaryngology, 47* (1999): 57–69.

Kenney, K., and E. Prather, "Articulation in preschool children: Consistency of productions." *Journal of Speech and Hearing Research, 29* (1986): 29–36.

Kent, R. D., "Anatomical and neuromuscular maturation of the speech mechanism: Evidence from acoustic studies." *Journal of Speech and Hearing Research, 19* (1976): 421–447.

Kent, R. D., and H. R. Bauer, "Vocalizations of one year olds." *Journal of Child Language, 12* (1985): 491–526.

Kent, R. D., and L. L. Forner, "Speech segment durations in sentence recitations by children and adults." *Journal of Phonetics, 8* (1980): 157–168.

Kent, R. D., J. F. Kent, and J. C. Rosenbek, "Maximum performance tests of speech production." *Journal of Speech and Hearing Disorders, 52* (1987): 367–387.

Kent, R. D., R. E. Martin, and R. L. Sufit, "Oral sensation: A review and clinical prospective." In H. Winitz (Ed.), *Human Communication and Its Disorders: A Review—1990* (pp. 135–191). Norwood, NJ: Ablex, 1990.

Kent, R. D., and F. D. Minifie, "Coarticulation in recent speech production models." *Journal of Phonetics, 5* (1977): 115–133.

Kent, R. D., G. Miolo, and S. Bloedel, "The intelligibility of children's speech: A review of evaluation procedures." *American Journal of Speech-Language Pathology, 3* (1994): 81–95.

Kent, R. D., and K. L. Moll, "Vocal-tract characteristics of the stop cognates." *Journal of the Acoustical Society of America, 46* (1969): 1549–1555.

Kent, R. D., and K. L. Moll, "Cinefluorographic analyses of selected lingual consonants." *Journal of Speech and Hearing Research, 15* (1972): 453–473.

Kent, R. D., and K. L. Moll, "Articulatory timing in selected consonant sequences." *Brain and Language, 2* (1975): 304–323.

Kent, R. D., and R. Netsell, "Effects of stress contrasts on certain articulatory parameters." *Phonetica, 24* (1972): 23–44.

Kent, R. D., M. J. Osberger, R. Netsell, and C. G. Hustedde, "Phonetic development in identical twins differing in auditory function." *Journal of Speech and Hearing Disorders, 52* (1987): 64–75.

Kent, R. D., and C. Tilkens, "Oromotor foundations of speech acquisition." In S. McLeod (Ed.), *International Guide to Speech Acquisition* (pp. 8–13) Clifton Park, NY: Thomson Delmar Learning, 2007.

Khan, L. M., "Major phonological processes." *Language, Speech, and Hearing Services in Schools, 13* (1982): 77–85.

Khan, L. M., *Basics of Phonological Analysis: A Programmed Learning Test.* San Diego, CA: College Hill, 1985.

Khan, L. M., and N. P. Lewis, *Khan-Lewis Phonological Analysis.* Circle Pines, MN: American Guidance Service, 1986, 2002.

Khinda, V., and N. Grewal, "Relationship of tongue-thrust swallowing and anterior open bite with articulation disorders: A clinical study." *Journal of the Indian Society of Pedodontia and Preventive Dentistry, 17* (1999): 33–39.

Kilminster, M. G. E., and E. M. Laird, "Articulation development in children aged three to nine years." *Australian Journal of Human Communication Disorders, 6* (1978): 23–30.

Kindler, A., "Survey of the states' LEP students 2000–2001 summary report." Washington, DC: National Clearinghouse for English Language Acquisition, 2001.

Kiparsky, P., and L. Menn, "On the acquisition of phonology." In J. MacNamara (Ed.), *Language Learning and Thought* (pp. 47–78). New York: Academic Press, 1977.

Kirk, C., and G. T. Gillon, "Longitudinal effects of phonological awareness intervention on morphological awareness in children with speech impairment." *Language, Speech, and Hearing Services in Schools* (in press).

Kirtley, C., P. Bryant, M. MacLean, and L. Bradley, "Rhyme, rime, and the onset of reading." *Journal of Experimental Child Psychology, 48* (1989): 224–245.

Kisatsky, T., "The prognostic value of Carter-Buck tests in measuring articulation skills in selected kindergarten children." *Exceptional Children, 34* (1967): 81–85.

Klaiman, P., M. A. Witzel, F. Margar-Bacal, and I. R. Munro, "Changes in aesthetic appearance and intelligibility of speech after partial glossectomy in patients with Down Syndrome." *Plastic and Reconstructive Surgery, 82* (1988): 403–408.

Klatt, D. H., "Linguistic uses of segmental duration in English: Acoustic and perceptual evidence." *Journal of the Acoustical Society of America, 59* (1976): 1208–1221.

Kleffner, F., "A comparison of the reactions of a group of fourth grade children to recorded examples of defective and nondefective articulation." Ph.D. Thesis, University of Wisconsin, 1952.

Klein, E. S., "Phonological/traditional approaches to articulation therapy: A retrospective group comparison." *Language, Speech, and Hearing Services in Schools, 27* (1996): 314–323.

Koch, H., "Sibling influence on children's speech." *Journal of Speech and Hearing Disorders, 21* (1956): 322–329.

Koegel, L. K., R. L. Koegel, and J. C. Ingham, "Programming rapid generalization of correct articulation through self-monitoring procedures." *Journal of Speech and Hearing Disorders, 51* (1986): 24–32.

Koegel, R., L. Koegel, K. Van Voy, and J. Ingham, "Within-clinic versus outside-of-clinic self-monitoring of articulation to promote generalization." *Journal of Speech and Hearing Disorders, 53* (1988): 392–399.

Kohnert, K., and A. Derr, "Language intervention with bilingual children." In B. Goldstein (Ed.), *Bilingual Language Development and Disorders in Spanish-English Speakers* (pp. 311–342). Baltimore, MD: Brookes, 2004.

Kohnert, K., D. Yim, K. Nett, P. F. Kan, and L. Duran, "Intervention with linguistically diverse preschool children: A focus on developing home language(s)." *Language, Speech, and Hearing Services in Schools, 36* (2005): 251–263.

Kronvall, E., and C. Diehl, "The relationship of auditory discrimination to articulatory defects of children with no known organic impairment." *Journal of Speech and Hearing Disorders, 19* (1954): 335–338.

Kumin, L., "Intelligibility of speech in children with Down Syndrome in natural settings: Parents' perspective." *Perceptual and Motor Skills, 78* (1994): 307–313.

Kumin, L., C. Council, and M. Goodman, "A longitudinal study of emergence of phonemes in children with Down syndrome." *Journal of Communication Disorders, 27* (1994): 293–303.

Labov, W., "The three dialects of English." In P. Eckert (Ed.), *New Ways of Analyzing Sound Change* (pp. 1–44). New York: Academic Press, 1991.

Ladefoged, P., *Preliminaries to Linguistic Phonetics.* Chicago: University of Chicago Press, 1971.

Ladefoged, P., *A Course in Phonetics.* New York: Harcourt Brace Jovanovich, 1975.

Ladefoged, P., *A Course in Phonetics* (3rd ed.). New York: Harcourt Brace, 1993.

Ladefoged, P., *Vowels and Consonants* (2nd ed.) Oxford, UK: Blackwell, 2005.

Laine, T., M. Jaroma, and A. L. Linnasalo, "Relationships between interincisal occlusion and articulatory components of speech." *Folia Phoniatrica, 39* (1987): 78–86.

Langdon, H., and L. R. L. Cheng, *Collaborating with Interpreters and Translators*. Eau Claire, WI: Thinking Publications, 2002.

Lanza, J. R., and L. K. Flahive, *Articulation*. East Moline, IL: LinguiSystems, 2000.

Lapko, L., and N. Bankson, "Relationship between auditory discrimination, articulation stimulability and consistency of misarticulation." *Perceptual and Motor Skills, 40* (1975): 171–177.

Lapointe, L., and R. Wertz, "Oral-movement abilities and articulatory characteristics of brain-injured adults." *Perceptual Motor Skills, 39* (1974): 39–46.

LaRiviere, C., H. Winitz, J. Reeds, and E. Herriman, "The conceptual reality of selected distinctive features." *Journal of Speech and Hearing Research, 17* (1974): 122–133.

Larrivee, L., and H. Catts, "Early reading achievement in children with expressive phonological disorders." *American Journal of Speech-Language Pathology, 8*, 2 (1999): 118–128.

Lasky, R. E., and A. L. Williams, "The development of the auditory system from conception to term." *Neoreviews, 6*, 3 (2005): e141–e152.

Lau v. *Nichols*, 414 U.S. 563 (1974).

Lau Remedies, Office of Civil Rights, task force findings specifying remedies available for eliminating past educational practices rules unlawful under *Lau* v. *Nichols*, IX, pt. 5, 1975.

Law, J., J. Boyle, F. Harris, A. Harkness, and C. Nye, "Screening for speech and language delay: A systematic review of the literature." *Health Technology and Assessment, 2*, 9 (1998): 1–183.

Law, J., Z. Garrett, and C. Nye, "The efficacy of treatment for children with developmental speech and language delay disorders: A meta-analysis." *Journal of Speech and Hearing Research, 47* (2004): 924–943.

Leap, W. "American Indian languages." In C. Ferguson and S. Heath (Eds.), *Language in the USA* (pp. 116–144). Cambridge: Cambridge University Press, 1981.

Lebrun, Y., "Tongue thrust, tongue tip position at rest, and stigmatism: A review." *Journal of Communication Disorders, 18* (1985): 305–312.

Lehiste, I., *Suprasegmentals*. Cambridge, MA: M.I.T. Press, 1970.

Leitão, S., and J. Fletcher, "Literacy outcomes for students with speech impairment: Long-term follow-up." *International Journal of Language and Communication Disorders, 39* (2004): 245–256.

Lenchner, O., and B. Podhajski, *The Sounds Abound Program*. East Moline, IL: Linguisystems, 1998.

Lenden, J. M., and P. Flipsen Jr., "Prosody and voice characteristics of children with cochlear implants." *Journal of Communication Disorders, 40* (2007): 66–81.

Leonard, L., "The nature of deviant articulation." *Journal of Speech and Hearing Disorders, 38* (1973): 156–161.

Leonard, L. B., and J. S. Leonard, "The contribution of phonetic context to an unusual phonological pattern: A case study." *Language, Speech, and Hearing Services in Schools, 16* (1985): 110–118.

Leonard, L. B., L. E. Rowan, B. Morris, and M. E. Fey, "Intra-word phonological variability in young children." *Journal of Child Language, 9* (1982): 55–69.

Leonard, R. J., "Characteristics of speech in speakers with oral/oralpharyngeal ablation." In J. Bernthal and N. Bankson (Eds.), *Child Phonology: Characteristics, Assessment, and Intervention with Special Populations* (pp. 54–78). New York: Thieme Medical Publishers, 1994.

Leopold, W., *Speech Development of a Bilingual Child: A Linguist's Record*. Vol. 1: Vocabulary growth in the first two years (1939), Vol. 2: Sound learning in the first two years (1947), Vol. 3: Grammar and general problems in the first two years (1949), Vol. 4: Diary from age two (1949). Evanstown, IL: Northwestern University Press, 1939–1949.

Leopold, W., *Speech Development of a Bilingual Child: A Linguist's Record*. Vol. 2: Sound Learning in the First Two Years. Evanstown, IL: Northwestern University Press, 1947.

Levi, G., F. Capozzi, A. Fabrizi, and E. Sechi, "Language disorders and prognosis for reading disabilities in developmental age." *Perceptual and Motor Skills, 54* (1982): 1119–1122.

Levitt, H., and H. Stromberg, "Segmental characteristics of speech of hearing-impaired children: Factors affecting intelligibility." In I. Hochberg, H. Levitt, and M. Osberger (Eds.), *Speech of the Hearing Impaired* (pp. 53–73). Baltimore, MD: University Park Press, 1983.

Lewis, B. A., B. Ekelman, and D. Aram, "A familial study of severe phonological disorders." *Journal of Speech and Hearing Research, 32* (1989): 713–724.

Lewis, B. A., L. A. Freebairn, A. J. Hansen, Miscimarra, S. K. Iyengar, and H. G. Taylor, "Speech and language skills of parents of children with speech sound disorders." *American Journal of Speech-Language Pathology, 16* (2007): 108–118.

Lewis, B. A., L. A. Freebairn, A. J. Hansen, C. M. Stein, L. D. Shriberg, S. K. Iyengar, and H. G. Taylor. "Dimensions of early speech sound disorders: A factor analytic study." *Journal of Communication Disorders, 39* (2006): 139–157.

Lewis, B. A., L. A. Freebairn, and H. G. Taylor. "Follow-up of Children with Early Expressive Phonology Disorders." *Journal of Learning Disabilities 33* (2000): 433–444.

Lewis, B. A., and L. Freebairn-Farr, "Preschool phonology disorders at school age, adolescence, and adulthood." Paper presented at the annual convention of the American Speech-Language-Hearing Association, Atlanta, 1991.

Lewis, B. A., B. O'Donnell, L. Freebairn, and H. Taylor, "Spoken language and written expression-interplay of delays." *American Journal of Speech-Language Pathology, 7,* 3 (1998): 77–84.

Li, C., and S. Thompson, "The acquisition of tone in Mandarin-speaking children." *Journal of Child Language, 4* (1977): 185–199.

Liberman, I., and D. Shankweiler, "Phonology and problems of learning to read and write." *Remedial and Special Education, 6* (1985): 8–17.

Lieberman, P., *Intonation, Perception and Language.* Cambridge, MA: M.I.T. Press, 1967.

Lindamood, C., and P. Lindamood, *Lindamood Auditory Conceptualization Test.* Boston: Teaching Resources, 1971.

Lindblom, B., "Spectrographic study of vowel reduction." *Journal of the Acoustical Society of America, 35* (1963): 1773–1781.

Lindblom, B., "Explaining phonetic variation: A sketch of the H&H theory." In W. J. Hardcastle and A. Marchal (Eds.), *Speech Production and Speech Modeling* (pp. 403–439). Amsterdam, The Netherlands: Kluwer, 1990.

Lindblom, B., and R. Zetterström (Eds.), *Precursors of Early Speech Development.* New York: Stockton, 1986.

Ling, D., *Foundations of Spoken Language for Hearing-Impaired Children.* Washington, DC: Alexander Graham Bell Association for the Deaf, 1989.

Lleo, C., "Homonymy and reduplication: On the extended availability of two strategies in phonological acquisition." *Journal of Child Language, 17* (1990): 267–278.

Lleo, C., and M. Prinz, "Consonant clusters in child phonology and the directionality of syllable structure assignment." *Journal of Child Language, 23* (1996): 31–56.

Locke, J., "Oral perception and articulation learning." *Perceptual and Motor Skills, 26* (1968): 1259–1264.

Locke, J., "The inference of speech perception in the phonologically disordered child. Part I: A rationale, some criteria, the conventional tests." *Journal of Speech and Hearing Disorders, 45* (1980a): 431–444.

Locke, J., "The inference of speech perception in the phonologically disordered child. Part II: Some clinically novel procedures, their use, some findings." *Journal of Speech and Hearing Disorders, 45* (1980b): 445–468.

Locke, J., "Vocal development in the human infant: Functions and phonetics." In F. Windsor, M. L. Kelly, and N. Hewlett (Eds.), *Investigations in Clinical Phonetics and Linguistics* (pp. 243–256). Hillsdale, NJ: Erlbaum, 2002.

Locke, J., and K. Kutz, "Memory for speech and speech for memory." *Journal of Speech and Hearing Research, 18* (1975): 179–191.

Locke, J., and P. Mather, "Genetic factors in phonology. Evidence from monozygotic and dizygotic twins." Paper presented at the annual convention of the American Speech-Language-Hearing Association, New Orleans, 1987.

Lof, G., "A study of phoneme perception and speech stimulability." Ph.D. Thesis, University of Wisconsin–Madison, 1994.

Lof, G., "Logic, theory and evidence against the use of nonspeech oral motor exercises to change speech sound productions." Invited presentation at the Annual Convention of the American Speech-Language-Hearing Association, Miami, 2006.

Lof, G., and S. Synan, "Is there a speech discrimination/perception link to disordered articulation and phonology? A review of 80 years of literature." *Contemporary Issues in Communication Science and Disorders, 24* (1997): 63–77.

Lonigan, C. J., S. R. Burgess, J. L. Anthony, and T. A. Barker, "Development of phonological sensitivity in 2- to 5-year-old children." *Journal of Educational Psychology, 90* (1998): 294–311.

Long, S., "About time: A comparison of computerized and manual procedures for grammatical and phonological analysis." *Clinical Linguistics and Phonetics, 15* (2001): 399–426.

Long, S. H., M. E. Fey, and R. W. Channell, "Computerized profiling (Version CP941.exe)." Cleveland, OH: Case Western Reserve University, 2002.

Lowe, R. J., *Assessment Link Between Phonology and Articulation (ALPHA)*. Moline, IL: LinguiSystems, 1986.

Lowe, R. J., P. J. Knutson, and M. A. Monson, "Incidence of fronting in preschool children." *Language, Speech, and Hearing Services in Schools, 16* (1985): 119–123.

Lundberg, I., J. Frost, and O. Peterson, "Effects of an extensive program for stimulating phonological awareness in preschool children." *Reading Research Quarterly, 23* (1988): 263–284.

Lynch, E. "Developing cross-cultural competence." In E. Lynch and M. Hanson (Eds.), *Developing Cross-Cultural Competence: A Guide for Working with Children and Their Families* (3rd ed., pp. 41–77). Baltimore, MD: Brookes, 2004.

Maassen, B., L. Nijland, and S. van der Meulen. "Coarticulation within and between syllables by children with developmental apraxia of speech." *Clinical Linguistics and Phonetics, 15* (2001): 145–150.

Macken, M., "Phonological acquisition." In J. A. Goldsmith (Ed.), *The Handbook of Phonological Theory* (pp. 671–696). Cambridge, MA: Blackwell, 1995.

Macken, M. A., "The child's lexical representation: The 'puzzle, puddle, pickle' evidence." *Journal of Linguistics, 16* (1980a): 1–17.

Macken, M. A., "Aspects of the acquisition of stop systems: A cross-linguistic perspective." In G. H. Yeni-Komshian, J. F. Kavanagh, and C. A. Ferguson (Eds.), *Child Phonology Vol 1: Production* (pp. 143–168) New York: Academic Press, 1980b.

Maclagan, M., and G. T. Gillon, "New Zealand English speech acquisition." In S. McLeod (Ed.), *The International Guide to Speech Acquisition* (pp. 257–268) Clifton Park, NY: Thomson Delmar Learning, 2007.

MacNeilage, P. F., "Speech physiology." In H. H. Gilbert (Ed.), *Speech and Cortical Functioning* (pp. 1–72). New York: Academic Press, 1972.

Madell, J. R., N. Sislian, and R. Hoffman, "Speech perception for cochlear implant patients using hearing aids on the unimplanted ear." *International Congress Series, 1273* (2004): 223–226.

Magnusson, E., and K. Naucler, "The development of linguistic awareness in language-disordered children." *First Language, 13* (1993): 93–111.

Majnemer, A., and B. Rosenblatt. "Reliability of parental recall of developmental milestones." *Pediatric Neurology, 10* (1994): 304–308.

Major, E. M., and B. H. Bernhardt, "Metaphonological skills of children with phonological disorders before and after phonological and metaphonological intervention." *International Journal of Language and Communication Disorders 33* (1998): 413–444.

Marchant, C. D., P. A. Shurin, V. A. Turczyk, D. E. Wasikowski, M. A. Tutihasi, and S. E. Kinney. "Course and outcome of otitis media in early infancy: A prospective study." *The Journal of Pediatrics, 104* (1984): 826–831.

Marder, L, and C. N. Cholmain, "Promoting language development for children with Down's syndrome." *Current Pediatrics, 16* (2006): 495–500.

Margar-Bacal, F., M. A. Witzel, and I. Munro, "Speech intelligibility after partial glossectomy in children with Down's Syndrome." *Plastic and Reconstructive Surgery, 79* (1987): 44–47.

Marquardt, T. P., A. Jacks, and B. L. Davis, "Token-to-token variability in developmental apraxia of speech: Three longitudinal case studies." *Clinical Linguistics and Phonetics, 18* (2004): 127–144.

Marquardt, T. P., H. M. Sussman, T. Snow, and A. Jacks, "The integrity of the syllable in developmental apraxia of speech." *Journal of Communication Disorders 35* (2002): 31–49.

Marshall, P., "Oral-motor techniques in articulation therapy." Videotapes. Seattle, WA: Innovative Concepts, 1992.

Marshalla, P., *Oral-Motor Techniques in Articulation Therapy*. Temecula, CA: Speech Dynamics, 1996.

Marunick, M., and N. Tselios, "The efficacy of palatal augmentation prostheses for speech and swallowing in patients undergoing glossectomy: A review of the literature." *The Journal of Prosthetic Dentistry, 91* (2004): 67–74.

Mase, D., "Etiology of articulatory speech defects." *Teacher's College Contribution to Education, No. 921*. New York: Columbia University, 1946.

Mason, R., "Orthodontic perspectives on orofacial myofunctional therapy." *International Journal of Orofacial Myology, 14* (1988): 49–55.

Mason, R., and W. Proffit, "The tongue-thrust controversy: Background and recommendations." *Journal of Speech and Hearing Disorders, 39* (1974): 115–132.

Mason, R., and N. Wickwire, "Examining for orofacial variations." *Communiqué, 8* (1978): 2–26.

Massengill, R., S. Maxwell, and K. Picknell, "An analysis of articulation following partial and total glossectomy."

Journal of Speech and Hearing Disorders, 35 (1970): 170–173.

Masterson, J., "Classroom-based phonological intervention." *American Journal of Speech-Language Pathology, 2* (1993): 5–9.

Masterson, J., and B. H. Bernhardt, *CAPES: Computerized Articulation and Phonology Evaluation System* (Version 1.0.1). San Antonio, TX: Psychological Corporation, 2001.

Masterson, J., and L. Crede, "Learning to spell: Implications for assessment and intervention." *Language, Speech, and Hearing Services in Schools, 30* (1999): 243–254.

Masterson, J., S. Long, and E. Buder, "Instrumentation in clinical phonology." In J. Bernthal and N. Bankson (Eds.), *Articulation and Phonological Disorders* (4th ed., pp. 378–406). Boston: Allyn and Bacon, 1998.

Masterson, J., and F. Pagan, *Interactive System for Phonological Analysis (ISPA)*. San Antonio, TX: The Psychological Corporation, 1993.

Matheny, A., and C. Bruggeman, "Children's speech: Heredity components and sex differences." *Folia Phoniatrica, 25* (1973): 442–449.

Matheny, N., and J. Panagos, "Comparing the effects of articulation and syntax programs on syntax and articulation improvement." *Language, Speech, and Hearing Services in Schools, 9* (1978): 57–61.

Maxwell, E. M., "On determining underlying phonological representations of children: A critique of the current theories." *Phonological Theory and the Misarticulating Child, ASHA Monograph 22* (pp. 18–29). Rockville, MD: ASHA, 1984.

Mayo, C., J. M. Scobbie, N. Hewlett, and D. Waters, "The influence of phonemic awareness development on acoustic cue weighting strategies in children's speech perception." *Journal of Speech, Language, and Hearing Research, 46*, 5 (2003): 1184–1196.

McCarthy, L., "Feature geometry and dependency: A review." *Journal of Phonetics, 43* (1988): 84–108.

McCauley, R. *Assessment of language disorders in children*. Mahwah, NJ: Lawrence Erlbaum.

McCormack, P., "New approaches to the assessment of children's speech." *Australian Communication Quarterly* (Autumn 1997): 3–5.

McCormack, P. F., and T. Knighton, "Gender differences in the speech patterns of two and a half year old children." In P. McCormack and A. Russell (Eds.), *Speech Science and Technology: Sixth Australian International Conference* (pp. 337–341).

Adelaide: Australian Speech Science and Technology Association, 1996.

McDermot, K. D., E. Bonora, N. Sykers, A. M. Coupe, C. S. Lai, S. C. Vernes, F. Vargha-Khadem, F. McKenzie, R. L. Smith, A. P. Monaco, and S. E. Fisher. "Identification of FOXP2 truncation as a novel cause of developmental speech and language deficits." *American Journal of Human Genetics, 76* (2005): 1074–1080.

McDonald, E. T., *Articulation Testing and Treatment: A Sensory Motor Approach*. Pittsburgh, PA: Stanwix House, 1964a.

McDonald, E. T., *A Deep Test of Articulation*. Pittsburgh, PA: Stanwix House, 1964b.

McDonald, E. T., and L. Aungst, "Apparent impedence of oral sensory functions and articulatory proficiency." In J. Bosma (Ed.), *Second Symposium on Oral Sensation and Perception*. Springfield, IL: Charles Thomas, 1970.

McEnery, E., and F. Gaines, "Tongue-tie in infants and children." *Journal of Pediatrics, 18* (1941): 252–255.

McGlaughlin, A., and A. Grayson, "A cross sectional and prospective study of crying in the first year of life." In S. P. Sohov (Ed.), *Advances in Psychology Research* (Vol. 22, pp. 37–58). New York: Nova Science, 2003.

McGregor, K. K., and R. G. Schwartz, "Converging evidence for underlying phonological representation in a child who misarticulates." *Journal of Speech and Hearing Research, 35* (1992): 596–603.

McKinnon, D. H., S. McLeod, and S. Reilly, "The prevalence of stuttering, voice and speech-sound disorders in primary school students in Australia." *Language, Speech, and Hearing Services in Schools, 38*, 1 (2007): 5–15.

McLaughlin, S., *Introduction to Language Development*. San Diego, CA: Singular, 1998.

McLeod, S., "Part I: The plethora of available data on children's speech development." *ACQuiring Knowledge in Speech, Language and Hearing, 4* (2002): 141–147.

McLeod, S., "General trends and individual differences: Perspectives on normal speech development." In F. Columbus (Ed.), *Advances in Psychology Research* (pp. 189–202) Happauge, NY: Nova Science, 2003.

McLeod, S., "Australian English speech acquisition." In S. McLeod (Ed.), *The International Guide to Speech Acquisition* (pp. 241–256) Clifton Park, NY: Thomson Delmar Learning, 2007.

McLeod, S. (Ed.), *The International Guide to Speech Acquisition.* Clifton Park, NY: Thomson Delmar Learning, 2007a.

McLeod, S., and S. R. Hewett, "Variability in the production of words containing consonant clusters by typical two- and three-year-old children." *Folia Phoniatrica et Logopaedica, 60* (2008): 163–172.

McLeod, S., J. van Doorn, and V. A. Reed, "Homonyms in children's productions of consonant clusters." In W. Ziegler and K. Deger (Eds.), *Clinical Phonetics and Linguistics* (pp. 108–114) London: Whurr, 1998.

McLeod, S., J. van Doorn, and V. A. Reed, "Normal acquisition of consonant clusters." *American Journal of Speech-Language Pathology, 10* (2001a): 99–110.

McLeod, S., J. van Doorn, and V. A. Reed, "Consonant cluster development in two-year-olds: General trends and individual difference." *Journal of Speech, Language, Hearing Research, 44* (2001b): 1144–1171.

McLeod, S., J. van Doorn, and V. A. Reed, "Typological description of the normal acquisition of consonant clusters." In F. Windsor, L. Kelly, and N. Hewlett (Eds.), *Investigations in Clinical Phonetics and Linguistics* (pp. 185–200). Hillsdale, NJ: Erlbaum, 2002.

McNeill, B., "Advancing spoken and written language development in children with childhood apraxia of speech." Unpublished doctoral dissertation. Christchurch, NZ: University of Canterbury, 2007.

McNeill, D., "The two-fold way for speech." In *Problèmes Actuels en Psycholinguistique.* Paris: Editions du Centre National de la Recherche Scientifique, 1974.

McNutt, J., "Oral sensory and motor behaviors of children with /s/ or /r/ misarticulations." *Journal of Speech and Hearing Research, 20* (1977): 694–703.

McNutt, J., "Generalization of /s/ from English to French as a result of phonological remediation." *Journal of Speech-Language Pathology and Audiology, 18* (1994): 109–114.

McReynolds, L. V., "Articulation generalization during articulation training." *Language and Speech, 15* (1972): 149–155.

McReynolds, L. V., and S. Bennett, "Distinctive feature generalization in articulation training." *Journal of Speech and Hearing Disorders, 37* (1972): 462–470.

McReynolds, L. V., and M. Elbert, "An experimental analysis of misarticulating children's generalization." *Journal of Speech and Hearing Research, 21* (1978): 136–150.

Menn, L., "Phonotactic rules in beginning speech." *Lingua, 26* (1971): 225–241.

Menn, L., "Phonological units in beginning speech." In A. Bell and J. B. Hooper (Eds.), *Syllables and Segments* (pp. 157–171). Amsterdam: North Holland, 1978.

Menn, L., "Development of articulatory, phonetic, and phonological capabilities." In B. Butterworth (Ed.), *Language Production* (Vol. 2, pp. 3–50). London: Academic Press, 1983.

Menn, L., "Perspective on research in first language developmental phonology." In M. Yavaş (Ed.), *First and Second Language Pathology* (pp. 3–8). San Diego, CA: Singular Publishing, 1994.

Menn, L., K. Markey, M. Mozer, and C. Lewis, "Connectionist modeling and the microstructure of phonological development: A progress report." In B. de Boysson-Bardies, S. de Schonen, P. Jusczyk, P. McNeilage, and J. Morton (Eds.), *Developmental Neurocognition: Speech and Face Processing in the First Year of Life* (pp. 421–433). Dordrecht: Kluwer Academic, 1993.

Menn, L., and E. Matthei, "The 'two lexicon' account of child phonology looking back, looking ahead." In C. A. Ferguson, L. Menn, and C. Stoel-Gammon (Eds.), *Phonological Development: Models, Research, Implications* (pp. 211–247). Timonium, MA: York, 1992.

Menn, L., and C. Stoel-Gammon, "Phonological development." In P. Fletcher and B. MacWhinney (Eds.), *The Handbook of Child Language* (pp. 335–359) Oxford: Blackwell, 1995.

Menyuk, P., J. Liebergott, and M. Schultz, "Predicting phonological development." In B. Lindblom and R. Zetterström (Eds.), *Precursors of Early Speech* (pp. 79–93). Basingstoke, Hampshire (UK): MacMillan, 1986.

Messner, A. H., and M. L. Lalakea, "The effect of ankyloglossia on speech in children." *Otolaryngology—Head and Neck Surgery, 127* (2002): 539–545.

Meyer, P. G., "Tongue, lip, and jaw differentiation and its relationship to orofacial myofunctional treatment." *International Journal of Orofacial Myology, 26* (2000): 44–52.

Meza, P. "Phonological analysis of Spanish utterances of highly unintelligible Mexican-American children." Unpublished master's thesis, San Diego State University, San Diego, CA, 1983.

Miccio, A., and M. Elbert, "Enhancing stimulability: A treatment program." *Journal of Communication Disorders, 29* (1996): 335–363.

Miccio, A. W., M. Elbert, and K. Forrest, "The relationship between stimulability and phonological acquisition in children with normally developing and disordered phonologies." *American Journal of Speech-Language Pathology, 8* (1999): 347–363.

Mills, A., and H. Streit, "Report of a speech survey, Holyoke, Massachusetts." *Journal of Speech Disorders, 7* (1942): 161–167.

Mines, M., B. Hanson, and J. Shoup, "Frequency of occurrence of phonemes in conversational English." *Language and Speech, 21* (1978): 221–241.

Mitchell, P. R., "Prelinguistic vocal development: A clinical primer." *Contemporary Issues in Communication Science and Disorders, 24* (1997): 87–92.

Moats, L., *Speech to Print.* Baltimore, MD: Brookes, 2000.

Moll, K. L., and R. G. Daniloff, "Investigation of the timing of velar movements during speech." *Journal of the Acoustical Society of America, 50* (1971): 678–684.

Moon, S. J., and B. Lindblom, "Formant undershoot in clear and citation-form speech: A second progress report." Royal Institute of Technology (Stockholm, Sweden). *Speech Transmission Laboratory, Quarterly Progress and Status Reports, 1* (1989): 121–123.

Morais, J., L. Cary, J. Alegria, and P. Bertelson, "Does awareness of speech as a sequence of phones arise spontaneously?" *Cognition, 7* (1979): 323–331.

Moran, M., "Final consonant deletion in African American English: A closer look." *Language, Speech, and Hearing Services in Schools, 24* (1993): 161–166.

Morgan, R., "Structural sketch of Saint Martin Creole." *Anthropological Linguistics, 1*, 8 (1959): 20–24.

Morley, D., "A ten-year survey of speech disorders among university students." *Journal of Speech and Hearing Disorders, 17* (1952): 25–31.

Morrison, J. A., and L. D. Shriberg, "Articulation testing versus conversational speech sampling." *Journal of Speech and Hearing Research, 35* (1992): 259–273.

Mowrer, D. E., *Methods of Modifying Speech Behaviors.* Columbus, OH: Merrill, 1977.

Mowrer, D. E., *Methods of Modifying Speech Behaviors* (2nd ed.). Columbus, OH: Merrill, 1982.

Mowrer, D., R. Baker, and R. Schutz, "Operant procedures in the control of speech articulation." In H. Sloane and B. MacAulay (Eds.), *Operant Procedures in Remedial Speech and Language Training.* Boston: Houghton Mifflin, 1968.

Munson, B., E. M. Bjorum, and J. Windsor, "Acoustic and perceptual correlates of stress in nonwords produced by children with suspected developmental apraxia of speech and children with phonological disorder." *Journal of Speech, Language, and Hearing Research, 46* (2003): 189–202.

Murray, B. A., K. A. Smith, and G. G. Murray, "The test of phoneme identities: Predicting alphabetic insight in prealphabetic readers." *Journal of Literacy Research, 32* (2000): 421–447.

Muter, V., C. Hulme, M. J. Snowling, and J. Stevenson. "Phonemes, Rimes, Vocabulary, and Grammatical Skills as Foundations of Early Reading Development: Evidence from a Longitudinal Study." *Developmental Psychology, 40* (2004): 665–681.

Muyksen, P., and N. Smith, "The study of pidgin and creole languages." In J. Arends, P. Muyksen, and N. Smith (Eds.), *Pidgins and Creoles: An Introduction* (pp. 3–14). Amsterdam: John Benjamins Publishing, 1995.

Muyksen, P., and T. Veenstra, "Haitian." In J. Arends, P. Muyksen, and N. Smith (Eds.), *Pidgins and Creoles: An Introduction* (pp. 153–164). Amsterdam: John Benjamins Publishing, 1995.

Naeser, M. A., "The American child's acquisition of differential vowel duration." Technical Report No. 144, Wisconsin Research and Development Center for Cognitive Learning, University of Wisconsin, Madison, 1970.

Nagy, J., *5–6 Éves Gyermekeink Iskolakészültsége (Preparedness for School of Five to Six Year Old Children).* Budapest: Akadémiai Kiadó, 1980.

Nakanishi, Y., K. Owada, and N. Fujita, "Kōonkensa to sono kekka ni kansuru kōsatsu." *Tokyo Gakugei Daigaku Tokushu Kyoiku Shisetsu Hokoku, 1* (1972): 1–19.

Nathan, L., J. Stackhouse, N. Goulandris, and M. Snowling, "The development of early literacy skills among children with speech difficulties: A test of the 'critical age hypothesis.'" *Journal of Speech, Language and Hearing Research, 47* (2004): 377–391.

Nathani, S., D. J. Ertmer, and R. E. Stark, "Assessing vocal development in infants and toddlers." *Clinical Linguistics and Phonetics, 20*, 5 (2006): 351–369.

Nation, K., and C. Hulme, "Phonemic segmentation, not onset-rime segmentation, predicts early reading and spelling skills." *Reading Research Quarterly, 32* (1997): 154–167.

Neils, J., and D. Aram, "Family history of children with developmental language disorders," *Perceptual and Motor Skills, 63* (1986): 655–658.

Neiva, F. S., and H. F. Wertzner, "A protocol for oral myofunctional assessment: For application with children." *International Journal of Orofacial Myology, 2* (1996): 8–19.

Nelson, L. "Establishing production of speech sound contrasts using minimal 'triads.'" *The Clinical Connection, 8,* 4 (1995): 16–19.

Nemoy, E. M., and S. F. Davis, *The Correction of Defective Consonant Sounds.* Magnolia, MA: Expression Company, 1954.

Netsell, R., *A Neurobiologic View of Speech Production and the Dysarthrias.* Boston: College-Hill Press, 1986.

Netsell, R., W. K. Lotz, J. E. Peters, and L. Schulte, "Developmental patterns of laryngeal and respiratory function for speech production." *Journal of Voice, 8* (1994): 123–131.

Newcomer, P., and E. Barenbaum, *Test of Phonological Awareness Skills.* Austin, TX: Pro-Ed, 2003.

Nichols, P., "Creoles of the USA." In C. Ferguson and S. Heath (Eds.), *Language in the USA* (pp. 69–91). Cambridge: Cambridge University Press, 1981.

Nittrouer, S. "The Relationship between Speech Perception and Phonological Awareness: Evidence from Low SES Children and Children with Chronic OM." *Journal of Speech and Hearing Research, 39* (1996): 1059–1070.

Nittrouer, S., "Challenging the notion of innate phonetic boundaries." *Journal of the Acoustical Society of America, 110,* 3 (2001): 1598–1605.

Norris, J., and P. Hoffman, "Language intervention within naturalistic environments." *Language, Speech, and Hearing Services in Schools, 2* (1990): 72–84.

Norris, J. A., and P. R. Hoffman, "Goals and targets: Facilitating the self-organizing nature of a neuro-network." In A. Kamhi and K. Pollack (Eds.), *Phonological Disorders in Children: Clinical Decision Making in Assessment and Intervention* (pp. 77–87). Baltimore, MD: Brookes, 2005.

Notari-Syverson, A., R. O'Connor, and P. F. Vadasy, *Ladders to Literacy: A Preschool Activity Book.* Baltimore, MD: Brookes, 1998.

Nuffield Centre Dyspraxia Programme. London, England: Royal National Throat Nose and Ear Hospital, 1994.

Núñez-Cedeño, R., and Morales-Front, A., *Fonología generativa contemporánea de la lengua española (Contemporary generative phonology of the Spanish language).* Washington, DC: Georgetown University Press, 1999.

O'Conner, R., and J. R. Jenkins, "Prediction of reading disabilities in kindergarten and first grade." *Scientific Studies of Reading, 3* (1999): 159–197.

O'Connor, R., A. Notari-Syverson, and P. F. Vadasy, *Ladders to Literacy: A Kindergarten Activity Book.* Baltimore, MD: Brookes, 2005.

Oetting, J., "Cajun English speech acquisition." In S. McLeod (Ed.), *The International Guide to Speech Acquisition* (pp. 169–176). Clifton Park, NY: Thomson Delmar Learning, 2007.

O'Grady, W., M. Dobrovolsky, M. Aranoff, and J. Rees-Miller, *Contemporary Linguistics: An Introduction* (5th ed.). New York: St. Martin's Press, 2004.

Ohala, D., "The influence of sonority on children's cluster reductions." *Journal of Communication Disorders, 32* (1999): 397–421.

Oller, D. K., "Metaphonology of infant vocalizations." In B. Lindblom and R. Zetterström (Eds.), *Precursors of Early Speech* (pp. 21–35). Basingstoke, Hampshire (UK): Macmillan, 1986.

Oller, D. K., *The Emergence of the Speech Capacity.* Mahwah, NJ: Erlbaum, 2000.

Oller, D. K., and R. Eilers, "Similarity of babbling in Spanish- and English-learning babies." *Journal of Child Language, 9* (1982): 565–577.

Oller, D. K., and R. E. Eilers, "The role of audition in infant babbling." *Child Development, 59*(2) (1988): 441–449.

Oller, D. K., R. E. Eilers, A. R. Neal, and H. K. Schwartz, "Precursors to speech in infancy: The prediction of speech and language disorders." *Journal of Communication Disorders, 32* (1999): 223–245.

Oller Jr., J. W., S. D. Oller, and L. C. Badon, *Milestones: Normal Speech and Language Development Across the Lifespan.* San Diego, CA: Plural Publishing, 2006.

Olmsted, D., *Out of the Mouth of Babes: Earliest Stages in Language Learning.* The Hague: Mouton, 1971.

Olswang, L. B., and B. A. Bain, "The natural occurrence of generalization articulation treatment." *Journal of Communication Disorders, 18* (1985): 109–129.

Olswang, L. B., and B. Bain, "Data collection: Monitoring children's progress." *American Journal of Speech-Language Pathology, 3* (1994): 55–66.

Otomo, K., and C. Stoel-Gammon, "The acquisition of unrounded vowels in English." *Journal of Speech and Hearing Research, 35* (1992): 604–616.

Overby, M., "Relationships among speech sound perception, speech sound production, and phonological spelling in second grade children." Unpublished doctoral dissertation, University of Nebraska–Lincoln, 2007.

Owens, R. E., *Language Development: An Introduction* (4th ed.). Boston: Allyn and Bacon, 1994.

Ozanne, A. E., "Normative data for sequenced oral movements and movements in context for children aged three to five years." *Australian Journal of Human Communication Disorders, 20* (1992): 47–63.

Pahkala, R., T. Laine, and S. Lammi, "Developmental stage of the dentition and speech sound production in a series of first-grade schoolchildren." *Journal of Craniofacial Genetics and Developmental Biology, 11* (1991): 170–175.

Palin, M., *Contrast Pairs for Phonological Training.* Austin, TX: Pro-Ed, 1992.

Palmer, J., "Tongue-thrusting: A clinical hypothesis." *Journal of Speech and Hearing Disorders, 27* (1962): 323–333.

Panagos, J., and P. Prelock, "Phonological constraints on the sentence productions of language disordered children." *Journal of Speech and Hearing Research, 25* (1982): 171–176.

Panagos, J., M. Quine, and R. Klich, "Syntactic and phonological influences on children's articulation." *Journal of Speech and Hearing Research, 22* (1979): 841–848.

Pandolfi, A. M., and M. O. Herrera, "Producción fonologica diastratica de niños menores de tres años (Phonological production in children less than three-years-old)." *Revista Teorica,* 1990.

Parker, F., "Distinctive features in speech pathology: Phonology or phonemics?" *Journal of Speech and Hearing Disorders, 41* (1976): 23–39.

Parker, F., and K. Riley, *Linguistics for non-linguists: A primer with exercises* (3rd ed.). Boston: Allyn and Bacon, 2000.

Parker, R. G., "Phonological process use in the speech of children fitted with cochlear implants." Unpublished Thesis, University of Tennessee, Knoxville, 2005.

Parlour, S., and P. Broen, "Environmental factors in familial phonological disorders: Preliminary home scale results." Paper presented at the annual convention of the American Speech-Language-Hearing Association, Atlanta, 1991.

Parsons, C. L., T. A. Iacono, and L. Rozner, "Effect of tongue reduction on articulation in children with Down Syndrome." *American Journal of Mental Deficiency, 91* (1987): 328–332.

Pascoe, M., J. Stackhouse, and B. Wells, "Phonological therapy within a psycholinguistic framework: Promoting change in a child with persisting speech difficulties." *International Journal of Language and Communication Disorders, 40* (2005): 189–220.

Pascoe, M., B. Wells, and J. Stackhouse, *Persisting Speech Difficulties in Children: Children's Speech and Literacy Difficulties Book 3.* London: Wiley and Sons, 2006.

Paterson, M., "Articulation and phonological disorders in hearing-impaired school-aged children with severe and profound sensorineural losses." In J. Bernthal and N. Bankson (Eds.), *Child Phonology: Characteristics, Assessment, and Intervention with Special Populations* (pp. 199–224). New York: Thieme Medical Publishers, 1994.

Paul, R., *Language Disorders from Infancy Through Adolescence* (2nd ed.). Philadelphia, PA: Mosby, 2001.

Paul, R., and P. Jennings, "Phonological behavior in toddlers with slow expressive language development." *Journal of Speech and Hearing Research, 35* (1992): 99–107.

Paul, R., and L. D. Shriberg, "Associations between phonology and syntax in speech delayed children." *Journal of Speech and Hearing Research, 25* (1982): 536–546.

Paul, R., and L. D. Shriberg, "Reply to Panagos and Prelock (Letter)." *Journal of Speech and Hearing Research, 27* (1984): 319–320.

Paynter, E. T., and N. A. Petty, "Articulatory sound acquisition of two-year-old children." *Perceptual and Motor Skills, 39* (1974): 1079–1085.

Paynter, W., and T. Bumpas, "Imitative and spontaneous articulatory assessment of three-year-old children." *Journal of Speech and Hearing Disorders, 42* (1977): 119–125.

Pearson, B. Z., S. L. Velleman, T. J. Bryant, and T. Charko, "Contrastive and non-contrastive phonological development in African American English-learning children." Paper submitted for publication.

Perfetti, C. A., I. Beck, L. C. Bell, and C. Hughes, "Phonemic knowledge and learning to read are reciprocal:

A longitudinal study of first grade children." *Merrill-Palmer Quarterly, 33* (1987): 283–319.

Peña, E. D., T. J. Spaulding, and E. Plante, "The composition of normative groups and diagnostic decision making: Shooting ourselves in the foot." *American Journal of Speech-Language Pathology, 15* (2006): 247–254.

Peña-Brooks, A., and M. N. Hegde, *Assessment and Treatment of Articulation and Phonological Disorders in Children.* Austin, TX: Pro-Ed, 2000.

Perez, E., "Phonological differences among speakers of Spanish-influenced English." In J. Bernthal and N. Bankson (Eds.), *Child phonology: Characteristics, Assessment, and Intervention with Special Populations* (pp. 245–254). New York: Thieme Medical Publishers, 1994.

Perkell, J. S., *Physiology of Speech Production.* Cambridge, MA: M.I.T. Press, 1969.

Perkins, W., *Speech Pathology: An Applied Behavioral Science.* St. Louis: Mosby, 1977.

Picheny, M. A., N. I. Durlach, and L. D. Braida, "Speaking clearly for the hard of hearing. II: Acoustic characteristics of clear and conversational speech." *Journal of Speech and Hearing Research, 29* (1986): 434–446.

Pigott, T., J. Barry, B. Hughes, D. Eastin, P. Titus, H. Stensil, K. Metcalf, and B. Porter, *Speech-Ease Screening Inventory (K–1).* Austin, TX: Pro-Ed, 1985.

Polka, L., and O. Bohn, "Asymmetries in vowel perception." *Speech Communication, 41* (2003): 221–231.

Pollock, K., "The identification of vowel errors using transitional articulation or phonological process test stimuli." *Language, Speech, and Hearing Services in Schools, 22* (1991): 39–50.

Pollock, K., "Identification of vowel errors: Methodological issues and preliminary data from the Memphis Vowel Project." In M. J. Ball and F. E. Gibbon (Eds.), *Vowel Disorders* (pp. 83–113) Boston: Butterworth Heinemann, 2002.

Pollock, K., G. Bailey, M. Berni, D. Fletcher, L. Hinton, I. Johnson, and R. Weaver, "Phonological characteristics of African American English Vernacular (AAVE): An updated feature list." Seminar presented at the convention of the American Speech-Language Hearing Association, San Antonio, TX, 1998.

Pollock, K., and M. C. Berni, "Incidence of non-rhotic vowel errors in children: Data from the Memphis Vowel Project." *Clinical Linguistics and Phonetics, 17* (2003): 393–401.

Poole, E., "Genetic development of articulation of consonant sounds in speech." *Elementary English Review, 11* (1934): 159–161.

Poplack, S. "Dialect acquisition among Puerto Rican bilinguals." *Language in Society, 7* (1978): 89–103.

Poplack, S. "Introduction." In S. Poplack (Ed.), *The English History of African American English* (pp. 1–32). Oxford, England: Blackwell, 2000.

Porter, J. H., and B. W. Hodson, "Collaborating to obtain phonological acquisition data for local schools." *Language, Speech, and Hearing Services in Schools, 32* (2001): 165–171.

Powell, T., and L. McReynolds, "A procedure for testing position generalization from articulation training." *Journal of Speech and Hearing Research, 12* (1969): 625–645.

Powell, T. W., and M. Elbert, "Generalization following the remediation of early-and later-developing consonant clusters." *Journal of Speech and Hearing Disorders, 49* (1984): 211–218.

Powell, T. W., M. Elbert, and D. A. Dinnsen, "Stimulability as a factor in the phonologic generalization of misarticulating preschool children." *Journal of Speech and Hearing Research, 34* (1991): 1318–1328.

Powers, M., "Functional disorders of articulation-symptomatology and etiology." In L. Travis (Ed.), *Handbook of Speech Pathology and Audiology.* Englewood Cliffs, NJ: Prentice-Hall, 1957, 1971.

Prather, E. M., D. L. Hedrick, and C. A. Kern, "Articulation development in children aged two to four years." *Journal of Speech and Hearing Disorders, 60* (1975): 179–191.

Preisser, D. A., B. W. Hodson, and E. P. Paden, "Developmental phonology: 18–29 months." *Journal of Speech and Hearing Disorders, 53* (1988): 125–130.

Price, E., and M. Scarry-Larkin, *Phonology* (CD-ROM). San Luis Obispo, CA: LocuTour Multimedia, 1999.

Prince, A. S., and P. Smolensky, *Optimality Theory: Constraint Interaction in Generative Grammar. RUCCS Technical Report #2.* New Brunswick, NJ: Rutgers University Center for Cognitive Science, 1993.

Prins, D., "Analysis of correlations among various articulatory deviations." *Journal of Speech and Hearing Research, 5* (1962a): 151–160.

Prins, D., "Motor and auditory abilities in different groups of children with articulatory deviations."

Journal of Speech and Hearing Research, 5 (1962b): 161–168.

Proffit, W. R., *Contemporary Orthodontics.* St. Louis: Mosby, 1986.

Prosek, R., and A. House, "Intraoral air pressure as a feedback cue in consonant production." *Journal of Speech and Hearing Research, 18* (1975): 133–147.

Rabiner, L., H. Levitt, and A. Rosenberg, "Investigation of stress patterns for speech synthesis by rule." *Journal of the Acoustical Society of America, 45* (1969): 92–101.

Ramirez, A., and R. Milk, "Notions of grammaticality among teachers of bilingual pupils." *TESOL Quarterly, 20* (1986): 495–513.

Read, C., and P. A. Schreiber, "Why short subjects are harder to find than long ones." In E. Wanner and L. Gleitman (Eds.), *Language Acquisition: The State of the Art.* Cambridge (UK): Cambridge University Press, 1982.

Reid, G., "The efficiency of speech re-education of functional articulatory defectives in elementary school." *Journal of Speech and Hearing Disorders, 12* (1947a): 301–313.

Reid, G., "The etiology and nature of functional articulatory defects in elementary school children." *Journal of Speech and Hearing Disorders, 12* (1947b): 143–150.

Rickford, J. (1999). *African American Vernacular English: Features, Evolution, Educational Implications.* Oxford, England: Blackwell.

Ringel, R., K. Burk, and C. Scott, "Tactile perception: Form discrimination in the mouth." In J. Bosma (Ed.), *Second Symposium on Oral Sensation and Perception.* Springfield, IL: Charles Thomas, 1970.

Ringel, R., and S. Ewanowski, "Oral perception: I. Two-point discrimination." *Journal of Speech and Hearing Research, 8* (1965): 389–400.

Ringel, R., A. House, K. Burk, J. Dolinsky, and C. Scott, "Some relations between orosensory discrimination and articulatory aspects of speech production." *Journal of Speech and Hearing Disorders, 35* (1970): 3–11.

Robb, M. P., and K. M. Bleile, "Consonant inventories of young children from 8 to 25 months." *Clinical Linguistics and Phonetics, 8* (1994): 295–320.

Robb, M., H. Gilbert, V. Reed, and A. Bisson, "Speech rates in young Australian English-speaking children: A preliminary study." *Contemporary Issues in Communication Science and Disorders, 30* (2003): 84–91.

Robb, M. P., and G. T. Gillon, "Speech rates of New Zealand English- and American English-speaking children." *Advances in Speech-Language Pathology, 9,* 2 (2007): 173–180.

Robbins, J., and T. Klee, "Clinical assessment of oropharyngeal motor developement in young children." *Journal of Speech and Hearing Disorders, 52* (1987): 271–277.

Roberts, J., S. H. Long, C. Malkin, E. Barnes, M. Skinner, E. A. Hennon, and K. Anderson, "A comparison of phonological skills of boys with Fragile X syndrome and Down syndrome." *Journal of Speech, Language, and Hearing Research, 48* (2005): 980–995.

Roberts, J. E., M. Burchinal, and M. M. Footo, "Phonological process decline from 2;6 to 8 years." *Journal of Communication Disorders, 23* (1990): 205–217.

Roberts, J. E., R. M. Rosenfeld, and S. A Zeisel, "Otitis media and speech and language: A meta-analysis of prospective studies." *Pediatrics, 113* (2004): e238–e248.

Robertson, C., and W. Salter, *The Phonological Awareness Test 2.* East Moline, IL: Linguisystems, 2007.

Robin, D. A., L. B. Somodi, and E. S. Luschei, "Measurement of tongue strength and endurance in normal and articulation disordered subjects." In C. A. Moore, K. M. Yorkston, and D. R. Beukelman (Eds.), *Dysarthria and Apraxia of Speech: Perspectives on Management* (pp. 173–184). Baltimore, MD: Brookes, 1991.

Roca, I., and W. Johnson, *A Course in Phonology.* Oxford: Blackwell, 1999.

Roe, V., and R. Milisen, "The effect of maturation upon defective articulation in elementary grades." *Journal of Speech Disorders, 7* (1942): 37–50.

Rosenbeck, J. C., R. D. Kent, and L. L. LaPointe, "Apraxia of speech: An overview and some perspectives." In J. C. Rosenbeck, M. R. McNeil, and A. E. Aronson (Eds.), *Apraxia of Speech: Physiology, Acoustics, Linguistics Management* (pp. 1–72). San Diego, CA: College Hill Press, 1984.

Rosin, M., E. Swift, D. Bless, and D. K. Vetter, "Communication profiles of adolescents with Down's Syndrome." *Journal of Childhood Communication Disorders, 12* (1988): 49–62.

Roth, F. P., and D. R. Paul, "Partnerships for Literacy: Principles and Practices—Foreword." *Topics in Language Disorders 26* (2006): 2–4.

Roulstone, S., S. Loader, K. Northstone, M. Beveridge, and the ALSPAC team, "The speech and language of children aged 25 months: Descriptive data from the Avon Longitudinal Study of Parents and Children." *Early Child Development and Care, 172,* 3 (2002): 259–268.

Ruben, R. J., "A time frame of critical/sensitive periods of language development." *Acta Otolaryngology, 117* (1997): 202–205.

Ruffoli, R., M. A. Giambellica, M. C. Scavuzzo, D. Bonfigli, R. Cristofani, M. Gabriele, M. R. Giuca, and F. Giannessi, "Ankyloglossia: Amorphofunctional investigation in children." *Oral Diseases, 11* (2005): 170–174.

Ruscello, D., "Articulation improvement and oral tactile changes in children." Thesis, University of West Virginia, 1972.

Ruscello, D., "The importance of word position in articulation therapy." *Language, Speech, and Hearing Services in Schools, 6* (1975): 190–196.

Ruscello, D., "Motor learning as a model for articulation instruction." In J. Costello (Ed.), *Speech Disorders in Children.* San Diego, CA: College-Hill Press, 1984.

Ruscello, D., and R. Shelton, "Planning and self-assessment in articulatory training." *Journal of Speech and Hearing Disorders, 44* (1979): 504–512.

Rvachew, S., "Speech perception training can facilitate sound production learning." *Journal of Speech and Hearing Research, 37* (1994): 347–357.

Rvachew, S., "Perceptual foundations of speech acquisition." In S. McLeod (Ed.), *The International Guide to Speech Acquisition* (pp. 26–30). Clifton Park, NY: Thomson Delmar Learning, 2007a.

Rvachew, S., "Phonological processing and reading in children with speech sound disorders." *American Journal of Speech-Language Pathology, 16* (2007b): 260–270.

Rvachew, S., and M. Nowak, "The effect of target-selection strategy on phonological learning." *Journal of Speech, Language, and Hearing Research, 44* (2001): 610–623.

Rvachew, S., M. Nowak, and G. Cloutier, "Effect of phonemic perception training on the speech production and phonological awareness skills of children with expressive phonological delay." *American Journal of Speech-Language Pathology, 13* (2004): 250–263.

Rvachew, S., A. Ohberg, M. Grawburg, and J. Heyding, "Phonological Awareness and Phonemic Perception in 4-Year-Old Children with Delayed Expressive Phonology Skills." *American Journal of Speech-Language Pathology 12* (2003): 463–471.

Rvachew, S., S. Rafaat, and M. Martin, "Stimulability, speech perception skills, and the treatment of phonological disorders." *American Journal of Speech-Language Pathology, 8* (1999): 33–43.

Sagey, E., "The representation of features and relations in non-linear phonology." Unpublished Ph.D. thesis, Massachusetts Institute of Technology, Cambridge, MA, 1986.

SAILS: Speech Assessment and Interactive Learning System (Computer Software). London, Ontario, Canada: AVAAZ Innovations, 1995.

Samuelsson, S., R. Olson, S. Wadsworth, R. Corley, J. C. DeFries, E. Willcutt, J. Hulslander, and B. Byrne, "Genetic and Environmental Influences on Prereading Skills and Early Reading and Spelling Development in the United States, Australia, and Scandinavia." *Reading and Writing 20,* (2007): 51–75.

Sander, E. K., "When are speech sounds learned?" *Journal of Speech and Hearing Disorders, 37* (1972): 55–63.

Sawyer, D., *Test of Awareness of Language Segments.* Austin, TX: Pro-Ed, 1987.

Sayler, H., "The effect of maturation upon defective articulation in grades seven through twelve." *Journal of Speech and Hearing Disorders, 14* (1949): 202–207.

Scarry-Larkin, M., *Articulation I: Consonant Phonemes.* Austin, TX: Pro-Ed, 2001.

Schiavettei, N., "Scaling procedures for the measurement of speech intelligibility." In R.D. Kent (Ed.), *Intelligibility in Speech Disorders.* Philadelphia: John Benjamin, 1992.

Schlanger, B., "Speech examination of a group of institutionalized mentally handicapped children." *Journal of Speech and Hearing Disorders, 18* (1953): 339–349.

Schlanger, B., and R. Gottsleben, "Analysis of speech defects among the institutionalized mentally retarded." *Journal of Speech and Hearing Disorders, 22* (1957): 98–103.

Schmauch, V., J. Panagos, and R. Klich, "Syntax influences the accuracy of consonant production in language-disordered children." *Journal of Communication Disorders, 11* (1978): 315–323.

Schmitt, L. S., B. H. Howard, and J. F. Schmitt, "Conversational speech sampling in the assessment of articulation proficiency." *Language, Speech, and Hearing Services in Schools, 14* (1983): 210–214.

Schuele, C. M., "The impact of developmental speech and language impairments on the acquisition of literacy skills." *Mental Retardation and Developmental Disabilities Research Reviews, 10* (2004): 176–183.

Schuele, C. M., and N. D. Dayton, *Intensive Phonological Awareness Program.* Cleveland, OH: Authors, 2000.

Schuele, C. M., K. Paul, and K. Mazzaferri, "Phonological awareness training: Is it worth the time?" Paper presented at the annual convention of the American Speech-Language-Hearing Association, San Antonio, TX, 1998.

Schuele, C. M., L. Justice, S. Cabell, K. Knighton, B. Kingery, and M. Lee, "Field-based evaluation of two-tiered instruction for enhancing kindergarten phonological awareness." *Early Education and Development*, in press.

Schuele, C. M., L. Skibbe, and P. Rao, "Assessing phonological awareness." In K. Pence (Ed.), *Assessment in emergent literacy* (pp. 275–326). San Diego: Plural Publishing.

Schwartz, A., and R. Goldman, "Variables influencing performance on speech sound discrimination tests." *Journal of Speech and Hearing Research, 17* (1974): 25–32.

Schwartz, R. G., "Nonlinear phonology as a framework for phonological acquisition." In R. S. Chapman (Ed.), *Processes in Language Acquisition and Disorders.* Chicago: Mosby-Year Book, 1992.

Schwartz, R. G., and L. B. Leonard, " 'Do children pick and choose?' An examination of phonological selection and avoidance in early lexical acquisition." *Journal of Child Language, 9* (1982): 319–336.

Schwartz, R. G., L. Leonard, M. K. Folger, and M. J. Wilcox, "Evidence for a synergistic view of linguistic disorders: Early phonological behavior in normal and language disordered children." *Journal of Speech and Hearing Disorders, 45* (1980): 357–377.

Schwartz, R. G., L. B. Leonard, M. J. Wilcox, and M. K. Folger, "Again and again: Reduplication in child phonology." *Journal of Child Language, 7* (1980): 75–87.

Scobbie, J. M., O. Gordeeva, and B. Matthews, "Scottish English speech acquisition." In S. McLeod (Ed.), *The International Guide to Speech Acquisition* (pp. 221–240) Clifton Park, NY: Thomson Delmar Learning, 2007.

Scott, C., and R. Ringel, "Articulation without oral sensory control." *Journal of Speech and Hearing Research, 14* (1971): 804–818.

Scripture, M. K., and E. Jackson, *A Manual of Exercises for the Correction of Speech Disorders.* Philadelphia, PA: F. A. Davis, 1927.

Secord, W., "The traditional approach to treatment." In N. Creaghead, P. Newman, and W. Secord (Eds.), *Assessment and Remediation of Articulatory and Phonological Disorders.* Columbus, OH: Merrill, 1989.

Secord, W., S. E. Boyce, J. S. Donahue, R. A. Fox, and R. E. Shine, *Eliciting Sounds: Techniques and Strategies for Clinicians* (2nd ed.). Greenville, SC: Super Duper Publications, 2007.

Secord, W., and R. Shine, *Secord Contextual Articulation Tests (S-CAT).* Sedona, AZ: Red Rock Educational Publications, 1997a.

Secord, W. A., and R. E. Shine, *Target Words for Contextual Training.* Sedona, AZ: Red Rock Educational Publications, 1997b.

Selby, J. C., M. P. Robb, and H. R. Gilbert, "Normal vowel articulations between 15 and 36 months of age." *Clinical Linguistics and Phonetics, 14* (2000): 255–266.

Seymour, H., and C. Seymour, "A therapeutic model for communicative disorders among children who speak Black English Vernacular." *Journal of Speech and Hearing Disorders, 42* (1977): 247–256.

Seymour, H., and C. Seymour, "Black English and Standard American English contrasts in consonantal development of four- and five-year-old children." *Journal of Speech and Hearing Disorders, 46* (1981): 274–280.

Shafer, V. L., D. W. Shucard, J. L. Shucard, and L. Gerken, "An electrophysiological study of infants' sensitivity to the sound patterns of English speech." *Journal of Speech, Language, and Hearing Research, 41* (1998): 874–886.

Shahidullah, S., and P. G. Hepper, "Hearing in the fetus: Prenatal detection of deafness." *International Journal of Prenatal and Perinatal Studies, 4* 3/4 (1992): 235–240.

Sheahan, P., I. Miller, J. N. Sheahan, M. J. Earley, and A. W. Blayney, "Incidence and outcome of middle ear disease in cleft lip and/or cleft palate." *International Journal of Pediatric Otorhinolaryngology, 67* (2003): 758–793.

Shelton, R., "Disorders of articulation." In P. Skinner and R. Shelton (Eds.), *Speech, Language, and Hearing.* Reading, MA: Addison-Wesley, 1978.

Shelton, R., personal communication, 1986.

Shelton, R., "Science, clinical art, and speech pathology." Paper presented at Kansas University, Spring 1989.

Shelton, R., A. F. Johnson, and W. B. Arndt, "Monitoring and reinforcement by parents as a means of automating articulatory responses." *Perceptual and Motor Skills, 35* (1972): 759–767.

Shelton, R., A. Johnson, and W. Arndt, "Delayed judgment speech sound discrimination and /r/ or /s/ articulation status and improvement." *Journal of Speech and Hearing Research, 20* (1977): 704–717.

Shelton, R., A. F. Johnson, V. Willis, and W. B. Arndt, "Monitoring and reinforcement by parents as a means of automating articulatory responses: II. Study of pre-school children." *Perceptual and Motor Skills, 40* (1975): 599–610.

Shelton, R., V. Willis, A. F. Johnson, and W. B. Arndt, "Oral form recognition training and articulation change." *Perceptual and Motor Skills, 36* (1973): 523–531.

Sherman, D., and A. Geith, "Speech sound discrimination and articulation skill." *Journal of Speech and Hearing Disorders, 10* (1967): 277–280.

Shprintzen, R. J. *Genetics, Syndromes, and Communication Disorders.* San Diego, CA: Singular Publishing, 1997.

Shriberg, L. D., "A response evocation program for /ɝ/." *Journal of Speech and Hearing Disorders, 40* (1975): 92–105.

Shriberg, L. D., "Toward classification of developmental phonological disorders" (pp. 1–18). In N. J. Lass (Ed.), *Speech and Language: Advances in Basic Research and Practice, Vol. 8.* Philadelphia: Saunders, 1982.

Shriberg, L. D., *Programs to Examine Phonetic and Phonologic Evaluation Records (PEPPER).* Hillsdale, NJ: Erlbaum, 1986.

Shriberg, L. D., "Directions for research in developmental phonological disorders." In J. Miller (Ed.), *Research on Child Language Disorders: A Decade of Progress* (pp. 267–276). Austin, TX: Pro-Ed, 1991.

Shriberg, L. D., "Four new speech and prosody-voice measures for genetics research and other studies in developmental phonological disorders." *Journal of Speech and Hearing Research, 36* (1993): 105–140.

Shriberg, L. D., D. M. Aram, and J. Kwiatkowski, "Developmental apraxia of speech: I. Descriptive and theoretical perspecives." *Journal of Speech, Language, and Hearing Research, 40* (1997a): 273–285.

Shriberg, L. D., D. M. Aram, and J. Kwiatkowski, "Developmental apraxia of speech: II. Toward a diagnostic marker." *Journal of Speech, Language, and Hearing Research, 40* (1997b): 286–312.

Shriberg, L. D., and D. Austin, "Comorbidity of speech-language disorder. Implications for a phenotype marker for speech delay." In R. Paul (Ed.) *Exploring the Speech-Language Connection* (pp. 73–117). Baltimore, MD: Brookes. 1998.

Shriberg, L. D., D. Austin, B. A. Lewis, J. L. McSweeny, and D. L. Wilson, "The percentage of consonants correct (PCC) metric: Extensions and reliability data." *Journal of Speech, Language and Hearing Research, 40* (1997a): 708–722.

Shriberg, L. D., D. Austin, B. A. Lewis, J. L. McSweeney, and D. L. Wilson, "The speech disorders classification system (SDCS): Extension and lifespan reference data." *Journal of Speech, Language, Hearing Research, 40* (1997b): 723–740.

Shriberg, L. D., K. J. Ballard, J. B. Tomblin, J. R. Duffy, K. H. Odell, and C. A. Williams, "Speech, prosody, and voice characteristics of a mother and daughter with a 7:13 translocation affecting FOXP2." *Journal of Speech, Language, and Hearing Research, 49* (2006): 500–525.

Shriberg, L. D., P. Flipsen Jr., H. B. Karlsson, and J. L. McSweeny. "Acoustic phenotypes for speech-genetics studies: An acoustic marker for residual /ɝ/ distortions. *Clinical Linguistics and Phonetics, 15* (2001): 631–650.

Shriberg, L. D., P. Flipsen Jr., J. Kwiatkowski, and J. L. McSweeny, "A diagnostic marker for speech delay associated with otitis media with effusion: The intelligibility-speech gap." *Clinical Linguistics and Phonetics, 17* (2003): 507–528.

Shriberg, L. D., P. Flipsen Jr., H. Thielke, J. Kwiatkowski, M. Kertoy, R. Nellis, and M. Block, "Risk for speech disorder associated with early recurrent otitis media with effusion: two retrospective studies." *Journal of Speech, Language, and Hearing Research, 43* (2000): 79–99.

Shriberg, L. D., S. Friel-Patti, P. Flipsen Jr., and R. L. Brown, "Otitis media, fluctuant hearing loss and speech-language delay: A preliminary structural equation model." *Journal of Speech, Language, and Hearing Research, 43* (2000): 100–120.

Shriberg, L. D., R. D. Kent, H. B. Karlsson, C. J. Nadler, and R. L. Brown, "A diagnostic marker for speech delay associated with otitis media with effusion:

backing of obstruents." *Clinical Linguistics and Phonetics, 17* (2003): 529–547.

Shriberg, L. D., and J. Kwiatkowski, *Natural Process Analysis.* New York: Wiley, 1980.

Shriberg, L. D., and J. Kwiatkowski, "Phonological disorders III: A procedure for assessing severity of involvement." *Journal of Speech and Hearing Disorders, 42* (1982a): 242–256.

Shriberg, L. D., and J. Kwiatkowski, "Phonological disorderss II: A conceptual framework for management." *Journal of Speech and Hearing Disorders, 42* (1982b): 242–256.

Shriberg, L. D., and J. Kwiatkowski, "Computer-assisted natural process analysis (NPA): Recent issues and data." In J. Locke (Ed.), *Assessing and Treating Phonological Disorders: Current Approaches*, Seminars in Speech and Language, 4. New York: Thieme-Stratton, 1983.

Shriberg, L. D., and J. Kwiatkowski, "A retrospective study of spontaneous generalization in speech-delayed children." *Language, Speech and Hearing Services in Schools, 18* (1987): 144–157.

Shriberg, L. D., and J. Kwiatkowski, "Self-monitoring and generalization in preschool speech-delayed children." *Language, Speech and Hearing Services in Schools, 21* (1990): 157–170.

Shriberg, L. D., and J. Kwiatkowski, "Developmental phonological disorders I: A clinical profile." *Journal of Speech and Hearing Research, 37* (1994): 1100–1126.

Shriberg, L. D., J. Kwiatkowski, S. Best, J. Hengst, and B. Terselic-Weber, "Characteristics of children with phonologic disorders of unknown origin." *Journal of Speech and Hearing Disorders, 51* (1986): 140–161.

Shriberg, L. D., J. Kwiatkowski, and F. A. Gruber, "Developmental phonological disorders II: Short-term speech-sound normalisation." *Journal of Speech and Hearing Research, 37* (1994): 1127–1150.

Shriberg, L. D., J. Kwiatkowski, and K. Hoffman, "A procedure for phonetic transcription by consensus." *Journal of Speech and Hearing Research, 27* (1984): 456–465.

Shriberg, L. D., B. A. Lewis, J. B. Tomblin, J. L. McSweeny, H. B. Karlsson, and A. R. Scheer, "Toward diagnostic and phenotype markers for genetically transmitted speech delay." *Journal of Speech, Language, and Hearing Research, 48* (2005): 834–852.

Shriberg, L. D., and G. L. Lof, "Reliability studies in broad and narrow phonetic transcription." *Clinical Linguistics and Phonetics, 5* (1991): 225–279.

Shriberg, L. D., and C. Widder, "Speech and prosody characteristics of adults with mental retardation." *Journal of Speech and Hearing Research, 33* (1990): 627–653.

Shriner, T., M. Holloway, and R. Daniloff, "The relationship between articulatory deficits and syntax in speech defective children." *Journal of Speech and Hearing Research, 12* (1969): 319–325.

Shuy, R. (1972). "Social dialect and employability: Some pitfalls of good intentions." In L. Davis (Ed.), *Studies in Linguistics.* Birmingham: University of Alabama Press.

Siegel, R., H. Winitz, and H. Conkey, "The influence of testing instruments in articulatory responses of children." *Journal of Speech and Hearing Disorders, 28* (1963): 67–76.

Silverman, E., "Listeners' impressions of speakers with lateral lisps." *Journal of Speech and Hearing Disorders, 41* (1976): 547–552.

Siqueland, E. R., and C. A. Delucia, "Visual reinforcement of non-nutritive sucking in human infants." *Science, 165* (1969): 1144–1146.

Skelly, M., D. Spector, R. Donaldson, A. Brodeur, and F. Paletta, "Compensatory physiologic phonetics for the glossectomee." *Journal of Speech and Hearing Disorders, 36* (1971): 101–114.

Skinner, B. F., *Cumulative Record: A Selection of Papers* (3rd ed.). New York: Appleton-Century-Crofts, 1972.

Sloat, C., S. H. Taylor, and J. E. Hoard, *Introduction to Phonology.* Englewood Cliffs, NJ: Prentice-Hall, 1978.

Small, L. (2004). *Fundamentals of Phonetics: A Practical Guide for Students* (2nd ed.). Boston: Allyn and Bacon.

Smit, A. B., "Ages of speech sound acquisition: Comparisons and critiques of several normative studies." *Language, Speech, and Hearing Services in Schools, 17* (1986): 175–186.

Smit, A. B., "Phonologic error distributions in the Iowa-Nebraska articulation norms project: Consonant singletons." *Journal of Speech and Hearing Research, 36* (1993a): 533–547.

Smit, A. B., "Phonologic error distributions in the Iowa-Nebraska articulation norms project: Word-initial consonant clusters." *Journal of Speech and Hearing Research, 36* (1993b): 931–947.

Smit, A. B., *Articulation and Phonology Resource Guide for School-Age Children and Adults.* Clifton Park, NY: Delmar Learning, 2004.

Smit, A. B., "General American English speech acquisition." In S. McLeod (Ed.), *The International Guide to Speech Acquisition* (pp. 128–147) Clifton Park, NY: Thomson Delmar Learning, 2007.

Smit, A. B., and J. Bernthal, "Voicing contrasts and their phonological implications in the speech of articulation-disordered children." *Journal of Speech and Hearing Research, 26* (1983): 19–28.

Smit, A. B., and L. Hand, *Smit-Hand Articulation and Phonology Evaluation (SHAPE)*. Los Angeles: Western Psychological Services, 1972, 1997.

Smit, A. B., L. Hand, J. J. Freilinger, J. E. Bernthal, and A. Bird, "The Iowa articulation norms project and its Nebraska replication." *Journal of Speech and Hearing Disorders, 55* (1990): 779–798.

Smith, A. B., L. Goffman, H. N. Zelaznik, G. Ying, and C. McGillem, "Spatiotemporal stability and patterning of speech movement sequences." *Experimental Brain Research, 104* (1995): 493–501.

Smith, B. L., "Temporal aspects of English speech production: A developmental perspective." *Journal of Phonetics, 6* (1978): 37–67.

Smith, B. L., K. K. McGregor, and D. Demille, "Phonological development in lexically precocious 2-year-olds." *Applied Psycholinguistics, 27* (2006): 355–375.

Smith, B. L., and C. Stoel-Gammon, "A longitudinal study of the development of stop consonant production in normal and Down's Syndrome children." *Journal of Speech and Hearing Disorders, 48* (1983): 114–118.

Smith, M. W., and S. Ainsworth, "The effect of three types of stimulation on articulatory responses of speech defective children." *Journal of Speech and Hearing Research, 10* (1967): 333–338.

Smith, N. V., *The Acquisition of Phonology: A Case Study*. New York: Cambridge University Press, 1973.

Snow, D., "Phrase-final syllable lengthening and intonation in early child speech." *Journal of Speech and Hearing Research, 37* (1994): 831–840.

Snow, J., and R. Milisen, "The influences of oral versus pictorial representation upon articulation testing results." *Journal of Speech and Hearing Disorders. Monograph Supplement, 4* (1954): 29–36.

Snow, K., "Articulation proficiency in relation to certain dental abnormalities." *Journal of Speech and Hearing Disorders, 26* (1961): 209–212.

Snowling, M., D. V. M. Bishop, and S. E. Stothard, "Is Preschool Language Impairment a Risk Factor for Dyslexia in Adolescence?" *Journal of Child Psychology and Psychiatry and Allied Disciplines 41* (2000): 587–600.

So, L., and B. Dodd, "Phonologically disordered Cantonese-speaking children." *Clinical Linguistics and Phonetics, 8* (1994): 235–255.

So, L. K. H., and B. J. Dodd, "The acquisition of phonology by Cantonese-speaking children." *Journal of Child Language, 22* (1995): 473–495.

Sommers, R. K., "Factors in the effectiveness of mothers trained to aid in speech correction." *Journal of Speech and Hearing Disorders, 27* (1962): 178–186.

Sommers, R. K., "The therapy program." In R. Van Hattum (Ed.), *Clinical Speech in the Schools*. Springfield, IL: Charles Thomas, 1969.

Sommers, R. K., A. K. Furlong, F. H. Rhodes, G. R. Fichter, D. C. Bowser, F. H. Copetas, and Z. G. Saunders, "Effects of maternal attitudes upon improvement in articulation when mothers are trained to assist in speech correction." *Journal of Speech and Hearing Disorders, 29* (1964): 126–132.

Sommers, R. K., R. Leiss, M. Delp, A. Gerber, D. Fundrella, R. Smith, M. Revucky, D. Ellis, and V. Haley, "Factors related to the effectiveness of articulation therapy for kindergarten, first- and second-grade children." *Journal of Speech and Hearing Research, 10* (1967): 428–437.

Sommers, R. K., R. Reinhart, and D. Sistrunk, "Traditional articulation measures of Down's Syndrome speakers, ages 13–22." *Journal of Childhood Communication Disorders, 12* (1988): 93–108.

Sommers, R. K., M. H. Schaeffer, R. H. Leiss, A. J. Gerber, M. A. Bray, D. Fundrella, J. K. Olson, and E. R. Tomkins, "The effectiveness of group and individual therapy." *Journal of Speech and Hearing Research, 9* (1966): 219–225.

Sonderman, J., "An experimental study of clinical relationships between auditory discrimination and articulation skills." Paper presented at the annual convention of the American Speech and Hearing Association, San Francisco, 1971.

Sowell, E. R., P. M. Thompson, C. M. Leonard, S. E. Welcome, E. Kan, and A. W. Toga, "Longitudinal mapping of cortical thickness and brain growth in normal children." *Journal of Neuroscience, 24*, 38 (2004): 8223–8231.

Sowell, E. R., P. M. Thompson, and A. W. Toga, "Mapping changes in the human cortex throughout the span of life." *Neuroscientist, 10*, 4 (2004): 372–392.

Spector, J., "Predicting progress in beginning reading: Dynamic assessment of phonemic awareness." *Journal of Educational Psychology, 84* (1992): 353–363.

Speirs, R. L., and M. A. Maktabi, "Tongue skills and clearance of toffee in two age-groups and in children with problems of speech articulation." *Journal of Dentistry for Children, 57* (1990): 356–360.

Spencer, A., "A nonlinear analysis of phonological disability." *Journal of Communication Disorders, 17* (1984): 325–348.

Spencer, A., "Towards a theory of phonological development." *Lingua, 68* (1986): 3–38.

Spencer, A., "A phonological theory of phonological development." In M. J. Ball (Ed.), *Theoretical Linguistics and Disordered Language* (pp. 115–151). London: Croom Helm, 1988.

Spencer, A., *Phonology.* Oxford, UK: Blackwell, 1996.

Square, P., "Treatment of developmental apraxia of speech: Tactile-kinesthetic, rhythmic, and gestural approaches." In A. Caruso and E. Strand (Eds.), *Clinical Management of Motor Speech Disorders in Children.* New York: Thieme, 1999.

St. Louis, K., and D. Ruscello, *The Oral Speech Screening Examination.* Baltmore, MD: University Park Press, 2000.

Stackhouse, J., "Barriers to literacy development in children with speech and language difficulties." In D. Bishop and L. Leonard (Eds.), *Speech and Language Impairments in Children: Causes, Characteristics, Intervention and Outcome* (pp. 73–98). Hove, UK: Psychology Press, 2000.

Stackhouse, J., and B. Wells, "Psycholinguistic assessment of developmental speech disorders." *European Journal of Disorders of Communication, 28* (1993): 331–348.

Stackhouse, J., and B. Wells, *Children's Speech and Literacy Difficulties I: A Psycholinguistic Framework.* London: Whurr Publishers, 1997.

Stackhouse, J., and B. Wells, *Children's Speech and Literacy Difficulties: Identification and Intervention.* London: Whurr, 2001.

Stackhouse, J., M. Pascoe, and H. Gardner, "Intervention for a child with persisting speech and literacy difficulties: A psycholinguistic approach." *Advances in Speech-Language Pathology, 8*(3) (2006): 231–244.

Stackhouse, J., M. Vance, M. Pascoe, and B. Wells, *Compendium of auditory and speech tasks. Children's speech and literacy difficulties 4.* Chichester: John Wiley and Sons, 2007.

Stahl, S. A., and B. A. Murray, "Defining phonological awareness and its relationship to early reading." *Journal of Educational Psychology, 86* (1994): 221–234.

Stampe, D., "The Acquisition of Phonetic Representation." Paper presented at the Papers from the Fifth Regional Meeting of the Chicago Linguistic Society, Chicago, 1969.

Stampe, D. *A Dissertation on Natural Phonology.* New York: Garland, 1979.

Stanovich, K., "Matthew effects in reading: Some consequences of individual differences in the acquisition of literacy." *Reading Research Quarterly, 21* (1986): 360–407.

Stanovich, K., *Progress in Understanding Reading. Scientific Foundations and New Frontiers.* New York: Guilford Press, 2000.

Stark, R. E., L. E. Bernstein, and M. E. Demorest, "Vocal communication in the first 18 months of life." *Journal of Speech and Hearing Research, 36* (1983): 548–558.

Starr, C., "Dental and occlusal hazards to normal speech production." In K. Bzoch (Ed.), *Communicative Disorders Related to Cleft Lip and Palate.* Boston: Little, Brown, 1972.

Stelcik, J., "An investigation of internal versus external discrimination and general versus phoneme-specific discrimination." Unpublished Thesis, University of Maryland, 1972.

Stemberger, J. P., "Between-word processes in child phonology." *Journal of Child Language, 15* (1988): 39–61.

Stemberger, J. P., "Speech errors in early child language production." *Journal of Memory and Language, 28* (1989):164–188.

Stemberger, J. P., and B. H. Bernhardt, "Optimality theory." In M. J. Ball and R. D. Kent (Eds.), *The New Phonologies: Developments in Clinical Linguistics* (pp. 211–245). San Diego, CA: Singular Publishing, 1997.

Stepanof, E. R. "Procesos phonologicos de niños Puertorriqueños de 3 y 4 años evidenciado en la prueba APP-Spanish (Phonological processes evidenced on the APP-Spanish by 3- and 4-year-old Puerto Rican children)." *Opphla, 8* 2 (1990): 15–20.

Stephens, M. I., P. Hoffman, and R. Daniloff, "Phonetic characteristics of delayed /s/ development." *Journal of Phonetics, 14* (1986): 247–256.

Steriade, D., "Greek Prosodies and the Nature of Syllabification." Unpublished doctoral dissertation, Massachusetts Institute of Technology, 1990.

Stewart, S. R., and G. Weybright, "Articulation norms used by practicing speech-language pathologists in

Oregon: Results of a survey." *Journal of Speech and Hearing Disorders, 45* (1980): 103–111.

Stewart, W., "Continuity and change in American Negro dialects." In W. Wolfram and N. Clarke (Eds.), *Black-White speech relationships* (pp. 51–73). Washington, DC: Center for Applied Linguistics, 1971.

Stockman, I., "Phonological development and disorders in African American children." In A. Kamhi, K. Pollock, and J. Harris (Eds.), *Communication Development and Disorders I in African American Children* (pp. 117–154). Baltimore, MD: Brookes, 1996a.

Stockman, I., "The promises and pitfalls of language sample analysis as an assessment tool for linguistic minority children." *Language, Speech, and Hearing Services in Schools, 27* (1996b): 355–366.

Stockman, I., "Evidence for a minimal competence core of consonant sounds in the speech of African American children: A preliminary study." *Clinical Linguistics and Phonetics, 20* (2006a): 723–749.

Stockman, I., "Alveolar bias in the final consonant deletion patterns of African American children." *Language, Speech, and Hearing Services in Schools, 37* (2006b): 85–95.

Stockman, I. J., and L. W. Stephenson, "Children's articulation of medial consonant clusters: Implications for syllabification. *Language and Speech, 24* (1981): 185–204.

Stoel-Gammon, C., "Phonetic inventories, 15–24 months: A longitudinal study." *Journal of Speech and Hearing Research, 28* (1985): 505–512.

Stoel-Gammon, C., "Phonological skills of 2-year-olds." *Language, Speech, and Hearing Services in Schools, 18* (1987): 323–329.

Stoel-Gammon, C., "Prespeech and early speech development of two late talkers." *First Language, 9* (1989): 207–224.

Stoel-Gammon, C., "Normal and disordered phonology in two-year-olds." *Topics in Language Disorders, 11* (1991): 21–32.

Stoel-Gammon, C., "Normal and disordered phonology in two-year olds." In K. Butler (Ed.), *Early Intervention: Working with Infants and Toddlers* (pp. 110–121). Rockville, MD: Aspen, 1994.

Stoel-Gammon, C., "Variability in the productions of young typically-developing children." Paper presented the meeting of the International Clinical Linguistics and Phonetics Association, Lafayette, LA, 2004.

Stoel-Gammon, C., "Variability in speech acquisition." In S. McLeod (Ed.), *The International Guide to Speech Acquisition* (pp. 55–60). Clifton Park, NY: Thomson Delmar Learning, 2007.

Stoel-Gammon, C., and C. Dunn, *Normal and Disordered Phonology in Children*. Baltimore, MD: University Park Press, 1985.

Stoel-Gammon, C. and P. B. Herrington, "Vowel systems of normally developing and phonologically disordered children." *Clinical Linguistics and Phonetics, 4* (1990): 145–160.

Stoel-Gammon, C., and M. Kehoe, "Hearing impairment in infants and toddlers: Identification, vocal development, and intervention in child phonology." In J. Bernthal and N. Bankson (Eds.), *Child Phonology: Characteristics, Assessment, and Intervention with Special Populations* (pp 163–181). New York: Thieme Medical Publishers, 1994.

Stoel-Gammon, C., and K. Otomo, "Babbling development of hearing-impaired and normally hearing subjects." *Journal of Speech and Hearing Disorders, 51*, 1 (1986): 33–41.

Stokes, S. F., T. Klee, C. P. Carson, and D. Carson, "A phonemic implicational feature hierarchy of phonological contrasts for English-speaking children." *Journal of Speech, Language, and Hearing Research, 48*, 4 (2005): 817–833.

Stokes, T. F., and D. M. Baer, "An implicit technology of generalization." *Journal of Applied Behavior Analysis, 10* (1977): 349–367.

Storch, S. A., and G. J. Whitehurst, "Oral Language and Code-Related Precursors to Reading: Evidence from a Longitudinal Structural Model." *Developmental Psychology 38* (2002): 934–947.

Storkel, H. L., "The emerging lexicon of children with phonological delays: Phonotactic constraints and probability in acquisition." *Journal of Speech, Language, and Hearing Research, 47* (2005): 1194–1212.

Storkel, H. L., "Do children still pick and choose? The relationship between phonological knowledge and lexical acquisition beyond 50 words." *Clinical Linguistics and Phonetics, 20*, 7/8 (2006): 523–529.

Storkel, H. L., and M. L. Morrisette, "The lexicon and phonology: Interactions in language acquisition." *Language, Speech, and Hearing Services in Schools, 33* (2002): 24–37.

Strand, E., and R. McCauley, "Assessment procedures for treatment planning in children with phonologic and motor speech disorders." In A. Caruso and E. Strand (Eds.), *Clinical Management of Motor*

Speech Disorders in Children. New York: Thieme, 1999.

Strand, E., and A. Skindner, "Treatment of developmental apraxia of speech: Integral stimulation methods." In A. Caruso and E. Strand (Eds.), *Clinical Management of Motor Speech Disorders in Children*. New York: Thieme, 1999.

Strange, W., and P. Broen, "Perception and production of approximant consonants by 3 year olds: A first study." In G. Yeni-Komshian, J. Kavanaugh, and C. A. Ferguson (Eds.), *Child Phonology, Vol. 2, Perception*. New York: Academic Press, 1980.

Subtelny, J., "Malocclusions, orthodontic corrections and orofacial muscle adaptation." *Angle Orthodontist, 40* (1970): 170.

Subtelny, J., J. Mestre, and J. Subtelny, "Comparative study of normal and defective articulation of /s/ as related to malocclusion and deglutition." *Journal of Speech and Hearing Disorders, 29* (1964): 269–285.

Subtelny, J., J. Worth, and M. Sakuda, "Intraoral pressure and rate of flow during speech." *Journal of Speech and Hearing Research, 9* (1966): 498–518.

Sullivan, M., C. Gaebler, D. Beukelman, G. Mahanna, J. Marshall, D. Lydiatt, and W. Lydiatt, "Impact of palatal prosthodontic intervention on communication performance of patients' maxillectomy defects: A multi-level outcome study." *Head and Neck, 24*, 6 (2002): 530–538.

Sutherland, D., and G. T. Gillon, "Assessment of phonological representations in children with speech impairment." *Language Speech and Hearing Services in Schools, 36* (2005): 294–307.

Sutherland, D., and G. T. Gillon, "Development of phonological representations and phonological awareness in children with speech impairment." *International Journal of Language and Communication Disorders, 42* 2 (2007): 229–250.

Swank, L., and H. Catts, "Phonological awareness and written word decoding." *Language, Speech, and Hearing Services in Schools, 25* (1994): 9–14.

Swanson, T. J., B. W. Hodson, and M. Schommer-Aikins, "An examination of phonological awareness treatment outcomes for 7th grade poor readers from a bilingual community." *Language, Speech and Hearing Services in Schools, 36* (2005): 336–345.

Tang, G., and J. Barlow, "Characteristics of the sound systems of monolingual Vietnamese-speaking children with phonological impairment." *Clinical Linguistics and Phonetics, 20* (2006): 423–445.

Taylor, O., "Teaching standard English as a second dialect." In O. Taylor (Ed.), *Treatment of Communication Disorders in Culturally and Linguistically Diverse Populations* (pp. 153–178). San Diego, CA: College-Hill Press, 1986.

Taylor, O., K. Payne, and N. Anderson, "Distinguishing between communication disorders and differences." *Seminars in Speech and Language, 8* (1987): 45–427.

Teele, D. W., J. O. Klein, B. A. Rosner, and the Greater Boston Otitis Media Study Group, "Otitis media with effusion during the first three years of life and development of speech and language." *Pediatrics, 74* (1984): 282–287.

Terai, H., and M. Shimahara, "Evaluation of speech intelligibility after a secondary dehiscence operation using an artificial graft in patients with speech disorders after partial glossectomy." *British Journal of Oral and Maxillofacial Surgery, 42* (2004): 190–194.

Templin, M., "Spontaneous vs. imitated verbalization in testing pre-school children." *Journal of Speech and Hearing Disorders, 12* (1947): 293–300.

Templin, M., "Certain language skills in children." *Institute of Child Welfare Monograph Series 26*. Minneapolis: University of Minnesota, 1957.

Templin, M., "Development of speech." *Journal of Pediatrics, 62* (1963): 11–14.

Templin, M., "Longitudinal study through the 4th grade of language skills of children with varying speech sound articulation in kindergarten" (Final Report, Project 2220). Washington, DC: U.S. Department of Health, Education, and Welfare, Office of Education, 1968.

Templin, M., and G. Glaman, "A longitudinal study of correlations of predictive measures obtained in prekindergarten and first grade with achievement measures through eleventh grade" (Unpublished report #101). Washington, DC: U.S. Department of Health, Education, and Welfare, Office of Education, 1976.

Terrell, S., and F. Terrell, "Effects of speaking Black English upon employment opportunities." *ASHA, 25* (1983): 27–29.

Thomas, R. M., *Comparing Theories of Child Development* (5th ed.). Belmont, CA: Wadsworth, 2000.

Thompson, A. E., and T. J. Hixon, "Nasal air flow during speech production." *Cleft Palate Journal, 16* (1979): 412–420.

Tiffany, W., "Effects of syllable structure on diadochokinetic and reading rates." *Journal of Speech and Hearing Research, 23* (1980): 894–908.

Tingley, B. M., and G. D. Allen, "Development of speech timing control in children." *Child Development, 46* (1975): 186–194.

Tipton, G., "Non-cognate consonants of Mandarin and Cantonese." *Journal of the Chinese Language Teachers Association, 10,* 1 (1975): 1–13.

Torgesen, J., "Assessment and instruction for phonemic awareness and word recognition skills." In H. Catts and A. Kamhi (Eds.), *Language and Reading Disabilities* (pp. 128–153). Boston: Allyn and Bacon, 1999.

Torgesen, J., and B.Bryant, *Test of phonological awareness-Second Edition: PLUS.* Austin, TX: Pro-Ed.

Torgesen, J., and P. Mathes, *A Basic Guide to Understanding, Assessing, and Teaching Phonological Awareness.* Austin, TX: Pro-Ed, 2000.

Torgesen, J., S. T. Morgan, and C. Davis, "Effects of two types of phonological awareness training on word learning in kindergarten children." *Journal of Educational Psychology, 84* (1992): 364–370.

Torgesen, J., R. Wagner, and C. Rashotte, "Longitudinal studies of phonological processing and reading." *Journal of Learning Disabilities, 27* (1994): 276–286.

Torgesen, J., R. Wagner, C. Rashotte, A. Alexander, and T. Conway, "Preventative and remedial interventions for children with severe reading disabilities." *Learning Disabilities: An Interdisciplinary Journal, 81* (1997): 51–62.

Travis, L., and B. Rasmus, "The speech sound discrimination ability of cases with functional disorders of articulation." *Quarterly Journal of Speech, 17* (1931): 217–226.

Trehub, S., "Infants' sensitivity to vowel and tonal contrasts." *Developmental Psychology, 9* (1973): 91–96.

Treiman, R. "Children's spelling errors on syllable-initial consonant clusters." *Journal of Educational Psychology, 83* (1991): 346–360.

Treiman, R., "The structure of spoken syllables: Evidence from novel word games." *Cognition, 15* (1983): 49–74.

Treiman, R., C. A. Fowler, J. Gross, D. Berch, and S. Weatherston, "Syllable structure or word structure? Evidence for onset and rime units with disyllabic and trisyllabic stimuli." *Journal of Memory and Language, 34* (1995): 132–155.

Treiman, R., and A. Zukowski, "Toward an understanding of English syllabification." *Journal of Memory and Language, 29* (1990): 66–85.

Treiman, R., and A. Zukowski, "Children's sensitivity to syllables, onsets, rimes, and phonemes." *Journal of Experimental Child Psychology, 61* (1996): 193–215.

Tse, J., "Tone acquisition in Cantonese: A longitudinal case study." *Journal of Child Language, 5* (1978): 191–204.

Ttofari Eecen, K., S. Reilly, and P. Eadie, "Parent report of speech sound development at 12 months of age: Evidence from a cohort study. Manuscript submitted for publication, 2007.

Turton, L. J., "Development bases of articulation assessment." In W. D. Wolfe and D. J. Goulding (Eds.), *Articulation and Learning* (2nd ed., pp. 129–155). Springfield, IL: Charles Thomas, 1980.

Tyler, A., "Planning and monitoring intervention programs." In K. E. Pollock and A. G. Kamhi (Eds.), *Phonological Disorders in Children: Clinical Decision Making in Assessment and Intervention* (pp. 123–138). Baltimore, MD: Brookes, 2005.

Tyler, A., M. Edwards, and J. Saxman, "Acoustic validation of phonological knowledge and its relationship to treatment." *Journal of Speech and Hearing Disorders, 55* (1990): 251–261.

Tyler, A., and G. R. Figurski, "Phonetic inventory changes after treating distinctions along an implicational hierarchy." *Clinical Linguistics and Phonetics, 8* (1994): 91–107.

Tyler, A., K. E. Lewis, A. Haskill, and L. C. Tolbert, "Efficacy of cross-domain effects of a morphosyntax and a phonologic intervention." *Language, Speech, and Hearing Services in Schools, 33* (2002): 52–66.

Tyler, A., K. Lewis, A. Haskill, and L. Tolbert, "Outcomes of different speech and language goal attack strategies." *Journal of Speech, Language, and Hearing Research, 46* (2003): 1077–1094.

Tyler, A., and K. T. Sandoval, "Preschoolers with phonological and language disorders: Treating different linguistic domains." *Language, Speech, and Hearing Services in Schools, 25* (1994): 215–234.

Tyler, A., and K. Watterson, "Effects of phonological versus language intervention in preschoolers with both phonological and language impairment." *Child Language Teaching and Therapy, 7* (1991): 141–160.

Ukrainetz, T. A., M. H. Cooney, S. K. Dyer, A. J. Kysar, and T. J. Harris. "An investigation into teaching phonemic awareness through shared reading and writing." *Early Childhood Research Quarterly 15* (2000): 331–355.

Umberger, F. G., and R. G. Johnston, "The efficacy of oral myofunctional and coarticulation therapy." *International Journal of Orofacial Myology, 23* (1997): 3–9.

U.S. Bureau of the Census, *Age by Language Spoken at Home by Ability to Speak English for the Population 5 Years and Over* (2000). Retrieved January 25, 2007, from www.census.gov/.

Vandervelden, M. C., and L. S. Siegel, "Phonological recording and phoneme awareness in early literacy: A developmental approach." *Reading Research Quarterly, 30* (1995): 854–875.

Van Hattum, R. J., "Program scheduling." In R. Van Hattum (Ed.), *Clinical Speech in the Schools*. Springfield, IL: Charles Thomas, 1969.

van Kleeck, A., "Preliteracy domains and stages: Laying the foundations for beginning reading." *Journal of Children's Communication Development, 20* (1998): 33–51.

van Kleeck, A., R. Gillam, and T. McFadden, "A study of classroom-based phonological awareness training for preschoolers with speech and/or language disorders." *American Journal of Speech-Language Pathology, 7,* 3 (1998): 65–76.

Van Riper, C., *Speech Correction: Principles and Methods*. Englewood Cliffs, NJ: Prentice-Hall, 1939.

Van Riper, C., *Speech Correction: Principles and Methods* (5th ed.). Englewood Cliffs, NJ: Prentice-Hall, 1972.

Van Riper, C., and L. Emerick, *Speech Correction: An Introduction to Speech Pathology and Audiology* (7th ed.). Englewood Cliffs, NJ: Prentice-Hall, 1984.

Van Riper, C., and R. Erickson, *Speech Correction: An Introduction to Speech Pathology and Audiology* (9th ed.). Englewood Cliffs, NJ: Prentice-Hall, 1996.

Van Riper, C., and J. V. Irwin, *Voice and Articulation*. Englewood Cliffs, NJ: Prentice-Hall, 1958.

Veatch, J., "An experimental investigation of a motor theory of auditory discrimination." Ph.D. Dissertation, University of Idaho, 1970.

Velleman, S., "Children's production and perception of English voiceless fricatives." Unpublished Ph.D. Dissertation, University of Texas at Austin, 1983.

Velleman, S., *Childhood Apraxia of Speech, Resource Guide*. Clifton Park, NY: Thomson Delmar Learning, 2003.

Velleman, S., B. Z. Pearson, T. J. Bryant, and T. Charko, "Phonotactic versus phonetic development in African American English." Manuscript submitted for publication.

Velleman, S., and K. Strand, "Developmental verbal dyspraxia." In J. Bernthal, and N. Bankson (Eds.), *Child Phonology: Characteristics, Assessment, and Intervention with Special Populations* (pp. 110–139). New York: Thieme Publishers, 1994.

Velten, H., "The growth of phonemic and lexical patterns in infant language." *Language, 19* (1943): 281–292.

Veltman, C., *The Future of the Spanish Language in the United States*. Washington, DC: Hispanic Policy Development Project, 1988.

Vihman, M. M., "Early phonological development." In J. Bernthal and N. Bankson (Eds.), *Articulation and Phonological Disorders* (2nd ed.). Baltimore, MD: Williams and Wilkins, 1988.

Vihman, M. M., *Early Syllables and the Construction of Phonology*. Timonium, MD: York, 1992.

Vihman, M. M., *Phonological Development: The Origins of Language in the Child*. Cambridge, MA: Blackwell, 1996.

Vihman, M. M., "Early phonological development." In J. Bernthal and N. Bankson (Eds.), *Articulation and Phonological Disorders* (5th ed.). Boston: Allyn and Bacon, 2004.

Vihman, M. M., and M. Greenlee, "Individual differences in phonological development: Ages one and three years." *Journal of Speech and Hearing Research, 30* (1987): 503–521.

Vogel Sosa, A., and C. Stoel-Gammon, "Patterns of intraword phonological variability during the second year of life." *Journal of Child Language, 33* (2006): 31–50.

Vorperian, H., R. D. Kent, L. R. Gentry, and B. S. Yandell, "Magnetic resonance imaging procedures to study the concurrent anatomic development of vocal tract structures: Preliminary results." *International Journal of Pediatric Otorhinolaryngology, 49,* 3 (1999): 197–206.

Wadsworth, S. D., C. A. Maul, and E. J. Stevens, "The prevalence of orofacial myofunctional disorders among children identified with speech and language disorders in grades kindergarten through six." *International Journal of Orofacial Myology, 24* (1998): 1–19.

Wagner, R., and J. K. Torgesen, "The nature of phonological processing and its causal role in the acquisition of reading skills." *Psychological Bulletin, 101* (1987): 192–212.

Wagner, R., J. Torgesen, and C. Rashotte, *Comprehensive Test of Phonological Processing.* Austin, TX: Pro-Ed, 1999.

Walker, J. F., and L. M. D. Archibald, "Articulation rate in preschool children: A 3-year longitudinal study." *International Journal of Language and Communication Disorders, 41*, 5 (2006): 541–565.

Walsh, B., and A. Smith, "Articulatory movements in adolescents: Evidence for protracted development of speech motor control processes." *Journal of Speech, Language, and Hearing Research, 45*, 6 (2002): 1119–1133.

Walsh, H., "On certain practical inadequacies of distinctive feature systems." *Journal of Speech and Hearing Disorders, 39* (1974): 32–43.

Wang, W., *Languages and Dialects of Chinese.* Palo Alto, CA: Stanford University Press, 1989.

Wang, W., "Theoretical issues in studying Chinese dialects." *Journal of the Chinese Language Teachers Association, 25*, (1990): 1–34.

Waring, R., J. Fisher, and N. Atkin, "The articulation survey: Putting numbers to it." In L. Wilson and S. Hewat (Eds.), *Proceedings of the 2001 Speech Pathology Australia National Conference: Evidence and innovation* (pp. 145–151). Melbourne: Speech Pathology Australia, 2001.

Warrick, N., and H. Rubin, "Phonological awareness: Normally developing and language delayed children." *Journal of Speech-Language Pathology and Audiology, 16*, 1 (1992): 11–20.

Warrick, N., H. Rubin, and S. Rowe-Walsh, "Phoneme awareness in language-delayed children: Comparative studies and intervention." *Annals of Dyslexia, 43* (1993): 153–173.

Washington, J., and H. Craig, "Articulation test performances of low-income African American preschoolers with communication impairments." *Language, Speech, and Hearing Services in Schools, 23* (1992): 201–207.

Washington, J., and H. Craig, "Socioeconomic status and gender influences on children's dialectal variations." *Journal of Speech, Language, and Hearing Research, 41* (1998): 618–626.

Watson, J. B., "Psychology as a behaviorist views it." *Psychological Review, 101* (1913/1994): 248–253.

Watson, M. M., and G. P. Scukanec, "Phonological changes in the speech of two-year olds: A longitudinal investigation." *Infant-Toddler Intervention, 7* (1997a): 67–77.

Watson, M. M., and G. P. Scukanec, "Profiling the phonological abilities of 2-year-olds: A longitudinal investigation." *Child Language Teaching and Therapy, 13* (1997b): 3–14.

Weaver, C., C. Furbee, and R. Everhart, "Paternal occupational class and articulatory defects in children." *Journal of Speech and Hearing Disorders, 25* (1960) 171–175.

Weaver-Spurlock, S., and J. Brasseur, "Position training on the generalization training of [s]." *Language, Speech, and Hearing Services in Schools, 19* (1988): 259–271.

Weber, J., "Patterning of deviant articulation behavior." *Journal of Speech and Hearing Disorders, 35* (1970): 135–141.

Weikum, W. M., A. Vouloumanos, J. Navarra, S. Soto-Faraco, N. Sebastián-Gallés, and J. F. Werker, "Visual language discrimination in infancy." *Science, 316*, 25 (2007): 1159.

Weiner, F., *Phonological Process Analysis.* Baltimore, MD: University Park Press, 1979.

Weiner, F., "Systematic sound preference as a characteristic of phonological disability." *Journal of Speech and Hearing Disorders, 46* (1981a): 281–286.

Weiner, F., "Treatment of phonological disability using the method of meaningful minimal contrast: Two case studies." *Journal of Speech and Hearing Disorders, 46* (1981b): 97–103.

Weiner, F., and N. Bankson, "Teaching features." *Language, Speech, and Hearing Services in Schools, 9* (1978): 29–34.

Weiner, P., "Auditory discrimination and articulation." *Journal of Speech and Hearing Disorders, 32* (1967): 19–28.

Weismer, G., D. Dinnsen, and M. Elbert, "A study of the voicing distinction associated with omitted, word-final stops." *Journal of Speech and Hearing Disorders, 46* (1981): 91–103.

Weiss, C. E., *Weiss Intelligibility Test.* Tigard, OR: CC Publications, 1982.

Wellman, B., I. Case, I. Mengert, and D. Bradbury, "Speech sounds of young children." *University of Iowa Studies in Child Welfare, 5* (1931).

Wells, B., and S. Peppé, "Intonation abilities of children with speech and language impairments." *Journal of Speech, Language, and Hearing Research, 46* (2003): 5–20.

Wells, B., and Peppé, S. and Goulandris, N., Intonation development from five to thirteen *Journal of Child Language, 31,* 4 (2004): 749–778.

Weston, A., and J. V. Irwin, "Use of paired-stimuli in modification of articulation." *Perceptual and Motor Skills, 32* (1971): 947–957.

Weston, A., and Irwin, J. "Paired stimuli treatment. " In P. Newman, N. Creaghead, and W. Secord (Eds.), *Assessment and Remediation of Articulatory and Phonological Disorders* (pp. 337–368). Columbus, OH: Merrill, 1985.

Whitehurst, G. J., and C. J. Lonigan, "Child development and emergent literacy." *Child Development, 69* (1998): 848–872.

Wilcox, K., and S. Morris, "Speech outcomes of the language-focused curriculum." In M. Rice and K. Wilcox (Eds.), *Building a Language-Focused Curriculum for the Preschool Classroom: A Foundation for Lifelong Communication* (pp. 73–79). Baltimore, MD: Brookes, 1995.

Wilcox, K., and S. Morris, *Children's Speech Intelligibility Measure.* San Antonio, TX: The Psychological Corporation, 1999.

Wilcox, L., and R. Anderson, "Distinguishing between phonological difference and disorder in children who speak African-American Vernacular English: An experimental testing instrument." *Journal of Communication Disorders, 31,* (1998): 315–335.

Wilhelm, C. L., "The effects of oral form recognition training on articulation in children." Dissertation, University of Kansas, 1971.

Williams, A. L., "Generalization patterns associated with training least phonological knowledge." *Journal of Speech and Hearing Research, 34* (1991): 722–733.

Williams, A. L., "Phonological reorganization: A qualitative measure of phonological improvement." *American Journal of Speech-Language Pathology, 2* (1993): 44–51.

Williams, A. L., "Multiple oppositions: Case studies of variables in phonological intervention." *American Journal of Speech-Language Pathology, 9* (2000a): 289–299.

Williams, A. L., "Multiple oppositions: Theoretical foundations for an alternative contrastive intervention approach." *American Journal of Speech-Language Pathology, 9* (2000b): 282–288.

Williams, A. L., "Phonological assessment of child speech." In D. Ruscello (Ed.), *Tests and Measurements in Speech-Language Pathology* (pp. 31–76). Boston: Butterworth-Heinemann, 2001.

Williams, A. L., *Speech Disorders Resource Guide for Preschool Children.* Clifton Park, NY: Singular Publishing, 2003.

Williams, A. L., *SCIP: Sound Contrasts in Phonology* (Version 1.0). Greenville, SC: Super-Duper Publications, 2006.

Williams, F., *Language and Speech: Introductory Perspectives.* Englewood Cliffs, NJ: Prentice-Hall, 1972.

Williams, G., and L. McReynolds, "The relationship between discrimination and articulation training in children with misarticulations." *Journal of Speech and Hearing Research, 18* (1975): 401–412.

Williams, P., and J. Stackhouse, "Diadochokinetic skills: Normal and atypical performance in children aged 3–5 years." *International Journal of Language and Communication Disorders, 33* (1998): 481–486.

Williams, P., and J. Stackhouse, "Rate, accuracy and consistency: Diadochokinetic performance of young, normally developing children." *Clinical Linguistics and Phonetics, 14* (2000): 267–294.

Wilson, F., "Efficacy of speech therapy with educable mentally retarded children." *Journal of Speech and Hearing Research, 9* (1966): 423–433.

Winitz, H., "Language skills of male and female kindergarten children." *Journal of Speech and Hearing Research, 2* (1959a): 377–386.

Winitz, H., "Relationship between language and nonlanguage measures of kindergarten children." *Journal of Speech and Hearing Research, 2* (1959b): 387–391.

Winitz, H., *Articulatory Acquisition and Behavior.* Englewood Cliffs, NJ: Prentice-Hall, 1969.

Winitz, H., *From Syllable to Conversation.* Baltimore, MD: University Park Press, 1975.

Winitz, H., "Auditory considerations in articulation training." In H. Winitz (Ed.), *Treating Articulation Disorders: For Clinicians By Clinicians.* Baltimore, MD: University Park Press, 1984.

Wise, C. M., *Introduction to Phonetics.* Englewood Cliffs, NJ: Prentice-Hall, 1957a.

Wise, C. M., *Applied Phonetics.* Englewood Cliffs, NJ: Prentice-Hall, 1957b.

Wolfe, V., S. D. Blocker, and N. J. Prater, "Articulatory generalization in two word-medial and ambisyllabic contexts." *Language, Speech, and Hearing Services in Schools, 19* (1988): 251–258.

Wolfe, V., and R. Irwin, "Sound discrimination ability of children with misarticulation of the /r/ sound." *Perceptual and Motor Skills, 37* (1973): 415–420.

Wolfram, W. *Sociolinguistic aspects of assimilation: Puerto Rican English in New York City.* Arlington, VA: Center for Applied Linguistics, 1974.

Wolfram, W., "Language Variation in the United States." In O. Taylor (Ed.), *Treatment of Communication Disorders in Culturally and Linguistically Diverse Populations* (pp. 73–116). San Diego, CA: College-Hill Press, 1986.

Wolfram, W., "The phonology of a sociocultural variety: The case of African American Vernacular English." In J. Bernthal and N. Bankson (Eds.), *Child Phonology: Characteristics, Assessment, and Intervention with Special Populations* (pp. 227–244). New York: Thieme Medical Publishers, 1994.

Wolfram, W., and N. Schilling-Estes, *American English: Dialects and Variation.* Oxford: Blackwell, 1998.

Woolf, G., and M. Pilberg, "A comparison of three tests of auditory discrimination and their relationship to performance on a deep test of articulation." *Journal of Communication Disorders, 3* (1971): 239–249.

Wright, V., R. Shelton, and W. Arndt, "A task for evaluation of articulation change: III. Imitative task scores compared with scores for more spontaneous tasks." *Journal of Speech and Hearing Research, 12* (1969): 875–884.

Wyllie-Smith, L., S. McLeod, and M. J. Ball, "Typically developing and speech impaired children's adherence to the sonority hypothesis." *Clinical Linguistics and Phonetics, 20,* 4/5 (2006): 271–291.

Yavaş, M., "Sonority effects of vowel nuclei in onset duration." Poster presented at VIIIth International Clinical Phonetics and Linguistics Association Conference, Edinburgh, 2000.

Yavaş, M., "Sonority and the acquisition of #sC clusters." *Journal of Multilingual Communication Disorders, 4,* 3 (2006): 159–168.

Yavaş, M., and C. Core, "Phonemic awareness of coda consonants and sonority in bi-lingual children." *Clinical Linguistics and Phonetics, 15* (2001): 35–39.

Yavaş, M., and L. Gogate, "Phoneme awareness in children: A function of sonority." *Journal of Psycholinguistic Research, 28* (1999): 245–260.

Yavaş, M., and B. Goldstein, "Phonological assessment and treatment of bilingual speakers." *American Journal of Speech-Language Pathology, 7* (1998): 49–60.

Yin, R., *Case Study Research Design and Methods.* Newbury Park, CA: Sage, 1989.

Yopp, H., "The validity and reliability of phonemic awareness tests." *Reading Research Quarterly, 23* (1988): 159–177.

Yorkston, K. M., D. R. Beukelman, E. A. Strand, and K. R. Bell, *Management of Motor Speech Disorders in Children and Adults* (2nd ed.). Austin, TX: Pro-Ed, 1999.

Young, E. C., "The effects of treatment on consonant cluster and weak syllable reduction processes in misarticulating children." *Language, Speech, and Hearing Services in Schools, 18* (1987): 23–33.

Zehel, Z., R. Shelton, W. Arndt, V. Wright, and M. Elbert, "Item context and /s/ phone articulation results." *Journal of Speech and Hearing Research, 15* (1972): 852–860.

Zhu, H., and B. Dodd, "The phonological acquisition of Putonghua (Modern Standard Chinese)." *Journal of Child Language, 27* (2000a): 3–42.

Zhu, H., and B. Dodd, "Putonghua (Modern Standard Chinese)-speaking children with speech disorder." *Clinical Linguistics and Phonetics, 14* (2000b): 165–191.

Ziegler, J. C., and U. Goswami, "Reading acquisition, developmental dyslexia, and skilled reading across languages: A psycholinguistic grain size theory." *Psychological Bulletin 131* (2005): 3–29.

Zimmerman, I., V. Steiner, and R. Pond, *Preschool Language Scale.* Columbus, OH: Merrill, 1992.

Subject Index